Anticoagulation Therapy

Joe F. Lau • Geoffrey D. Barnes
Michael B. Streiff
Editors

Anticoagulation Therapy

Springer

Editors
Joe F. Lau, MD, PhD
Associate Professor of Cardiology
Department of Cardiology
Zucker School of Medicine
at Hofstra/Northwell
Northwell Health
Manhasset, NY, USA

Geoffrey D. Barnes, MD, MSc
Assistant Professor
Division of Internal Medicine
Frankel Cardiovascular Center at the
University of Michigan
Ann Arbor, MI, USA

Michael B. Streiff, MD
Professor of Medicine and Pathology
Division of Hematology
Department of Medicine
The Johns Hopkins University
School of Medicine
Baltimore, MD, USA

ISBN 978-3-030-08840-8 ISBN 978-3-319-73709-6 (eBook)
https://doi.org/10.1007/978-3-319-73709-6

Softcover re-print of the Hardcover 1st edition 2018

Printed on acid-free paper

This Springer imprint is published by the registered company Springer International Publishing AG part of Springer Nature.
The registered company address is: Gewerbestrasse 11, 6330 Cham, Switzerland

Preface

Since the introduction of vitamin K antagonists in the 1950s, the field of anticoagulation has evolved considerably to include an ever-increasing number of new therapeutic agents and procedures for thromboembolic disease. The rapidity of change presents a challenge for busy healthcare providers to stay abreast of the latest developments in the management of thrombotic disease. This book outlines the current state of antithrombotic therapy which will serve as a foundation upon which the field will inevitably continue to grow and develop. We hope that the readers will find this book to be a valuable resource and reliable reference for patient care.

Manhasset, NY, USA — Joe F. Lau, MD, PhD
Ann Arbor, MI, USA — Geoffrey D. Barnes, MD, MSc
Baltimore, MD, USA — Michael B. Streiff, MD

Acknowledgments

For my parents, who sacrificed and gave their all so their children can succeed; for my wife, Nora, and my sons, Justin and Daniel, who have continued to inspire me through their unwavering and loving support; and to my mentors and colleagues over the years—I thank you for keeping doors open for the kid who dreamed big.—Joe F. Lau

For my parents, who nurtured my love of science and medicine; for my husband, Grant, and my daughter, Gillian, who give me endless support and encouragement; and to my mentors, colleagues, and patients who have taught me the true joy of medicine.—Geoffrey D. Barnes

I would like to acknowledge my wife, Lauren, and my children, Zachary and Madeline, who have been a source of pride and joy and who have been unbelievably supportive despite my crazy schedule and extremely patient and tolerant of my working vacations and weekends. I would also like to thank my parents, Richard and Jenny Streiff, as well as the mentors who taught and inspired me including Richard R. Streiff, MD; Craig S. Kitchens, MD; Richard Lottenberg, MD; William R. Bell, MD, PhD; Jerry L. Spivak, MD; and Thomas S. Kickler, MD.—Michael B. Streiff

Contents

Contributors

Ibrahim M. Ali Department of Cardiology, Northwell Health, Zucker School of Medicine at Hofstra/Northwell, Manhasset, NY, USA

Geoffrey D. Barnes Department of Internal Medicine, Division of Cardiovascular Medicine, Frankel Cardiovascular Center at the University of Michigan, Ann Arbor, MI, USA

Stuart J. Beldner Department of Cardiology, Northwell Health, Zucker School of Medicine at Hofstra/Northwell, Manhasset, NY, USA

Allison E. Burnett University of New Mexico College of Pharmacy, Albuquerque, NM, USA

Teresa L. Carman Division of Cardiovascular Medicine, University Hospitals Cleveland Medical Center, Cleveland, OH, USA

Department of Medicine, Case Western Reserve University School of Medicine, Cleveland, OH, USA

Nathan P. Clark Clinical Pharmacy Anticoagulation and Anemia Service, Kaiser Permanente Colorado, Aurora, CO, USA

Matthew T. Crim Department of Medicine, Division of Cardiology, Emory University School of Medicine, Atlanta, GA, USA

Emily Downs Department of Surgery, Division of Thoracic and Cardiovascular Surgery, University of Virginia Medical Center, University of Virginia, Charlottesville, VA, USA

Sammy Elmariah Division of Cardiology, Department of Medicine, Massachusetts General Hospital, Boston, MA, USA

Natalie S. Evans Department of Cardiovascular Medicine, Section of Vascular Medicine, Cleveland Clinic, Cleveland, OH, USA

John Fanikos Department of Pharmacy, Brigham and Women's Hospital, Boston, MA, USA

Meghan L. Fletcher Inpatient Pharmacy Department, University of New Mexico Hospital, Albuquerque, NM, USA

Svetlana Goldman Department of Pharmacy, University of Virginia Medical Center, University of Virginia, Charlottesville, VA, USA

Marcelo P. V. Gomes Department of Cardiovascular Medicine, Section of Vascular Medicine, Cleveland Clinic, Cleveland, OH, USA

Adriana Guigova Division of Hematology/Oncology, Department of Medicine, Zucker School of Medicine at Hofstra/Northwell, Northwell Health, Lake Success, NY, USA

Dipti Gupta Department of Medicine, Memorial Sloan Kettering Cancer Center, New York, NY, USA

Gregory C. Hadlock Inpatient Pharmacy Department, University of New Mexico Hospital, Albuquerque, NM, USA

Jonathan L. Halperin The Cardiovascular Institute, Mount Sinai Medical Center, New York, NY, USA

Ruchika Harisingani Department of Medicine, Northwell Health, Zucker School of Medicine at Hofstra/Northwell, Manhasset, NY, USA

Deborah Hornacek Department of Cardiovascular Medicine, Section of Vascular Medicine, Cleveland Clinic, Cleveland, OH, USA

Mansour Khaddr Department of Medicine, Memorial Sloan Kettering Cancer Center, New York, NY, USA

Jessica A. Kvasic Department of Medicine, Zucker School of Medicine at Hofstra/Northwell, Northwell Health, Manhasset, NY, USA

Kyla M. Lara Department of Medicine, The Icahn School of Medicine at Mount Sinai, New York, NY, USA

Joe F. Lau Department of Cardiology, Zucker School of Medicine at Hofstra/Northwell, Northwell Health, Manhasset, NY, USA

Suegene K. Lee Department of Medicine, Division of Cardiology, Emory University School of Medicine, Atlanta, GA, USA

Rhynn J. Malloy Department of Pharmacy, Brigham and Women's Hospital, Boston, MA, USA

Simon Mantha Department of Medicine, Memorial Sloan Kettering Cancer Center, New York, NY, USA

Edith A. Nutescu Department of Pharmacy Systems, Outcomes and Policy, Center for Pharmacoepidemiology and Pharmacoeconomic Research, The University of Illinois at Chicago College of Pharmacy, Chicago, IL, USA

Surabhi Palkimas Department of Pharmacy, University of Virginia Medical Center, University of Virginia, Charlottesville, VA, USA

Nilay K. Patel Division of Cardiology, Department of Medicine, Massachusetts General Hospital, Boston, MA, USA

Salonie Pereira Department of Medicine, Northwell Health, Zucker School of Medicine at Hofstra/Northwell, Manhasset, NY, USA

Tony Philip Division of Hematology/Oncology, Department of Medicine, Zucker School of Medicine at Hofstra/Northwell, Northwell Health, Lake Success, NY, USA

Elizabeth T. Renner Anticoagulation Service, Faculty Group Practice: Pharmacy Innovations and Partnerships, University of Michigan, Ann Arbor, MI, USA

Megan Rhoten Department of Pharmacy, Brigham and Women's Hospital, Boston, MA, USA

Jessica Rimsans Department of Pharmacy, Brigham and Women's Hospital, Boston, MA, USA

Chadi Salmane Department of Medicine, Memorial Sloan Kettering Cancer Center, New York, NY, USA

Steven A. Savella Department of Cardiology, Zucker School of Medicine at Hofstra/Northwell, Northwell Health, Manhasset, NY, USA

Maya Serhal Department of Cardiovascular Medicine, Section of Vascular Medicine, Cleveland Clinic, Cleveland, OH, USA

Bhakti Shah Department of Medicine, Northwell Health, Zucker School of Medicine at Hofstra/Northwell, Manhasset, NY, USA

Aditya M. Sharma Department of Medicine, Cardiovascular Medicine Division, Heart and Vascular Center, University of Virginia Medical Center, University of Virginia, Charlottesville, VA, USA

Supriya Shore Department of Medicine, Division of Cardiology, Emory University School of Medicine, Atlanta, GA, USA

Gerald A. Soff Department of Medicine, Memorial Sloan Kettering Cancer Center, New York, NY, USA

Richard Steingart Department of Medicine, Memorial Sloan Kettering Cancer Center, New York, NY, USA

David L. Stern Department of Cardiology, Northwell Health, Zucker School of Medicine at Hofstra/Northwell, Manhasset, NY, USA

Michael B. Streiff Division of Hematology, Department of Medicine, The Johns Hopkins University School of Medicine, Baltimore, MD, USA

Katelyn Sylvester Department of Pharmacy, Brigham and Women's Hospital, Boston, MA, USA

Alexander Volodarskiy Department of Cardiology, New York-Presbyterian/Queens, Flushing, NY, USA

Bryan J. Wells Department of Medicine, Division of Cardiology, Emory University School of Medicine, Atlanta, GA, USA

Daniel M. Witt University of Utah College of Pharmacy, Salt Lake City, UT, USA

About the Editors

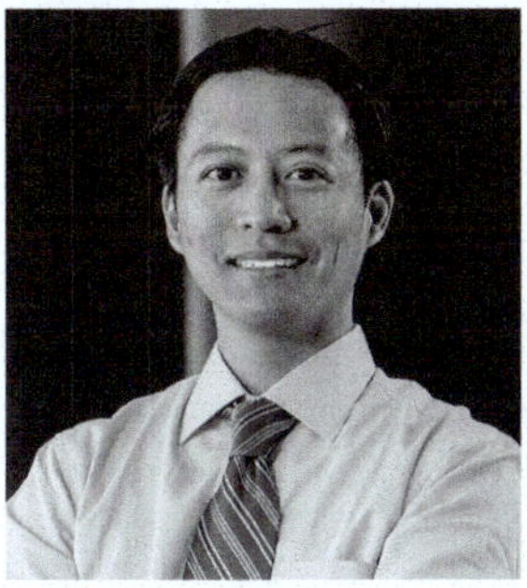

Joe F. Lau, MD, PhD, FACC, FASE, FSVM, RPVI is Associate Professor of Cardiology at the Zucker School of Medicine at Hofsta/Northwell. Dr. Lau is an attending cardiologist and vascular medicine specialist at Northwell Health, the largest integrated health system in New York State, where he serves as the Director of Vascular Medicine and Medical Director of the Non-Invasive Vascular Laboratory. Dr. Lau has an extensive clinical practice with research goals that focus on both cardiac and vascular diseases, while publishing and lecturing frequently within the field. His clinical practice emphasizes on caring for patients with thrombotic disorders such as atrial fibrillation and venous thromboembolism. Dr. Lau is also currently involved with numerous clinical trials, observational studies, and investigator-initiated trials. His research interests include evaluating the mechanisms of vascular and thrombotic complications associated with cancer and cancer therapies. Dr. Lau is actively involved with national vascular medicine and cardiovascular societies, with leadership roles in both the American Heart Association and the American College of Cardiology, for which he is currently a member of the ACC Scientific Sessions Program Committee and Peripheral Vascular Disease Section Leadership Council.

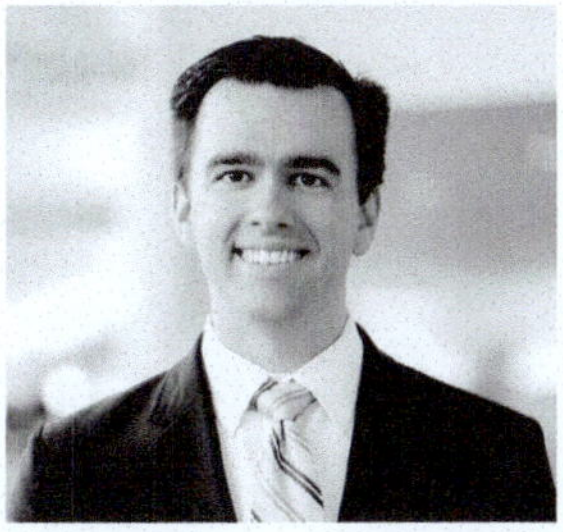

Geoffrey D. Barnes, MD, MSc, FACC, RPVI is a cardiologist and vascular medicine specialist at the University of Michigan. He has a long-standing interest in anticoagulation care and the care of patients with thrombotic disorders, including atrial fibrillation and venous thromboembolism. In addition to his clinical practice in vascular medicine, his research aims to improve systems of care for patients on anticoagulants and with thrombotic disorders, such as atrial fibrillation and venous thromboembolism. He is the co-director of the Michigan Anticoagulation Quality Improvement Initiative and has received funding from the NIH to improve anticoagulation care delivery. He is an active leader of many national and international thrombosis and cardiovascular societies and organizations, including the American College of Cardiology, the American Heart Association, the International Society on Thrombosis and Haemostasis, the Society for Vascular Medicine, the National PERT Consortium, and the Anticoagulation Forum.

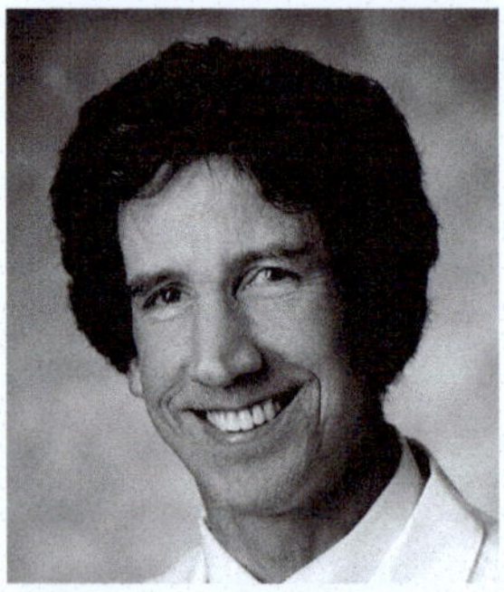

Michael B. Streiff, MD, FACP is a hematologist who specializes in the management of venous thromboembolism and anticoagulation. He is co-director of the Johns Hopkins Venous Thromboembolism Collaborative that has developed innovative information technology strategies that have led to dramatic improvements in VTE prevention and management at Johns Hopkins Medical Institutions. Their work has won awards from the North American Thrombosis Forum and the Centers for Disease Control and Prevention. He chairs the Venous Thromboembolism Guideline Committee for the National Comprehensive Cancer Network and has served on several international consensus panels to develop evidence-based guidelines for the management of VTE. He is a board member of the Anticoagulation Forum and the president of the Medical and Scientific Advisory Board for the National Blood Clot Alliance. Dr. Streiff and the Johns Hopkins Anticoagulation Management Service team have played a key role in developing evidence-based guidelines and electronic order sets for anticoagulation therapy at Johns Hopkins Medical Institutions. He has published over 150 articles and book chapters focusing on topics in VTE management and thrombosis and hemostasis and delivered over 300 lectures at local, national, and international meetings.

Abbreviations

ABC	Age, biomarkers, and clinical history score
ABW	Adjusted body weight
ACA	Anticardiolipin antibody
ACC	American College of Cardiology
ACCP	American College of Chest Physicians
ACF	Anticoagulation Forum
ACS	Acute coronary syndrome
ACT	Activated clotting time
ADP	Adenosine diphosphate
AERS	Adverse Event Report System
AF	Atrial fibrillation
AHA	American Heart Association
AMS	Anticoagulation Management Service
APC	Activated Protein C
APC-r	Activated protein C resistance
APS	Antiphospholipid antibody syndrome
aPTT	Partial thromboplastin time
ASA	Aspirin
ASD	Atrial septal defect
ASH	American Society of Hematology
AST	Aspartate aminotransferase
AT	Antithrombin
ATE	Arterial thromboembolism
AV	Atrioventricular
AVM	Arteriovenous malformation
AVR	Aortic valve replacement
BAL	Bronchoalveolar lavage
β2GP-1	β2-Glycoprotein-1 antibody
BID	Bis in die (twice a day)
BMI	Body mass index
CABG	Coronary artery bypass graft
CAD	Coronary artery disease
CBC	Complete blood count
CDC	Center for Disease Control and Prevention (USA)
CDTM	Collaborative drug therapy management
CFX	Chromogenic factor X
CI	Confidence interval

CKD	Chronic kidney disease
CKD-EPI	Chronic Kidney Disease Epidemiology Collaboration formula
CMR	Cardiac magnetic resonance imaging
CrCl	Creatinine clearance
COR	Class of recommendation
COX-1,2	Cyclooxygenase-1, 2
CPB	Cardiopulmonary bypass
CRRT	Continuous renal replacement therapy
DAPT	Dual antiplatelet therapy
DCCV	Direct current cardioversion
DCT	Direct clotting time
DDAVP	Desmopressin acetate
DES	Drug-eluting stent
DIC	Disseminated intravascular coagulation
dL	Deciliter
DOAC	Direct oral anticoagulant
dRVVT	Dilute Russell's viper venom time
DTI	Direct thrombin inhibitor
dTT	Dilute thrombin time
DVT	Deep vein thrombosis
DW	Dosing weight
EACTS	European Association for Cardio-Thoracic Surgery
ECG	Electrocardiogram
ECMO	Extracorporeal membrane oxygenation
ECT	Ecarin clotting time
EGD	Esophagogastroduodenoscopy
eGFR	Estimated glomerular filtration rate
ELISA	Enzyme-linked immunosorbent assay
ERCP	Endoscopic retrograde cholangiopancreatography
ESC	European Society of Cardiology
ESRD	End-stage renal disease
ET	Essential thrombocythemia (also known as essential thrombocytosis)
ETP	Endogenous thrombin potential
FDA	Food and Drug Administration (USA)
FIRM	Focal impulse and rotor modulation
FFP	Fresh frozen plasma
FSVM	Fellow of the Society of Vascular Medicine
FVa	Activated factor V
FVL	Factor V Leiden mutation
GFR	Glomerular filtration rate
GI	Gastrointestinal
GPI	Glycoprotein IIb/IIIa inhibitor
HAS-BLED	**H**ypertension, **a**bnormal renal/liver function, **s**troke, **b**leeding history or predisposition, **l**abile INRs, **e**lderly (> 65 years old), use of **d**rugs that promote bleeding excess, or alcohol

Hct	Hematocrit
HD	High dose
HEMORR2HAGES	**H**epatic or renal disease, **e**thanol abuse, **m**alignancy, **o**lder age (age > 75 years), **r**educed platelet count or function, **h**ypertension (uncontrolled), **a**nemia, **g**enetic factors, **e**xcessive fall risk, and **s**troke.
HEP	HIT Expert Probability
HERDOO2	**H**yperpigmentation, **e**dema, or **r**edness in either leg; **D**-dimer level ≥ 250 μg/L; **o**besity with body mass index ≥ 30; or **o**lder age, ≥ 65 years
HFS	Heart Failure Society
Hgb	Hemoglobin
HIT	Heparin-induced thrombocytopenia
HITTS	Heparin-induced thrombocytopenia thrombosis syndrome
HMW	High-molecular-weight
HR	Hazard ratio
HR	Heart rate
HRS	Heart Rhythm Society
HTN	Hypertension
IBW	Ideal body weight
ICD	Implantable cardioverter defibrillator
ICH	Intracranial hemorrhage, intracerebral hemorrhage
IM	Intramuscular
INR	International normalized ratio
IPC	Intermittent pneumatic compression
IQR	Interquartile range
ISHLT	International Society for Heart & Lung Transplantation
ISTH	International Society on Thrombosis and Haemostasis
IU	International units
IV	Intravenous
IVC	Inferior vena cava
LA	Lupus anticoagulant
LAA	Left atrial appendage
LAFB	Left anterior fascicular block
LBBB	Left bundle branch block
LBW	Lean body weight
LD	Low dose
LDL	Low-density lipoprotein
LMWH	Low-molecular-weight heparin
LOE	Level of evidence
LV	Left ventricular
LVAD	Left ventricular assist device
LVEF	Left ventricular ejection fraction
MACE	Major adverse cardiovascular events
MDRD	Modification of Diet in Renal Disease formula
mg	Milligrams
MI	Myocardial infarction

MRA	Magnetic resonance angiography
MRI	Magnetic resonance imaging
MRV	Magnetic resonance venography
MTHFR	Methylenetetrahydrofolate reductase
MVR	Mitral valve replacement
NCBAP	National Certification Board for Anticoagulation Providers
NBTE	Nonbacterial thrombotic endocarditis
NOAC	Novel oral anticoagulant, non-vitamin K antagonist oral anticoagulant
NPO	Nil per os—nothing by mouth
NSAID	Nonsteroidal anti-inflammatory drug
NSTE-ACS	Non-ST-segment acute coronary syndromes
NSTEMI	Non-ST-segment elevation myocardial infarction
NT-proBNP	N-terminal pro-B-type natriuretic peptide
NVAF	Non-valvular atrial fibrillation
OAC	Oral anticoagulation
OBRI	Outpatient bleeding risk index
OCP	Oral contraceptive pills
OD	Optical density
OR	Odds ratio
PAD	Peripheral artery disease
PaGIA	Particle gel immunoassay
PAI-1	Plasminogen activator inhibitor 1
PAR-1	Protease-activated receptor-1
PC	Protein C
PCC	Prothrombin complex concentrate
PCI	Percutaneous coronary intervention
PD	Pharmacodynamics
PE	Pulmonary embolism
PEO-CO	Polyethoxylated castor oil
PF4	Platelet factor 4
PFO	Patent foramen ovale
PGM	Prothrombin gene mutation
P-gp	P-glycoprotein
PICC	Peripherally inserted central catheters
PK	Pharmacokinetics
PNH	Paroxysmal nocturnal hemoglobinuria
PNP	Platelet neutralization procedure
PO	Per os (per oral)
POC	Point-of-care
PS	Protein S
PSM	Patient self-management
PST	Patient self-testing
PT	Prothrombin time
PTAV	Percutaneous transluminal aortic valvuloplasty
PV	Polycythemia vera
PVI	Pulmonary vein isolation

RBBB	Right bundle branch block
RCT	Randomized control/controlled trial
RR	Relative risk
RRR	Relative risk ratio
SC	Subcutaneous
SCD	Sequential compression devices
SD	Standard deviation
SLE	Systemic lupus erythematosus
SQ	Subcutaneous
SRA	Serotonin release assay
START/STOPP	Screening tool to alert doctors to right treatment/ screening tool of older persons' prescriptions
STEMI	ST-segment elevation myocardial infarction
STS	Society of Thoracic Surgeons
SVT	Superficial vein thrombosis
SVT	Supraventricular tachycardia
TAFI	Thrombin-activatable fibrinolysis inhibitor
TAVR	Transcatheter aortic valve replacement
TBW	Total body weight
TEE	Transesophageal echocardiogram
THA	Total hip arthroplasty
TIA	Transient ischemia attack
TKA	Total knee arthroplasty
TNK	Tenecteplase
TOAT	Triple oral anticoagulant therapy
TRALI	Transfusion-related acute lung injury
TSOAC	Target-specific oral anticoagulants
TT	Thrombin time
TTE	Transthoracic echocardiogram
TTR	Time-in-therapeutic range
UA	Unstable angina
UFH	Unfractionated heparin
USPTF	US Preventative Task Force
VATS	Video-assisted thoracoscopic surgery
Vd	Volume of distribution
VEGF	Vascular endothelial growth factor
VKA	Vitamin K antagonist
VKOR	Vitamin K epoxide reductase
VSD	Ventricular septal defect
VT	Ventricular tachycardia
VTE	Venous thromboembolism
vWF	von Willebrand factor
WHO	World Health Organization

Trial Abbreviations

ACUITY	Acute Catheterization and Urgent Intervention Triage Strategy trial
ACUTE	Assessment of Cardioversion Using Transesophageal Echocardiography (ACUTE) Multicenter Study
ADVANCE	Action in Diabetes and Vascular Disease: Preterax and Diamicron MR Controlled Evaluation trial
AFFIRM	Atrial Fibrillation Follow-up Investigation of Rhythm Management
AMPLIFY	Apixaban for the Initial Management of Pulmonary Embolism and Deep-Vein Thrombosis as First-Line Therapy trial
AMPLIFY-EXT	Apixaban for Extended Treatment of Venous Thromboembolism trial
ANNEXA-A	Andexanet Alfa, a Novel Antidote to the Anticoagulation Effects of FXA Inhibitors Apixaban
ANNEXA-R	Andexanet Alfa, a Novel Antidote to the Anticoagulation Effects of FXA Inhibitors Rivaroxaban
APEX	Acute Medically III VTE (Venous Thromboembolism) Prevention with Extended Duration Betrixaban trial
APOLLO	Fondaparinux combined with intermittent pneumatic compression vs. intermittent pneumatic compression alone for prevention of venous thromboembolism after abdominal surgery: a randomized, double-blind comparison
APPRAISE	Apixaban for Prevention of Acute Ischemic and Safety Events
ARISTOTLE	Apixaban for Reduction in Stroke and Other Thromboembolic Events in Atrial Fibrillation trial
AREVA	Anticoagulation et Remplacement Valvulaire (France)
ARTEMIS	Affordability and Real-world Antiplatelet Treatment Effectiveness After Myocardial Infarction Study
ASAP	ASA Plavix Feasibility Study with Watchman Left Atrial Appendage Closure Technology study

ASAP-TOO	Assessment of the Watchman Device in Patients Unsuitable for Oral Anticoagulation
ASPIRE	Low-Dose Aspirin for Preventing Recurrent Venous Thromboembolism
ATBAT	Anticoagulant Therapy with Bivalirudin to Assist in the performance of percutaneous coronary intervention in patients with heparin-induced Thrombocytopenia
ATLAS-TIMI-46	Rivaroxaban versus placebo in patients with acute coronary syndromes
ATLAS-TIMI-51	Rivaroxaban in patients with a recent acute coronary syndrome
ATLAS ACS 2-TIMI 51	Anti-Xa Therapy to Lower cardiovascular events in addition to Aspirin with or without thienopyridine therapy in Subjects with Acute Coronary Syndrome 2—Thrombolysis in Myocardial Infarction 51 Trial
ATOLL	Acute STEMI Treated with Primary PCI and IV Enoxaparin or UFH to Lower Ischemic and Bleeding Events at Short- and Long-Term Follow-up trial
ATRIA	Anticoagulation and Risk Factors in Atrial Fibrillation study
ATTRACT	Acute Venous Thrombosis: Thrombus Removal with Adjunctive Catheter-Directed Thrombolysis trial
AUGUSTUS	Apixaban in Patients With Atrial Fibrillation and ACS/PCI
AUREC	Austrian Study of Recurrent Venous Thromboembolism
AVERROES	Apixaban Versus Acetylsalicylic Acid to Prevent Stroke in Atrial Fibrillation trial
AXAFA	Apixaban During Atrial Fibrillation Catheter Ablation: Comparison to Vitamin K Antagonist Therapy
BRAVO-3	Bivalirudin Versus Heparin Anticoagulation in Transcatheter Aortic Valve Replacement
BRIDGE	Bridging Anticoagulation in Patients who Require Temporary Interruption of Warfarin Therapy for an Elective Invasive Procedure or Surgery
BRUISE CONTROL	Bridge or Continue Coumadin for Device Surgery Randomized Controlled Trial
CALISTO	Comparison of Arixtra in Lower Limb Superficial Vein Thrombosis with Placebo trial
CASSINI	Efficacy and Safety of Rivaroxaban Prophylaxis Compared with Placebo in Ambulatory Cancer Patients Initiating Systemic Cancer Therapy and at High Risk for Venous Thromboembolism

CATCH	Comparison of Acute Treatments in Cancer Haemostasis trial
CAVENT	Catheter-Directed Venous Thrombolysis in Acute Iliofemoral Vein Thrombosis study
CLOT	Randomized Comparison of Low-Molecular-Weight Heparin versus Oral Anticoagulant Therapy for the Prevention of Recurrent Venous Thromboembolism in Patients with Cancer
COMPASS	Cardiovascular Outcomes for People Using Anticoagulation Strategies trial
CRUSADE	Can Rapid Risk Stratification of Unstable Angina Patients Suppress Adverse Outcomes With Early Implementation of the ACC/AHA Guidelines study
DAWA	Dabigatran Versus Warfarin After Bioprosthesis Valve Replacement for the Management of Atrial Fibrillation Postoperatively study
EINSTEIN	Oral Rivaroxaban for Symptomatic Venous Thromboembolism
EINSTEIN CHOICE	Rivaroxaban or Aspirin for Extended Treatment of Venous Thromboembolism
EINSTEIN PE	Oral Direct Factor Xa Inhibitor Rivaroxaban in Patients With Acute Symptomatic Pulmonary Embolism
EINSTEIN DVT	Oral Direct Factor Xa Inhibitor Rivaroxaban in Patients With Acute Symptomatic Deep-Vein Thrombosis
EMANATE	Apixaban compared with parenteral heparin and/or vitamin K antagonist in patients with nonvalvular atrial fibrillation undergoing cardioversion
ENGAGE AF-TIMI 48	Effective Anticoagulation with Factor Xa Next Generation in Atrial Fibrillation – Thrombolysis in Myocardial Infarction 48
ENSURE-AF	Edoxaban Versus Enoxaparin–Warfarin in Patients Undergoing Cardioversion of Atrial Fibrillation Trial
ENTRUST-PCI	Edoxaban Treatment Versus Vitamin K Antagonist in Patients With Atrial Fibrillation Undergoing Percutaneous Coronary Intervention
EQUINOX	Bioequipotency Study of Idrabiotaparinux and Idraparinux in Patients With Deep Venous Thrombosis of the Lower Limbs
ESSENCE	Efficacy and Safety of Subcutaneous Enoxaparin in Unstable Angina and Non-Q-Wave MI trial
EUROMAX	European Ambulance Acute Coronary Syndrome Angiography Trial

FUTURA/OASIS 8	Fondaparinux Trial with Unfractionated Heparin During Revascularization in Acute Coronary Syndromes
GARFIELD	Global Anticoagulant Registry in the FIELD registry
GELIA	German Experience with Low Intensity Anticoagulation
GLORIA-AF	Global Registry on Long-Term Oral Antithrombotic Treatment in Patients with Atrial Fibrillation
GUSTO	Global Use of Strategies to Open Occluded Coronary Arteries
HEAT-PPCI	Unfractionated heparin versus bivalirudin in primary percutaneous coronary intervention
HOKUSAI-VTE	Edoxaban for the long-term treatment of *venous thromboembolism*
HOPE-2	(Heart Outcomes Prevention Evaluation) placebo-controlled randomized clinical trial
HORIZONS-AMI	Harmonizing Outcomes with Revascularization and Stents in Acute Myocardial Infarction trial
ISAR-TRIPLE	Triple Therapy in Patients on Oral Anticoagulation After Drug-Eluting Stent Implantation
LIWACAP	Low-intensity oral anticoagulant plus low-dose aspirin during the first six months versus standard-intensity oral anticoagulant therapy after mechanical heart valve replacement: a pilot study of low-intensity warfarin and aspirin in cardiac prostheses
LOWERING-IT	LOWERing the INtensity of oral anticoaGulant Therapy trial
MATISSE DVT	Mondial Assessment of Thromboembolism treatment Initiated by Synthetic pentasaccharide with Symptomatic Endpoints—Deep Vein Thrombosis
MATISSE PE	Mondial Assessment of Thromboembolism treatment Initiated by Synthetic pentasaccharide with Symptomatic Endpoints—Pulmonary Embolism
MOMENTUM	A Fully Magnetically Levitated Circulatory Pump for Advanced Heart Failure
OASIS	Organization to Assess Strategies in Acute Ischemic Syndromes
OASIS-5	Comparison of Fondaparinux and Enoxaparin in Acute Coronary Syndromes: The Fifth Organization to Assess Strategies in Acute Ischemic Syndromes Investigators
OASIS-6	The Effects of Fondaparinux on Mortality and Reinfarction in Patients with Acute ST-segment Elevation Myocardial Infarction: The Sixth Organization to Assess Strategies in Acute Ischemic Syndromes Investigators

OCEAN	Optimal Anticoagulation for Higher Risk Patients Post-Catheter Ablation for Atrial Fibrillation Trial
ORBIT	Outcomes Registry for Better Informed Treatment of Atrial Fibrillation registry
PEITHO	Pulmonary Embolism Thrombolysis trial
PEGASUS	Placebo on a Background of Aspirin-Thrombolysis in Myocardial Infarction
PENTHIFRA-Plus	Pentasaccharide in Hip-Fracture Surgery Plus
PERIOP 2	A Safety and Effectiveness of LMWH vs Placebo Bridging Therapy for Patients on Long Term Warfarin Requiring Temporary Interruption of Warfarin
PIONEER AF-PCI	A Study Exploring Two Strategies of Rivaroxaban and One of Oral Vitamin K Antagonist in Patients With Atrial Fibrillation Who Undergo Percutaneous Coronary Intervention trial
POPular TAVI	Antiplatelet Therapy for Patients Undergoing Transcatheter Aortic Valve Implantation
PREFER in AF	Prevention of Thromboembolic Events—European Registry in Atrial Fibrillation
PREPIC	Prevention du Risque d'Embolie Pulmonaire par Interruption Cave study
PREVENT-HIT	A Comparative Clinical and Pharmacoeconomic Study Comparing Argatroban® IV vs Desirudin SC for Patients With Suspected Heparin-Induced Thrombocytopenia (HIT)With or Without Thrombosis Syndrome (HIT/TS)
PREVAIL	Watchman LAA Closure Device in Patients With Atrial Fibrillation Versus Long-Term Warfarin Therapy
PROACT	Prospective Randomized On-X Anticoagulation Clinical Trial
PROTECT AF	Watchman Left Atrial Appendage System for Embolic Protection in Patients With Atrial Fibrillation
RE-ALIGN	Randomized, phase II study to Evaluate the sAfety and pharmacokinetics of oraL dabIGatran etexilate in patients after heart valve replacemeNt trial
RE-CIRCUIT	Randomized Evaluation of Dabigatran Etexilate Compared to warfarIn in pulmonaRy Vein Ablation: Assessment of an Uninterrupted periproCedUral antIcoagulation sTrategy
RECORD	REgulation of Coagulation in major Orthopedic surgery reducing the Risk of DVT and PE trial
RE-COVER	A Phase III, Randomized, Double Blind, Parallel-group Study of the Efficacy and Safety of Oral Dabigatran Etexilate 150 mg Twice Daily Compared

	to Warfarin (INR 2.0–3.0) for 6 Month Treatment of Acute Symptomatic Venous Thromboembolism (VTE), Following Initial Treatment (5–10 Days) With a Parenteral Anticoagulant Approved for This Indication
RE-DEEM	RandomizEd Dabigatran Etexilate Dose Finding Study in Patients With Acute Coronary Syndromes Post Index Event With Additional Risk Factors for Cardiovascular Complications Also Receiving Aspirin and Clopidogrel: Multi-centre, Prospective, Placebo Controlled, Cohort Dose Escalation Study
RE-DUAL	Randomized Evaluation of Dual Therapy with Dabigatran vs. Triple Therapy Strategy with Warfarin in Patients with NVAF that have undergone PCI with Stenting
RE-LY	Randomized Evaluation of Long-Term Anticoagulation Therapy trial
REMATCH	Long-Term Use of a Left Ventricular Assist Device for End-Stage Heart Failure
RE-MEDY	A Phase III, Randomised, Multicenter, Double-blind, Parallel-group, Active Controlled Study to Evaluate the Efficacy and Safety of Oral Dabigatran Etexilate (150 mg Bid) Compared to Warfarin (INR 2.0–3.0) for the Secondary Prevention of Venous Thromboembolism
RE-NOVATE	A Phase III Randomised, Parallel Group, Double-blind, Active Controlled Study to Investigate the Efficacy and Safety of Orally Administered 220 mg Dabigatran Etexilate Capsules (110 mg Administered on the Day of Surgery Followed by 220 mg Once Daily) Compared to Subcutaneous 40 mg Enoxaparin Once Daily for 28–35 Days, in Prevention of Venous Thromboembolism in Patients With Primary Elective Total Hip Arthroplasty Surgery
RE-SONATE	Twice-daily Oral Direct Thrombin Inhibitor Dabigatran Etexilate in the Long-Term Prevention of Recurrent Symptomatic VTE
REVERSE-AD	A Study of the RE-VERSal Effects of Idarucizumab on Active Dabigatran
RIETE	Registro Informatizado de Pacientes con Enfermedad TromboEmbólica (Spain)
ROCKET-AF	Rivaroxaban Once Daily Oral Direct Factor Xa Inhibition Compared with Vitamin K Antagonism for Prevention of Stroke and Embolism Trial in Atrial Fibrillation trial
SAVE-ONCO	Semuloparin for prevention of VTE in Cancer Patients Receiving Chemotherapy trial

SPORTIF	Stroke Prevention using ORal Thrombin Inhibitor in atrial Fibrillation
SYNERGY	Superior Yield of the New strategy of Enoxaparin, Revascularization and GlYcoprotein IIb/IIIa inhibitors trial
ULTIMA	ULTrasound Accelerated Thrombolysis of PulMonAry Embolism trial
VENTURE AF	A randomized, open-label, active-controlled multicenter study to evaluate the safety of rivaroxaban and vitamin K antagonists in subjects undergoing catheter ablation for atrial fibrillation
WARFASA	Aspirin for Preventing the Recurrence of Venous Thromboembolism
WOA	Comparing warfarin to aspirin after aortic valve replacement with the St. Jude Medical Epic heart valve bioprosthesis
WOEST	What is the Optimal antiplatElet and anticoagulant therapy in patients with oral anticoagulation and coronary StenTing trial
XANTUS	Xarelto for Prevention of Stroke in Patients with Atrial Fibrillation
X-VeRT	EXplore the efficacy and safety of once-daily oral riVaroxaban for the prEvention of caRdiovascular events in patients with nonvalvular aTrial fibrillation scheduled for cardioversion trial

1 Introduction

Joe F. Lau, Geoffrey D. Barnes,
and Michael B. Streiff

Anticoagulation Therapy: A Historical Perspective

Arterial and venous thromboembolism have long been recognized as common causes of morbidity and mortality. Hippocrates of Cos (460–370 BC), the ancient Greek physician often regarded as the "father of medicine," recognized stroke as a clinical syndrome 2400 years ago and, at the time, called it "apoplexy" [1]. In the mid-1600s, Swiss pathologist and pharmacologist Johann Jakob Wepfer noted that patients with apoplexy had either bleeding or vascular occlusions in their brains, marking the first accurate description of the pathophysiology for stroke [2].

The first historical description of deep vein thrombosis (DVT) dates back to the Middle Ages. In 1271, Guillaume de Saint Pathus described the case of Raoul, a 20-year-old French cobbler who presented with right calf pain and swelling. He went on to develop a leg ulcer which was healed when he applied dust from the floor next to the tomb of King Saint Louis [2, 3]. In 1676, the English surgeon Richard Wiseman was the first to suggest that DVT represented an alteration of the blood [4]. Scottish surgeon John Hunter suggested that blood clots occluding the vein were the cause of DVT, describing it as "inflammation of the internal coat of veins" in his 1793 paper—published the same year as his death [5]. To combat the propagation and extension of venous thrombi, Hunter performed venous ligation on his patients. In fact, prior to the development of anticoagulants, the primary treatment for DVT focused on surgical ligation, bed rest, extremity elevation, bloodletting to relieve venous congestion, and warm compresses to increase collateral circulation.

The Evolving Anticoagulant Armamentarium

Hippocrates might have been the first clinician to prescribe anticoagulation therapy. He believed that four humors—black bile, yellow bile, phlegm, and blood—directly regulated a patient's temperament and health and that an imbalance of

J. F. Lau (✉)
Department of Cardiology, Zucker School of Medicine at Hofstra/Northwell, Northwell Health, Manhasset, NY, USA
e-mail: JLau@northwell.edu

G. D. Barnes (✉)
Department of Internal Medicine, Division of Cardiovascular Medicine, Frankel Cardiovascular Center at the University of Michigan, Ann Arbor, MI, USA
e-mail: gbarnes@umich.edu

M. B. Streiff (✉)
Division of Hematology, Department of Medicine, The Johns Hopkins University School of Medicine, Baltimore, MD, USA
e-mail: mstreif@jhmi.edu

J. F. Lau et al. (eds.), *Anticoagulation Therapy*, https://doi.org/10.1007/978-3-319-73709-6_1

these humors led to disease or illness. Because blood was the dominant humor, Hippocrates believed that prescribing the use of medicinal leeches to remove blood from his patients was the critical step toward rebalancing these humors and therefore treating most maladies. Unbeknownst to Hippocrates, the secreted saliva from medicinal leeches contained the anticoagulant protein hirudin, a highly potent inhibitor of thrombin, which was later identified by English physiologist John Berry Haycraft in 1884. Recombinant biotechnological approaches have since led to the development of a number of commercially available hirudin-based anticoagulant products such as lepirudin [6].

Modern-day anticoagulation therapy took shape at the beginning of the 20th century, when in 1916, a second-year medical student, Jay McLean, worked with the Johns Hopkins physiologist William Henry Howell to successfully isolate a protein from canine liver that induced anticoagulant properties such as excessive bleeding in experimental animals. In 1918, a second medical student, L. Emmett Holt, Jr., worked with Howell to isolate another similar compound with anticoagulant properties, and Howell coined the term "heparin" from the Greek "hepar," or liver, from which it was isolated [7]. It was not until the early 1930s when heparin was successfully isolated in larger, purified quantities from bovine tissue, leading to its first documented clinical application in dogs for the prevention of thrombus formation in veins that have been chemically or mechanically distressed [8]. Heparin was subsequently tested in humans in April 1937, when it was infused into the brachial artery of a patient, leading to increased clotting time. It subsequently became the first anticoagulant to be widely applied to the treatment of thrombotic disease [9]. Over 80 years have since passed, and heparin—in both its unfractionated formulation and in low-molecular-weight heparins (LMWH) such as enoxaparin, developed much later in 1987—continues to be an indispensable anticoagulant therapeutic agent, particularly for a number of clinical indications such as the initial treatments for acute coronary syndrome, venous thromboembolic disease, and cancer-associated thrombosis.

The story behind the discovery of the first oral vitamin K antagonists (VKA) that include warfarin and acenocoumarol is even more captivating. During the Great Depression in the 1920s, Canadian and Northern Great Plains farmers allowed their cattle and sheep to graze on spoiled sweet clover hay when finances were tight. It was subsequently observed that these cattle developed a fatal hemorrhagic disease [10–12]. More than a decade had passed until the offending agent, coumarin, was first isolated by Karl Paul Link. In a moldy, damp environment, coumarin was noted to oxidize to dicoumarol, which is a competitive inhibitor of vitamin K epoxide reductase that recycles vitamin K into its active form that is required for hepatic synthesis of vitamin K-dependent coagulation proteins (this mechanism of action was discovered much later in 1978) [13]. Mark Stahmann, a biochemistry professor at Wisconsin, performed much of the initial work on isolating dicoumarol, with his work funded by the Wisconsin Alumni Research Foundation (WARF), which in 1941 received the patent rights for dicoumarol [14]. Renowned cardiologist and former president of the American Heart Association (AHA) Irving Wright, along with his research fellow Andrew Prandoni, obtained dicoumarol from the WARF group to treat patients with deep vein thrombosis at the now-defunct Goldwater Memorial Hospital in New York City in 1941, but widespread use as an anticoagulant did not occur until a decade later [15, 16]. In 1948, Karl Paul Link, who was also at Wisconsin and funded by WARF, developed a more potent derivative with the intent to use it as a rodenticide and called it warfarin [17]. In 1954, warfarin was approved for use in humans as an anticoagulant for the treatment of myocardial infarction and stroke. One of the first recipients of warfarin was the US President Dwight Eisenhower, who received the anticoagulant after suffering a myocardial infarction while still in office in 1955.

While the heparins and VKAs have remained the mainstay of anticoagulant therapy since their

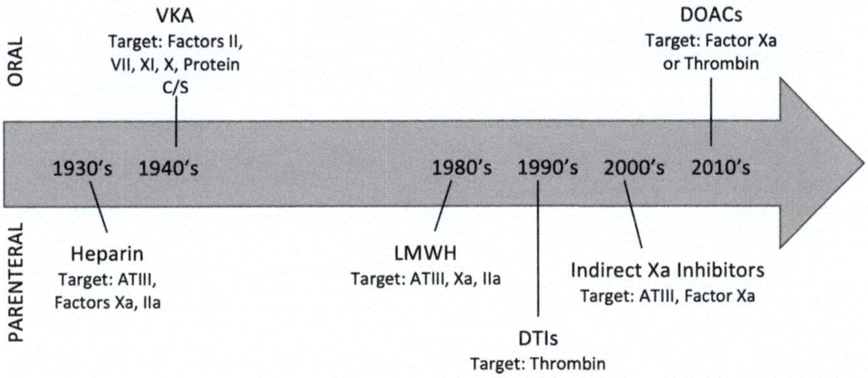

Fig. 1.1 The evolving anticoagulant armamentarium. Since the discovery of heparin in the 1930s and vitamin K antagonists in the 1940s, the number of anticoagulant agents available to clinicians have markedly increased since the 1990s. Newer anticoagulants have increased in target specificity and ease of use

inception, their perceived inconveniences drove the pharmaceutical industry to develop anticoagulants with greater specificity and ease of use. Direct thrombin inhibitors (DTI) were first introduced in the 1990s (see Fig. 1.1). The first synthetic indirect Xa inhibitor, fondaparinux, was approved in the early 2000s but still had the limitation of being available only in parenteral formulation. Ximelagatran, the first oral DTI, was never approved by the US Food and Drug Administration (FDA) and was ultimately withdrawn from the European market in 2006 because of severe liver toxicity in some patients. Dabigatran, another DTI, was approved for use in Europe in 2008, becoming the first approved "novel" oral anticoagulant since warfarin (see Figs. 1.1 and 1.2). Oral direct factor Xa inhibitors, which inhibit thrombin generation instead of inhibiting thrombin itself, include agents such as rivaroxaban, apixaban, and edoxaban (Fig. 1.2). With the oral direct thrombin inhibitor, dabigatran, these direct factor Xa inhibitors form the so-called direct oral anticoagulants (DOACs), which have been approved worldwide for use in both the prophylaxis and treatment of arterial and venous thromboembolic diseases. DOACs have continued to gain significant utilization, particularly following their recent expansion of indications for the treatment of venous thromboembolism [18].

Resources for Anticoagulation Management

With the rapid increase in the number of antithrombotic agents, it has become increasingly challenging for practitioners to keep abreast of the latest developments in the management of thromboembolic disease. No single provider can be expected to possess complete knowledge of all aspects of antithrombotic therapy. Therefore, it is essential for the prudent provider to have ready access to well-developed resources that can assist him/her when making anticoagulation-related decisions. This book is intended to be one such resource, with both the depth of detail and easy-to-use tables and figures for front line anticoagulation providers. In addition, many other resources should be used to supplement this text, especially as new findings and guidelines are developed.

Traditionally, the American College of Chest Physicians (www.chestnet.org) has produced evidence-based guidelines pertaining to a broad range of anticoagulation issues. The most recent comprehensive set of guidelines was published in 2012 [19]. They have issued one update in 2016 focused on the management of patients with venous thromboembolism (VTE) [20]. However, no timetable has been set for a future comprehensive update to the 2012 guidelines. The Anticoagulation Forum

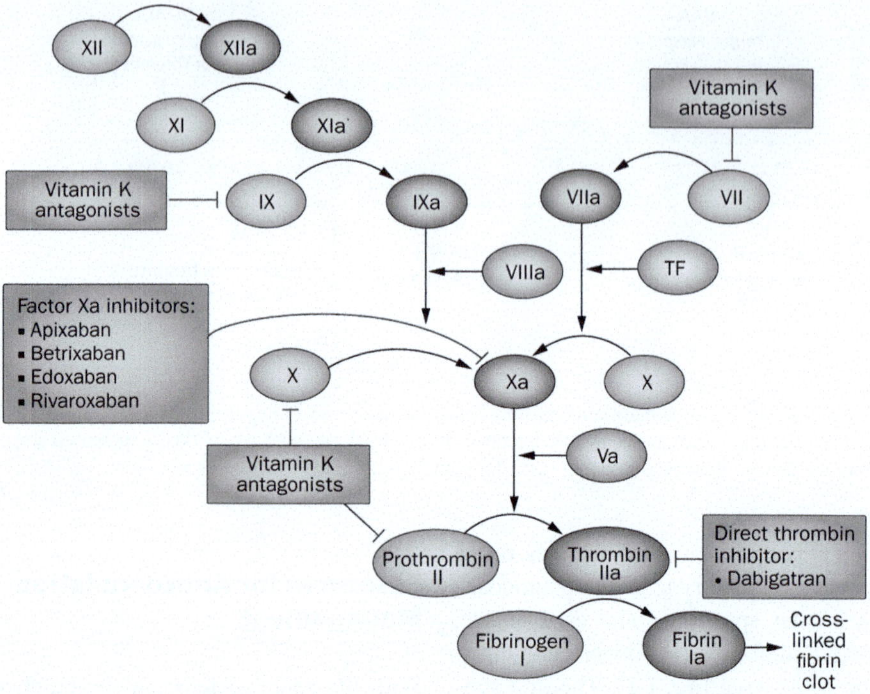

Fig. 1.2 Coagulation cascade and point of effect of the common oral anticoagulants. Vitamin K antagonists, such as warfarin, inhibit factors II, VII, IX, and X. Dabigatran directly inhibits factor IIa (thrombin). Apixaban, betrixaban, edoxaban, and rivaroxaban inhibit factor Xa. *TF* tissue factor [18]. Reprinted from Makaryus JN, Halperin JL, Lau JF, Oral anticoagulants in the management of venous thromboembolism, Nature Reviews Cardiology, © 2013, Vol. 10/No. 7, pages 397–409

(www.acforum.org) released a set of expert guidance documents on the management of VTE in 2016, which intend to provide guidance for practical, everyday situations, often when clear cut evidence is lacking or contradictory [21].

Further guideline and guidance documents have been produced by large cardiovascular societies in North America and Europe [22–32]. Many of these documents contain useful tables and figures that providers may reference when determining appropriate drug choices, doses, contraindications, and follow-up protocols. For patients with cancer, the American Society of Clinical Oncology (ASCO) and the National Comprehensive Cancer Network have published guidelines on the management of thrombotic disease in cancer patients [33, 34]. The National Comprehensive Cancer Network updates their guideline on an annual basis and posts it on their website (www.nccn.org) [34]. Finally, the Anticoagulation Forum Centers of Excellence website (www.excellence.acforum.org) [35] is a robust resource for patient- and provider-focused toolkits for both inpatient and outpatient anticoagulation management. This website contains tools focused on specific disease states, medications, and clinical settings. It also houses comprehensive toolkits, some of which are continually reviewed and updated (*e.g.*, www.anticoagulationtoolkit.org) [36].

Providers can rely on this book and the various online resources as they develop their own institutional protocols and procedures as well as for guidance in managing unique clinical situations. Of course, no book or published document can replace good clinical judgment. Instead, these tools are meant to provide ready access to important evidence and clinical data that may guide clinician decision making and ensure high-quality patient care.

Exploring the Future of Anticoagulation Care

As noted above, the field of anticoagulation has changed drastically in the last half century. From the introduction of vitamin K antagonists to direct oral anticoagulants, from the development of unfractionated heparin to the refinement of low-molecular-weight heparins, and from individual clinical management to the proliferation of robust anticoagulation management services, this field has continued to change and grow. Yet much work is still left to do. In fact, anticoagulants remain the leading cause of adverse drug events in emergency departments across the United States [37]. Efforts to improve the quality and safety of anticoagulation care are needed at both local and national levels.

Recounting the history of anticoagulation therapy in our Introduction is not merely an academic exercise but a reminder to us of how far we have come in preventing and treating thromboembolic diseases. The future holds many exciting possibilities and some challenges to overcome. New drug development will continue to offer patients more choice, more convenience, and (hopefully) a better balance between efficacy and side effect. To guide that process, regulatory bodies (e.g., the US Food and Drug Administration) must continue to ensure high-quality evidence guides their review process without unnecessarily preventing or delaying the introduction of these medications to the market. At the same time, the healthcare system must continue to grapple with the challenge of financing care for a growing population of patients at risk for thromboembolic complications. Potential solutions may include personalized therapies that improve the likelihood of treatment benefit as well as redesigning our clinical delivery systems to ensure safe care. The many anticoagulation clinics that have developed over the past few decades with great expertise in warfarin management may prove to be essential in the management of non-warfarin therapies [38].

This book outlines the current state of anticoagulation care. It also provides a foundation on which the field will inevitably continue to grow and develop. We hope that the readers will find this book to be a useful and reliable reference for patient care.

References

1. Pearce JM. Johann Jakob Wepfer (1620-95) and cerebral hemorrhage. J Neurol Neurosurg Psychiatry. 1997;62:387.
2. de Saint Pathus G. La vie et les Miracles de Saint Louis. Paris: Biblioth eque National de France.1271;1330–50.
3. Galanaud J-P, Laroche J-P, Righini M. The history and historical treatments of deep vein thrombosis. J Thromb Haemost. 2013;11:402–11.
4. Anning S. The historical aspects. In: Dodd H, Cockett F, editors. The pathology and surgery of the lower limbs. 2nd ed. Edinburgh: Churchill Livingston; 1976. p. 3–17.
5. Hunter H. Observations on the inflammation of the internal coats of veins. Trans Soc Improv Med Chir Knowledge. 1793;1:18–41.
6. Magner L. A history of medicine. New York: Marcel Dekker; 1992. 393 p.
7. Howell H, Holt E. Two new factors in blood coagulation - heparin and pro-antithrombin. Am J Phys. 1918;47:328–41.
8. Murray D, Jacques L, Perrett T, Best C. Heparin and the thrombosis of veins following injury. Surgery. 1937;2:163–87.
9. Wardrop D, Keeling D. The story of the discovery of heparin and warfarin. Br J Haematol. 2008;474:757–63.
10. Roderick L. The pathology of sweet clover disease in cattle. J Am Vet Med Assoc. 1929;74:314–25.
11. Roderick L. A problem in the coagulation of blood: "sweet clover disease of cattle". Am J Phys. 1931;96:413–25.
12. Schofield F. The cause of a new disease in cattle stimulating hemorrhagic septicaemia and blackleg. J Am Vet Med Assoc. 1924;64:553–75.
13. Whitlon D, Sadowski J, Suttie J. Mechanisms of coumarin action: significance of vitamin K epoxide reductase inhibition. Biochemistry. 1978;17(8):1371–7.
14. Stahmann M, Huebner C, Link K. Studies on the hemorrhagic sweet clover disease. J Biol Chem. 1941;138:513–27.
15. Wright I. Experience with anticoagulants. Circulation. 1959;19:110–3.
16. Prandoni A, Wright I. The anti-coagulants, heparin and the dicoumarin 3,3′ methylene-bis (4-hydroxy-coumarin). N Y Acad Med. 1942;18:433.
17. Link K. The discovery of dicoumarol and its sequels. Circulation. 1959;19:97–107.

18. Makaryus JN, Halperin JL, Lau JF. Oral anticoagulants in the management of venous thromboembolism. Nat Rev Cardiol. 2013;10(7):397–409.
19. Guyatt GH, Akl EA, Crowther M, Gutterman DD, Schuunemann HJ. American college of chest physicians Antithrombotic T, et al. executive summary: antithrombotic therapy and prevention of thrombosis, 9th ed: American College of Chest Physicians Evidence-Based Clinical Practice Guidelines. Chest. 2012;141(2 Suppl):7S–47S.
20. Kearon C, Akl EA, Ornelas J, Blaivas A, Jimenez D, Bounameaux H, et al. Antithrombotic therapy for VTE disease: CHEST guideline and expert panel report. Chest. 2016;149(2):315–52.
21. Ansell JE. Management of venous thromboembolism: clinical guidance from the Anticoagulation Forum. J Thromb Thrombolysis. 2016;41(1):1–2.
22. Konstantinides SV, Torbicki A, Agnelli G, Danchin N, Fitzmaurice D, Galie N, et al. 2014 ESC guidelines on the diagnosis and management of acute pulmonary embolism. Eur Heart J. 2014;35(43):3033–69, 69a-69k.
23. Heidbuchel H, Verhamme P, Alings M, Antz M, Diener HC, Hacke W, et al. Updated European Heart Rhythm Association Practical Guide on the use of non-vitamin K antagonist anticoagulants in patients with non-valvular atrial fibrillation. Europace. 2015;17(10):1467–507.
24. Cohen H, Arachchillage DR, Middeldorp S, Beyer-Westendorf J, Abdul-Kadir R. Management of direct oral anticoagulants in women of childbearing potential: guidance from the SSC of the ISTH. J Thromb Haemost. 2016;14(8):1673–6.
25. Martin K, Beyer-Westendorf J, Davidson BL, Huisman MV, Sandset PM, Moll S. Use of the direct oral anticoagulants in obese patients: guidance from the SSC of the ISTH. J Thromb Haemost. 2016;14(6):1308–13.
26. Ruff CT, Ansell JE, Becker RC, Benjamin EJ, Deicicchi DJ, Mark Estes NA, et al. North American Thrombosis Forum, AF action initiative consensus document. Am J Med. 2016;129(5 Suppl):S1–S29.
27. January CT, Wann LS, Alpert JS, Calkins H, Cigarroa JE, Cleveland JC Jr, et al. 2014 AHA/ACC/HRS guideline for the management of patients with atrial fibrillation: a report of the American College of Cardiology/American Heart Association Task Force on Practice Guidelines and the Heart Rhythm Society. Circulation. 2014;130(23):e199–267.
28. Task Force Members, Lip GY, Windecker S, Huber K, Kirchhof P, Marin F, Document Reviewers, et al. Management of antithrombotic therapy in atrial fibrillation patients presenting with acute coronary syndrome and/or undergoing percutaneous coronary or valve interventions: a joint consensus document of the European Society of Cardiology Working Group on Thrombosis, European Heart Rhythm Association (EHRA), European Association of Percutaneous Cardiovascular Interventions (EAPCI) and European Association of Acute Cardiac Care (ACCA) endorsed by the Heart Rhythm Society (HRS) and Asia-Pacific Heart Rhythm Society (APHRS). Eur Heart J. 2014;35(45):3155–79.
29. Verma A, Cairns JA, Mitchell LB, Macle L, Stiell IG, Gladstone D, et al. 2014 focused update of the Canadian Cardiovascular Society Guidelines for the management of atrial fibrillation. Can J Cardiol. 2014;30(10):1114–30.
30. Sticherling C, Marin F, Birnie D, Boriani G, Calkins H, Dan GA, et al. Antithrombotic management in patients undergoing electrophysiological procedures: a European Heart Rhythm Association (EHRA) position document endorsed by the ESC Working Group Thrombosis, Heart Rhythm Society (HRS), and Asia Pacific Heart Rhythm Society (APHRS). Europace. 2015;17(8):1197–214.
31. Heidenreich PA, Solis P, Estes NA 3rd, Fonarow GC, Jurgens CY, Marine JE, et al. 2016 ACC/AHA clinical performance and quality measures for adults with atrial fibrillation or atrial flutter: a report of the American College of Cardiology/American Heart Association Task Force on Performance Measures. J Am Coll Cardiol. 2016;68(5):525–68.
32. Kirchhof P, Benussi S, Kotecha D, Ahlsson A, Atar D, Casadei B, et al. 2016 ESC Guidelines for the management of atrial fibrillation developed in collaboration with EACTS. Europace. 2016;18(11):1609–78.
33. Lyman GH, Bohlke K, Khorana AA, Kuderer NM, Lee AY, Arcelus JI, et al. American Society of Clinical Oncology. Venous thromboembolism prophylaxis and treatment in patients with cancer: American Society of Clinical Oncology Clinical Practice Guideline update 2014. J Clin Oncol. 2015;33(6):654–6.
34. Streiff MB, Holmstrom B, Ashrani A, Bockenstedt PL, Chesney C, Eby C, et al. Cancer-associated venous thromboembolic disease, version 1.2015. J Natl Compr Cancer Netw. 2015;13(9):1079–95.
35. Anticoagulation forum centers of excellence. Website www.excellence.acforum.org.
36. Anticoagulation toolkit on anticoagulation forum of excellence. Website www.anticoagulationtoolkit.org.
37. Shehab N, Lovegrove MC, Geller AI, Rose KO, Weidle NJ, Budnitz DS. US emergency department visits for outpatient adverse drug events, 2013–2014. JAMA. 2016;316(20):2115–25.
38. Barnes GD, Nallamothu BK, Sales AE, Froehlich JB. Reimagining anticoagulation clinics in the era of direct oral anticoagulants. Circ Cardiovasc Qual Outcomes. 2016;9(2):182–5.

Part I

Anticoagulants

Warfarin

2

Gregory C. Hadlock, Allison E. Burnett, and Edith A. Nutescu

Clinical Vignette

AG is a 63-year-old woman presenting to the emergency department with a 4-day history of shortness of breath. 3 weeks prior to the onset of her symptoms, she had a left tibia fracture and has been largely immobile since. She has a past medical history of type 2 diabetes mellitus, hypertension, and stage 4 chronic kidney disease (CKD), with a baseline serum creatinine of 2.9 mg/dL. She is up-to-date on her cancer screenings, including for breast, colon, and cervical cancers, which all have been negative. A computed tomography angiogram of the chest revealed bilateral pulmonary emboli. The patient was initiated on therapeutic anticoagulation with a heparin infusion and bridged to warfarin for a 3-month treatment duration.

Introduction

Until recently, vitamin K antagonists, such as warfarin, were the only oral anticoagulants available for long-term or extended anticoagulation. Although very effective for prevention and treatment of venous and arterial thromboembolism, warfarin has a narrow therapeutic index; has many drug, disease, and dietary interactions; and requires frequent monitoring and dose adjustments [1–4]. These drawbacks have historically resulted in under treatment of patients that warrant anticoagulation therapy [5]. While direct oral anticoagulants (DOACs) have significantly changed approaches to anticoagulation therapy, are more convenient, and are easier to use, warfarin will continue to be a mainstay of therapy for many patients. Thus, clinicians must possess familiarity with this still widely used medication. In this chapter, we will discuss the pharmacology,

G. C. Hadlock
Inpatient Pharmacy Department, University of New Mexico Hospital, Albuquerque, NM, USA
e-mail: ghadlock@salud.unm.edu

A. E. Burnett (✉)
University of New Mexico College of Pharmacy, Albuquerque, NM, USA
e-mail: aburnett@salud.unm.edu

E. A. Nutescu
Department of Pharmacy Systems, Outcomes and Policy, Center for Pharmacoepidemiology and Pharmacoeconomic Research, The University of Illinois at Chicago College of Pharmacy, Chicago, IL, USA
e-mail: enutescu@uic.edu

J. F. Lau et al. (eds.), *Anticoagulation Therapy*, https://doi.org/10.1007/978-3-319-73709-6_2

clinical utility, and practical management aspects that promote optimized safety and efficacy of warfarin therapy.

Pharmacology

Mechanism of Action

Warfarin is an oral anticoagulant that acts as a vitamin K antagonist. Vitamin K is an essential cofactor in the γ-carboxylation of several glutamic acid residues in the hepatically produced vitamin K-dependent procoagulant factors II, VII, IX, and X, as well as the anticoagulant proteins C and S. Warfarin interferes with the hepatic recycling of vitamin K by inhibiting vitamin K epoxide reductase (VKOR), the enzyme that converts vitamin K epoxide to vitamin K. The accumulation of vitamin K epoxide reduces the effective concentration of vitamin K and reduces the synthesis of functional coagulation factors. Concentrations of functional clotting factors II, VII, IX, and X are diminished gradually at rates corresponding to their elimination half-lives (Table 2.1). As it has no effect on preexisting functional circulating clotting factors, the onset of the anticoagulant effect of warfarin is delayed. It takes approximately 5–7 days to reach a steady state of anticoagulation after warfarin therapy is initiated or after dosing changes. Protein C and its cofactor protein S are also vitamin K dependent, and these proteins are depleted by warfarin at rates dependent on their elimination half-lives. Due to its shorter half-life, protein C activity falls more rapidly than the procoagulant clotting factors II, IX, and X, which can lead to a paradoxical hypercoagulable state during the first few days of warfarin therapy. This can be managed through avoidance of excessive "loading" doses of warfarin (e.g., >10 mg) which may cause protein C to fall too precipitously and/or use of overlapping parenteral therapy during the first 5–7 days of warfarin initiation [1, 3, 6].

Table 2.1 Elimination half-lives of vitamin K-dependent clotting factors

Clotting factor	Half-life (h)
II (prothrombin)	42–72
VII	4–6
IX	21–30
X	27–48
Protein C	9
Protein S	60

Warfarin is administered orally as a racemic mixture of stereoisomers (*R* and *S* enantiomers), each with distinctive metabolic pathways, half-lives, and potencies. The S isomer is three to five times more potent than the R isomer, has a longer elimination half-life, and is primarily metabolized by cytochrome P450 (CYP) 2C9. The R isomer is metabolized primarily by CYP1A2 and CYP3A4. Many drugs, herbal, and nutritional products interact with warfarin by stereoselectively inhibiting the metabolism of either the R isomer or the S isomer (Table 2.2 and Table 2.3). Differences in metabolism, along with disease- and/or drug-induced alterations in metabolism, account for much of the variation in an individual's initial response to, and maintenance requirement for, warfarin. Genetic expression of CYP2C9 influences the rate of metabolism of warfarin and thus impacts dosing requirements to meet a particular therapeutic end point [7]. Variability in genetic expression of VKORC1 (the gene that encodes subunit 1 of the vitamin K epoxide reductase complex) also influences dosing requirements in patients taking warfarin [7]. Genetic testing for CYP2C9 genotype and VKORC1 haplotype can be incorporated with clinical and demographic information to predict warfarin dose requirements in individual patients, using dosing algorithms that have been developed and investigated. A practical example is available online at www.warfarindosing.org [8]. The prevalence of these polymorphisms varies in different populations. Current evidence does not support routine use of genetic information to guide warfarin dosing as it has not been shown to provide significant benefit above and beyond use of clinical information and dosing nomograms [9].

Pharmacokinetics

Absorption

Warfarin has almost 100% oral bioavailability and is rapidly absorbed in the upper gastrointestinal tract (GI). Peak plasma concentrations of warfarin occur in 90 min [10, 11].

Table 2.2 Clinically significant warfarin drug interactions[a]

Increase anticoagulation effect (↑ INR)	Decrease anticoagulation effect (↓ INR)	Increase bleeding risk
Alcohol binge	Azathioprine	Abciximab
Allopurinol	Barbiturates	Argatroban
Amiodarone	Carbamazepine	Aspirin
Azithromycin	Cholestyramine	Bivalirudin
Bactrim	Dicloxacillin	Clopidogrel
Ciprofloxacin	Griseofulvin	Dalteparin
Citalopram	Nafcillin	Danaparoid
Clarithromycin	Phenytoin	Dipyridamole
Clofibrate	Primidone	DOACs
Danazol	Rifampin	Enoxaparin
Disulfiram	Rifabutin	Eptifibatide
Doxycycline	Sucralfate	Fondaparinux
Erythromycin	Vitamin K	Nonsteroidal anti-inflammatory drugs (NSAIDs)
Fenofibrate		Prasugrel
Fluconazole		Ticagrelor
Fluorouracil		Ticlopidine
Fluoxetine		Tirofiban
Fluvoxamine		Unfractionated heparin
Gemfibrozil		
Isoniazid		
Itraconazole		
Levofloxacin		
Lovastatin		
Metronidazole		
Miconazole		
Neomycin		
Omeprazole		
Phenylbutazone		
Piroxicam		
Propafenone		
Sertraline		
Simvastatin		
Sulfamethoxazole		
Sulfinpyrazone		
Tamoxifen		
Testosterone		
Tetracycline		
Vitamin E		
Voriconazole		
Zafirlukast		

INR international normalized ratio
[a]List is not exhaustive

Distribution

Warfarin is approximately 99% bound to the plasma protein albumin, which leads to its relatively low volume of distribution (Vd) of 0.14 L/kg [11]. Also, because of its extensive protein binding, warfarin exhibits nonlinear pharmacokinetics, and small adjustments in dose can lead to large changes in anticoagulant response [1].

Table 2.3 Potential warfarin interactions with herbal and nutritional products[a]

Increased anticoagulation effect (increase bleeding risk or ↑ INR)		Decreased anticoagulation effect (↓ INR)
Amica flower	Ginkgo	Coenzyme Q_{10}
Angelica root	Horse chestnut	Ginseng
Anise	Licorice root	Green tea
Asafoetida	Lovage root	St. John's wort
Bogbean	Meadowsweet	
Borage seed oil	Onion	
Bromelain	Papain	
Capsicum	Parsley	
Celery	Passionflower herb	
Chamomile	Poplar	
Clove	Quassia	
Danshen	Red clover	
Devil's claw	Rue	
Dong quai	Sweet clover	
Fenugreek	Turmeric	
Feverfew	Vitamin E	
Garlic	Willow bark	
Ginger		

INR international normalized ratio
[a]List is not exhaustive

Metabolism

Racemic warfarin has an average plasma half-life of ~40 h (range of 15–60 h). Warfarin is extensively metabolized in the liver via several isoenzymes including CYP 1A2, 3A4, 2C9, 2C19, 2C8, and 2C18. Due to genetic variations in these isoenzymes, hepatic metabolism of warfarin varies greatly among patients, leading to potentially large interpatient differences in dose requirements [1, 3, 4, 10, 11].

Elimination

Warfarin and its metabolites are primarily excreted in the urine [3, 10, 11]. Renal impairment has no direct impact on warfarin pharmacodynamics since these metabolites have little or no anticoagulant activity. However, renal impairment may diminish the function of CYP2C9, leading to accumulation of warfarin, thus enhancing its effect [10].

Pharmacodynamics

Warfarin's *anticoagulant* effect is related to plasma depletion of vitamin K-dependent coagulation factors and manifests as an elevation in the international normalized ratio (INR) which is exquisitely sensitive to reductions in factor VII. The *antithrombotic* effect of warfarin relies on significant depletion of prothrombin (factor II) and factor X in the plasma that is delayed for at least 5–7 days after warfarin initiation due the long half-life of prothrombin and factor X. It is important to recognize that patients may achieve a therapeutic INR within the first few days of therapy (due to rapid depletion of factor VII that usually occurs in the setting of excessive warfarin doses) and appear to be anticoagulated but may still be at risk for propagation or recurrence of an acute thrombus since prothrombin and factor X levels are still close to normal. This provides rationale for continuing overlapping parenteral therapy for a full 5 days, even if a therapeutic INR is attained prior to day 5, in patients with an acute event [1, 3, 10]. Rapid increases in INR during the first few days of therapy warrant warfarin dose reductions to prevent supratherapeutic INR values early in warfarin therapy. Through its antithrombotic effects, warfarin reduces the likelihood of thrombus propagation in acute VTE and lowers the risk of thromboembolism in other indications associated with thrombosis, such as atrial fibrillation [1].

Clinical Utility

As the only oral anticoagulant for over 60 years, warfarin is widely used in the treatment and prevention of thromboembolic events across a broad range of disease states and conditions. In the past decade, the advent of direct oral anticoagulants (DOACs), including the factor Xa inhibitors apixaban, edoxaban, and rivaroxaban, and the direct thrombin inhibitor (DTI), dabigatran, has ushered in a new era of oral anticoagulant options for patients and clinicians. While research and experience with warfarin exceed that with DOACs, the advent of these non-vitamin K antagonist therapies is significantly and rapidly changing the therapeutic landscape and leading to a decline in warfarin use [12, 13]. Several large randomized controlled trials and meta-analyses have shown DOACs to be equally effective to warfarin, with significantly better safety profiles, in both non-valvular atrial fibrillation

(NVAF) and treatment of venous thromboembolism (VTE) [14, 15]. Importantly, these results have been confirmed in several phase IV, real-world analyses [16–23]. Based on these findings, DOACs have been placed on equal or better footing than warfarin in several national and international societal guidelines for NVAF [24, 25] and are preferred for treatment of VTE [26]. Additionally, DOACs are more convenient, are easier to use, and provide greater patient satisfaction [27–29]. Table 2.4 provides a comparison of the characteristics of warfarin and DOACs.

It is important to note that not all patients are eligible for treatment with a DOAC [30]. Additionally, warfarin has been extensively used for numerous clinical indications since its approval in the 1950s, providing a significant advantage of patient and clinician familiarity and experience. Thus, in many populations, warfarin will likely continue to serve an important role [4]. Table 2.5 lists characteristics of patients who are not optimal DOAC candidates and should likely be managed with warfarin therapy.

Practical Management

Regardless of the setting where an anticoagulation patient is to be managed, best practices suggest that it should be done "in a systematic and coordinated fashion, incorporating patient education, systematic INR testing, tracking, follow-up and patient communication of results and dosing decisions" [2]. Structured anticoagulation therapy management services (e.g., anticoagulation clinics) have been demonstrated to improve the efficacy and safety of warfarin therapy, and consideration for patient referral is recommended [33].

Patient Engagement and Education

Patient education is a vital component of warfarin therapy. Improved outcomes have been reported when patients take responsibility for, understand, and adhere to an anticoagulation plan of care [1, 2, 34]. National regulatory bodies, such as the Joint Commission, have mandated patient

Table 2.4 Comparison of oral anticoagulant pharmacokinetics and pharmacodynamics

	Warfarin	Dabigatran	Rivaroxaban	Apixaban	Edoxaban
Target(s)	IIa, VIIa, IXa, Xa	IIa	Xa	Xa	Xa
Prodrug	No	Yes	No	No	No
Bioavailability (%)	80–100	6.5 (pH dependent)	80	50	62
Volume of distribution (L)	10	50–70	50	23	> 300
Peak effect	4–5 days	1.5–3 h	2–4 h	1–3 h	1–2 h
Half-life[a]	40 h	12–17 h	5–9 h	9–14 h	10–14 h
Renal elimination	None	80%	33%	25%	35–50%
Protein binding (%)	> 99	35	90	87	55
Dialyzable	No	Yes	No	No	Possible
Drug interactions	Numerous	P-gp	CYP3A4, P-gp	CYP3A4, P-gp	P-gp
Routine coagulation monitoring	Yes	No	No	No	No
Antidote	Vitamin K	Idarucizumab	No	No	No
Lab measure	INR	aPTT* TT, dTT, ECT*	PT* Anti-Xa*	Anti-Xa*	Anti-Xa*
Dietary interactions/ considerations	Numerous	None	Take treatment doses with food	None	None

*For qualitative assessment only as these measures have not been correlated with pharmacodynamic effect

P-gp P-glycoprotein, *INR* international normalized ratio, *aPTT*, activated partial thromboplastin time, *TT* thrombin time, *dTT* dilute thrombin time, *ECT* ecarin clotting time, *PT* prothrombin time

aIn patients with normal renal function

Table 2.5 Patients that should be considered for warfarin therapy rather than a DOAC [4]

Characteristic	Comment/rationale
Suboptimal adherence	Compared to DOACs, warfarin has a long half-life (~40 h vs. ~12 h), and missed doses will result in less dramatic fluctuations in anticoagulant levels and increased risk for adverse events
Significant DOAC drug interactions	Warfarin drug interactions may be managed via increased frequency of INR monitoring and dose adjustment. With DOACs, there is no routine, readily available laboratory assay to aid in monitoring for accumulation or underexposure in the setting of possible drug interactions
Reduced renal or hepatic function	The DOACs are all at least partially reliant on renal elimination. In patients with severe renal impairment, warfarin would be the preferred oral anticoagulant until more data is available. Among patients with significant hepatic impairment, anticoagulant status and drug accumulation may be more readily assessed for warfarin (via INR testing) compared to DOACs
Financial constraints	Because it is available in generic form, warfarin (and its associated monitoring) may have less financial impact on patients compared to DOACs. All patients should be evaluated for longitudinal access to needed medications for the duration of therapy prior to prescribing
Mechanical cardiac valve	Based on negative results of the RE-ALIGN trial [31], which was terminated early due to an increased risk of thromboembolic and bleeding events in patients receiving dabigatran when compared to warfarin, patients with mechanical cardiac valves should be managed with warfarin therapy
Indication for anticoagulation or patient population in which DOACs have not been adequately studied	These include, but are not limited to: • Antiphospholipid antibody syndrome (APS) • Cancer-associated VTE • Extremes of weight (< 50 or >120 kg) • Indications other than NVAF or VTE • Require concomitant dual antiplatelet therapy • Pregnancy • Breastfeeding • Pediatrics Until more data is available, the above patient populations should receive conventional anticoagulant therapies, such as warfarin or LMWH, whenever possible
Express a preference for warfarin over a DOAC	• With multiple oral anticoagulant options now available, it is imperative to employ a shared decision-making approach with patients, families, and caregivers. • Some patients may prefer warfarin therapy and associated routine monitoring • Additionally, some patients may express concern over lack of an antidote for factor Xa inhibitors such as apixaban, edoxaban, and rivaroxaban • While evidence suggests an advantage for DOACs over warfarin in bleeding outcomes and mortality despite no antidote [32], patient preference must be considered in order to optimize adherence

DOAC direct oral anticoagulant, *INR* international normalized ratio, *VTE* venous thromboembolism, *NVAF* non-valvular atrial fibrillation

and family education prior to discharge from the hospital on key elements of warfarin therapy including, but not limited to, the importance of follow-up monitoring, compliance, interactions, and management of potential adverse events [35]. Effective methods of anticoagulation education for patients and caregivers include face-to-face interaction with a trained professional, group training sessions, audiovisual resources, and/or the use of written materials. Several web resources are available for warfarin education, including the video "Staying Active and Healthy with Blood Thinners" from the Agency for Healthcare Research and Quality (AHRQ) (Available at https://www.ahrq.gov/patients-consumers/diagnosis treatment/treatments/btpills/stayactive.html) [36].

Education provided to patients should be delivered at an appropriate health literacy and reading level and in the patient's preferred language. The use of the "teach back" method with open-ended questions aids in assessing the patient degree of understanding and should be routinely employed. Key elements should be discussed upon initiation of therapy, with reinforcement of education at each clinic visit [37] (Table 2.6).

Table 2.6 Key elements of warfarin patient education

• Identification of generic and brand names of warfarin
• Reasons they need anticoagulation therapy
• Expected duration of therapy
• Dosing and administration
• Visual recognition of warfarin tablet strength and color
• What to do if a dose is missed
• Importance of INR monitoring and compliance with medications and appointments
• Recognition of signs and symptoms of bleeding and thromboembolism
• What to do if bleeding or thromboembolism occurs
• Recognition of signs and symptoms of disease states that influence warfarin dosing requirements
• Potential for interactions with prescription and over-the-counter medications and natural/herbal products
• Dietary considerations and use of alcohol
• Avoidance of pregnancy
• Significance of informing other healthcare providers that warfarin has been prescribed
• Importance of obtaining and wearing a medical alert bracelet or necklace stating they are on anticoagulation therapy
• When, where, and with whom follow-up will be provided

INR international normalized ratio

Dosing: Initiation

When initiating warfarin therapy, it is challenging to predict the precise maintenance dose a patient will eventually require. The dose response to warfarin is influenced by several factors, including inherent patient characteristics, such as age and genetics, as well as drug/diet/disease state interactions and clinical status (Table 2.7). These should all be factored into decisions about what warfarin dose to administer.

Before initiating therapy, patients should be assessed for any contraindications to anticoagulation therapy (Table 2.8) and risk factors for major bleeding (Table 2.9). Clinicians should conduct a thorough medication history including the use of prescription and nonprescription drugs and any herbal supplements to detect interactions that may affect warfarin dosing requirements (Tables 2.2 and 2.3). A brief review of the vitamin K content of foods and the importance of maintaining a stable intake of vitamin K from week to week should be included in the initial patient visit with reinforcement during subsequent patient visits (Table 2.10).

Because warfarin does not follow linear kinetics, small dose adjustments can lead to large changes in anticoagulant response [3, 10]. Therefore, warfarin dose must be determined by frequent clinical and laboratory monitoring, and adjustments should be guided by dosing nomograms [38–41]. An example of a flexible dosing nomogram that allows for initiation of warfarin 5 or 10 mg is shown in Table 2.11. Although there are conflicting data regarding the optimal warfarin induction regimen, when the patient's genotype is not known, most patients can start with 5 mg daily, and subsequent doses are determined based on INR response. Younger (<55 years) and otherwise healthy patients may safely use higher warfarin initiation doses (e.g., 7.5 or 10 mg). Conversely, more conservative initiation doses (e.g., <5 mg) should be used in patients likely to be more warfarin sensitive, including elderly patients (≥75 years); patients with heart failure, liver disease, or poor nutritional status; and patients who are taking interacting prescription and herbal or over-the-counter medications (Tables 2.2 and 2.3) or are at high risk of bleeding [1, 2, 10]. Loading doses of warfarin (e.g., ≥15 mg) should be avoided, as they may provide a false impression that a therapeutic INR has been achieved in 2–3 days as well as lead to potential future overdosing [2, 4].

Dosing: Maintenance

When a patient's INR is out of range, an adjustment in warfarin dosing may be necessary. Table 2.12 describes suggested approaches to warfarin dosing adjustments for both regular-intensity (INR goal 2–3) and high-intensity (INR goal 2.5–3.5) maintenance therapy. Typically, dosing adjustments of 5–20% of the total daily dose (or the total weekly dose) are appropriate to reach the therapeutic range [1, 2, 10, 44]. Because warfarin does not follow linear kinetics, small

Table 2.7 Warfarin interactions with disease states and clinical conditions

Clinical condition	Effect on warfarin therapy
Advanced age	• Increased sensitivity to warfarin due to reduced vitamin K stores and/or lower plasma concentrations of vitamin K-dependent clotting factors (with decreasing hepatic function over time)
Pregnancy	• Teratogenic; avoid exposure during pregnancy whenever possible
Breastfeeding	• Not excreted in breast milk; can be used postpartum by nursing mothers
Alcohol	• Acute ingestion: Inhibits warfarin metabolism, with acute elevation in INR
	• Chronic ingestion: Induces warfarin metabolism, with higher dose requirements
Hepatic impairment	• May induce coagulopathy by decreased production of clotting factors, with baseline elevation in INR
	• May reduce clearance of warfarin
Renal impairment	• Reduced activity of CYP2C9, with lower warfarin dose requirements
Heart failure	• Reduced warfarin metabolism due to concomitant congestive hepatopathy
Cardiac valve replacement	• Enhanced sensitivity to warfarin postoperatively due to hypoalbuminemia, lower oral intake, decreased physical activity, and reduced clotting factor concentrations after cardiopulmonary bypass
Nutritional status	• Changes in dietary vitamin K intake (intentional or as the result of disease, surgery, etc.) alter response to warfarin
	• Reduced levels of serum albumin will potentiate warfarin effect
Use of tube feedings	• Decreased sensitivity to warfarin, possibly caused by warfarin binding to feeding tube, changes in absorption, or vitamin K content of nutritional supplements
Thyroid disease	• Hypothyroidism: Decreased catabolism of clotting factors requiring increased dosing requirements
	• Hyperthyroidism: Increased catabolism of clotting factors causing increased sensitivity to warfarin
Tobacco use	• Smoking: May induce CYP1A2, increasing warfarin dosing requirements
	• Chewing tobacco: May contain vitamin K, increasing warfarin dosing requirements
Fever/active infection	• Increased catabolism of clotting factors, causing acute increase in INR
Diarrhea	• Reduction in secretion of vitamin K by gut flora, as well as increased flushing of vitamin K from gut, causing acute increase in INR
Malignancy	• Increased sensitivity to warfarin by multiple factors (drug interactions, altered absorption, etc.)

INR international normalized ratio

Table 2.8 Contraindications to warfarin [1, 2]

General
Active bleeding
Hemophilia or other hemorrhagic tendencies
Severe liver disease with elevated baseline INR
Severe thrombocytopenia (platelet count <20 × 10^3/mm^3 [20 × 10^9/L])
Malignant hypertension
Inability to meticulously supervise and monitor treatment
Hypersensitivity to warfarin
Pregnancy
History of purple toe syndrome
Inability to obtain follow-up INR measurements
Inappropriate medication use or lifestyle behaviors

INR international normalized ratio

dose adjustments can lead to large INR changes; thus large dose adjustments (i.e., >20% of the total weekly dose) are not recommended. Maintenance dosing guidelines should only be applied to patients who have reached a steady-state dose and are not still in the initiation phase of therapy (Table 2.12).

Administration

Warfarin should be administered orally once a day at approximately the same time each day. In clinical practice, patients are often encouraged to take their dose later in the day so as to facilitate implementation of needed dose changes identified at daytime clinic visits. Warfarin may be crushed and given via feeding tubes [11]. However, bioavailability of warfarin given via this route will be significantly diminished and will require a dose increase.

Table 2.9 Risk factors for major bleeding while on warfarin therapy [42]

Anticoagulation intensity (e.g., INR > 5, aPTT >120 s)
Initiation of therapy (first few days and weeks)
Unstable anticoagulation response
Age > 65 years
Concurrent antiplatelet drug use
Concurrent nonsteroidal anti-inflammatory drug use
History of gastrointestinal bleeding
Recent surgery or trauma
High risk for fall/trauma
Heavy alcohol use
Renal failure
Hepatic impairment
Cerebrovascular disease
Malignancy

aPTT activated partial thromboplastin time, *INR* international normalized ratio

Monitoring

Before the initiation of any antithrombotic therapy, including warfarin, an assessment of baseline coagulation status is necessary. The clinician should obtain a baseline platelet count, hemoglobin (Hgb), and/or hematocrit (Hct), as well as evaluate the integrity of the extrinsic and intrinsic coagulation pathways with the prothrombin time (PT) and the activated partial thromboplastin time (aPTT).

Because warfarin has a narrow therapeutic index and significant inter- and intrapatient variability, it requires frequent laboratory monitoring to ensure optimal outcomes and minimize complications. The PT, which measures the biological activity of factors II, VII, and X, was initially the most frequently used test to monitor warfarin's anticoagulant effect. However, wide variation in sensitivity among commercially

Table 2.10 Vitamin K content of select foods[a]

Very high (>200 mcg)	High (100–200 mcg)	Medium (50–100 mcg)	Low (<50 mcg)
Brussels sprouts	Basil	Apple, green	Apple, red
Chickpea	Broccoli	Asparagus	Avocado
Collard greens	Canola oil	Cabbage	Beans
Coriander	Chive	Cauliflower	Breads and grains
Endive	Coleslaw	Mayonnaise	Carrot
Kale	Cucumber (unpeeled)	Pistachios	Celery
Lettuce, red leaf	Green onion/scallion	Squash, summer	Cereal
Parsley	Lettuce, butterhead		Coffee
Spinach	Mustard greens		Corn
Swiss chard	Soybean oil		Cucumber (peeled)
Tea, black			Dairy products
Tea, green			Eggs
Turnip greens			Fruit (varies)
Watercress			Lettuce, iceberg
			Meats, fish, poultry
			Pasta
			Peanuts
			Peas
			Potato
			Rice
			Tomato

[a]Approximate amount of vitamin K per 100 g (3.5 oz) serving

Table 2.11 Flexible warfarin initiation dosing nomogram [43]

Day	INR	10 mg initiation dose	5 mg initiation dose
1		10 mg	5 mg
2	<1.5	7.5–10 mg	5 mg
	1.5–1.9	2.5 mg	2.5 mg
	2.0–2.5	1.0–2.5 mg	1–2.5 mg
	>2.5	0	0
3	<1.5	5–10 mg	5–10 mg
	1.5–1.9	2.5–5 mg	2.5–5 mg
	2.0–2.5	0–2.5 mg	0–2.5 mg
	2.5–3.0	0–2.5 mg	0–2.5 mg
	>3.0	0	0
4	<1.5	10 mg	10 mg
	1.5–1.9	5–7.5 mg	5–7.5 mg
	2.0–3.0	0–5 mg	0–5 mg
	>3.0	0	0
5	<1.5	10 mg	10 mg
	1.5–1.9	7.5–10 mg	7.5–10 mg
	2.0–3.0	0–5 mg	0–5 mg
	>3.0	0	0
6	<1.5	7.5–12.5 mg	7.5–12.5 mg
	1.5–1.9	5–10 mg	5–10 mg
	2.0–3.0	0–7.5 mg	0–7.5 mg
	>3.0	0	0

INR international normalized ratio

available thromboplastin reagents was found to provide significantly different PT results across reference laboratories, potentially leading to inappropriate dosing decisions [1, 2, 10]. In the early 1980s, the World Health Organization (WHO) developed a system to standardize PT results. All commercially available thromboplastins are compared with an international reference thromboplastin and then assigned an International Sensitivity Index (ISI). This value is used to mathematically convert PT results to the international normalized ratio (INR) by exponentially multiplying the PT ratio to the power of the ISI of the thromboplastin being used in the laboratory to measure the test ($INR = [PT\ patient/PT\ mean\ normal]^{ISI}$), with the ISI of the international reference thromboplastin being 1.0. Thus, the INR has become the internationally recognized standard for monitoring warfarin therapy.

The goal or target INR for each patient is based on the indication for warfarin therapy [2, 10]. The therapeutic INR range was first developed empirically but has since been confirmed by a number of large prospective trials [10]. Standard-intensity warfarin therapy is defined as a goal INR of 2.5 (range, 2.0–3.0) and is appropriate for most clinical situations that require prevention and/or treatment of thromboembolic disease. High-intensity warfarin therapy is used in mechanical valve replacement and certain situations of thromboembolic recurrence, despite adequate anticoagulation, and is defined by a goal INR of 3.0 (range, 2.5–3.5) [2, 10].

After initiating warfarin therapy, the INR should be monitored at least every 2–3 days during the first week of therapy. Once a stable response to therapy is achieved, INR monitoring may be performed less frequently, once a week for the first 1–2 weeks, then every 2 weeks, and eventually monthly thereafter. Very stable patients may have their monitoring extended up to every 12 weeks. Highly motivated and well-trained patients may be good candidates for self-testing or self-management by using a point-of-care INR testing device approved for home use [2, 10].

At each encounter, the patient should be interviewed by use of open-ended questions about any factors that may impact the INR including general health status, use of interacting medications, adherence to therapy, dietary variances, and any issues with bleeding or clotting. Warfarin dose adjustments should take into account not only the INR result but also patient-related factors that influence the result.

Transitioning Between Warfarin and Other Anticoagulants

If a transition *from* warfarin to a DOAC or parenteral anticoagulant is indicated, we suggest stopping warfarin, trending the INR, and initiating the new anticoagulant once the INR is <2.5 and trending down [30].

If transitioning *to warfarin* from a DOAC or parenteral anticoagulant, consideration of the patient's underlying thromboembolic risk

Table 2.12 Warfarin maintenance dosing nomogram

Goal INR 2–3	Adjustment	Goal INR 2.5–3.5
INR < 1.5	• Increase maintenance dose by 10–20% • Consider a booster dose of 1.5–2x daily maintenance dose • Consider resumption of prior maintenance dose if factor causing decreased INR is considered transient (e.g., missed warfarin dose(s))	INR < 2.0
INR 1.5–1.8	• Increase maintenance dose by 5–15% • Consider a booster dose of 1.5–2x daily maintenance dose • Consider resumption of prior maintenance dose if factor causing decreased INR is considered transient (e.g., missed warfarin dose(s))	INR 2.0–2.3
INR 1.8–1.9	• No dosage adjustment may be necessary if the last two INRs were in range, if there is no clear explanation for the INR to be out of range, and if in the judgment of the clinician, the INR does not represent an increased risk of thromboembolism for the patient • If dosage adjustment needed, increase by 5–10% • Consider a booster dose of 1.5–2x daily maintenance dose • Consider resumption of prior maintenance dose if factor causing decreased INR is considered transient (e.g., missed warfarin dose(s))	INR 2.3–2.4
INR 2.0–3.0	Desired range—No adjustment needed	INR 2.5–3.5
INR 3.1–3.2	• No dosage adjustment may necessary if the last two INRs were in range, if there is no clear explanation for the INR to be out of range, and if in the judgment of the clinician, the INR does not represent an increased risk of hemorrhage for the patient • If dosage adjustment needed, decrease by 5–10% • Consider resumption of prior maintenance dose if factor causing elevated INR is considered transient (e.g., acute alcohol ingestion)	INR 3.6–3.7
INR 3.3–3.4	• Decrease maintenance dose by 5–10% • Consider resumption of prior maintenance dose if factor causing elevated INR is considered transient (e.g., acute alcohol ingestion)	INR 3.8–3.9
INR 3.5–3.9	• Consider holding one dose • Decrease maintenance dose by 5–15% • Consider resumption of prior maintenance dose if factor causing elevated INR is considered transient (e.g., acute alcohol ingestion)	INR 4.0–4.4
INR ≥ 4.0 but <9 and no bleeding	• Hold until INR < upper limit of therapeutic range • Decrease maintenance dose by 5–20% • Consider resumption of prior maintenance dose if factor causing elevated INR is considered transient (e.g., acute alcohol ingestion) • If patient considered to be at significant risk for bleeding, may consider low dose vitamin K 1–2.5 mg orally	INR ≥ 4.5 but <9 and no bleeding
INR ≥ 9 and no bleeding	• Hold until INR < upper limit of therapeutic range • Administer vitamin K 2.5–5 mg orally • Decrease maintenance dose by 5–20% • Consider resumption of prior maintenance dose if factor causing elevated INR is considered transient (e.g., acute alcohol ingestion)	INR ≥ 9 and no bleeding

INR international normalized ratio

should be undertaken. If the patient has an acute thrombotic event, the DOAC should be overlapped with the warfarin for at least 3 days and until the INR is >2. As the DOACs will impact the INR, it is important in patients transitioning from a DOAC to have their INR measured just prior to the next DOAC dose to minimize this lab interference [4]. Rapid-acting parenteral anticoagulants, such as LMWH, should be overlapped with warfarin for a minimum of 5 days and until the INR is >2. If the patient does not have an acute thrombotic event, it is reasonable to simply stop the DOAC or parenteral anticoagulant and initiate warfarin at a dose appropriate for the patient's clinical characteristics and current clinical status.

Management of Warfarin Around Elective Procedures

With perioperative warfarin management, the first question should be "Does the patient require interruption of warfarin therapy?" Minimally invasive procedures, such as minor dental procedures, cataract surgery, chest tube removal, catheter ablation, minor dermatologic procedures, etc., do not warrant interruption of warfarin therapy [4, 45, 46]. For more invasive procedures, it may be necessary to temporarily interrupt long-acting warfarin therapy to mitigate bleeding risk. Based primarily on expert opinion, it became common over the last two decades to employ a "bridging strategy" for patients requiring temporary warfarin interruption for a procedure. This is accomplished via suspending the warfarin for a number of days prior to the procedure to allow offset of anticoagulant effect and then utilizing a shorter-acting anticoagulant (most commonly LMWH) prior to and after the procedure to minimize the time the patient has subtherapeutic levels of anticoagulation. However, more recent evidence, both retrospective and prospective, has found that bridging is associated with a higher risk of major bleeding and does not significantly reduce thromboembolic events [47–49]. Thus, there is a paradigm shift away from bridging practices except for those patients at highest thromboembolic risk [50]. This may include patients with a thromboembolic event within the past 3 months, mechanical cardiac valve(s), known strong thrombophilia (e.g., antiphospholipid antibody syndrome), history of recurrent thromboembolic events, or history of a thromboembolic event during warfarin interruption. Warfarin bridging is not recommended for patients who are not at high thromboembolic risk [4, 45, 46, 50]. If patient is deemed to be at high risk for a thromboembolic event, this must be carefully weighed against their individual risk of bleeding as well as the bleed risk of the procedure itself. If the bleed risk outweighs the thromboembolic risk, it may be reasonable to forego bridging. For patients at high thromboembolic risk in whom a bridging strategy is to be employed around an elective procedure, it should be done in a standardized manner. For example, warfarin should be interrupted 4–5 days before the procedure but possibly for fewer days (i.e., 2–3 days) for less invasive procedures where some residual anticoagulant activity is acceptable. LMWH at a therapeutic dose should be started 2–3 days before the procedure and stopped ≥24 h before the start of surgery. The day prior to surgery, an INR should be checked to ensure it is at goal for the procedure. If the INR is above goal for the procedure, low-dose oral vitamin K 1–2.5 mg may be administered (see reversal section below for more information). If the patient is hemodynamically stable, and no further invasive procedures are anticipated, warfarin should be resumed the evening of the procedure. LMWH should be started no sooner than 24 h postoperatively for low bleed risk procedures and 48–72 h for high bleed risk procedures and continued until INR is therapeutic [4, 46]. A step-up approach wherein prophylactic dose LMWH is employed for 24–48 h prior to increasing to therapeutic dose LMWH is a reasonable approach to minimize risk for postoperative deep vein thrombosis (DVT) [49].

For management of warfarin around urgent or emergent procedures, see reversal section below.

Adverse Effects

Skin Necrosis

Warfarin-induced skin necrosis is an extremely rare but serious adverse effect that occurs in <0.1% of patients treated with warfarin [51]. It presents as an eggplant-colored skin lesion or a maculopapular rash within the first week of warfarin therapy and usually manifests in fatty areas such as the abdomen, buttocks, and breasts. The lesions may progress to frank necrosis with blackening and eschar as a result of microvascular thromboses within subcutaneous fat. Patients who receive large loading doses of warfarin or have protein C or S deficiency are at the highest risk of developing this complication [52]. In these patients, rapid depletion of protein C before depletion of vitamin K-dependent clotting factors during early warfarin therapy can result in an imbalance between procoagulant and anticoagulant activity, leading to initial hypercoagulability and thrombosis. Adequate heparinization during initiation of warfarin and/or avoidance of large loading doses can prevent the development of an early hypercoagulable state.

In patients who develop skin necrosis, warfarin therapy should be discontinued immediately. However, subsequent treatment with warfarin is not necessarily contraindicated if it is required for treatment or prevention of thromboembolic disease and there are no other viable options. In patients with protein C or protein S deficiency and a history of skin necrosis who are not candidates for alternative anticoagulants, warfarin therapy may be reinitiated at low dosages as long as therapeutic heparinization has been achieved. Heparin therapy should be maintained until the INR has been within the therapeutic range for at least 72 h [51, 52].

Purple Toe Syndrome

Purple toe syndrome is another rare side effect of warfarin. Patients typically present 1–2 months after warfarin initiation with a purplish, painful discoloration of their toes that blanches with pressure and fades with elevation. The pathophysiology of this syndrome has been related to cholesterol microembolization from atherosclerotic plaques, leading to arterial obstruction. Because cholesterol microembolization has been associated with renal failure and death, warfarin therapy should be discontinued in patients who develop purple toe syndrome, and an alternative anticoagulant should be initiated [53].

Other Adverse Effects

Other side effects of warfarin that have been reported include alopecia, calciphylaxis, and hypersensitivity reactions [11]. Alternative anticoagulant options should be considered in cases of calciphylaxis as warfarin is thought to increase the risk of this life-threatening skin complication of end-stage renal disease. Occasionally, patients have an allergy to the color dye in warfarin tablets. In these instances, if no other anticoagulant options are viable, white, dye-free 10 mg warfarin tablets may be used in appropriate dosing fractions (e.g., ½ tablet for 5 mg dose).

Bleeding

Similar to other anticoagulants, the primary side effect of warfarin is bleeding [42]. The incidence of warfarin-related bleeding appears to be highest during the first few weeks of therapy and ranges from 1% to 10% annually, with the gastrointestinal tract being the most common site of bleeding [54]. Intracranial hemorrhage (ICH) is the most concerning bleeding complication as it is associated with high morbidity and mortality [55]. It is important to counsel patients that warfarin will increase their likelihood of bruising, longer bleeding from cuts, increased menstrual flow, and occasional nosebleeds. Serious bleeding requires evaluation by a medical provider for potential intervention and to assess whether the bleeding is due to their warfarin therapy or another cause (e.g., cancer, injury, etc.). Signs and symptoms of serious bleeding that warrant medical attention include hematemesis, black and tarry stools, bright red blood in the stool or urine, altered mental status, severe headache, bleeding that will not stop, and head injury. While there are myriad risk factors for bleeding (see Table 2.7), the strongest risk factor for bleeding is the intensity of anticoagulation [1, 42]. A number of clinical tools have been developed to estimate a patient's bleeding risk, including the commonly used HAS-BLED score [56, 57]. Bleeding risk scores should never be used as the sole reason to avoid use of anticoagulation therapy. Conversely, such clinical tools should be routinely employed to identify, modify, and/or remove any factors that might contribute to anticoagulant-associated bleeding (e.g., concomitant antiplatelet therapy that may not be necessary). Growing evidence suggests that after patient experiences a significant bleed, the benefit of resuming anticoagulant therapy and avoidance of thromboembolic events far outweighs the risk of recurrent bleed. Thus, most patients should have their therapy reinitiated. The timing of resumption is less clear and depends on the location of the bleed and underlying indication for anticoagulation. In most instances, resuming sometime between 14 and 30 days is reasonable but may differ based on the clinical situation and patient preferences [58]. The risk versus benefit of anticoagulation therapy must be regularly assessed in an ongoing manner via a shared decision-making process between the clinician and the patient or caregiver.

Reversal

There may be clinical situations that require warfarin reversal, such as severe INR derangements, need for urgent or emergent procedures, or significant bleeding events [42]. Reversal of warfarin may be achieved by withholding warfarin, administration of the antidote vitamin K, repletion of functional clotting factors with fresh frozen plasma (FFP) or prothrombin complex concentrate (PCC), or some combination of these approaches [10, 11, 59, 60]. The reversal strategy employed should be based on both the severity of the patient's clinical status and the rapidity with which reversal needs to occur. Warfarin reversal should be performed judiciously and only in certain clinical situations, as normalization of the patient's underlying coagulation status may predispose them to thromboembolic events.

INR Derangements in Asymptomatic Patients

INR < 9

The 30-day risk of bleeding in patients with an INR between 5 and 9 is low (0.96%), and use of vitamin K is not common practice in the United States [61]. While administration of low-dose oral vitamin K 1.25 mg in asymptomatic (i.e., non-bleeding) patients with an INR between 5 and 9 has been shown to lower the INR more quickly than simply withholding warfarin, it is not associated with a decreased risk of major bleeding [60, 62]. Thus, in patients with an INR $\leq$ 9 with no active bleeding or imminent risk of bleeding, it is recommended to withhold warfarin until the INR decreases to within therapeutic range, reduce the weekly dose or address causative factors for the INR derangement, and employ more frequent monitoring until INR stability is regained. The time required for INR to return to the therapeutic range after warfarin is withheld depends on several patient characteristics. Advanced age, lower warfarin maintenance dose requirements, and higher INR are associated with increased time for INR correction. Other factors that can prolong the time for INR to return to the therapeutic range include decompensated heart failure, active malignancy, and recent use of medications known to potentiate warfarin. To shorten the time of INR correction to within the therapeutic range, an alternative approach is to withhold warfarin and administer a small dose of oral vitamin K (1–2.5 mg), which will correct over-anticoagulation in 24–48 h without causing prolonged resistance to warfarin therapy, a problem commonly seen with larger (e.g., 10 mg) doses of vitamin K [10, 59, 60].

INR > 9

In asymptomatic patients with an INR > 9, warfarin should be withheld for one to two doses along with investigation for cause of the derangement, administration of a higher dose of oral vitamin K (2.5–5 mg), and more frequent INR monitoring [10, 60], as these patients may be at higher risk for bleeding over 30 days [61].

Bleeding Events

Nonmajor Bleeding

Patients who experience a non-life-threatening bleeding event, such as bleeding into the oral cavity, should have their warfarin therapy temporarily held and be given low-dose IV vitamin K 1–2.5 mg, followed by monitoring for adequate response to interventions and hemostasis (Fig. 2.1).

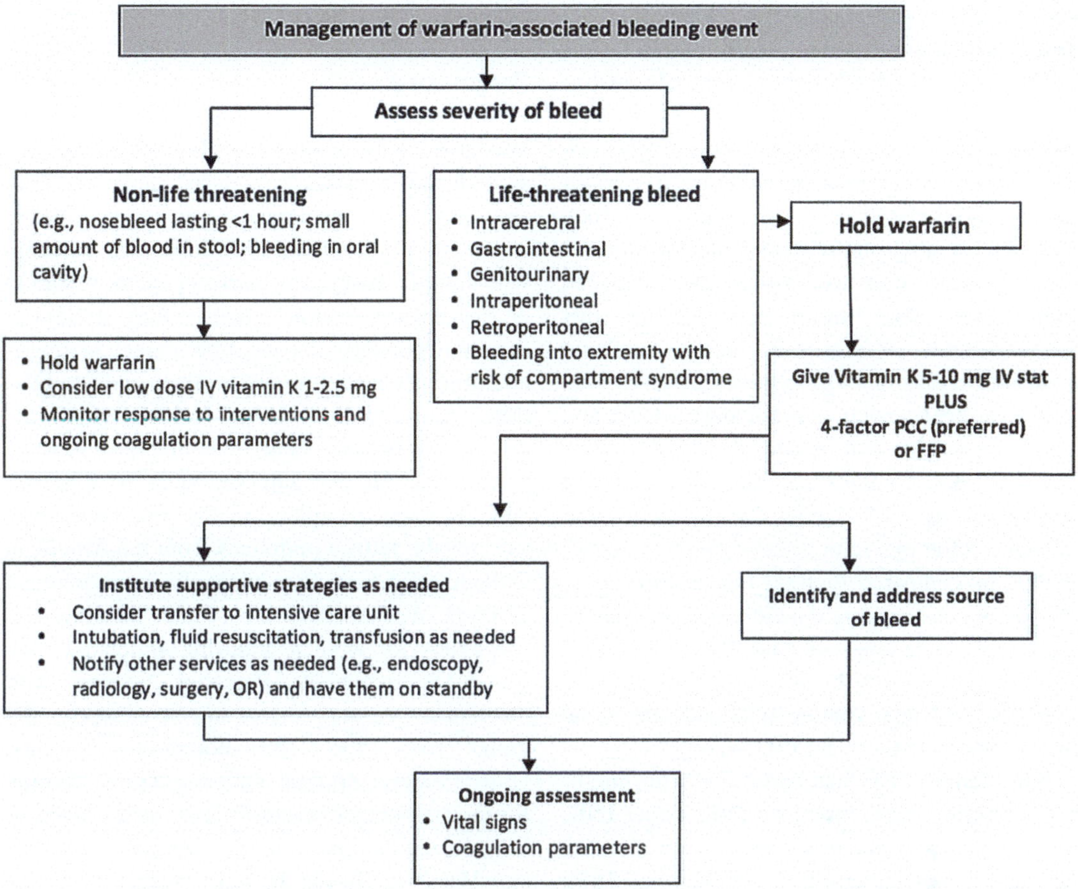

PCC, prothrombin complex concentrate; FFP, fresh frozen plasma

Fig. 2.1 Management of warfarin-associated bleeding event. *PCC* prothrombin complex concentrate, *FFP* fresh frozen plasma

Major Bleeding

Major bleeding may be life- or limb-threatening and often occurs in non-compressible areas such as the gastrointestinal tract, retroperitoneal space, or in the head. The 30-day mortality rate for major bleeding in warfarin patients is approximately 10%. Intracranial hemorrhage is the most concerning type of bleed, with a 30-day mortality rate of approximately 50%. Warfarin patients who experience a major bleed, regardless of their INR, require prompt and assertive intervention strategies. While there is no robust evidence toward better outcomes with rapid INR normalization, every attempt should be made to correct the coagulopathy as quickly as possible. Patients should have their warfarin held, receive 5–10 mg of vitamin K intravenously, and have their clotting factors aggressively replaced [10, 60]. Vitamin K will provide sustained reversal and avoid a rebound hypocoagulable state. Due to the delayed onset of intravenous vitamin K, rapid reversal of the INR is achieved through administration of either prothrombin complex concentrate (PCC) or fresh frozen plasma (FFP) [10, 11, 59, 60].

The PCC product that is available in the United States for warfarin reversal is the four-factor product, Kcentra®. It contains the vitamin K-dependent clotting factors II, VII, IX, and X, as well as small amounts of Proteins C and S and heparin to mitigate thrombotic potential. PCC is preferred over FFP in most clinical situations as it has numerous advantages [59]. FFP must be cross-matched to the patient to ensure ABO compatibility and must be thawed prior to administration, both of which can delay therapy. The biggest drawback of FFP is potential for volume overload. For effective INR reversal in the setting of a major bleed, it should be dosed at 15–30 mL/kg, which can often equate to more than a liter of fluid [4, 59]. In patients that need volume resuscitation, such as major gastrointestinal hemorrhage, this may be desirable. However, in other patients who are unable to tolerate large volumes, this may lead to adverse events such as pulmonary edema and sometimes transfusion-related acute lung injury (TRALI). PCC contains 25 times the amount of clotting factors of FFP [63]. Thus, an equivalent amount of clotting factors can be given in 40 mL of PCC as compared to 1000 mL of FFP. Also, PCC does not requiring thawing or cross-matching. Recent meta-analyses have shown that PCC provides more rapid reduction in the INR, reduced mortality, and less volume overload and is no more prothrombotic than FFP [64, 65].

Importantly, PCC has variable dosing methods, including those based on INR, target INR, bodyweight, and fixed dosages, with no one method showing superiority over the others [66]. Recombinant factor VII has also been used for warfarin reversal [11, 59, 60]. However, its safety and efficacy in restoring hemostasis is not well-defined [67] and should not be used first-line.

Urgent or Emergent Procedures

For warfarin patients who require urgent or emergent procedures, the reversal strategy depends on how quickly and how much the patient needs to be reversed.

- For procedures that need to occur within the next 6–8 h and cannot be delayed, PCC is preferred.
- For procedures that need to occur within the next 24 h, it is recommended to give IV vitamin K 0.5–2.5 mg.
- For procedures that are anticipated to occur between 24 and 72 h, the use of oral vitamin K 0.5–2.5 mg is recommended.
- For procedures that are to occur at >72 h, simply withholding warfarin and trending the INR are appropriate.

Special Considerations

Pregnancy

Warfarin freely crosses the placenta, and exposure during pregnancy is associated with fetal anomalies and late fetal loss in up to 10% of cases [68–70]. Women of childbearing potential who require long-term warfarin therapy should be instructed to use an effective form of contraception or undergo frequent pregnancy testing if attempting conception [71]. When anticoagulation is required during pregnancy, the safety and efficacy for both the mother and the fetus must be considered. Neither unfractionated (UFH) nor LMWH cross the placenta and are considered safe for the fetus. Guidelines from the American College of Chest Physicians [71] recommend LMWH over warfarin throughout all stages of pregnancy for women requiring anticoagulation for VTE treatment. Pregnant women with mechanical cardiac valves are at exceptionally high risk for thromboembolic events. Unfortunately, optimal anticoagulation therapy for mechanical valves during pregnancy, particularly during the first trimester, remains controversial. Warfarin affords the most protection for the mother against thromboembolic events (2–4% compared to 9–12% for LMWH and up to 33% for subcutaneous unfractionated heparin) in the setting of mechanical cardiac valves [68, 72]. However, this must be balanced against warfarin-associated fetal complications. The risk appears to be greatest during the first trimester and among women whose warfarin dosing requirement is ≥5 mg daily [68, 70, 73]. As such, anticoagulation for mechanical valves during pregnancy is a highly individualized choice. Pregnant patients with mechanical valves should be counseled regarding the risks of warfarin therapy, especially during the first trimester and at term [71]. National and international guidelines suggest it reasonable to continue warfarin during the first trimester if the daily dose requirement is ≤5 mg and there has been full disclosure of the risks and benefits through a shared decision-making process with the patient. For women whose warfarin requirement is >5 mg daily or place a higher value on avoiding embryopathies than avoiding valve thrombosis, anticoagulation with LMWH or UFH during the first trimester may be employed with the cognizance of a possible increased risk of thromboembolic complications with these agents. When used, LMWH should be administered twice daily with close monitoring to ensure adequate levels of anticoagulation. Unfractionated heparin should be administered intravenously via continuous infusion, as the subcutaneous route in pregnant women with mechanical valves is associated with a very high incidence of valve thrombosis. As with LMWH, close monitoring for adequate levels of anticoagulation is imperative. For the second and third trimesters, it is recommended to utilize warfarin, if the patient is amenable, along with low-dose concomitant aspirin 81 mg daily. At the 36th week of gestation, the patient should be transitioned from warfarin to LMWH or UFH in anticipation of delivery [74, 75].

Breastfeeding

Warfarin is not detectable in breast milk from lactating patients treated with warfarin and is thus a viable option in breastfeeding mothers [11, 76].

Pediatric Patients

Thromboembolic events in pediatric patients occur less frequently than in adults. Consequently, much of the anticoagulation clinical management practices in pediatric patients are based off adult evidence and recommendations [77]. Warfarin therapy is a commonly used long-term anticoagulant in children and can be successfully managed using INR goals similarly as with adults [77, 78]. Furthermore, warfarin is currently the only oral anticoagulant FDA-approved for use in pediatric patients; however, several clinical trials of DOACs in pediatric populations are currently underway [79, 80].

While the management of warfarin is similarly performed with INR monitoring and goals as with adults [77], warfarin use in pediatric patients can be more challenging [81]. In pediatric patients, warfarin is initiated using weight-based dosing (e.g., 0.2 mg/kg/day) and requires more frequent monitoring and dose adjustments than in adults. For instance, in neonates, plasma levels of vitamin K-dependent coagulation factors are much lower than in adults. Further, infant formula is often supplemented with vitamin K, but breast milk has very low levels of vitamin K, and consequently the primary source of nutrition in neonates and infants will dramatically affect their warfarin sensitivity [77]. Additionally, as a child ages, their hemostatic system changes and subsequently may alter their warfarin requirements, with infants generally requiring more warfarin than older pediatric patients to achieve their INR goal [11, 78].

Conclusion

Although the therapeutic landscape of anticoagulation is rapidly changing with the advent of the DOACs, warfarin will continue to be a mainstay of therapy for many patient populations and in numerous clinical indications. Optimized safety and efficacy depends on active participation of knowledgeable patients as well as clinician familiarity with the unique, and sometimes challenging, pharmacokinetics, pharmacodynamics, and practical management aspects of warfarin.

Key Points

- Due to the hypercoagulable state during the first few days of warfarin therapy, along with delayed antithrombotic effect, patients with acute thrombosis should receive a rapid-acting anticoagulant (heparin, low-molecular-weight heparin (LMWH), or fondaparinux) while transitioning to warfarin therapy [1, 6, 10].
- Warfarin is metabolized by multiple hepatic cytochrome P450 isoenzymes and has many clinically significant drug-drug interactions that may warrant dose adjustment or increased frequency

of monitoring to avoid adverse events (Tables 2.2 and 2.3).

- Warfarin is prone to numerous clinically significant drug-drug and drug-food interactions, and patients on warfarin should be questioned at every encounter to assess for any potential interactions with foods, drugs, herbal products, and nutritional supplements. More frequent monitoring should be instituted when interacting medications are changed to avoid clinically significant hemorrhagic or thromboembolic complications.
- Patients on warfarin may experience changes in the INR due to fluctuating intake of dietary vitamin K (Table 2.10). However, patients should be instructed to maintain a consistent diet rather than strictly avoiding vitamin K-rich foods.
- Most patients may be initiated on a dose of warfarin 5 mg daily with frequent monitoring and dose adjustment until their response to warfarin is known. Small dosage adjustments (5–20%) should be made, if indicated, recognizing that the full effect of any dose adjustment will not be seen for 2–3 days.
- Vitamin K is the antidote for warfarin. It should be given either orally (PO) or intravenously (IV), depending on the clinical situation. Both routes are equally effective in reversing warfarin, but the IV route provides more rapid reversal.
- All warfarin patients with major bleeding should receive IV vitamin K 5–10 mg.
- PCC is preferred over FFP for factor replenishment in warfarin-associated major hemorrhage.

Self-Assessment Questions

1. A 73-year-old woman with a past medial history of heart failure presents with new onset atrial fibrillation. Her renal function and drug interactions preclude her from being a good DOAC candidate, and she is initiated on warfarin 5 mg PO every evening. Which of the following is the most appropriate counseling point regarding her dietary intake?
   (a) She does not have to avoid healthy foods, such as leafy green vegetables, but rather should strive to maintain consistency in her diet.
   (b) She should avoid leafy green vegetables, such as spinach, as this will antagonize the warfarin and make it difficult to keep her INR in the therapeutic range.
   (c) She should take her warfarin with food to promote absorption.
   (d) She should take warfarin on an empty stomach to promote absorption.
2. A 75-year-old woman with a history of heart failure and atrial fibrillation on chronic warfarin therapy presents to the emergency department with a chief complaint of significant blood in her stools and fatigue. She is hypotensive (BP 83/50) and has decreased mental status. Her hemoglobin is 4.6 g/dL, down from 11.2 g/dL at last visit. Her INR is 3.3.

   What is the most appropriate action at this time in regard to managing her anticoagulation?
   (a) Withhold any anticoagulation, administer vitamin K 2.5 mg PO, and have her follow up at the anticoagulation clinic.
   (b) Withhold any anticoagulation and administer FFP 6–8 units.
   (c) Withhold any anticoagulation, and administer IV vitamin K 10 mg stat along with PCC.
   (d) Withhold warfarin, trend the INR, and resume once it is in the therapeutic range.
3. A 68-year-old man is diagnosed with bilateral pulmonary emboli 1 week after he underwent a total knee arthroplasty. His past medical history is significant for a gastrointestinal bleed 4 months ago, cirrhosis, heart failure, and hypertension. His baseline INR is 1.4 and his renal function is normal. His insurance will not cover a DOAC, and the decision is made to start warfarin. What would be the most appropriate starting dose of warfarin?

   (a) 10 mg PO daily as he may be warfarin resistant.
   (b) 5 mg PO daily as he should not be warfarin sensitive.
   (c) 2.5 mg PO daily as he may be warfarin sensitive.
   (d) His risk for bleeding precludes the use of anticoagulation.
4. How long should enoxaparin be overlapped with his warfarin therapy during warfarin initiation?
   (a) Until the INR is >2.
   (b) For a minimum of 5 days and until the INR is within the target range.
   (c) Enoxaparin bridging is not indicated in this patient.
   (d) For 3 days or until the INR is >2.
5. Which of the following patients would require warfarin therapy rather than a DOAC?
   (a) A 77-year-old woman with a past medical history of hypertension, hyperlipidemia, mechanical aortic valve, and atrial fibrillation
   (b) A 35-year-old man with an upper extremity DVT secondary to his hemodialysis catheter
   (c) Neither
   (d) Both

Self-Assessment Answers

1. (a) She does not have to avoid healthy foods, such as leafy green vegetables, but rather should strive to maintain consistency in her diet.

   Because warfarin inhibits vitamin K-dependent factor development, it is important to maintain a consistent level of dietary vitamin K every day to reduce fluctuations in INR levels. Patients should not be counseled to avoid dietary vitamin K, but rather they should be counseled to keep the dietary vitamin K intake relatively consistent.
2. (c) Withhold any anticoagulation, and administer IV vitamin K 10 mg stat along with PCC.

   Given her acute drop in hemoglobin, altered mental status, and bloody stools, she likely requires rapid reversal of warfarin's effect. This is best achieved with IV vitamin K as well as PCCs. Oral vitamin K will not achieve a sufficiently rapid effect. FFP may rapidly reverse her INR, but the high volume required for administration puts her at risk for a heart failure exacerbation.
3. (c) 2.5 mg PO daily as he may be warfarin sensitive

   Given his known cirrhosis comorbidity and prior gastrointestinal bleed, initiation of low-dose warfarin is most appropriate to avoid INR levels above the therapeutic range.
4. (b) For a minimum of 5 days and until the INR is within the target range

   Due to the half-life of various factors (II, VII, IX, and X) along with protein C and protein S, enoxaparin should be overlapped with warfarin for a minimum of 5 days and until the INR is within the target range.
5. (d) Both

   Warfarin is preferred of DOAC therapy in any patient with a mechanical cardiac valve replacement due to high rates of valve thrombosis with DOAC therapy. Patients on hemodialysis are generally not good DOAC candidates because each of the DOAC medications is partially excreted by the kidneys.

References

1. Ageno W, Gallus AS, Wittkowsky A, Crowther M, Hylek EM, Palareti G. Oral anticoagulant therapy: antithrombotic therapy and prevention of thrombosis, 9th ed: American College of Chest Physicians Evidence-Based Clinical Practice Guidelines. Chest. 2012;141(2 Suppl):e44S–88S.
2. Holbrook A, Schulman S, Witt DM, Vandvik PO, Fish J, Kovacs MJ, et al. Evidence-based management of anticoagulant therapy: antithrombotic therapy and prevention of thrombosis, 9th ed: American College of Chest Physicians Evidence-Based Clinical Practice Guidelines. Chest. 2012;141(2 Suppl):e152S–84S.
3. Nutescu EA, Burnett A, Fanikos J, Spinler S, Wittkowsky A. Erratum to: pharmacology of anticoagulants used in the treatment of venous thromboembolism. J Thromb Thrombolysis. 2016; 42(2):296–311.
4. Witt DM, Clark NP, Kaatz S, Schnurr T, Ansell JE. Guidance for the practical management of warfa-

rin therapy in the treatment of venous thromboembolism. J Thromb Thrombolysis. 2016;41:187–205.
5. Ogilvie IM, Newton N, Welner SA, Cowell W, Lip GYH. Underuse of oral anticoagulants in atrial fibrillation: a systematic review. Am J Med. 2010;123(7):638–645.e4.
6. Brandjes DP, Heijboer H, Büller HR, de Rijk M, Jagt H, ten Cate JW. Acenocoumarol and heparin compared with acenocoumarol alone in the initial treatment of proximal-vein thrombosis. N Engl J Med. 1992;327(21):1485–9.
7. Limdi NA, Veenstra DL. Warfarin pharmacogenetics. Pharmacotherapy. 2008;28(9):1084–97.
8. www.warfarindosing.org. Last accessed 07/12/2017.
9. Kimmel SE. Warfarin pharmacogenomics: current best evidence. J Thromb Haemost. 2015;13(Suppl 1): S266–71.
10. Ansell J, Hirsh J, Hylek E, Jacobson A, Crowther M, Palareti G. Pharmacology and management of the vitamin k antagonists*: American college of chest physicians evidence-based clinical practice guidelines (8th edition). Chest. 2008;133(6_Suppl):160S–98S.
11. pi_coumadin.pdf [Internet]. [cited 2017 July 9]. Available from: https://packageinserts.bms.com/pi/pi_coumadin.pdf.
12. Alalwan AA, Voils SA, Hartzema AG. Trends in utilization of warfarin and direct oral anticoagulants in older adult patients with atrial fibrillation. Am J Health Syst Pharm. 2017;74(16):1237–44.
13. Olesen JB, Sørensen R, Hansen ML, Lamberts M, Weeke P, Mikkelsen AP, et al. Non-vitamin K antagonist oral anticoagulation agents in anticoagulant naïve atrial fibrillation patients: danish nationwide descriptive data 2011–2013. Europace. 2015;17(2):187–93.
14. Ruff CT, Giugliano RP, Braunwald E, Hoffman EB, Deenadayalu N, Ezekowitz MD, et al. Comparison of the efficacy and safety of new oral anticoagulants with warfarin in patients with atrial fibrillation: a meta-analysis of randomised trials. Lancet. 2014;383(9921):955–62.
15. van der Hulle T, Kooiman J, den Exter PL, Dekkers OM, Klok FA, Huisman MV. Effectiveness and safety of novel oral anticoagulants as compared with vitamin K antagonists in the treatment of acute symptomatic venous thromboembolism: a systematic review and meta-analysis. J Thromb Haemost. 2014;12(3):320–8.
16. Beyer-Westendorf J, Förster K, Pannach S, Ebertz F, Gelbricht V, Thieme C, et al. Rates, management, and outcome of rivaroxaban bleeding in daily care: results from the Dresden NOAC registry. Blood. 2014;124(6):955–62.
17. Jacobs V, May HT, Bair TL, Crandall BG, Cutler MJ, Day JD, et al. Long-term population-based cerebral ischemic event and cognitive outcomes of direct oral anticoagulants compared with warfarin among long-term anticoagulated patients for atrial fibrillation. Am J Cardiol. 2016;118(2):210–4.
18. Noseworthy PA, Yao X, Abraham NS, Sangaralingham LR, McBane RD, Shah ND. DIrect comparison of dabigatran, rivaroxaban, and apixaban for effectiveness and safety in nonvalvular atrial fibrillation. Chest. 2016;150(6):1302–12.
19. Raschi E, Bianchin M, Ageno W, De Ponti R, De Ponti F. Risk–benefit profile of direct-acting oral anticoagulants in established therapeutic indications: an overview of systematic reviews and observational studies. Drug Saf. 2016;39(12):1175–87.
20. Tamayo S, Frank Peacock W, Patel M, Sicignano N, Hopf KP, Fields LE, et al. Characterizing major bleeding in patients with nonvalvular atrial fibrillation: a pharmacovigilance study of 27 467 patients taking rivaroxaban. Clin Cardiol. 2015;38(2):63–8.
21. Villines TC, Peacock WF. Safety of direct oral anticoagulants: insights from postmarketing studies. Am J Med. 2016;129(11):S41–6.
22. Xu Y, Schulman S, Dowlatshahi D, Holbrook AM, Simpson CS, Shepherd LE, et al. Direct oral anticoagulant- or warfarin-related major bleeding: characteristics, reversal strategies and outcomes from a multi-center observational study. Chest. 2017;152(1):81–91. https://doi.org/10.1016/j.chest.2017.02.009.
23. Yao X, Abraham NS, Sangaralingham LR, Bellolio MF, McBane RD, Shah ND, et al. Effectiveness and safety of dabigatran, rivaroxaban, and apixaban versus warfarin in nonvalvular atrial fibrillation. J Am Heart Assoc. 2016;5(6):e003725.
24. January CT, Wann LS, Alpert JS, Calkins H, Cigarroa JE, Cleveland JC, et al. 2014 AHA/ACC/HRS guideline for the management of patients with atrial fibrillation. Circulation. 2014;130(23):e199–267.
25. Kirchhof P, Benussi S, Kotecha D, Ahlsson A, Atar D, Casadei B, et al. 2016 ESC guidelines for the management of atrial fibrillation developed in collaboration with EACTS. Eur Heart J. 2016;37(38):2893–962.
26. Kearon C, Akl EA, Ornelas J, Blaivas A, Jimenez D, Bounameaux H, et al. Antithrombotic therapy for VTE disease: chest guideline and expert panel report. Chest. 2016;149(2):315–52.
27. Hanon O, Chaussade E, Gueranger P, Gruson E, Bonan S, Gay A. Patient-reported treatment satisfaction with rivaroxaban for stroke prevention in atrial fibrillation. A French observational study, the SAFARI study. PLoS One. 2016;11(12):e0166218.
28. Toth PP. Considerations for long-term anticoagulant therapy in patients with venous thromboembolism in the novel oral anticoagulant era. Vasc Health Risk Manag. 2016;12:23–34.
29. Coleman CI, Haas S, Turpie AGG, Kuhls S, Hess S, Evers T, et al. Impact of switching from a vitamin K antagonist to rivaroxaban on satisfaction with anticoagulation therapy: the XANTUS-ACTS substudy. Clin Cardiol. 2016;39(10):565–9.
30. Burnett AE, Mahan CE, Vazquez SR, Oertel LB, Garcia DA, Ansell J. Guidance for the practical management of the direct oral anticoagulants (DOACs) in VTE treatment. J Thromb Thrombolysis. 2016;41:206–32.
31. Eikelboom JW, Connolly SJ, Brueckmann M, Granger CB, Kappetein AP, Mack MJ, et al. Dabigatran versus

warfarin in patients with mechanical heart valves. N Engl J Med. 2013;369(13):1206–14.
32. Chai-Adisaksopha C, Hillis C, Isayama T, Lim W, Iorio A, Crowther M. Mortality outcomes in patients receiving direct oral anticoagulants: a systematic review and meta-analysis of randomized controlled trials. J Thromb Haemost. 2015;13(11):2012–20.
33. Garcia DA, Witt DM, Hylek E, Wittkowsky AK, Nutescu EA, Jacobson A, et al. Delivery of optimized anticoagulant therapy: consensus statement from the anticoagulation forum. Ann Pharmacother. 2008;42(7):979–88.
34. Garcia DA, Schwartz MJ. Warfarin therapy: tips and tools for better control. J Fam Pract. 2011;60(2):70–5.
35. Hospital: 2017 National patient safety goals [Internet]. Available from: http://www.jointcommission.org/hap_2017_npsgs/.
36. Staying Active and Healthy with Blood Thinners" from the Agency for Healthcare Research and Quality (AHRQ). Available at https://www.ahrq.gov/patients-consumers/diagnosis-treatment/treatments/btpills/stayactive.html.
37. Nutescu EA, Wittkowsky AK, Burnett A, Merli GJ, Ansell JE, Garcia DA. Delivery of optimized inpatient anticoagulation therapy: consensus statement from the anticoagulation forum. Ann Pharmacother. 2013;47(5):714–24.
38. Pengo V, Biasiolo A, Pegoraro C. A simple scheme to initiate oral anticoagulant treatment in outpatients with nonrheumatic atrial fibrillation. Am J Cardiol. 2001;88(10):1214–6.
39. Tait RC, Sefcick A. A warfarin induction regimen for out-patient anticoagulation in patients with atrial fibrillation. Br J Haematol. 1998;101(3):450–4.
40. Siguret V, Gouin I, Debray M, Perret-Guillaume C, Boddaert J, Mahé I, et al. Initiation of warfarin therapy in elderly medical inpatients: a safe and accurate regimen. Am J Med. 2005;118(2):137–42.
41. Kovacs MJ, Anderson DA, Wells PS. Prospective assessment of a nomogram for the initiation of oral anticoagulation therapy for outpatient treatment of venous thromboembolism. Pathophysiol Haemost Thromb. 2002;32(3):131–3.
42. Schulman S, Beyth RJ, Kearon C, Levine MN. Hemorrhagic complications of anticoagulant and thrombolytic treatment: American College of Chest Physicians Evidence-Based Clinical Practice Guidelines (8th Edition). Chest. 2008;133(6 Suppl):257S–98S.
43. Harrison L, Johnston M, Massicotte MP, Crowther M, Moffat K, Hirsh J. Comparison of 5-mg and 10-mg loading doses in initiation of warfarin therapy. Ann Intern Med. 1997;126(2):133–6.
44. Gage BF, Fihn SD, White RH. Management and dosing of warfarin therapy. Am J Med. 2000;109(6):481–8.
45. Rechenmacher SJ, Fang JC. Bridging anticoagulation: Primum Non Nocere. J Am Coll Cardiol. 2015;66(12):1392–403.
46. Doherty JU, Gluckman TJ, Hucker WJ, Januzzi JL, Ortel TL, Saxonhouse SJ, et al. 2017 ACC expert consensus decision pathway for periprocedural management of anticoagulation in patients with nonvalvular atrial fibrillation. J Am Coll Cardiol. 2017; 69(7):871–98.
47. Siegal D, Yudin J, Kaatz S, Douketis JD, Lim W, Spyropoulos AC. Periprocedural heparin bridging in patients receiving vitamin K antagonists: systematic review and meta-analysis of bleeding and thromboembolic rates. Circulation. 2012;126(13):1630–9.
48. Clark NP, Witt DM, Davies LE, Saito EM, McCool KH, Douketis JD, et al. Bleeding, recurrent venous thromboembolism, and mortality risks during warfarin interruption for invasive procedures. JAMA Intern Med. 2015;175(7):1163–8.
49. Douketis JD, Spyropoulos AC, Kaatz S, Becker RC, Caprini JA, Dunn AS, et al. Perioperative bridging anticoagulation in patients with atrial fibrillation. N Engl J Med. 2015;373(9):823–33.
50. Rose AJ, Allen AL, Minichello T. A call to reduce the use of bridging anticoagulation. Circ Cardiovasc Qual Outcomes. 2016;9(1):64–7.
51. Nazarian RM, Van Cott EM, Zembowicz A, Duncan LM. Warfarin-induced skin necrosis. J Am Acad Dermatol. 2009;61(2):325–32.
52. Kozac N, Schattner A. Warfarin-induced skin necrosis. J Gen Intern Med. 2014;29(1):248–9.
53. Hirschmann JV, Raugi GJ. Blue (or purple) toe syndrome. J Am Acad Dermatol. 2009;60(1):1–20. quiz 21–22.
54. Landefeld CS, Beyth RJ. Anticoagulant-related bleeding: clinical epidemiology, prediction, and prevention. Am J Med. 1993;95(3):315–28.
55. Fang MC, Go AS, Chang Y, Hylek EM, Henault LE, Jensvold NG, et al. Death and disability from warfarin-associated intracranial and extracranial hemorrhages. Am J Med. 2007;120(8):700–5.
56. Pisters R, Lane DA, Nieuwlaat R, de Vos CB, Crijns HJGM, Lip GYH. A novel user-friendly score (HAS-BLED) to assess 1-year risk of major bleeding in patients with atrial fibrillation: the Euro Heart Survey. Chest. 2010;138(5):1093–100.
57. Zhu W, He W, Guo L, Wang X, Hong K. The HAS-BLED score for predicting major bleeding risk in anticoagulated patients with atrial fibrillation: a systematic review and meta-analysis. Clin Cardiol. 2015;38(9):555–61.
58. Witt DM. What to do after the bleed: resuming anticoagulation after major bleeding. Hematology Am Soc Hematol Educ Program. 2016;2016(1):620–4.
59. Dentali F, Crowther MA. Management of excessive anticoagulant effect due to vitamin K antagonists. Hematology Am Soc Hematol Educ Program. 2008;2008:266–70.
60. Garcia DA, Crowther MA. Reversal of warfarin. Circulation. 2012;125(23):2944–7.
61. Garcia DA, Regan S, Crowther M, Hylek EM. The risk of hemorrhage among patients with warfarin-associated coagulopathy. J Am Coll Cardiol. 2006;47(4):804–8.

62. Crowther MA, Ageno W, Garcia D, Wang L, Witt DM, Clark NP, et al. Oral vitamin K versus placebo to correct excessive anticoagulation in patients receiving warfarin: a randomized trial. Ann Intern Med. 2009;150(5):293–300.
63. Franchini M, Lippi G. Prothrombin complex concentrates: an update. Blood Transfus. 2010;8(3):149–54.
64. Chai-Adisaksopha C, Hillis C, Siegal DM, Movilla R, Heddle N, Iorio A, et al. Prothrombin complex concentrates versus fresh frozen plasma for warfarin reversal. A systematic review and meta-analysis. Thromb Haemost. 2016;116(5):879–90.
65. Brekelmans MPA, van Ginkel K, Daams JG, Hutten BA, Middeldorp S, Coppens M. Benefits and harms of 4-factor prothrombin complex concentrate for reversal of vitamin K antagonist associated bleeding: a systematic review and meta-analysis. J Thromb Thrombolysis. 2017;44(1):118–29.
66. Khorsand N, Kooistra HAM, van Hest RM, Veeger NJGM, Meijer K. A systematic review of prothrombin complex concentrate dosing strategies to reverse vitamin K antagonist therapy. Thromb Res. 2015;135(1):9–19.
67. Logan AC, Goodnough LT. Recombinant factor VIIa: an assessment of evidence regarding its efficacy and safety in the off-label setting. Hematology Am Soc Hematol Educ Program. 2010;2010:153–9.
68. Chan WS, Anand S, Ginsberg JS. Anticoagulation of pregnant women with mechanical heart valves: a systematic review of the literature. Arch Intern Med. 2000;160(2):191–6.
69. Cotrufo M, De Feo M, De Santo LS, Romano G, Della Corte A, Renzulli A, et al. Risk of warfarin during pregnancy with mechanical valve prostheses. Obstet Gynecol. 2002;99(1):35–40.
70. Vitale N, De Feo M, De Santo LS, Pollice A, Tedesco N, Cotrufo M. Dose-dependent fetal complications of warfarin in pregnant women with mechanical heart valves. J Am Coll Cardiol. 1999;33(6):1637–41.
71. Bates SM, Greer IA, Middeldorp S, Veenstra DL, Prabulos A-M, Vandvik PO. VTE, thrombophilia, antithrombotic therapy, and pregnancy: antithrombotic therapy and prevention of thrombosis, 9th ed: American College of Chest Physicians Evidence-Based Clinical Practice Guidelines. Chest. 2012;141(2 Suppl):e691S–736S.
72. Oran B, Lee-Parritz A, Ansell J. Low molecular weight heparin for the prophylaxis of thromboembolism in women with prosthetic mechanical heart valves during pregnancy. Thromb Haemost. 2004;92(4):747–51.
73. De Santo LS, Romano G, Della Corte A, D'Oria V, Nappi G, Giordano S, et al. Mechanical aortic valve replacement in young women planning on pregnancy: maternal and fetal outcomes under low oral anticoagulation, a pilot observational study on a comprehensive pre-operative counseling protocol. J Am Coll Cardiol. 2012;59(12):1110–5.
74. Nishimura RA, Otto CM, Bonow RO, Carabello BA, Erwin JP, Guyton RA, et al. AHA/ACC guideline for the management of patients with valvular heart disease. Circulation. 2014;129: CIR.0000000000000031.
75. European Society of Gynecology (ESG), Association for European Paediatric Cardiology (AEPC), German Society for Gender Medicine (DGesGM), Regitz-Zagrosek V, Blomstrom Lundqvist C, Borghi C, et al. ESC guidelines on the management of cardiovascular diseases during pregnancy: the task force on the management of cardiovascular diseases during pregnancy of the European Society of Cardiology (ESC). Eur Heart J. 2011;32(24):3147–97.
76. Shoup J, Carson DS. Anticoagulant use during lactation. J Hum Lact. 1999;15(3):255–7.
77. Monagle P, Chan AKC, Goldenberg NA, Ichord RN, Journeycake JM, Nowak-Göttl U, et al. Antithrombotic therapy in neonates and children: antithrombotic therapy and prevention of thrombosis, 9th ed: American College of Chest Physicians Evidence-Based Clinical Practice Guidelines. Chest. 2012;141(2 Suppl):e737S–801S.
78. Streif W, Andrew M, Marzinotto V, Massicotte P, Chan AK, Julian JA, et al. Analysis of warfarin therapy in pediatric patients: a prospective cohort study of 319 patients. Blood. 1999;94(9):3007–14.
79. Gillespie MA, Lyle CA, Goldenberg NA. Updates in pediatric venous thromboembolism. Curr Opin Hematol. 2015;22(5):413–9.
80. von Vajna E, Alam R, So T-Y. Current clinical trials on the use of direct oral anticoagulants in the pediatric population. Cardiol Ther. 2016;5(1):19–41.
81. Radulescu VC. Anticoagulation therapy in children. Semin Thromb Hemost. 2017. https://doi.org/10.1055/s-0036-1598004. [Epub ahead of print].

3 Unfractionated Heparin and Low-Molecular-Weight Heparin

Rhynn J. Malloy, Jessica Rimsans, Megan Rhoten, Katelyn Sylvester, and John Fanikos

Clinical Vignettes

Case 1: *A 51-year-old obese woman with a history of hypertension, hyperlipidemia, and bipolar disorder presents to the emergency department with sudden onset of dyspnea. She is diagnosed with a submassive bilateral pulmonary embolism (PE). She denies a history of venous thromboembolism, but her sister has a history of deep vein thrombosis (DVT). She denies smoking, use of oral contraceptives, and recent travel or surgery. The patient is admitted to medicine service. The Pulmonary Vascular Service would like him initiated on unfractionated heparin. What would be the best recommendation?*

The patient's pertinent examination results follow:
Weight: 124 kg
Height: 60.2 in
Body mass index (BMI): 53 kg/m2
Serum creatinine: 0.93 mg/dL
D-dimer: >4000 ng/mL.

Case 2: *This same 51-year-old obese woman is now to be discharged on enoxaparin as a bridge to warfarin. What dose should be recommended based on the patient's profile?*
Weight: 124 kg
Height: 60.2 in
Body mass index (BMI): 53 kg/m2
Serum creatinine: 0.93 mg/dL
Please describe the best monitoring strategy for enoxaparin using anti-Xa levels (i.e. when levels should be drawn and what is the appropriate target anti-Xa level).

R. J. Malloy (✉) · J. Rimsans · M. Rhoten
K. Sylvester · J. Fanikos
Department of Pharmacy, Brigham and Women's Hospital, Boston, MA, USA
e-mail: rmalloy@partners.org; rimsans@partners.org; mrhoten@partners.org; ksylvester3@partners.org; jfanikos@partners.org

Introduction

Anticoagulants are the cornerstone of therapy for venous and arterial thrombosis prevention and treatment. Unfractionated heparin (UFH) remains the primary choice for treatment of acute coronary

J. F. Lau et al. (eds.), *Anticoagulation Therapy*, https://doi.org/10.1007/978-3-319-73709-6_3

syndromes (ACS). Although the use of direct-acting oral anticoagulants has increased since their approval, initial use of intravenous (IV) and subcutaneous (SC) anticoagulation with UFH and/or low-molecular-weight heparin (LMWH) continues to play an important role in the treatment of acute thrombosis due to their rapid onset of antithrombotic activity and the availability of reversal agents. Clinicians must be familiar with these anticoagulants, their pharmacological properties, pharmacodynamics, dosing, monitoring, and toxicity.

Unfractionated Heparin

UFH is one of the most commonly used parenteral anticoagulants to treat or prevent thromboembolism and has been utilized for nearly a century. It is used in a wide variety of settings; including systemically, catheter instillation, extracorporeal circuits, or coating of artificial surfaces of medical devices to prevent thrombotic complications. Since heparins are dependent on the presence of antithrombin (AT) for clotting factor inhibition, they are considered indirect-acting anticoagulants. Heparins have no intrinsic fibrinolytic activity and will not lyse existing thrombi. They contain an active pentasaccharide sequence that binds to AT (Fig. 3.1). The active pentasaccharide sequence responsible for catalyzing AT is found on one-third and one-fifth of the chains of UFH and LMWH, respectively. Once heparin binds and activates AT, it can readily dissociate and bind to additional AT, providing a continuous anticoagulant effect. This binding produces a conformational change, accelerating AT binding and inactivation of coagulation factors XIIa, XIa, Xa, and IXa and thrombin (IIa). Thrombin and factor Xa are the most sensitive to inhibition by the heparin/AT complex, with thrombin being approximately tenfold more sensitive to inhibition than factor Xa. UFH's inhibition of thrombin requires binding to both the coagulation enzyme and AT through the high-affinity pentasaccharide, whereas inhibition of factor Xa requires that heparin bind only to AT. By inactivating thrombin, heparin not only prevents fibrin formation but also inhibits thrombin-induced activation of platelets and coagulation factors V and VIII. In addition to its

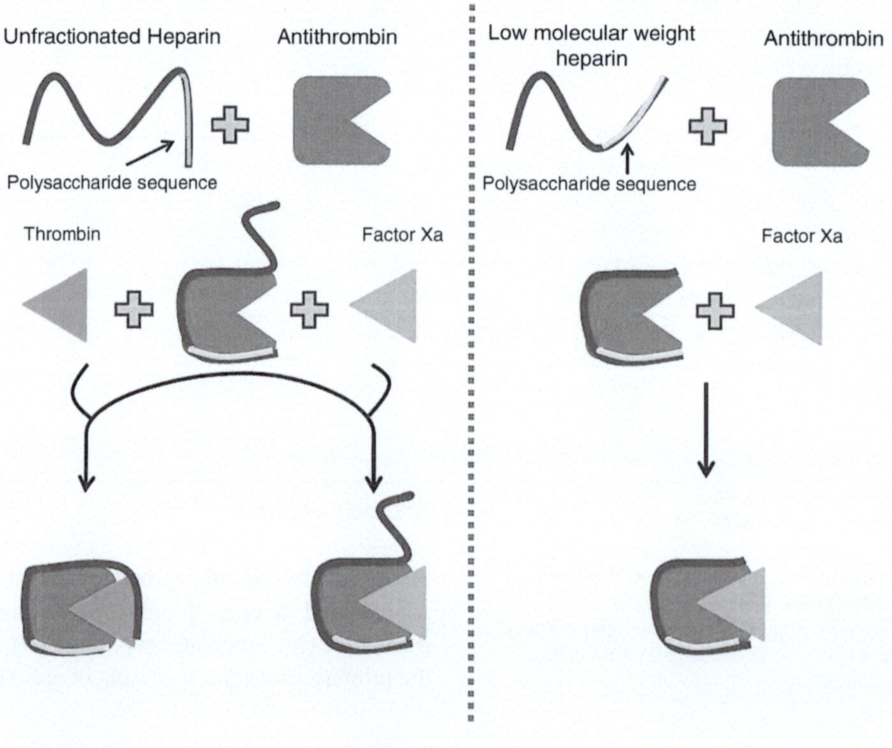

Fig. 3.1 Mechanism of action of UFH and LMWH

anticoagulant effects, heparin increases vessel wall permeability, suppresses the proliferation of vascular smooth muscle cells, suppresses osteoblast formation, and activates osteoclasts [1].

Pharmacokinetics and Pharmacodynamics

UFH is derived from porcine intestines and structurally consists of highly sulfated, linked disaccharide chains that vary in size and length. Intravenous infusion or SC injections are the available routes for UFH administration, with IV being the preferred route. When given via SC injection for therapeutic anticoagulation, doses need to be large enough (30,000 units/day) to overcome UFH's low bioavailability (Table 3.1). UFH readily binds to plasma proteins, which contributes to its variable anticoagulant response after parenteral administration. Despite these limitations, IV administration rapidly achieves therapeutic plasma concentrations that can be effectively monitored and adjusted based on infusion rates [2].

Systemic UFH clearance is dose dependent and occurs through two independent mechanisms. The initial phase is the rapid and saturable binding to endothelial cells, macrophages, and local proteins where UFH is depolymerized. The second phase is a slower, nonsaturable, renal-mediated clearance. At therapeutic doses, UFH is cleared primarily via depolymerization, with the higher-molecular-weight chains being cleared faster than lower-weight counterparts. As clearance becomes renally dependent, increased or prolonged UFH dosing provides a disproportionate increase in both the intensity and the duration of the anticoagulant effect. The anticoagulant response to UFH administration is typically monitored using the activated partial thromboplastin time (aPTT). The aPTT should be measured every 6 h with IV administration and doses adjusted accordingly, until the patient has achieved stable therapeutic levels. Once steady state is reached, the frequency of monitoring can be extended [3–6].

Table 3.1 Pharmacologic features of UFH versus LMWH [3]

Feature	Heparin	LMWH
Source	Biological-porcine intestines	Biological-porcine intestines
Molecular weight (daltons)	15,000	5000
Target	Xa:IIa	Xa > IIa
Bioavailability (%)	30	90
Half-life (hours)[a]	IV: dose dependent 1–3 SQ: dose dependent 2–5	3–7
Protamine reversal	Complete	Partial (60–80%)
Renal excretion	Dose dependent	Yes
Incidence of heparin-induced thrombocytopenia (%)	<5.0	<1.0

LMWH low-molecular-weight heparin
[a]In normal renal function

Clinical Indications and Dosing

Indications for UFH use include the treatment of ACS, treatment or prevention of venous thromboembolism (VTE), bridge therapy to chronic oral anticoagulation, and prevention of thrombotic events during cardioversion or invasive surgical procedures (Table 3.2), among others. Due to UFH's short half-life and reversibility, it remains the best anticoagulant option in patients at a higher bleeding risk or organ dysfunction. When used for thromboprophylaxis in medical patients, three times daily UFH dosing provides better efficacy in reducing VTE events compared to twice daily dosing but is associated with more major bleeding episodes [7].

To overcome the variable effect of UFH, weight-based dosing nomograms are recommended for treatment of thromboembolic disease. Dosing UFH for the treatment of VTE should be weight-based and titrated to reach a goal aPTT range [6]. Doses of UFH in ACS are much lower than those used to treat VTE, with dosing maximums placed on both bolus and infusion rates [8]. Table 3.2 reviews dosing for VTE and ACS treatment, bridging, and VTE prophylaxis. The applicability of weight-based heparin dosing recommendations in the obese and morbidly obese population is uncertain, as limited data are available (see "Special Population Considerations").

Table 3.2 Unfractionated heparin (UFH) dosing

Indication	Dose	Considerations
VTE treatment	LD: 80 units/kg bolus 18 units/kg/h infusion adjusted per institution heparin nomogram Target aPTT, 1.5–2.5 × control Target anti-Xa, 0.3–0.7 units/mL	Monitoring: • aPTT every 6 h until therapeutic and then at least once daily (dependent upon clinical scenario) • Anti-Xa levels every 6 h and after each rate changes • Complete blood count, repeat every 3–5 days during therapy (including platelet count) • Heparin-induced thrombocytopenia (HIT) antibody testing for thrombocytopenia, thrombosis, heparin-induced skin lesions, or other signs pointing to a potential diagnosis of immune-mediated response • Bleeding Precautions: • Prior allergic or hypersensitivity-type reactions • Congenital or acquired bleeding disorders • Hepatic disease with altered baseline coagulation assays • Hereditary antithrombin III deficiency and concurrent use of antithrombin Contraindications: • Severe thrombocytopenia • Positive assay for immune-mediated HIT (PF4/SRA) • Patients within a remote history of HIT (>100 days) could be considered for a rechallenge with heparin provided a negative antibody test
ACS treatment	LD: 60 units/kg (maximum 4000 units) 12 units/kg/h (maximum initial dosing 1000 units/h) specifically adjusted to maintain aPTT 1.5–2 × control Target anti-Xa, 0.3–0.7 units/mL	
Bridge therapy to oral anticoagulation for atrial fibrillation, cardioversion, invasive procedure	IV infusion: 80 units/kg bolus 18 units/kg/h infusion adjusted per institution heparin nomogram Target aPTT 1.5–2.5 × control Target anti-Xa, 0.3–0.7 units/mL	
Prophylaxis of VTE in the medically ill or surgical population	5000 units SC Q8–12 h No routine monitoring 5000 units SC Q8–12 h	

LD loading dose, *h* hour, *kg* kilogram, *s* seconds, *Q* every, *anti-Xa* antifactor-Xa, *PF4* platelet factor 4, *SRA* serotonin release assay

Monitoring

UFH anticoagulant response is monitored using the aPTT, a measurement sensitive to inhibition of thrombin and factor Xa. Since different aPTT reagents (and even different lots of the same reagent) have variable sensitivity to the anticoagulant effects of UFH, it is incumbent on each laboratory to ensure that their aPTT therapeutic range is based upon heparin levels measured by anti-Xa assays (target range 0.3–0.7 units/mL) or protamine titration (0.2–0.4 units/mL). The aPTT should be measured every 6 h based on the half-life of UFH, and doses are adjusted until the patient achieves therapeutic levels based on the target aPTT range. Once two consecutive aPTT values are within the therapeutic range, testing may be extended to once or twice daily depending upon the clinical scenario. Weight-based dosing nomograms, comprised of a bolus dose and infusion rate with periodic monitoring utilizing aPTT, are recommended for treatment of thromboembolic disease (Table 3.3).

Nomograms have been associated with a shorter time to reach therapeutic levels without an increase in bleeding events. UFH dosing nomograms differ between hospitals due to differences in thromboplastin reagents, calibration, and interlaboratory standards in aPTT measurements. This has led to assessments of alternative monitoring strategies. The functional heparin assay, also known as the anti-Xa assay, has been promoted as a more reliable measure of UFH as it is insensitive to factors

Table 3.3 Unfractionated heparin (UFH) monitoring [8–10]

Acute coronary syndromes [8]		Venous thromboembolism [9]		Venous thromboembolism [10]	
Assay result (aPTT in seconds)	Dose adjustment	Assay result (aPTT in seconds)	Dose adjustment	Assay result (anti-Xa concentration in units/mL)	Dose adjustment
Initial dose	60 units/kg bolus, then 12 units/kg/h	Initial dose	80 units/kg bolus, then 18 units/kg/h	Initial dose	80 units/kg bolus, then 15 units/kg/h
aPTT <1× control	60 units/kg bolus, then increase 2 units/kg/h	aPTT <35 s	80 units/kg bolus, then increase 4 units/kg/h	<0.20	26 units/kg bolus, then increase by 4 units/kg/h
aPTT 1–1.5× control	Increase 2 units/kg/h	aPTT 35–45 s	40 units/kg bolus, then increase 2 units/kg/h	0.20–0.29	No bolus, increase by 2 units/kg/h
aPTT 1.5–2× control	No change	aPTT 46–70 s	No change	0.30–0.70	No change
aPTT 2–3× control	Decrease infusion rate by 2 units/kg/h	aPTT 71–90 s	Decrease infusion rate by 2 units/kg/h	0.1–0.80	Decrease by 1 unit/kg/h
aPTT >3× control	Stop infusion, recheck aPTT, start treatment again based on repeat aPTT	aPTT >90 s	Hold infusion for 1 h, and then decrease infusion rate by 3 units/kg/h	0.81–0.99	Decrease by 2 units/kg/h
				≥1.00	Hold infusion for 1 h, and then decrease by 3 units/kg/h

aPTT activated partial thromboplastin time, *h* hour, *kg* kilograms

other than UFH, such as concomitant warfarin use, sodium citrate in collection tubes, interference from the presence of lupus anticoagulants (LA), elevated factor VIII activity, and liver disease. Acquired inhibitors, such as LA, cause prolongation of the aPTT making it impossible to accurately measure the level of anticoagulation due to UFH. In these cases, if the aPTT is maintained within the usual therapeutic range, it may result in subtherapeutic doses of UFH and progression or recurrence of thrombosis. Institutions with limited access to anti-Xa testing or a long lab-processing time require simultaneous testing of aPTT and anti-Xa levels to estimate patient-specific therapeutic aPTT values on heparin [11]. Weight-based UFH protocols utilizing anti-Xa levels to monitor UFH are now used in many hospitals and have been associated with fewer dose changes and a greater time in the therapeutic range.

Considerations in Special Populations

Populations with potentially altered pharmacodynamic and pharmacokinetic profiles are less well studied and remain an area of clinical controversy when considering appropriate dosing strategies. These populations include elderly patients, those with extremes of body weight, and patients with liver and renal dysfunction. In these cases, there are no formal guidelines or recommendations for alternative dosing strategies. Instead, clinicians must individually evaluate each patient before initially dosing them based on underlying bleeding and thrombotic risk and make timely dose adjustments based on coagulation monitoring tests.

Obesity

Obesity has become a national epidemic and is a risk factor for cardiovascular events. It is important to understand the impact of obesity on heparin dosing due to variable pharmacokinetic changes in the volume of distribution and clearance [12, 13]. UFH has a small volume of distribution (0.07 L/kg; range 0.04–0.014 L/kg) that is generally limited to the intravascular space. However, larger doses may have some distribution into the tissue [14]. Adipose tissue is less vascular than lean muscle tissue, making the volume of distribution difficult to assess in obese patients. Since the volume of distribution of UFH is largely intravascular, a nonlinear relationship exists between weight and heparin requirements at extreme BMIs (BMI < 20 kg/m^2 and ≥35 kg/m^2) [15]. Dosing controversies include choosing the appropriate weight for dosing (total body weight (TBW), adjusted body weight (ABW), dosing weight (DW), ideal body weight (IBW)) and whether to set maximum initial bolus and continuous infusion dose rates to ensure patients do not exceed target therapeutic monitoring levels, thereby increasing bleeding risk.

Studies consistently show that weight is one of the most important predictors of anticoagulant dosing requirements. The altered volume of distribution from excess adipose tissue supports using TBW for UFH dosing. Alternatively, measurement of lean muscle argues for a dosing strategy based on ABW. Retrospective reviews of dosing strategies indicate that obese and morbidly obese patients are frequently underdosed with the use of the weight-based recommended guidelines, putting them at risk of recurrent thromboembolism [16]. Several published studies assess the appropriate dosing strategy in this patient population (Table 3.4). Although a general consensus is lacking for the optimal dosing strategy for UFH in obese patients, it is reasonable to use TBW with maximum initial bolus and continuous infusion rates for very obese patients (considered a BMI ≥ 35) or alternatively to use TBW with an empirically reduced weight-based initial dosing regimen (e.g., 12–15 units/kg/h instead of 18 units/kg/h in morbidly obese and very obese patients, respectively) [14, 17]. Regardless of the strategy selected, all patients will require diligent monitoring with both aPTT and anti-Xa levels and prompt adjustments to ensure their levels of anticoagulation do not exceed threshold targets. Appropriate monitoring of aPTT and anti-Xa levels will be discussed below.

Pregnancy

The incidence of thrombosis is increased by twofold to fourfold during pregnancy as compared with the nonpregnant population [23–25]. Risk increases further in the immediate post-delivery period (defined as 6–12 weeks post-delivery), especially following delivery via cesarean section [23, 26]. Anticoagulant considerations during the peripartum period are further confounded by fetal/maternal risk factors, delivery schedule, efficacy, cost, convenience, patient characteristics, anesthesia modality, and breastfeeding compatibility [23, 26]. The pharmacokinetic and pharmacodynamic profile of UFH changes throughout pregnancy due to alterations in blood volume, renal function, coagulation factor levels (FVIII, fibrinogen, and von Willebrand factor), and plasma concentrations of heparin-binding proteins, making frequent monitoring a necessity [23, 27]. Despite the well-documented incidence of thromboembolism during the peripartum period, well-designed, randomized, controlled trials have been rarely conducted in this population. Most recommendations are based on either observational studies or data extrapolated from other populations [28]. Historically, UFH has been the treatment of choice for both prevention and treatment of venous and arterial thrombi, though literature shows that LMWH is at least as effective and safer in many cases [29–33]. Recent consensus guidelines recommend LMWH over UFH [28]. Despite being largely replaced by LMWH, UFH remains the treatment of choice in patients with reduced renal function (CrCl < 30 mL/min), requiring rapid reversal, at extremes of body weight, and in those patients for whom LMWH is either cost prohibitive or unavailable [24, 34].

UFH is large molecule that does not cross the placenta and is not secreted into breast milk. Therefore, it is considered safe to the fetus and the breastfeeding infant [23, 25, 35]. Risks to the mother include heparin-induced thrombocytopenia

Table 3.4 Evidence for dosing UFH in obesity [15, 18–22]

Population	Dosing strategy	Conclusion
Case report of 388 kg male with VTE; also includes a review of current literature [15]	• Due to protocol maximum rates: 5000 unit initial bolus and initial rate of 1500 units/h Goal aPTT reached 55 h later with an infusion rate of 3650 units/h	Weight-based heparin nomograms with capped maximum doses lead to delays in time to therapeutic range; recommend to use DW in morbidly obese patients
UFH infusions in nonobese, obese, and morbidly obese critically ill patients [18]	• TBW • No bolus • Initial dosing continuous infusion: – Nonobese: 18 units/kg/h – Obese: 16 units/kg/h – Morbidly obese: 12 units/kg/h	TBW with a reduced initial body weight is associated with similar time to the first therapeutic aPTT and steady state with no difference in bleeding
UFH infusions in obese patients with VTE [19]	• Recommended dosing based on actual body weight with 80 units/kg bolus and 18 units/kg/h continuous infusion • Retrospective based on provider dosing choice	More than 75% of obese patients received less than the recommended dosing of heparin resulting in delays in time to therapeutic aPTT
All patients admitted to the cardiac care unit for unstable angina, acute myocardial infarction, pulmonary embolism, or rule-out myocardial infarction [20]	• Weight – TBW if < IBW – If TBW > IBW, dosing weight = IBW + 0.3 (TBW—IBW) • Initial nomogram 80 units/kg bolus and 18 units/kg/h continuous infusion for all indications • Later modified initial bolus to 75 units/kg	After the third aPTT measurement, 77% (65/84) of obese patients were in the therapeutic range, 5% (4/84) were subtherapeutic, and 18% (15/84) were supratherapeutic
All patients on UFH for all indications [21]	• Weight – DW for patients if TBW was > IBW + 10 kg – All others used TBW • Initial nomogram 80 units/kg bolus and 18 units/kg/h continuous infusion for all indications; however, data of 80% of patients would reach therapeutic aPTT with 15 units/kg/h	Infusion rates deviated less from dosing guidelines when TBW was used (rather than IBW or DW), especially in obese patients Recommend TBW in all patients with maximum loading dose of 10,000 units and maximum initial infusion rate of 1500 units/h
Morbidly obese patients receiving therapeutic UFH infusion for greater than 24 h compared to overweight/class I and II obesity and normal/underweight patients [22]	• Protocol based on TBW • Initial bolus 80 units/kg for VTE and 60 units/kg ACS Initial continuous infusion 14 units/kg/h (options to increase to 18 units/kg/h or decrease to 12 units/kg/h depending on indication)	Morbidly obese patients require smaller UFH infusion rates per kilogram TBW compared to patients with lower body mass indices Recommend maximum initial infusion rates of 14 units/kg/h if BMI >/= 40 kg/m^2

UFH unfractionated heparin, *CI* continuous infusion, *TBW* total body weight, *VTE* venous thromboembolism, *aPTT* activated prothrombin time, *CCU* cardiac care unit, *IBW* ideal body weight, *DW* dosing weight, *BMI* body mass index

(HIT), osteoporosis, and bleeding, especially during labor and delivery. All of these risks are higher with UFH when compared to LMWH [23, 24]. Other limitations of UFH include the need for continuous infusion or multiple daily SC doses and the requirement of frequent monitoring due to the unpredictable pharmacokinetics.

While UFH is typically monitored via the aPTT, this test may not be a reliable measure of anticoagulation during pregnancy, and some patients will require monitoring via anti-Xa levels [27]. Elevated levels of FVIII during pregnancy may impact the aPTT, leading to what may appear as "heparin resistance." The administration of very

Table 3.5 Unfractionated heparin (UFH) dosing for treatment and prevention of thromboembolism during pregnancy [28]

Indication for anticoagulation	Treatment options	Lab monitoring
VTE treatment doses	• Bolus: 5000 units IV (or 80 units/kg) • Continuous infusion: 1250 units/h (18 units/kg/h) for 5 days and then convert total daily dose into BID-TID SC dosing • Adjusted per institution heparin nomogram targeting aPTT 1.5–2.5 × control *Alternative*: 250 units/kg SC Q12H adjusted to mid-interval PTT 1.5–2.5 × control • Consider 333 units/kg loading dose for acute VTE • Not to be used in arterial thrombosis	For continuous infusion dosing, draw aPTT or anti-Xa 6 h after initial dose and all adjustments Draw anti-Xa levels at mid-interval (6 h after a dose for Q12H/BID dosing)
VTE prophylactic doses	First trimester: 5000–10,00 units SC BID Second trimester: 7500–10,000 units SC BID Third trimester: 10,000 units SC BID *Alternative*: Titrate to anti-Xa levels of 0.1–0.3 units/mL	For fixed prophylactic dosing of UFH, monitoring is typically not required Draw anti-Xa levels at mid-interval (6 h after a dose for Q12H/BID dosing)

BID twice daily, *TID* three times daily, *aPTT* activated prothrombin time, *SC* subcutaneously, *Q* every, *h* hours, *VTE* venous thromboembolism

high UFH doses may not result in appropriate or expected increases in the aPTT. Patients with "heparin resistance" are at a high risk of over-anticoagulation; though data does not correlate this phenomenon with higher bleeding rates. These patients should be switched to LMWH or be monitored with anti-Xa levels while receiving UFH [23, 28].

The aPTT target for IV UFH anticoagulation is 1.5–2.5 times the institution lab control (or whatever range is determined therapeutic for the individual laboratory's aPTT reagent). The goal anti-Xa level is 0.3–0.7 anti-Xa units/milliliter [28]. For patients on twice daily SC UFH, levels should be checked mid-interval (6 h post dose for twice daily dosing) with goal anti-Xa levels of 0.5–1.2 units/mL or a goal aPTT of 2–2.5 times the control value [27] (Table 3.5). For patients on UFH for prophylaxis, fixed doses can be used without monitoring, or, alternatively, anti-Xa levels of 0.1–0.3 units/mL can be targeted 6 h after the dose [23, 28].

Recommendations for treatment duration differ based on indication. Guidelines suggest continuing anticoagulation through at least the first 6 weeks postpartum, for a total of 3–6 months from the onset of thromboembolism for a first occurrence or longer for patients at high risk of recurrence after their first VTE [24, 28]. For patients receiving therapeutic UFH SC at the time of planned delivery (i.e., an induction or scheduled cesarean section), the UFH should be discontinued at least 24 h prior to delivery to minimize the risk of bleeding and allow for spinal or epidural anesthesia [24, 25]. Patients at high risk of thromboembolism, such as those with mechanical heart valves or recent VTE, should switch to IV UFH and continue up to 4–6 h prior to delivery [36]. For patients undergoing spontaneous delivery, neuraxial anesthesia should not be used, and consideration should be given to the reversal of anticoagulation with protamine, depending on the aPTT/anti-Xa level at the time of labor [28]. Prophylactic SC UFH should be discontinued at the onset of labor and should not be considered a contraindication to neuraxial anesthesia [25]. Anticoagulation should be resumed 4–6 h after a vaginal delivery or 6–12 h post-cesarean delivery, assuming hemostasis has been achieved [37]. See Chap. 18 for more detailed information.

Strategies for Reversal of Unfractionated Heparin

Major bleeding is a serious and possibly fatal complication associated with heparin therapy. Major bleeding occurs in 0–7% of patients with 0–3% of these cases resulting in fatal bleeding [3]. Bleeding risk increases with treatment-related factors (i.e., route of administration, anticoagulation intensity, concomitant antiplatelet, and fibrinolytic agents) and patient-specific factors (i.e., age, gender, end-organ function, body weight, and excessive alcohol consumption) [38]. As anticoagulation intensity increases, the rate of intracranial hemorrhage, mortality, stroke, major bleeding, and reinfarction increase; this is especially true in the elderly [39–41]. Although analysis of major clinical trials has shown a correlation with increased therapeutic levels, there is no well-defined relationship between a threshold aPTT or anti-Xa level and risk of bleeding. Notably, patients within therapeutic ranges still experience bleeding complications [3].

In the case of clinically significant bleeding or emergency surgery, UFH reversal can be accomplished by a combination of the following: holding the medication (particularly for IV administration due to its short half-life), administering protamine, blood product transfusions, and supportive care. Protamine sulfate is a strongly basic low-molecular-weight protein. When administered alone, it is a weak anticoagulant with clinically insignificant effects; however, when it binds to heparin, which is acidic, the two form a stable salt complex that renders them both pharmacologically inactive. The onset of action is rapid, generally neutralizing heparin within 5 min, and the duration of effect can persist up to 2 h. The required dose of protamine depends on the amount of heparin administered and the time since the last dose. For immediate reversal of heparin administered within the last hour, 1 mg of protamine is typically required for every 100 units of heparin administered. Less protamine is required for heparin administered more than 1 h previously (Table 3.6). For subcutaneous (SC) heparin administration, due to the extended half-life, repeat doses or prolonged infusions of protamine may be required [1]. Regardless of the dose given, assessment of reversal effect should be done by evaluating clinical signs and symptoms of bleeding and via lab monitoring with either the aPTT or anti-Xa assay. The maximum dose of protamine recommended is 50 mg. If the dose of heparin administered is unknown, 50 mg of protamine can be administered and assessed with lab monitoring [42]. Based on institution-specific protocols, larger doses of protamine may be administered in select cases such as during heparin reversal following cardiac surgery.

Table 3.6 Reversal of heparin with protamine sulfate [42]

Time from heparin exposure	Protamine dose
Less than 1 h	1 mg protamine for every 100 units of heparin
1–2 h	0.5 mg protamine for every 100 units of heparin
More than 2 h	0.25 mg protamine for every 100 units of heparin

Examples

1. A patient receives IV bolus of 5000 units of heparin within the last hour but has not yet started the continuous infusion:

   Protamine required for complete reversal: 50 mg

   100% heparin in the last hour: 5000 units
2. A patient has been receiving a heparin infusion at 1500 units/h without any recent bolus doses. To calculate the amount of heparin received in the last 3 h:

Protamine required for complete reversal: 26.25 mg

100% heparin in the last hour: 1500 units

50% heparin in the preceding hour: 750 units

25% heparin in an hour before that: 375 units

Total heparin: 1500 + 750 + 375 units = 2625 units

Protamine dose to be administered: 2625 units of heparin/100 = 26.25 mg

High doses or rapid administration of protamine can cause severe hypotension, bradycardia, cardiovascular collapse, pulmonary hypertension, and/or anaphylactic reactions. To minimize this risk, protamine should be administered slowly and not exceed 50 mg over 10 min [42]. Although rare, patients who have previously received protamine or protamine-containing insulin, those with a fish allergy (although not supported by data), or those who have undergone a vasectomy may be at higher risk of developing anaphylactic reactions due to existing anti-protamine antibodies [1]. Pretreatment with corticosteroids or antihistamines may mitigate some of this risk [43].

Complications

Heparin Resistance

Patients requiring escalating UFH doses, without corresponding prolongation of the aPTT, are deemed to be heparin resistant (generally defined as a daily UFH requirement exceeding 35,000 units in 24 h) [1, 44]. True heparin resistance may be caused by AT deficiency, increased clearance, or increases in heparin-binding proteins due to physiologic stress or high clot burdens. In these patients, frequent monitoring and dose adjustments are required to ensure patients are adequately anticoagulated. Correction of the underlying cause of resistance, if possible, may reduce the requirement for large UFH doses.

Alternatively, other patients may have an artificial heparin resistance related to altered coagulation factors and their effect on the aPTT rather than a decrease in the anticoagulant effect of UFH. Common contributors include elevations in factor VIII and fibrinogen, conditions that are frequently seen in pregnant and burn injury patients [1, 44]. Utilizing UFH boluses and assessing a response in aPTT values 1–2 h post administration may be helpful in patients with suspected heparin resistance. Additionally, monitoring the effect of anticoagulation with anti-Xa levels instead of aPTT levels may allow for lower UFH doses while still maintaining the same clinical outcomes and theoretically reducing the risk of bleeding [45]. Alternative anticoagulation may be continued with a direct thrombin inhibitor (DTI), such as bivalirudin, given it does not require AT to produce its anticoagulant effects.

Osteopenia

In addition to its anticoagulant effects, UFH suppresses osteoblast formation and activates osteoclasts which eventually can lead to heparin-induced osteoporosis with prolonged use [1]. This is caused by non-specific binding of UFH to osteoblasts which leads to the downstream activation of osteoclasts resulting in both decreased bone formation and increased bone resorption [46]. The majority of data on osteopenia associated with UFH come from case reports of patients requiring long-term treatment or prevention of VTE during pregnancy as these effects are rarely seen with short-term UFH use. The risk of developing osteopenia and the degree of bone degeneration do not consistently appear to be correlated with either the UFH dose or treatment, and the effects may be reversible after treatment cessation [47, 48]. One of the largest observational studies of pregnant women on long-term prophylactic UFH determined that 2–3% of patients developed vertebral fractures, which is noteworthy since this young population generally has limited risk factors for osteoporosis [49].

Heparin-Induced Thrombocytopenia

Heparin-induced thrombocytopenia (HIT) is an immune-mediated response that leads to the activation of platelets through an IgG antibody-platelet factor 4 (PF4) complex. Heparin binds to plasma proteins including PF4 [50]. IgG antibodies bind to this PF4-heparin complex and in turn activate platelets, endothelial cells, and monocytes. This leads to the release of procoagulant platelet microparticles, tissue factor expression on monocytes and endothelial cells, and ultimately activation of the clotting cascade, thrombin generation, and clot formation. Patients with HIT are highly prothrombotic, such that over 50% develop thromboembolism in the absence of treatment within 30 days of diagnosis. Patients receiving UFH are at tenfold greater risk of developing HIT than those receiving LMWH. Patients undergoing major surgeries which are associated with significant platelet activation (and therefore PF4 production) and exposure to large amounts of UFH (i.e., cardiac surgery) are at higher risk of developing HIT (1–5%) compared to medically ill patients [51, 52].

	Score = 2	Score = 1	Score = 0
Thrombocytopenia Compare the highest platelet count within the sequence of declining platelet counts with the lowest count to determine the % of platelet fall. **(Select only 1 option)**	o > 50% platelet fall AND nadir of ≥ 20 AND no surgery within preceding 3 days	o > 50% platelet fall BUT surgery within preceding 3 days OR o any combination of platelet fall and nadir that does not fit criteria for Score 2 or Score 0 (eg, 30-50% platelet fall or nadir 10-19)	o < 30% platelet fall o any platelet fall with nadir < 10
Timing (of platelet count fall or thrombosis*) Day 0 = first day of most recent heparin exposure **(Select only 1 option)**	o platelet fall day 5-10 after start of heparin o platelet fall within 1 day of start of heparin AND exposure to heparin within past 5-30 days	o consistent with platelet fall days 5-10 but not clear (eg, missing counts) o platelet fall within 1 day of start of heparin AND exposure to heparin in past 31-100 days o platelet fall after day 10	o platelet fall ≤ day 4 without exposure to heparin in past 100 days
Thrombosis (or other clinical sequelae) **(Select only 1 option)**	o confirmed new thrombosis (venous or arterial) o skin necrosis at injection site o anaphylactoid reaction to IV heparin bolus o adrenal hemorrhage	o recurrent venous thrombosis in a patient receiving therapeutic anticoagulants o suspected thrombosis (awaiting confirmation with imaging) o erythematous skin lesions at heparin injection sites	o thrombosis suspected
oTher cause for Thrombocytopenia** **(Select only 1 option)**	o no alternative explanation for platelet fall is evident	**Possible other cause is evident:** o sepsis without proven microbial source o thrombocytopenia associated with initiation of ventilator o other	**Probable other cause present:** o within 72 h of surgery o confirmed bacteremia/ fungemia o chemotherapy or radiation within past 20 days o DIC due to non-HIT cause o posttransfusion purpura (PTP) o platelet count < 20 AND given a drug implicated in causing D-ITP (see list) o non-necrotizing skin lesions at LMWH injection site (presumes DTH) o other

Drugs implicated in drug-induced immune thrombocytopenia (D-ITP)

Relatively Common: glycoprotein IIb/IIIa antagonists (abciximab, eptifibatide, tirofiban); quinine, quinidine, sulfa antibiotics, carbamazepine, vancomycin
Less Common: actinomycin, amitriptyline, amoxicillin/piperacillin/nafcillin, cephalosporins (cefazolin, ceftazidime, ceftriaxone), celecoxib, ciprofloxacin, esomeprazole, fexofenadine, fentanyl, fucidic acid, furosemide, gold salts, levofloxacin, metronidazole, naproxen, oxaliplatin, phenytoin, propranolol, propoxyphene, ranitidine, rifampin, suramin, trimethoprim. Note: This is a partial list.

Fig. 3.2 The "4T score" for diagnosis of heparin-induced thrombocytopenia [50]. (Reprinted from CHEST, Vol. 141/ Issue 2 Supp, Linkins LA, Dans AL, Moores LK, Bona R, Davidson BL, Schulman S, Crowther M, Treatment and prevention of heparin-induced thrombocytopenia: antithrombotic therapy and prevention of thrombosis 9th ed.: American College of Chest Physicians Evidence-based Clinical Practice Guidelines, pages e495s–e530s, © 2012, with permission from Elsevier)

The "4T score" is a validated pretest probability assessment tool that is useful for determining the risk of HIT in a patient with thrombocytopenia (Fig. 3.2). Patients with a low 4T score are considered unlikely to have HIT, and laboratory testing is not necessary. For patients at moderate or high risk, objective laboratory testing is required. The most widely available test for HIT is the PF4 enzyme-linked immunosorbent assay. In patients with intermediate 4T score and an inconclusive PF4 (depending on the assay, an ELISA optical density <1 or as high as <2 can be considered inconclusive), a confirmatory serotonin release assay (SRA) is recommended. A confirmatory SRA should also be sent when the clinical picture, and immunoassay results are discordant (e.g., patient with very high probability 4T score and negative immunoassay). In patients with high 4T scores or those with intermediate 4T scores and PF4 optical densities ≥1.5, an SRA is not required to confirm the diagnosis of HIT [50, 53–55]. The SRA remains the gold standard for the diagnosis of HIT [56]. There is controversial evidence correlating the "4T score" to a positive SRA. The literature suggests that there is a very low correlation of a positive SRA to a low "4T score," while correlation varies once a patient receives a moderate-high score. As a general rule, as the "4T score" increases, the relationship between the score and the SRA becomes more accurate [57, 58].

If a patient is suspected to have HIT, all heparin-containing products, such as LMWH or UFH, should be discontinued, and anticoagulation with a direct thrombin inhibitor such as bivalirudin or argatroban should be initiated. In the acute setting, parenteral DTIs are the preferred agents. Argatroban and bivalirudin should be dosed according to an aPTT-based algorithm. If oral vitamin K antagonists (warfarin) were initiated prior to the diagnosis of HIT, they should be discontinued and reversed with phytonadione to prevent progressive thrombosis and venous gangrene associated with protein C depletion. Once platelets have been recovered to be greater than 150 K/mcL or to the patient's baseline, warfarin should be initiated targeting an INR of 2–3 and continued for 3–6 months. If bridging therapy is required and the patient has good renal function, fondaparinux, though not FDA approved, may be used. Fondaparinux is an alternative synthetic factor Xa inhibitor that is injected SC once daily [50] (Fig. 3.3) (see Chap. 17).

Low-Molecular-Weight Heparin

LMWH is a porcine-derived polysaccharide that contains the same active pentasaccharide sequence required for anticoagulant activity as UFH. It is generated from UFH via chemical or

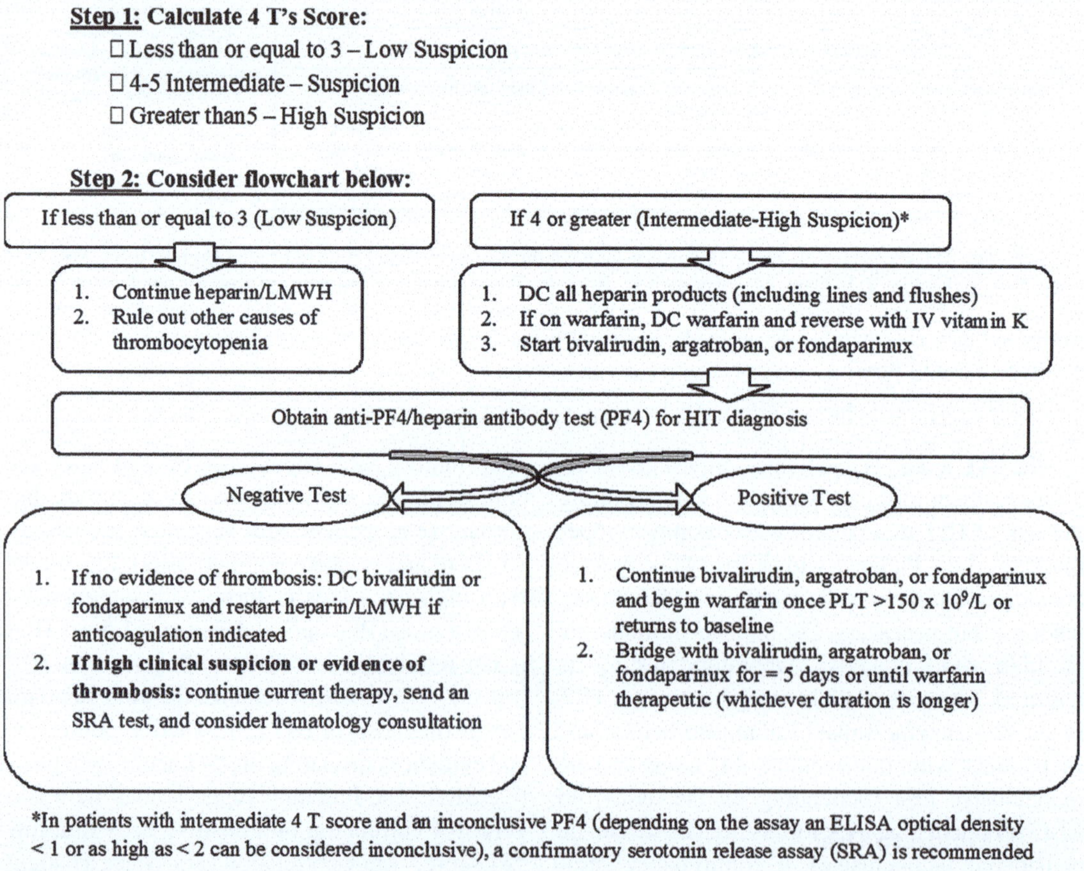

Fig. 3.3 A stepwise approach to the management of patients with suspected heparin-induced thrombocytopenia (HIT) [51, 57]

enzymatic degradation. Each LMWH product undergoes a different method of preparation. The clinical development of LMWH was driven by certain observations including a reduction in thrombin activity in relation to anti-factor Xa activity, a more favorable benefit/risk ratio in animal studies, and superior pharmacokinetic properties. Several products exist internationally (Table 3.7). LMWHs are approximately one-third the molecular weight of UFH (4000–5000 daltons). Due to their smaller size, LMWHs have a decreased affinity for thrombin since they cannot bind both AT and thrombin simultaneously; however, they maintain the same affinity for factor Xa. Factor Xa does not require heparin to stabilize its interaction with AT; thus, smaller molecules like LMWH inactivate factor Xa as well as larger molecules like UFH. In contrast, a polysaccharide chain length of at least 18 saccharides, including the active pentasaccharide sequence, is required to create the bridge between AT and thrombin. Approximately 25–50% of LMWH molecules are above this chain length. Conversely, all LMWH chains contain the active pentasaccharide sequence such that 100% can mediate inactivation of factor Xa [1].

Pharmacodynamics

There are several biological consequences of the reduced size of LMWH as compared to UFH (Table 3.8). There is decreased LMWH binding to other plasma proteins, macrophages, and endothelial cells. This results in a more predictable dose-response relationship and a longer plasma half-life for LMWH. Therefore, unlike UFH, no routine plasma monitoring is required which facilitates outpatient management. Furthermore, a lower incidence of HIT has been observed due to decreased binding to PF4 and platelets. LMWH also has reduced binding to

Table 3.7 LMWH product profiles [59–62]

	Enoxaparin	Dalteparin	Tinzaparin
Brand name	Lovenox™	Fragmin™	Innohep™
Manufacturing process	Benzylation followed by alkaline hydrolysis	Controlled nitrous acid depolymerization	Heparinase digestion
Mean molecular weight (daltons)	4500	6000	6500
Elimination half-life (hours)	4.5–7	3–5	3.4
Metabolism	Hepatic desulfation/ depolymerization	–	Non-hepatic desulfation/ depolymerization
Excretion	Renal	Renal	Renal
Bioavailability (%)	90–92	87	87
Anti-Xa/anti-IIa ratio	3.8	2.7	2.8
Anti-Xa activity (international units/mg)	100	156	100

Table 3.8 Biological consequences of reduced binding to proteins and cells of LMWH compared to UFH [1]

Binding target	Biologic effects	Clinical consequences
Proteins	More predictable anticoagulant response	Monitoring of anticoagulant effect is unnecessary
Macrophages	Cleared through renal mechanism	Longer plasma half-life. Once daily SC treatment is effective
Platelets	Reduced incidence of heparin-dependent antibody	Reduced incidence of HIT
Osteoblasts	Reduced activation of osteoclasts	Lower incidence of osteopenia

SC subcutaneously, *HIT* heparin-induced thrombocytopenia

osteoblasts resulting in a lower incidence of osteoclast activation and lower levels of bone loss [1].

Pharmacokinetics

All LMWH products have an elimination half-life ranging from 3 to 7 h and are 87–90% bioavailable (Table 3.7). Peak anti-Xa activity occurs 3–5 h after SC injection with a predictable dose response. All agents are metabolized via desulfation or depolymerization, and all agents are excreted renally. Enoxaparin, dalteparin, and tinzaparin are the agents available in the United States. Enoxaparin is the only LMWH available in the United States for IV use in ST-segment elevation myocardial infarction (STEMI) managed medically or with subsequent percutaneous coronary intervention (PCI) [59–62].

Clinical Indications and Dosing

LMWHs are often not considered a first-line agent for critically ill patients due to their prolonged duration of action and renal clearance. They play an important role in the stable medically ill patients, as well as patients transitioning to an ambulatory phase of care, and specific ambulatory patient populations. Enoxaparin has the largest number of indications as compared to dalteparin or tinzaparin (Table 3.9) [59–62]. Often, these agents are used outside of their approved indications. Enoxaparin is often recommended as an option to bridge patients who may be undergoing a procedure or starting warfarin therapy as it has a wide array of indications, has been extensively studied, and provides specific dose adjustments for renal dysfunction [63, 64].

Most acute treatment dosing regimens are weight-based, while thromboprophylaxis typically employs fixed dosing (Table 3.9). However, the recent literature supports the consideration of weight under certain circumstances (see LMWH special populations) [65, 66]. All weight-based dosing should be done according to TBW or, when dealing with the obese population, using ABW [1, 67]. Controversy still exists when determining the appropriate weight limit for adjusted dosing in obese patients. Ultimately, age, weight, renal function, and comorbidities must be considered when selecting the appropriate agent and dose for patients.

Considerations in Special Populations

The use of LMWH in patients with altered renal function or those with altered volumes of distribution must be carefully managed. LMWHs are renally eliminated, and the risks of bleeding and prolonged exposure in patients with altered clearance should be weighed prior to utilizing these agents. In contrast, LMWHs have superior pharmacokinetic properties as compared to UFH, including high bioavailability, making them a desirable alternative. Their use may facilitate expedited discharges for patients who would otherwise need to remain hospitalized while receiving continuous infusion UFH. However, alternative dosing strategies and close monitoring are required in patients with altered volumes of distribution, the elderly, and those with renal dysfunction.

Table 3.9 Dosing of LMWH [60–62]

Drug	Indication	Dose, route, frequency	Dose adjustments	Considerations
Enoxaparin [60] (Lovenox™)	Treatment of VTE	1 mg/kg SC every 12 h *Or* 1.5 mg/kg SC every 24 h	*CrCl < 30 mL/min*: 1 mg/kg SC every 24 h *CrCl < 15 mL/min*: not recommended	*Monitoring*: • Anti-Xa level recommended with renal impairment, obese or low-weight patients, children, pregnancy, bleeding or hypercoagulable states • Renal function • Signs and symptoms of bleeding • If bridging with warfarin, monitor daily INR and use appropriate bridging strategy [bridge for a minimum of 5 days and until INR is ≥2.0 for at least 24 h] • Signs of HIT [thrombocytopenia, thrombosis, bleeding, skin lesions, or other signs] *Precautions*: • History of bleeding or thrombosis • Renal impairment • Liver disease • History of HIT • Concomitant use of antithrombotic agents • Recent spinal or ophthalmologic surgery • Indwelling epidural • *Tinzeparin*: Increased risk of death in elderly patients with renal insufficiency (≥70 years with CrCl < 30 mL/min OR ≥ 75 years with CrCl ≤ 60 mL/min)
	Treatment of ACS • STEMI • UA/NSTEMI	• 30 mg IV bolus plus 1 mg/kg with tenecteplase followed by 1 mg/kg SC every 12 h • 1 mg/k SC every 12 h	*CrCl < 30 mL/min*: not recommended	
	Prophylaxis/bridge therapy for AF or VTE/cardioversion	1 mg/kg SC every 12 h *Or* 1.5 mg/kg every 24 h	*CrCl < 30 mL/min*: 1 mg/kg SC every 24 h *CrCl < 15 mL/min*: not recommended	
	Prophylaxis of VTE in the medically ill or surgical population	40 mg SC every 24 h *Or* 30 mg SC every 12 h	*CrCl < 30 mL/min*: 30 mg SC every 24 h *CrCl < 15 mL/min*: not recommended	
	Prophylaxis of VTE in trauma patients	40 mg SC every 24 h *Or* 30 mg SC every 12 h	*CrCl < 30 mL/min*: 30 mg SC every 24 h *CrCl < 15 mL/min*: not recommended	
Dalteparin [61] (Fragmin™)	Treatment of VTE	<56 kg: 10,000 units SC every 24 h 57–68 kg: 18,000 units SC every 24 h 83–98 kg: 18,000 units SC every 24 h >99 kg: 18,000 units SC every 24 h	N/A	
	Treatment of UA/NSTEMI	120 IU/kg SC every 12 h (MAX 10,000 IU/dose)	N/A	
	Prophylaxis of VTE after hip or other major surgeries (first month)	Initial dose: 2500 units once Maintenance: 2500–5000 units SC every 24 h	N/A	
	Prophylaxis of VTE in the medically ill or surgical population	5000 units SC every 24 h	N/A	
Tinzaparin [62] (Innohep™)	Treatment of DVT in addition to warfarin	175 units/kg SC every 24 h	N/A	

h hours, *CrCl* creatinine clearance, *ACS* acute coronary syndrome, *STEMI* ST-segment elevation myocardial infarction, *UA/NSTEMI* unstable angina or non-ST-segment elevation myocardial infarction, *INR* international normalized ratio, *HIT* heparin-induced thrombocytopenia, *CBC* complete blood count, *NA* not available

Obesity

Obesity is considered an independent risk factor for the development of VTE, and appropriate dosing strategies of LMWHs need to be employed in this high-risk patient population [67]. Obesity alters the volume of distribution of many medications, including LMWHs, and has a direct effect on the pharmacokinetic properties of these agents. Studies have suggested that dosing of individual LMWHs do not need to be adjusted for the following patients: (1) enoxaparin if ≤144 kg, (2) dalteparin if ≤190 kg, and (3) tinzaparin if ≤165 kg [68–72].

Ultimately, the effectiveness of LMWH depends on appropriate dosing and monitoring considerations. One such method of laboratory monitoring includes measuring anti-Xa levels (Table 3.10). Guidelines currently recommend monitoring anti-Xa levels only in certain populations, including obese patients [18]. Anti-Xa levels theoretically correlate with both efficacy and bleeding risk, although the literature supporting this conclusion is lacking. Studies have shown that body weight can have a negative correlation with anti-Xa activity in healthy volunteers receiving prophylactic doses of LMWHs. This supports the concept that guideline-directed, fixed thromboprophylaxis dosing strategies employed for nonobese patients may not be sufficient for obese patients [17, 75] (Table 3.11).

There are numerous published studies evaluating the efficacy and safety of therapeutic dosing of LMWH in obese patients. It has been shown that a TBW-based dosing regimen with LMWH

Table 3.10 Anti-factor Xa monitoring for LMWHs [17, 60–62, 73, 74]

Agent	Population	Dosing in VTE	Target anti-Xa level	Timing
Enoxaparin	Obese (>120 kg)	1 mg/kg Q12 h	Peak: 0.6–1.0 units/mL	4–6 h after the first dose
	Renal dysfunction (CrCl < 30 mL/min)[a]	1 mg/kg Q24 h	Peak: 0.6–1.0 units/mL	4–6 h after the third dose
		1.5 mg/kg Q24 h	Peak: 1–2 units/mL	
Dalteparin	Obese (>120 kg)	200 units/kg daily	Peak: 0.5–1.0 units/mL	4–6 h after the first dose
	Renal dysfunction (CrCl < 30 mL/min)[a]		Peak: 0.5–1.5 units/mL	4–6 h after the third dose

CrCl creatinine clearance, *Q* every, *h* hour

[a]In patients where there is concern for accumulation of enoxaparin or dalteparin, trough levels should be drawn just prior to the next dose (target trough <0.4 units/mL)

Table 3.11 LMWHs dosing in obesity [17, 28, 76]

Agent	Treatment dose	Prophylaxis dose
Enoxaparin	VTE: • Total body weight (dose capping not recommended) • Twice daily dosing ACS: • STEMI: – Total body weight (max of 100 mg for the first two doses) • UA/NSTEMI: – Total body weight (dose capping not recommended)	Increase dose by ~30% (BMI ≥ 40 kg/m^2)
Dalteparin	VTE: • Use total body weight (consider dose cap at 18,000 units) ACS: • Use total body weight (dose cap at 10,000 units)	Increase dose by ~30% (BMI ≥ 40 kg/m^2)
Tinzaparin	Use total body weight (dose capping not recommended)	Increase dose by ~30% (BMI ≥ 40 kg/m^2)

VTE venous thromboembolism, *BID* twice daily, *ACS* acute coronary syndrome, *STEMI* ST-segment elevation myocardial infarction, *UA/NSTEMI* unstable angina or non-ST-segment elevation myocardial infarction, *BMI* body mass index

may result in overdosing of patients when used for therapeutic indications. Patients with lean body mass may have higher rates of blood flow when compared to those with excess adipose tissue [77, 78]. This may lead to dose alterations with LMWH. Multiple regimens have been proposed, such as enoxaparin 1 mg/kg SC every 8 h (based on lean body weight (LBW)) (see Table 3.11) [78]. This strategy has achieved the desired anti-Xa levels for the treatment of both ACS and VTE. Another dosing strategy recommended the use of enoxaparin 1.5 mg/kg SC daily. They found that this dosing regimen has similar pharmacokinetic properties in both obese and nonobese healthy volunteers (see Table 3.12) [79]. Currently, guidelines recommend enoxaparin 1 mg/kg SC BID (based on TBW) in obese patients [17].

Table 3.12 LMWH in obesity: summary of evidence [78, 79, 81–84]

Population	Dosing Strategy	Conclusion
Treatment with LMWH		
Patients requiring anticoagulant treatment for ACS, VTE, or prophylaxis and were stratified based on BMI ($n = 96$) [78]	Dosing strategies were evaluated to achieve peak anti-Xa levels • Strategy 1 based on LBW: enoxaparin 1 mg/kg Q8h • Strategy 2 (total body weight (TBW): enoxaparin 1 mg/kg Q12 h For patients <90 kg (>50 years old) or >120 kg (<50 years old)	The use of either of the two proposed treatment strategies in the respective patient populations would be expected to maintain a therapeutic anti-Xa level throughout the dosing interval
Obese and nonobese volunteers stratified by BMI matched based on age, sex, and height ($n = 48$) [79]	• Regimen 1: enoxaparin 1.5 mg/kg SC daily for 4 days • Regimen 2: enoxaparin 1.5 mg/kg infusion (over 6 h) • Patients were crossed over into the other regimen after a 7-day washout	• Enoxaparin administered as a SC injection increased levels of anti-factor X a activity in obese patients in comparison with nonobese patients only marginally • Enoxaparin 1.5 mg/kg SC daily had similar levels of exposure in both groups of patients and can be considered as a treatment regimen in obese patients with a BMI up to 40 kg/m^2
Thromboprophylaxis with LMWH		
Primary or revisional bariatric surgery patients with an average BMI of 50–51 kg/m^2 ($n = 481$) [81]	• Group 1: enoxaparin 30 mg SC Q12 h • Group 2: enoxaparin 40 mg SC Q12 h	• Group 1 patients had a significantly longer hospital length of stay • VTE complications and rates were higher in patients in group 1 compared to group 2 • There was one bleeding event that occurred in each group • Enoxaparin 40 mg SC Q12 h had improve effectiveness without an increased risk of bleeding
Medically ill, hospitalized patients that were both obese and elderly ($n = 1118$) [82, 83]	• Group 1: dalteparin 5000 units SC daily • Group 2: placebo	• The composite of symptomatic VTE, fatal PE, sudden death, or asymptomatic proximal DVT were similar between dalteparin and placebo • The risk of major hemorrhage was not increased in obese patients
Hospitalized, medically ill patients with extreme obesity (average BMI ≥ 60 kg/m^2) ($n = 31$) [84]	• Group 1: enoxaparin 40 mg SC daily (control group) • Group 2: enoxaparin 0.4 mg/kg SC daily (LD) • Group 3: enoxaparin 0.5 mg/kg SC daily (HD)	• Peak anti-Xa levels (goal 0.2–0.5 IU/mL) were significantly higher in the HD groups vs. the control or LD group • HD enoxaparin was found to be superior in achieving target anti-Xa levels when compared to standard or low-dose regimens and did not result in an increased risk of complications, such as bleeding

BMI body mass index, *SC* subcutaneously, *ACS* acute coronary syndrome, *VTE* venous thromboembolism, *LBW* lean body weight, *Q* every, *h* hour, *LD* low dose, *HD* high dose

Another controversial topic with limited reliable data is whether obese patients should receive the same fixed LMWH thromboprophylaxis doses as nonobese patients. Standard thromboprophylactic doses of LMWH may not be adequate in obese patients, thus putting them at increased risk for VTE [80]. Scholten and colleagues evaluated obese patients undergoing bariatric surgery who received either LMWH 30 or 40 mg SC every 12 h postoperatively (Table 3.12). Patients receiving the 40 mg regimen had significantly lower rates of VTE without an increased risk of bleeding [81]. Other trials evaluating the use of dalteparin found similar efficacy profiles compared with placebo with no significantly increased risk of major hemorrhage in both obese and elderly patients (see Table 3.11) [82, 83].

Evidence supports the use of anti-Xa monitoring in obese or morbidly obese patients requiring therapeutic treatment with LMWH, often identified as weighing more than 190 kg or having a BMI greater than 40 kg/m^2 [65]. Peak anti-Xa levels should be monitored routinely in these patients to ensure adequate dosing [84]. In obese patients requiring thromboprophylaxis, it may be justified to consider a weight-based dosing strategy (Table 3.10). Patients require close monitoring in order to prevent VTE without increasing the risk of significant bleeding.

Renal Dysfunction and Elderly Patients

Renal dysfunction and older age both individually and collectively contribute to patients' risk of bleeding and thromboembolic events. LMWH accumulates in patients with impaired kidney function. Many large randomized studies evaluating the efficacy and safety of LMWH have specifically excluded patients with renal dysfunction. Thorevska and colleagues assessed hospitalized patients with impaired renal function receiving full therapeutic doses of UFH or enoxaparin twice daily. Major bleeding rates were similar between the two groups despite varying degrees of renal impairment. However, minor bleeding rates were significantly increased in those with severe renal dysfunction who were receiving enoxaparin as compared to UFH [85]. Monitoring anti-Xa levels should be considered when treating renally impaired patients with prolonged courses of LMWH (Table 3.10).

There have been several studies evaluating the use of LMWHs in elderly, renal-impaired patients (Table 3.13). Chow and colleagues studied patients with severe renal dysfunction (CrCl $\leq$ 30 mL/min) and discovered that patients had elevated anti-Xa levels after three doses of enoxaparin, indicating the risk of accumulation of these agents [86]. Fox and colleagues evaluated patients with ACS on dose-adjusted enoxaparin. In a subgroup of elderly patients with severe renal dysfunction (CrCl < 30 mL/min), they found that enoxaparin was associated with an insignificantly increased risk of the major bleeding events when compared to UFH [87].

Guidelines support dose reduction of LMWH in patients with renal dysfunction (CrCl < 30 mL/min) whether their indication is for treatment or thromboprophylaxis (see Table 3.14) [17]. In this subset of patients, enoxaparin is the most widely used LMWH, at a dose of 1 mg/kg daily. Because studies have demonstrated that up to one-fourth of patients on dose-adjusted enoxaparin therapy can be underdosed (defined as anti-Xa levels <0.5 IU/mL), patients with severe renal dysfunction on LMWH therapy should undergo anti-Xa monitoring [91].

Pregnancy

Similarly to UFH, evidence is lacking with regard to evaluating the safety and efficacy of LMWH in pregnancy. Recommendations from guidelines are largely extrapolated from evidence supporting the use of LMWH in nonpregnant patients with VTE and ACS. LMWH, like UFH, does not cross the placenta leading to a generally low risk of fetal bleeding as shown in retrospective observational studies [31, 92] (Table 3.15).

Based on several retrospective studies, thromboprophylactic dosing of enoxaparin 40 mg SC daily appears to be safe and effective for prevention of VTE during pregnancy [93]. Depending upon the risk of VTE, consensus guidelines suggest thromboprophylaxis dosing strategies of enoxaparin 40 mg SC daily, dalteparin 5000 units SC daily, or dose-adjusted enoxaparin to achieve peak anti-Xa levels of 0.6–1 units/mL [28].

Table 3.13 LMWH in renal dysfunction and elderly: summary of evidence [86–89]

Population	Dosing strategy	Conclusion
Enoxaparin		
Prospective open-label study of patients with varying degrees of renal function (mean age 75 years) [86]	• All patients received enoxaparin 1 mg/kg Q12 h • Group 1: CrCl > 61 mL/min • Group 2: CrCl 31–60 mL/min • Group 3: CrCl ≤ 30 mL/min • Peak blood levels of anti-Xa concentrations were drawn at 4 ± 0.5 after three doses	The adjusted anti-Xa levels after three doses were as follows: • CrCl > 30 mL/min: 0.91 • CrCl ≤ 30 mL/min: 1.34 Dose adjustments should be made for patients with CrCl ≤ 30 mL/min
RCT subgroup analysis of ACS patients who were stratified according to renal function [87]	• Enoxaparin 1 mg/kg SC daily • UFH continuous infusion	Results of patients with CrCl < 30 mL/min: There was a significant difference in the composite of death from any cause or recurrent nonfatal MI in the enoxaparin vs. UFH groups at 30 days, respectively • No significant difference in death from any cause • Rates of major bleeding were increased in the enoxaparin vs. UFH group, respectively, risk but was not statistically significant
Dalteparin		
Prospective observational study of patients who were hospitalized and stratified based on GFR [88]	All patients received dalteparin 100 units/kg SC Q12 h • Group 1: GFR ≥ 60 mL/min • Group 2: GFR 30–59 mL/min • Group 3: GFR < 30 mL/min • Peak plasma anti-Xa activity was measured and adjusted to applied dose and body weight after the first dose, on day 2, and every second day after	Median anti-Xa levels were as follows (after 6 days): • Group 1: 0.57 • Group 2: 0.66 • Group 3: 1.21 there was a significant different between anti-Xa levels in group 1 vs. group 3, but no significant difference between group 1 and group 2 • Anti-Xa levels should be monitored in patients taking dalteparin who have severe renal dysfunction due to the risk for bioaccumulation
Tinzaparin		
Prospective study of patients who were >70 years old with a mean CrCl of 40.6 mL/min [89]	Tinzaparin 175 anti-Xa units/kg SC daily for 10 days	• There was no increase in the anti-Xa and anti-IIa activities after 10 days of treatment with tinzaparin • No accumulation occurred • No major bleeding and only one minor bleed occurred • No VTE events or deaths occurred • No need to adjust doses of tinzaparin in patients with CrCl > 20 mL/min

RCT randomized controlled trial, *CrCl* creatinine clearance, *GFR* glomerular filtration rate, *MI* myocardial infarction

Table 3.14 Dose reductions for LMWHs (CrCl < 30 mL/min) [17, 60–62, 83, 90]

Agent	Dose
Enoxaparin	VTE treatment: • 1 mg/kg SC daily • Monitor anti-Xa VTE prophylaxis: • 30 mg SC daily STEMI: • <75 years old—30 mg IV x1 followed by 1 mg/kg SC daily • ≥75 years old—No IV bolus, start with 1 mg/kg SC daily • Monitor anti-Xa Unstable angina/NSTEMI: • 1 mg/kg SC daily • Monitor anti-Xa[a]
Dalteparin	VTE treatment: • Anti-Xa monitoring recommended, but no specific dose adjustments given per manufacturer VTE prophylaxis: • No specific adjustments required
Tinzaparin	VTE treatment: • No specific adjustments per manufacturer • Use with caution

[a]Not recommended for use in hemodialysis patients

However, since these agents have not been directly compared in clinical trials, the optimal dosing strategy is largely unknown and based on observational studies (Table 3.15).

Guidelines recommend that pregnant women requiring therapeutic anticoagulation for treatment of VTE use LMWHs over UFH or vitamin K antagonists (VKA) during the peripartum period [28]. Therapeutic dosing strategies with LMWHs remain controversial in the pregnant population (Table 3.16). Both once and twice daily regimens of LMWHs have been employed in pregnant women in observational studies (Table 3.15). Some studies suggest the need for dose adjustment based on the expected weight gain throughout pregnancy. Others recommend the use of anti-Xa levels as a monitoring strategy at 1–3-month intervals [97]. Currently, it is not recommended to adjust LMWH doses as weight changes or to periodically monitor anti-Xa levels [28]. Rodie and colleagues evaluated pregnant women receiving enoxaparin twice daily (based on early pregnancy weight). The majority of patients did not require a dose increase to maintain adequate anti-Xa levels. Contrary to popular belief, three women required a dose reduction due to anti-Xa levels higher than the intended range (target range 0.4–1 units/mL) [94]. Weight-based LMWH for treatment of acute VTE is recommended during pregnancy for at least 6 weeks postpartum with a recommended duration of 3–6 months, depending on the risk of recurrence [28].

Strategies for Reversal of Low-Molecular-Weight Heparins

LMWH is associated with a lower incidence of major bleeding as compared to UFH. Several pooled analyses have demonstrated a reduced frequency of both major and minor bleeding with LMWH as compared to UFH [29, 98, 99]. In contrast, there was an increased rate of Thrombolysis in Myocardial Infarction (TIMI) and Global Use of Strategies to Open Occluded Arteries (GUSTO)-defined major bleeding with LMWH as compared to UFH in patients with ACS [72, 100, 101].

There is no proven method for complete reversal of LMWH. Protamine cannot completely reverse LMWH, but it neutralizes the AT effect [3]. All anti-IIa activity is reversed, but only 60–80% of anti-Xa is reversed (enoxaparin 60%, dalteparin 80%) [60, 61]. For non-urgent, elective discontinuation for impending procedures or surgery, the last dose should be 12–24 h prior to the procedure. Consideration must be given to the patient's other comorbidities such as renal function, which may require a longer washout period [3]. With urgent, life-threatening bleeding, IV protamine should be given in conjunction with resuscitation with blood products (i.e., platelets and packed red blood cells). Recombinant activated factor VIIa is a consideration for patients with refractory bleeding or bleeding in critical sites (i.e., intracranial) (Table 3.17).

Table 3.15 LMWHs in pregnancy [31, 93–95]

Population	Treatment strategy	Conclusion
Retrospective study of high-risk pregnant women who received enoxaparin [31]	• Therapeutic LMWH group: enoxaparin 1 mg/kg SC BID for an average of 85 days • Prophylactic LMWH group: enoxaparin 20 mg SC daily or 40 mg once daily for an average of 49 days • Therapy was initiated in the first, second, and third trimester in 7.7%, 25.2%, and 67.1% of cases, respectively	• Serious maternal hemorrhage occurred in 11 patients during pregnancy with only 1 case being reasonably attributable to enoxaparin; 8 VTEs occurred. There were no fetal or neonatal complications or adverse events that were a result of enoxaparin exposure
Retrospective case series of 57 pregnancies in 50 women with an indication for enoxaparin (previous VTE or thrombophilia) [93]	Thromboprophylaxis groups: • Previous VTE: enoxaparin 40 mg SC daily • Previous VTE and thrombophilia: enoxaparin 40 mg SC daily • No current or previous VTE: enoxaparin 40 mg SC daily Treatment groups: • Enoxaparin 1 mg/kg SC BID enoxaparin 40 mg SC daily	• No VTEs occurred in any patients receiving thromboprophylaxis • There were four cases of postpartum hemorrhage and one antepartum hemorrhage • Peak anti-Xa levels (units/mL): – 40 mg SC daily: 0.23 – 40 mg SC BID: 0.38 – 60 mg SC BID: 0.68 – 80 mg SC BID: 0.68
Prospective observational study of women with an acute VTE diagnosed during pregnancy or immediately postpartum [94]	Enoxaparin 1 mg/kg SC BID (based on early pregnancy weight) for a median duration of 6 weeks	• In 30/36 women, the original dose of enoxaparin resulted in acceptable peak anti-Xa levels throughout treatment (despite increasing weight) (median anti-Xa level 0.8 units/mL) • Three women required a dose decrease due to elevated anti-Xa levels • There were no reports of thrombocytopenia, hemorrhage, or recurrent VTE in this study
Prospective case control study of women with pulmonary embolism (PE) during pregnancy who were matched to pregnant women without a PE during pregnancy [95]	Once or twice daily (doses not reported) • Enoxaparin (*n* = 83) • Dalteparin (*n* = 25) • Tinzaparin (*n* = 26)	• There were five deaths that occurred from PE • There were two recurrent PEs (one receiving enoxaparin once daily, one receiving twice daily) • There were no reports of hemorrhage, thrombocytopenia, or fractures related to osteoporosis

BID twice daily

Protamine dosing is based on the timing of LMWH dosing (Table 3.17). If any of the agents have been administered within the past 8 h, protamine may be given. Enoxaparin has a 1:1 mg dosing ratio with protamine, while dalteparin and tinzaparin have a 1 mg:100 unit ratio. The maximum dose of protamine that may be given at any time is 50 mg. It is recommended that an anti-Xa level be drawn every 3 h with possible repeated doses of protamine (0.5 mg/required amount of LMWH) [37].

Table 3.16 LMWHs dosing in pregnancy [17, 28, 96]

Agent	Treatment dosing	Anti-Xa levels (4–6 h postinjection)
Enoxaparin	• 1 mg/kg SC Q12 h[a] • 1.5 mg/kg SC daily	• BID dosing target: 0.6–1 units/mL • Daily dosing target: 1–2 units/mL • Mechanical valve: 0.8–1.2 units/mL[b]
Dalteparin	• 100 units/kg SC Q12 h • 200 units/kg SC daily	• 0.5–1.5 units/mL • Mechanical valve: 0.8–1.2 units/mL[b]
Tinzaparin	• 175 units/kg SC Q24 h	• 0.85[c]

Q every, *h* hours, *BID* twice daily
[a]Twice daily enoxaparin is preferred over once daily
[b]Anti-Xa levels are recommended for pregnant women with mechanical heart valves (should be monitored at least monthly)
[c]No specific recommendation per manufacturer, based on recommendations from Garcia et al. [17]

Table 3.17 Reversal of LMWH with protamine sulfate [37]

Enoxaparin protamine dosing	Dalteparin protamine dosing	Tinzaparin protamine dosing
1 mg per 1 mg enoxaparin in the past 8 h	1 mg per 100 units dalteparin in the past 8 h	1 mg per 100 units tinzaparin in the past 8 h

Summary

Unfractionated heparin and LMWH both play pivotal roles when a patient is indicated for anticoagulation. There are multiple patient factors that must be considered when initiating these agents that include obesity, renal function, and considerations of special populations. Additionally, appropriate monitoring is essential to prevent both underdosing and overdosing patients. Lastly, it is important to consider the route of administration of these medications as patients receive these agents in both the inpatient and outpatient setting. These agents often remain first-line options when initiating anticoagulation, and it is important that the clinician be appropriately acquainted with these agents prior to using them.

Examples

1. Patient receives 70 mg of enoxaparin at 0600. It is currently 1200 and a dose of protamine must be given.
   Time passed: 6 h.
   Protamine required for complete reversal: 50 mg
2. Patient has received 18,000 units of dalteparin at 0800. It is currently 2000. What does of protamine should the patient receive?
   Time passed: 12 h.
   Protamine dose to be administered: 0 mg as it has been >8 h.

Key Points

- UFH and LMWH exert their anticoagulant effect by binding antithrombin.
- UFH dosing varies by indication and should be adjusted based on the aPTT or anti-Xa level.
- LMWH heparin provides more consistent weight-based dosing than UFH and can be administered without routine monitoring. When laboratory monitoring is desired, anti-Xa levels can be checked.
- LMWH has a lower risk of HIT than UFH. Use the 4T score guides HIT testing and diagnosis.

Self-Assessment Questions

1. Which of the following statements regarding UFH is *true*?
   (a) UFH is rapidly and completely absorbed when administered subcutaneously in doses of less than 7500 U.
   (b) UFH molecules with fewer than 18 saccharide units possess no anticoagulant activity.
   (c) UFH has a 15-h half-life and should be given in significantly lower doses to patients with liver disease.
   (d) Despite weight-based dosing, UFH produces an unpredictable degree of anticoagulation.

2. Which of the following drug regimens would be the most appropriate initial treatment for a 57-year-old, 100 kg man who has a proximal DVT and no other comorbid conditions?
   (a) Unfractionated heparin 5000 U IV bolus followed by 1000 U/h given by continuous IV infusion
   (b) Dalteparin 5000 U IV bolus followed by 1000 U SQ Q24 h
   (c) Unfractionated heparin 8000 U IV boluses followed by 1800 U/h given by continuous infusion
   (d) Enoxaparin 30 mg SQ Q12 h
3. Heparin must first bind to ________to exert its anticoagulant activity.
   (a) Antithrombin
   (b) Thrombin
   (c) Factor X
   (d) Protein C
4. Which of the following statements is correct for the diagnosis of heparin-induced thrombocytopenia (HIT)?
   (a) Thrombocytopenia generally presents as severe with platelet counts <10 ×109/L in most cases.
   (b) Patients will generally demonstrate a fall in platelets 5–10 days after their first exposure to heparin or within 1 day if they have had previous exposure to heparin within the past 5–30 days.
   (c) The frequency of HIT is similar for unfractionated heparin and low-molecular-weight heparin.
   (d) The platelet factor 4 (PF4) enzyme-linked immunosorbent assay is considered the gold standard for diagnosing HIT.
5. AJ is a 31-year-old pregnant woman at 29 weeks' gestation who presents to her obstetrician with dull left-sided chest pain and acute-onset shortness of breath. She denies calf or thigh tenderness. Physical examination and imaging reveal a deep vein thrombosis in the pelvic vein. The team decides to initiate anticoagulation, which option is best for AJ:
   (a) Warfarin 10 mg targeting INR goal 2–3 with a continuous infusion heparin bridge targeting aPTT 60–80
   (b) Enoxaparin 1 mg/kg Q12 h
   (c) Dalteparin 200 units/kg units Q12 h
   (d) Heparin 333 units/kg Q12 h targeting aPTT 60–80
6. A.B. is a 39-year-old male with an inferior wall non-ST-segment-elevation MI. He has a history of poorly controlled HTN and diabetes mellitus (DM). You initiate aspirin, clopidogrel, and atorvastatin. His baseline serum creatinine is 3.4 mg/dL, and you estimate his creatinine clearance to be 25 mL/min. What dose of enoxaparin would you choose?
   (a) 1 mg/kg every 12 h.
   (b) 1 mg/kg daily.
   (c) Enoxaparin is not indicated at this time.
   (d) Fondaparinux is safer to use in patients with chronic kidney disease.

Self-Assessment Answers

1. (d) Despite weight-based dosing, UFH produces an unpredictable degree of anticoagulation.

   Even with weight-based dosing, frequent laboratory monitoring is needed to safely dose UFH in most patients. LMWH, on the other hand, is much more predictable and can be safely dosed based on weight and renal function without the need for routine laboratory monitoring.
2. (c) Unfractionated heparin 8000 U IV boluses followed by 1800 U/h given by continuous infusion

   Treatment of acute DVT is usually accomplished with intravenous UFH or weight-based full (treatment) dose LMWH. Based on the patient's weight, 8000 U IV bolus followed by 1800 U/h as an IV infusion is the most appropriate.
3. (a) antithrombin

   Both UFH and LMWH exhibit their effect through binding to antithrombin, which is why they are known as "indirect anticoagulants."
4. (b) Patients will generally demonstrate a fall in platelets 5–10 days after their first exposure to heparin or within 1 day if they have had previous exposure to heparin within the past 5–30 days.

   A fall in platelets 5–10 days following initial heparin exposure, or within 1 day with prior to heparin exposure, is a central component to the 4T score.
5. (b) Enoxaparin 1 mg/kg Q12 h

Use of LMWH is preferred over UFH given unreliable aPTT levels during pregnancy. Dosing for pregnant patients with acute VTE is enoxaparin 1 mg/kg Q12 h and dalteparin 200 units/kg daily (not Q12 h). Warfarin doses >5 mg daily are not preferred in pregnant patients.

6. (c) Enoxaparin is not indicated at this time.
   Enoxaparin is not recommended for patients with CrCl < 30 mL/min.

Disclosures The authors have nothing to disclose.

References

1. Hirsh J, Raschke R. Heparin and low molecular weight heparin. The seventh ACCP conference on antithrombotic and thrombolytic therapy. Chest. 2004;126:188S–203S.
2. Weitz DS, Weitz JI. Update on heparin: what do we need to know? J Thromb Thrombolysis. 2010;29:199–207.
3. Alquwaizani M, Buckley L, Adams C, Fanikos J. Anticoagulants: a review of the pharmacology, dosing, and complications. Curr Emerg Hosp Med Rep. 2013;1:83–97.
4. Bussey H, Francis J. Heparin consensus group. Heparin overview and issues. Pharmacotherapy. 2004;24:103S–7S.
5. Hull RD, Raskob GE, Hirsh J, Jay RM, Leclerc JR, Geerts WH, et al. Continuous intravenous heparin compared with intermittent subcutaneous heparin in the initial treatment of proximal-vein thrombosis. N Engl J Med. 1986;315:1109–14.
6. Raschke RA, Reilly BM, Guidry JR, Fontana JR, Srinvas S. The weight-based heparin dosing nomogram compared with a "standard care" nomogram: a randomized controlled trial. Ann Intern Med. 1993;119:874–81.
7. King CS, Holley AB, Jackson JL, Shorr AF, Moores LK. Twice vs three times daily heparin dosing for thromboembolism prophylaxis in the general medical population: a metaanalysis. Chest. 2007;131:507–16.
8. Braunwald E, Antman EA, Beasley JW, Califf RM, Cheitlin MD, Hochman JS, et al. ACC/AHA guidelines for the management of patients with unstable angina, and non-ST-segment elevation myocardial infarction. A report of the American College of Cardiology/American Heart Association task force on practice guidelines (committee on the management of patients with unstable angina). J Am Coll Cardiol. 2000;36:970–1062.
9. Raschke R, Gollihare B, Peirce J. The effectiveness of implementing the weight-based heparin nomogram as a practice guideline. Arch Intern Med. 1996;156:1645–9.
10. Smith ML, Wheeler KE. Weight-based heparin protocol using antifactor Xa monitoring. Am J Health-Syst Pharm. 2010;67:371–4.
11. Gehrie E, Laposata M. Test of the month: the chromogenic antifactor Xa assay. Am J Hematol. 2012;87:194–6.
12. World Heart Federation. Obesity. http://www.world-heart-federation.org/cardiovascular-health/cardiovascular-disease-risk-factors/obesity/. Accessed 11/3/2016.
13. Patel JP, Roberts LN, Arya R. Anticoagulating obese patients in the modern era. Br J Haematol. 2011;155:137–49.
14. Dager WE, Gulseth MP, Nutescu EA. Anticoagulation therapy: a point-of-care guide. Bethesda, MD: American Society of Health-System Pharmacists; 2011. p. 33–59.
15. Myzienski AE, Lutz M, Smythe M. Unfractionated heparin dosing for venous thromboembolism in morbidly obese patients: case report and review of the literature. Pharmacotherapy. 2010;3:324.
16. Buehler KS, Yancey AM. Underdosing in obesity—an epidemic: focus on anticoagulation. Formul J Anticoagulat. 2013. http://formularyjournal.modernmedicine.com.
17. Garcia DA, Baglin TP, Weitz JI, Samama MM. Parenteral anticoagulants antithrombotic therapy and prevention of thrombosis, 9th ed: American College of Chest Physicians Evidence-Based Clinical Practice Guidelines. Chest. 2012;1(Suppl):e24S–43S. https://doi.org/10.1378/chest.11-2291.
18. Gerlach AT, Folino J, Morris BN, Murphy CV, Stawicki SP, Cook CH. Comparison of heparin dosing based on actual body weight in non-obese, obese and morbidly obese critically ill patients. Int J Crit Illn Inj Sci. 2013;3:195–9.
19. Hurewitz AN, Khan SU, Groth ML, Patrick PA, Brand DA. Dosing of unfractionated heparin in obese patients with venous thromboembolism. J Gen Intern Med. 2010;26:487–91.
20. Pinder T, Daughtry W, Shah Z, Vailoces TO. A weight-based heparin protocol for improved anticoagulation in a coronary care unit. J Clin Outcomes Manag. 1999;6:27–33.
21. Yee W, Norton LL. Optimal weight base for a weight-based heparin dosing protocol. Am J Health Syst Pharm. 1998;55:159–62.
22. Riney JN, Hollands JM, Smith JR, Deal EN. Identifying optimal infusion rates for unfractionated heparin in morbidly obese patients. Ann Pharmacother. 2010;44:1141–51.
23. Bates SM, Ginsberg JS. How we manage venous thromboembolism during pregnancy. Blood. 2002;100:3470–8.

24. Dresang L, Fontaine P, Leeman L, King VJ. Venous thromboembolism during pregnancy. Am Fam Physician. 2008;77:1709–916.
25. Gibson PS, Powrie R. Anticoagulants and pregnancy: when are they safe? Cleve Clin J Med. 2009;79:113–27.
26. Kamel H, Navi BB, Sriram N, Hovsepian BS, Devereux RB, Elkind M. Risk of a thrombotic event after the 6-week postpartum period. N Engl J Med. 2014;370:1307–15. 1–9.
27. Casele HL. The use of unfractionated heparin and low molecular weight heparin in pregnancy. Clin Obstet Gynecol. 2006;49:895–905.
28. Bates SM, Greer IA, Middeldorp S, Veenstra DL, Prabulos AM, Vandvik PO, et al. VTE, thrombophilia, antithrombotic therapy and pregnancy. Antithrombotic therapy and prevention of thrombosis, 9th ed: American College of Chest Physicians Evidence-Based Clinical Practice Guidelines. Chest. 2012;141:e691S–736S.
29. Gould MK, Dembitzer AD, Doyle RL, Hastie TJ, Garber AM. Low-molecular-weight heparins compared with unfractionated heparin for treatment of acute deep venous thrombosis. A meta-analysis of randomized, controlled trials. Ann Intern Med. 1999;130(10):800–9.
30. Quinlan DJ, McQuillan A, Eikelboom JW. Low-molecular-weight heparin compared with intravenous unfractionated heparin for treatment of pulmonary embolism: a meta-analysis of randomized, controlled trials. Ann Intern Med. 2004;140(3):175–83.
31. Lepercq J, Conard J, Borel-Derlon A, Darmon JY, Boudignat O, Francoual C, et al. Venous thromboembolism during pregnancy: a retrospective study of enoxaparin safety in 624 pregnancies. BJOG. 2001;108(11):1134–40.
32. Sanson BJ, Lensing AWA, Prins MH, Ginsberg JS, Barkagan ZS, Lavenne-Pardonge E, et al. Safety of low-molecular-weight heparin in pregnancy: a systematic review. Thromb Haemost. 1999;81(5):668–72.
33. Greer IA, Nelson-Piercy C. Low-molecular-weight heparins for thromboprophylaxis and treatment of venous thromboembolism in pregnancy: a systematic review of safety and efficacy. Blood. 2005;106(2):401–7.
34. Springel EH. Thromboembolism in pregnancy medicine [Internet]. Obstetrics and Gynecology: Medscape Ref Drugs Dis Proced. [Updated 2016 Jan 20; cited 2016 Apr 12]. Available from: https://emedicine.medscape.com/article/2056380-overview#a1
35. Ginsberg JS, Hirsh J. Anticoagulants during pregnancy. Annu Rev Med. 1989;40:79–86.
36. American College of Obstetricians and Gynecologists (ACOG). Thromboembolism in pregnancy. Washington, DC: American College of Obstetricians and Gynecologists (ACOG); 2011. (ACOG practice bulletin; 123). https://doi.org/10.1097/AOG.0b013e3182310c4c.
37. Cushman M, Lim W, Zakai NA. Clinical Practice Guide on Antithrombotic Drug Dosing and Management of Antithrombotic Drug-Associated Bleeding Complications in Adults: 9th edition American College of Chest Physicians Evidence-Based Clinical Practice Guidelines. Am Soc Hematol. 2014(2):1–4.
38. Sylvester K, Rimsans J, Fanikos J. Anticoagulant therapy; Chapter 254. In: McKean S, Dressler D, Ross J, Schurer D, editors. Principles and practice of hospital medicine. 2nd ed. New York: McGraw-Hill; 2017. [In Press; expected publication Spring 2017].
39. Menon V, Berkowitz SD, Antman EM, Fuchs RM, Hochman JS. New heparin dosing recommendations for patient with acute coronary syndromes. Am J Med. 2001;110:641–50.
40. Granger CB, Hirsh J, Califf RM, Col J, White HD, Betriu A, et al. Activated partial thromboplastin time and outcomes after thrombolytic therapy for acute myocardial infarction: results from the GUSTO-I trial. Circulation. 1996;93:870–8.
41. Arnand SS, Yusuf S, Pogue J, Ginsberg JS, Hirsh J. Organization to assess strategies for ischemic syndromes investigators. Relationship of activated partial thromboplastin time to coronary events and bleeding in patients with acute coronary syndromes who receive heparin. Circulation. 2003;107:2884–8.
42. Protamine Package Insert. APP Pharmaceuticals, LLC. Revised January 2008.
43. McEvoy GK, editor. Protamine sulfate. In: AHFS drug information 2008. Bethesda, MD: American Society of Health-System Pharmacists; 2008; p. 1595–1597.
44. Krishnaswamy A, Lincoff M, Cannon C. The use and limitations of unfractionated heparin. Crit Pathw Cardiol. 2010;9(1):35–40.
45. Levine MN, Hirsh J, Gent M, Turpie AG, Cruickshank M, Weitz J, et al. A randomized trial comparing activated thromboplastin time with heparin assay in patients with acute venous thromboembolism requiring large daily doses of heparin. Arch Intern Med. 1994;154(1):49–56.
46. Wolinsky-Friedland M. Drug-induced metabolic bone disease. Endocrinol Metab Clin N Am. 1995;24(2):395–420.
47. Dahlman T, Lindvall N, Hellgren M. Osteopenia in pregnancy during long-term heparin treatment: a radiological study post partum. Br J Obstet Gynaecol. 1990;97(3):221–8.
48. Dahlman TC, Sjöberg HE, Ringertz H. Bone mineral density during long-term prophylaxis with heparin in pregnancy. Am J Obstet Gynecol. 1994;170(5 Pt 1):1315.
49. Dahlman TC. Osteoporotic fractures and the recurrence of thromboembolism during pregnancy and the puerperium in 184 women undergoing thromboprophylaxis with heparin. Am J Obstet Gynecol. 1993;168(4):1265–70.
50. Linkins LA, Dans AL, Moores LK, Bona R, Davidson BL, Schulman S, et al. Treatment and

prevention of heparin-induced thrombocytopenia: antithrombotic therapy and prevention of thrombosis 9th ed: American College of Chest Physicians Evidence-Based Clinical Practice Guidelines. Chest. 2012;141(2 Suppl):e495S–530S.
51. Greinacher A, Alban S, Omer-Adam MA, Weitschies W, Warkentin TE. Heparin induced thrombocytopenia: a stoichiometry-based model to explain the differing immunogenicities of unfractionated heparin, low-molecular-weight heparin, and fondaparinux in different clinical settings. Thromb Res. 2008;122(2):211–20.
52. Warkentin TE, Cook RJ, Marder VJ, Greinacher A. Anti-PF4/heparin antibody formation postorthopedic surgery thromboprophylaxis: the role of non-drug risk factors and evidence for a stoichiometry-based model of immunization. J Thromb Haemost. 2010;8(3):504–12.
53. Warkentin TE, Sheppard JI, Moore JC, Sigouin CS, Kelton JG. Quantitative interpretation of optical density measurements using PF4-dependent enzyme-immunoassays. J Thromb Haemost. 2008; 6(8):1304–12.
54. Warkentin TE, Arnold DM, Nazi I, Kelton JG. The platelet serotonin-release assay. Am J Hematol. 2015;90:564–72.
55. McFarland J, Lochowicz A, Aster R, Chappell B, Curtis B. Improving the specificity of the PF4 ELISA in diagnosing heparin-induced thrombocytopenia. Am J Hematol. 2012;87(8):776–81.
56. Warkentin TE, Linkins LA. Non-necrotizing heparin-induced skin lesions and the 4Ts score. J Thromb Haemost. 2010;8:1483–5.
57. Lo GK, Juhl D, Warkentin TE, Sigouin CS, Eichler P, Greinacher A. Evaluation of pretest clinical score (4 T's) for the diagnosis of heparin-induced thrombocytopenia in two clinical settings. J Thromb Haemost. 2006;4(4):759–65.
58. Passero F, Xavier M. Retrospective analysis of heparin-induced thrombocytopenia management at a large tertiary hospital. J Hematol. 2014;3(2):2–33.
59. Merli GJ, Groce JB. Pharmacological and clinical differences between low-molecular-weight heparins: implications for prescribing practice and therapeutic interchange. P T. 2010;35(2):95–105.
60. Lovenox [package insert]. Bridgewater (NJ): Sanofi Aventis; 2008.
61. Fragmin [package insert]. New York (NY): Pfizer, Inc.; 2016.
62. Innohep [package insert]. Boulder (CO): Celgene; 2008.
63. Kearon C, Akl E, Comerota AJ, Prandoni P, Bounameaux H, Goldbaher SZ, et al. Antithrombotic therapy for VTE disease: antithrombotic therapy and prevention of thrombosis 9th ed: American College of Chest Physicians Evidence-Based Clinical Practice Guidelines. Chest. 2012;141(2 Suppl):e419S–e94S.
64. You JJ, Singer DE, Howard PA, Lane DA, Eckman MH, Fang MC, et al. Antithrombotic therapy for atrial fibrillation: antithrombotic therapy and prevention of thrombosis 9th ed: American College of Chest Physicians Evidence-Based Clinical Practice Guidelines. Chest. 2012;141(2 Suppl):e531S–75S.
65. Nutescu EA, Spinler SA, Wittkowsky A, Dager WE. Low-molecular-weight heparins in renal impairment and obesity: available evidence and clinical practice recommendations across medical and surgical settings. Ann Pharmacother. 2009;43(6):1064–83.
66. Wang TF, Milligan PE, Wong CA, Deal EN, Thoelke MS, Gage BF. Efficacy and safety of high-dose thromboprophylaxis in morbidly obese inpatients. Thromb Haemost. 2014;111(1):88–93.
67. Ageno W, Becattini C, Brighton T, Selby R, Kamphuisen PW. Cardiovascular risk factors and venous thromboembolism: a meta-analysis. Circulation. 2008;117(1):93–102.
68. Al-Yaseen E, Wells PS, Anderson J, Martin J, Kovacs MJ. The safety of dosing dalteparin based on actual body weight for the treatment of acute venous thromboembolism in obese patients. J Thromb Haemost. 2005;3(1):100–2.
69. Hainer JW, Barrett JS, Assaid CA, Fossler MJ, Cox DS, Leathers T, et al. Dosing in heavy-weight/obese patients with the LMWH, tinzaparin: a pharmacodynamic study. Thromb Haemost. 2002;87:817–23.
70. Becker RC, Spencer FA, Gibson M, Rush JE, Sanderink G, Murphy SA, et al. TIMI 11A investigators. Influence of patient characteristics and renal function on factor Xa inhibition pharmacokinetics and pharmacodynamics after enoxaparin administration in non-ST-segment elevation acute coronary syndromes. Am Heart J. 2002;143(5):753–9.
71. Freeman AL, Pendleton RC, Rondina MT. Prevention of venous thromboembolism in obesity. Expert Rev Cardiovasc Ther. 2010;8(12):1711–21.
72. Wilson SJ, Wilbur K, Burton E, Anderson DR. Effect of patient weight on the anticoagulant response to adjusted therapeutic dosage of low-molecular-weight heparin for the treatment of venous thromboembolism. Haemostasis. 2001;31(1):42–8.
73. Schmid P, Fischer AG, Wuillemin WA. Low-molecular-weight heparin in patients with renal insufficiency. Swiss Med Wkly. 2009;139(31–32):438–52.
74. Harenberg J. Is laboratory monitoring of low-molecular-weight heparin therapy necessary? Yes. J Thromb Haemost. 2004;2:547–50.
75. Frederiksen SG, Hedenbro JL, Norgren L. Enoxaparin effect depends on body-weight and current doses may be inadequate in obese patients. Br J Surg. 2003;90:547–8.
76. Yee J, Duffull S. The effect of body weight on dalteparin pharmacokinetics. Eur J Clin Pharmacol. 2000;56:293–7.
77. Cheymol G. Effects of obesity on pharmacokinetics implications for drug therapy. Clin Pharmacokinet. 2000;39(3):215–31.
78. Green B, Duffull S. Development of a dosing strategy for enoxaparin in obese patients. Br J Clin Pharmacol. 2003;56(1):96–103.

79. Sanderink GJ, Le Liboux A, Jariwala N, Harding N, Ozoux ML, Shukla U, et al. The pharmacokinetics and pharmacodynamics of enoxaparin in obese volunteers. Clin Pharmacol Ther. 2002;72:308–18.
80. Shelkrot M, Miraka J, Perez ME. Appropriate enoxaparin dose for venous thromboembolism prophylaxis in patients with extreme obesity. Hosp Pharm. 2014;49(8):740–7.
81. Scholten DJ, Hoedema RM, Scholten SE. A comparison of two different prophylactic dose regimens of low molecular weight heparin in bariatric surgery. Obes Surg. 2002;12:19–24.
82. Kucher N, Leizorovicz A, Vaitkus PT, Cohen AT, Turpie AG, Osson CG, et al. Efficacy and safety of fixed low-dose dalteparin in preventing venous thromboembolism among obese or elderly hospitalized patients: a subgroup analysis of the PREVENT trial. Arch Intern Med. 2005;165:341–5.
83. Vaitkus PT, Leizorovicz A, Goldhaber SZ. The PREVENT Investigator Group. Rationale and design of a clinical trial of a low-molecular-weight heparin in preventing clinically important venous thromboembolism in medical patients: the prospective evaluation of dalteparin efficacy for prevention of venous thromboembolism in immobilized patients trial (the PREVENT study). Vasc Med. 2002;7(4):269–73.
84. Freeman A, Horner T, Pendleton RC, Rondina MT. Prospective comparison of three enoxaparin dosing regimens to achieve target anti-factor Xa levels in hospitalized, medically ill patients with extreme obesity. Am J Hematol. 2012;87:740.
85. Thorevska N, Amoateng-Adjepong Y, Sabahi R, Schiopescu I, Salloum A, Muralidharan V, et al. Anticoagulation in hospitalized patients with renal insufficiency: a comparison of bleeding rates with unfractionated heparin vs enoxaparin. Chest. 2004;125(3):856–63.
86. Chow SL, Zammit K, West K, Dannenhoffer M, Lopez-Candales A. Correlation of antifactor xa concentrations with renal function in patients on enoxaparin. J Clin Pharmacol. 2003;43(6):586–90.
87. Fox KAA, Antman EM, Montalescot G, Agewall S, SomaRaju B, Verheugt FW, et al. The impact of renal dysfunction on outcomes in the ExTRACT-TIMI 25 trial. J Am Coll Cardiol. 2007;49(23):2249–55.
88. Schmid P, Brodmann D, Odermatt Y, Fischer AG, Wuillemin WA. Study of bioaccumulation of dalteparin at a therapeutic dose in patients with renal insufficiency. J Thromb Haemost. 2009;7:1629–32.
89. Siguret V, Pautas E, Fevrier M, Wipff C, Durand-Gasselin B, Laurent M, et al. Elderly patients treated with tinzaparin (Innohep®) administered once daily (175 anti-Xa IU/kg): anti-Xa and anti-IIa activities over 10 days. Thromb Haemost. 2000;84:800–4.
90. Hughes S, Szeki I, Nash MJ, Thachil J. Anticoagulation in chronic kidney disease patients—the practical aspects. Clin Kidney J. 2014;7(5):442–9.
91. Montalescot G, Collet JP, Tanguy ML, et al. Anti-Xa activity relates to survival and efficacy in unselected acute coronary syndrome patients treated with enoxaparin. Circulation. 2004;110:392–8.
92. Forestier F, Daffos F, Rainaut M, Toulemonde F. Low molecular weight heparin (CY 216) does not cross the placenta during the third trimester of pregnancy. Thromb Haemost. 1987;57(2):234.
93. Ellison J, Walker ID, Greer IA. Antenatal use of enoxaparin for prevention and treatment of thromboembolism during pregnancy. BJOG. 2000;107(9):1116–21.
94. Rodie VA, Thomson AJ, Stewart FM, Quinn AJ, Walker ID, Greer IA. Low molecular weight heparin for the treatment of venous thromboembolism in pregnancy: a case series. BJOG. 2002;1099:1020–4.
95. Knight M, UKOSS. Antenatal pulmonary embolism: risk factors, management and outcomes. BJOG. 2008;1154:453–61.
96. Egan G, Ensom MHH. Measuring anti–factor Xa activity to monitor low-molecular-weight heparin in obesity: a critical review. Can J Hosp Pharm. 2015;68(1):33–47.
97. Jacobsen AF, Qvigstad E, Sandset PM. Low molecular weight heparin (dalteparin) for the treatment of venous thromboembolism in pregnancy. BJOG. 2003;1102:139–44.
98. Dolovich LR, Ginsberg JS, Douketis JD, Holbrook AM, Cheah G. A meta-analysis comparing low- molecular-weight heparins with unfractionated heparin in the treatment of venous thromboembolism: examining some unanswered questions regarding location of treatment, product type, and dosing frequency. Arch Intern Med. 2000;160(2):181–8.
99. van Dongen CJ, van den Belt AG, Prins MH, Lensing AW. Fixed dose subcutaneous low molecular weight heparins versus adjusted dose unfractionated heparin for venous thromboembolism. Cochrane Database Syst Rev. 2004;(4):CD001100.
100. Blazing MA, de Lemos JA, White HD, Fox KA, Verheugt FW, Ardissino D, et al. Safety and efficacy of enoxaparin vs unfractionated heparin in patients with non-ST-segment elevation acute coronary syndromes who receive tirofiban and aspirin: a randomized controlled trial. JAMA. 2004;292 (98):55–64.
101. Ferguson JJ, Califf RM, Antman EM, Cohen M, Grines CL, Goodman S, et al. Enoxaparin vs unfractionated heparin in high risk patients with non-ST-segment elevation acute coronary syndromes managed with an intended early invasive strategy: primary results of the SYNERGY randomized trial. JAMA. 2004;292:45–54.

4 Parenteral Anticoagulants: Direct Thrombin Inhibitors and Pentasaccharides

Meghan L. Fletcher and Allison E. Burnett

Clinical Vignettes

Case 1: *RD is a 49-year-old admitted to the hospital for pancreatitis. His past medical history is significant for chronic alcohol use, diabetes mellitus, hypertension, and chronic kidney disease with a baseline serum creatinine of 2.3 mg/dL. Unfractionated heparin for deep vein thrombosis (DVT) prophylaxis was initiated on hospital day 1. Baseline platelet count was 180,000/μL. On hospital day 4, the patient was incidentally found to have a splenic vein thrombosis during abdominal ultrasound examination of a peripancreatic fluid collection concerning for an infected pseudocyst. Prophylactic heparin was discontinued, and a heparin infusion was initiated to treat the splenic vein thrombosis. 3 days later, the patient developed a precipitous drop in his platelets to 27,103/μL. A 4T pretest probability score for heparin-induced thrombocytopenia (HIT) was determined to be 6 (high risk). The heparin infusion was stopped; an ELISA HIT antibody was sent, and bivalirudin was immediately started. Both the ELISA and a confirmatory serotonin-release assay returned positive. The patient was successfully bridged to warfarin with bivalirudin for a 3-month course of therapeutic anticoagulation.*

Case 2: VS *is a 56-year-old woman who presents to the urgent care clinic with a chief complaint of 5–6 days of increasing pain in her thigh. She reports that she returned home from an*

M. L. Fletcher
Inpatient Pharmacy Department, University of New Mexico Hospital, Albuquerque, NM, USA
e-mail: mefletcher@salud.unm.edu

A. E. Burnett (✉)
University of New Mexico College of Pharmacy, Albuquerque, NM, USA
e-mail: aburnett@salud.unm.edu

J. F. Lau et al. (eds.), *Anticoagulation Therapy*, https://doi.org/10.1007/978-3-319-73709-6_4

international business trip last week. Shortly after returning home, she noticed some tenderness on the inside of her right thigh and states that the area has gradually become more red and swollen. She decided to come to urgent care today after the pain continued to worsen, and she noticed what she describes as a "knot" running vertically along the inside of her thigh up toward her groin. She has a past medical history significant for obesity, varicose veins, and tobacco use. She does not take any chronic medications and has no allergies. Compression ultrasonography reveals a thrombus within the right greater saphenous vein near its junction with the common femoral vein. Further imaging of the deep venous system of both legs reveals no clot burden. She is diagnosed with superficial thrombophlebitis, also known as superficial venous thrombosis. Given the severity of her presentation and the extent of the clot, it is recommended to initiate anticoagulant therapy. The patient is amenable and receives a prescription for fondaparinux 2.5 mg subcutaneously once daily for 45 days.

Parenteral Direct Thrombin Inhibitors (Argatroban and Bivalirudin)

Pharmacology

Mechanism of Action

Thrombin (factor IIa) has several procoagulant roles including platelet activation, activation of factors V and VIII, conversion of fibrinogen to fibrin, and clot stabilization via activation of factor XIII. Thus, its inhibition effectively prevents thrombus formation. Conversely, thrombin also contributes to endogenous anticoagulation when bound to thrombomodulin by activating protein C (Fig. 4.1). Hirudin is a naturally occurring direct thrombin inhibitor (DTI) derived from leech saliva which has high affinity for thrombin. Two synthetic hirudin analogs, argatroban and bivalirudin, are currently available for clinical use. Unlike indirect anticoagulants such as heparins and pentasaccharides whose inhibition of thrombin and factor Xa is mediated via binding to antithrombin (AT), DTIs bind specifically and directly to thrombin [1, 2]. Thrombin has multiple binding sites including an active (or catalytic) site, exosite 1 which binds substrates such as fibrin and exosite 2, the heparin-binding site. Bivalirudin is a bivalent DTI that reversibly binds to thrombin at both the active site and exosite 1. Argatroban, a monovalent DTI, reversibly binds thrombin at the active site only. Heparins are unable to bind to clot-bound thrombin due to inaccessibility of exosite 2 and thus can only inhibit free-floating thrombin. Conversely, DTIs are able to inhibit both clot-bound and free-floating thrombin, preventing both initiation and propagation of clot formation. Additionally, DTIs exert antiplatelet effects by reducing thrombin-mediated platelet activation [2].

Pharmacokinetics

Absorption

Argatroban and bivalirudin are administered parenterally and thus do not require absorption. Due to their short half-lives, they are administered via continuous infusion. Both agents produce an immediate anticoagulant effect, and steady-state plasma concentrations are achieved within a few hours of initiation of therapy [3–7].

Distribution

The parenteral direct thrombin inhibitors do not bind to plasma proteins or cells and thus produce a more linear and predictable anticoagulant response than unfractionated heparin [1, 2, 4]. They are distributed primarily in the extracellular space with volumes of distribution of approximately 240 mL/kg and 170 mL/kg for bivalirudin and argatroban, respectively [3, 5–7].

Metabolism

Argatroban is metabolized primarily in the liver via hydroxylation and aromatization to four minimally active, clinically nonrelevant metabolites. Patients with impaired hepatic function have a

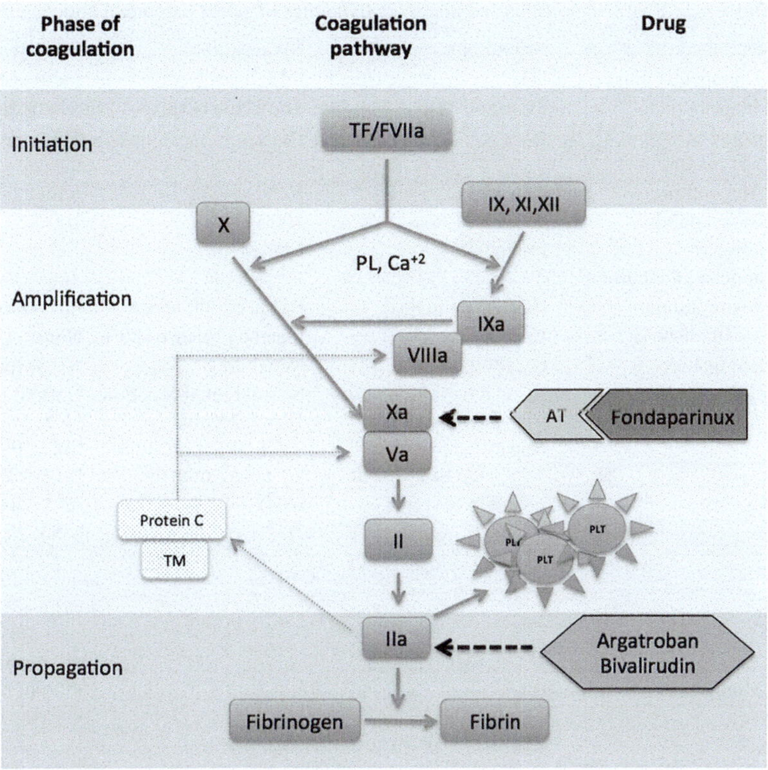

Fig. 4.1 Site of action of DTIs and fondaparinux within the coagulation cascade. Fondaparinux, an indirect anticoagulant, binds to antithrombin (AT) inducing a conformational change in AT that facilitates AT binding and inactivation of FXa, which results in inhibition of thrombin (FIIa) formation. The parenteral direct thrombin inhibitors (DTIs), argatroban and bivalirudin, do not require a cofactor and bind directly to thrombin (FIIa). They are able to bind both free-floating and clot-bound thrombin

fourfold decrease in clearance and therefore require dose adjustments [6].

Bivalirudin is metabolized primarily via blood proteases and broken down into the amino acid pool [3]. Thrombin itself cleaves bivalirudin, resulting in reversible binding and restoration of thrombin activity [2, 4, 5].

Elimination

Argatroban is excreted primarily in the feces through biliary secretion [6, 7]. Approximately 20% of bivalirudin is excreted via the kidneys as unchanged drug. Thus, in diminished renal function, the half-life will be prolonged, and dose adjustments are indicated [4, 8].

The pharmacokinetics of bivalirudin and argatroban are summarized in Table 4.1.

Pharmacodynamics

Both bivalirudin and argatroban affect coagulation parameters in a dose-dependent fashion, including the activated clotting time (ACT), activated partial thromboplastin time (aPTT), prothrombin time (PT)/international normalized ratio (INR), and thrombin time (TT). Bivalirudin only mildly affects the INR, with a mean increase of 0.6 [12], whereas argatroban imparts a more pronounced effect. It should be noted this is only a lab artifact and does not convey the same increased bleed risk as an elevated INR with warfarin therapy [13]. It can, however, make transitioning to warfarin very challenging (see section on transitioning to oral anticoagulation below). Because they are anticoagulants, the most common adverse effect of these parenteral DTIs is bleeding. There is no specific antidote for argatroban or bivalirudin. In healthy subjects, coagulation parameters return to baseline 1–2 h after stopping a parenteral DTI infusion [5, 6, 14]. The parenteral DTIs have no pharmacokinetic drug interactions since they are not metabolized in the liver. However, concomitant use of other antithrombotics (such as antiplatelet agents) poses a pharmacodynamic interaction that may potentiate bleed risk.

Table 4.1 Pharmacokinetics and pharmacodynamics of select parenteral anticoagulants [5, 7, 9–11]

Parameter	Argatroban	Bivalirudin	Fondaparinux
Therapeutic class	DTI	DTI	Indirect FXa inhibitor/pentasaccharide
Target	Thrombin (FIIa)	Thrombin (FIIa)	Factor Xa
Route of administration	IV	IV	SQ
Absorption	N/A	N/A	Rapid and complete
Bioavailability	100%	100%	100%
Onset of anticoagulant effect	Immediate	Immediate	2–3 h
Distribution	Extracellular space	Extracellular space	Intravascular space
Metabolism	Hepatic	Plasma proteases 80%	None
Elimination	Fecal/biliary	Renal 20%	>75% renal as unchanged drug
*t*1/2	Normal hepatic function • 39–51 min Hepatic impairment • Up to 181 min	Normal renal function • 25 min CrCl 10–29 mL/min • 57 min Dialysis • 3.5 h	Normal renal function • 17–21 h CrCl 50–80 ml/min • 25% reduced clearance • Monitor for s/sx of accumulation CrCl 30–49 ml/min • 40% reduced clearance • Consider alternative anticoagulant CrCl <30 ml/min • 55% reduced clearance • Avoid use
Monitoring	Hit • aPTT Coronary reperfusion (PCI or CABG) • ACT		• Not routinely done • May consider anti-Xa activity assay if – Changing renal function – Elderly – Extremes of weight • Anti-Xa assay must be calibrated to fondaparinux
Drug interactions	Concomitant antithrombotics and NSAIDs		
Adverse effect(s)	Bleeding		
Reversal	• No antidote • Discontinuation of infusion • May consider rFVIIa		• No antidote • May consider rFVIIa

ACS acute coronary syndromes, *CABG* coronary artery bypass grafting, *DTI* direct thrombin inhibitor, *FXa* activated factor X, *HIT* heparin-induced thrombocytopenia, *IV* intravenous, *PCI* percutaneous coronary intervention, *rFVIIa* recombinant-activated FVII, *SQ* subcutaneous, *s/sx* signs/symptoms, *t1/2* half-life

Clinical Utility

Parenteral DTIs have been most extensively studied in niche settings that either preclude the use of heparin products, such as heparin-induced thrombocytopenia (HIT), or in conditions where DTIs would have theoretical clinical advantages over UFH, such as coronary reperfusion.

Heparin-Induced Thrombocytopenia (HIT)

Immune-mediated heparin-induced thrombocytopenia (HIT) is a potentially fatal, prothrombotic condition in which UFH or LMWH binds to platelet factor 4 (PF4) and stimulates production of IgG antibodies that can promote platelet activa-

	Score = 2	Score = 1	Score = 0
Thrombocytopenia Compare the highest platelet count within the sequence of declining platelet counts with the lowest count to determine the % of platelet fall. **(Select only 1 option)**	o > 50% platelet fall AND nadir of ≥ 20 AND no surgery within preceding 3 days	o > 50% platelet fall BUT surgery within preceding 3 days OR o any combination of platelet fall and nadir that does not fit criteria for Score 2 or Score 0 (eg, 30-50% platelet fall or nadir 10-19)	o < 30% platelet fall o any platelet fall with nadir < 10
Timing (of platelet count fall or thrombosis*) Day 0 = first day of most recent heparin exposure **(Select only 1 option)**	o platelet fall day 5-10 after start of heparin o platelet fall within 1 day of start of heparin AND exposure to heparin within past 5-30 days	o consistent with platelet fall days 5-10 but not clear (eg, missing counts) o platelet fall within 1 day of start of heparin AND exposure to heparin in past 31-100 days o platelet fall after day 10	o platelet fall ≤ day 4 without exposure to heparin in past 100 days
Thrombosis (or other clinical sequelae) **(Select only 1 option)**	o confirmed new thrombosis (venous or arterial) o skin necrosis at injection site o anaphylactoid reaction to IV heparin bolus o adrenal hemorrhage	o recurrent venous thrombosis in a patient receiving therapeutic anticoagulants o suspected thrombosis (awaiting confirmation with imaging) o erythematous skin lesions at heparin injection sites	o thrombosis suspected
oTher cause for Thrombocytopenia** **(Select only 1 option)**	o no alternative explanation for platelet fall is evident	**Possible other cause is evident:** o sepsis without proven microbial source o thrombocytopenia associated with initiation of ventilator o other	**Probable other cause present:** o within 72 h of surgery o confirmed bacteremia/ fungemia o chemotherapy or radiation within past 20 days o DIC due to non-HIT cause o posttransfusion purpura (PTP) o platelet count < 20 AND given a drug implicated in causing D-ITP (see list) o non-necrotizing skin lesions at LMWH injection site (presumes DTH) o other

Drugs implicated in drug-induced immune thrombocytopenia (D-ITP)
Relatively Common: glycoprotein IIb/IIIa antagonists (abciximab, eptifibatide, tirofiban); quinine, quinidine, sulfa antibiotics, carbamazepine, vancomycin **Less Common:** actinomycin, amitriptyline, amoxicillin/piperacillin/nafcillin, cephalosporins (cefazolin, ceftazidime, ceftriaxone), celecoxib, ciprofloxacin, esomeprazole, fexofenadine, fentanyl, fucidic acid, furosemide, gold salts, levofloxacin, metronidazole, naproxen, oxaliplatin, phenytoin, propranolol, propoxyphene, ranitidine, rifampin, suramin, trimethoprim. Note: This is a partial list.

Fig. 4.2 The "4T score" for diagnosis of heparin-induced thrombocytopenia [15]. (Reprinted from CHEST, Vol. 141/ Issue 2 Supp, Linkins LA, Dans AL, Moores LK, Bona R, Davidson BL, Schulman S, Crowther M, Treatment and prevention of heparin-induced thrombocytopenia: antithrombotic therapy and prevention of thrombosis 9th ed.: American College of Chest Physicians Evidence-based Clinical Practice Guidelines, pages e495s–e530s, © 2012, with permission from Elsevier)

tion and thrombus formation. HIT is a rare condition, occurring in <5% of patients exposed to UFH and to a much lesser degree with LMWH [15]. To avoid misdiagnosis, clinicians are encouraged to use a pretest clinical probability score, such as the 4 T score, which has a 95% negative predictive value (see Fig. 4.2). For patients with a score ≤3, testing for HIT antibodies is not recommended. Patients with a score of ≥4 should undergo HIT testing and appropriate management based on test results [16]. As it can potentially lead to thrombus formation, HIT requires administration of an alternative anticoagulant during diagnostic evaluation in suspected cases or for the duration of therapy in confirmed cases. Due to their mechanism of action, argatroban and bivalirudin have become the mainstays of initial HIT treatment. They do not interact with PF4, and their direct inhibition of thrombin reduces platelet activation and prevents thrombus formation [15].

Argatroban

Argatroban has been shown to be effective in the treatment of immune-mediated HIT in two non-randomized, single-arm, open-label studies, ARG-911 and ARG-915 [17, 18]. Prospective patients with diagnosed or suspected HIT were treated with argatroban titrated to an aPTT ratio of 1.5–

3.0 times baseline. These patients were then compared to historical controls treated with the local standard of care (either discontinuation of heparin or discontinuation of heparin plus initiation of an oral anticoagulant). Serologic confirmation of HIT was not required for study inclusion, and over one-third of patients had no evidence of HIT antibodies in post hoc testing [19]. Argatroban patients were found to have a significantly decreased incidence of the composite endpoint, which included all-cause death, all-cause amputation, and new thrombosis compared to control patients (HR 0.3), with no difference in bleeding. These trials led to the American College of Chest Physicians (ACCP) Grade 1C recommendation to utilize argatroban in treatment of immune-mediated HIT over continuation of heparin, a LMWH or a vitamin K antagonist (VKA), such as warfarin [15].

Bivalirudin

Off-label use of bivalirudin for immune-mediated HIT has increased over the last decade. Evidence for its use in this setting comes from retrospective studies comparing bivalirudin to other parenteral DTIs, such as argatroban [20, 21]. Collectively, these studies suggest that immune-mediated HIT patients treated with bivalirudin achieve the target aPTT more quickly than with other DTIs, with similar or reduced incidence of bleeding. Additionally, bivalirudin has several practical advantages over argatroban, including less impact on the INR, less reliance on organ elimination, and potentially lower cost. While bivalirudin is not specifically recommended as a treatment option for HIT in the most recent ACCP guidelines, it is noted that "other factors such as drug availability, cost, and ability to monitor the anticoagulant effect may influence the choice of agent" [15].

Coronary Reperfusion

During elective or emergent coronary reperfusion procedures including percutaneous coronary intervention (PCI) and coronary artery bypass grafting (CABG), patients are vulnerable to thrombotic events due to plaque disruption and endothelial damage, thus requiring anticoagulation [22]. Traditionally, UFH has been considered first-line therapy in this setting. However, parenteral DTIs have several potential advantages over UFH in this setting, including:

- More predictable dose-dependent anticoagulant effect
- Shorter half-life with faster offset
- Lack of platelet activation and associated HIT
- Ability to inhibit clot-bound thrombin

As such, both argatroban and bivalirudin have been studied in patients, with or without HIT, that require coronary reperfusion.

Percutaneous Coronary Intervention (PCI) in Patients without HIT

Argatroban

In a multicenter, prospective, open-label, non-comparator pilot study of 152 patients undergoing PCI, argatroban was administered as a bolus followed by infusion, along with a glycoprotein IIb/IIIa inhibitor (GPI), either abciximab or eptifibatide [23]. Argatroban was monitored via the ACT with a target range of 275–325 s. The incidence of the composite primary outcome (death, myocardial infarction, urgent revascularization) and major bleeding was considered by investigators to be acceptably low (<3%). While argatroban may be effective in PCI, it is not recommended as the primary anticoagulant choice due to more robust evidence with other agents, including bivalirudin.

Bivalirudin

A meta-analysis of early clinical trials comparing bivalirudin plus provisional GPI to heparin or LMWH plus planned GPI therapy in patients undergoing elective or emergent PCI showed no difference between the groups in regard to major adverse cardiovascular events (OR 1.07; 95% CI 0.96–1.19), death (OR 0.93; 95% CI 0.72–1.21), or urgent revascularization (OR 1.06; 95% CI 0.86–1.3). However, patients in the bivalirudin arms experienced significantly less major bleeding (OR 0.55; 95% CI 0.44–

0.69) [24]. Based on these findings, recent iterations of both the American College of Cardiology/American Heart Association (ACC/AHA) and European Society of Cardiology (ESC) have recommended bivalirudin in patients with non-ST elevation (NSTEMI) and ST elevation (STEMI) myocardial infarction undergoing PCI with a higher level of evidence than UFH [25–28]. The ACC/AHA guidelines further recommend that in patients at higher risk of bleeding, it is reasonable to choose bivalirudin monotherapy over the use of UFH with provisional GPI use [25, 26].

The majority of evidence that supports the use of bivalirudin in PCI comes from trials utilizing heparin plus a GPI, a strategy that is no longer commonly employed. Two large, recently published meta-analyses included several contemporary trials comparing bivalirudin to UFH without systematic use of GPIs. Results showed the decreased bleeding risk associated with bivalirudin varies widely and is dependent on both the concomitant use of GPIs and the dose of UFH used. Results also suggest that the use of a bivalirudin-based anticoagulation regimen results in a significantly increased incidence of acute stent thrombosis compared to a heparin-based regimen, but with no difference in mortality [29, 30]. Theoretical reasons for the increased incidence of stent thrombosis include the faster offset of bivalirudin compared to UFH, lack of monitoring for anticoagulant effect (ACT) of bivalirudin as is done with UFH, or more potent platelet inhibition with UFH [30]. Based on these findings, the most recent European guidelines on coronary revascularization have been revised. Bivalirudin is still recommended over UFH patients with non-ST elevation myocardial infarction (NSTEMI). However, for patients with ST-elevation myocardial infarction (STEMI) at higher risk of ischemic events, UFH receives a Level I recommendation, whereas bivalirudin was downgraded from a Level I recommendation to Level IIa due to conflicting data [31].

Percutaneous Coronary Intervention (PCI) in Patients with HIT

Patients with active or recent HIT should not receive UFH or LMWH during PCI, and an alternate anticoagulation strategy should be employed. Both argatroban and bivalirudin have been shown to be effective in this setting, but they have never been compared in a head-to-head trial.

Argatroban

Three prospective, non-comparator, multicenter open-label studies ($N = 91$) have shown argatroban to be a viable alternative to heparin for patients with HIT undergoing PCI. At the time of these studies, there was no approved comparator for PCI with HIT, and a placebo comparator would have been considered unethical. Argatroban dosing consisted of a 350 mcg/kg bolus dose and initiation of a 25–30 mcg/kg/min infusion to achieve a goal ACT of 300–450 s. The primary endpoint was a positive outcome of the procedure (subjectively determined by the investigator) with adequate anticoagulation. Satisfactory outcomes were achieved in 94.5% of patients during initial treatment, and acute complications (death, emergency graft surgery, or myocardial infarction) occurred in <3% of patients. Major and minor bleeding rates were 1.1 and 32%, respectively [32].

Argatroban has also been studied in patients with suspected or confirmed HIT undergoing PCI with concomitant use of GPIIb/GPIIIa therapy (abciximab, eptifibatide, or tirofiban). This approach appears reasonable for patients who may need salvage therapy with concomitant GPIIb/GPIIIa, as there was no increased risk of bleeding compared to argatroban monotherapy, and clinical outcomes were similar [33].

Bivalirudin

Bivalirudin has also been shown to be a safe and effective alternative to UFH in HIT patients undergoing PCI. In the ATBAT trial, a total of 52 patients were treated with bivalirudin prior to PCI at a higher dose of 1 mg/kg bolus followed by 2.5 mg/kg/h infusion or the conventional lower dose of 0.75 mg/kg bolus followed by a 1.75 mg/kg/h infusion. Procedural success was achieved in 98% of patients with minimal adverse clinical events including death, acute myocardial infarction, stroke, or major bleeding [34].
Both ACC/AHA and ESC guidelines recommend either argatroban or bivalirudin over UFH or LMWH for patients with HIT who require PCI [15, 31, 35].

Acute Myocardial Infarction (NSTEMI or STEMI) in Patients Who Cannot Undergo PCI

In institutions without immediate PCI capability, patients with acute myocardial infarction (MI) generally receive a thrombolytic and a heparin infusion. Parenteral DTIs are not recommended by current guidelines for use in acute MI patients who are medically managed. However, in acute MI patients with HIT that cannot undergo PCI nor receive heparin products, consideration for their use seems reasonable. Argatroban has been shown to be a viable alternative to heparin in the medically managed population, achieving similar reperfusion rates and a comparable safety profile [36, 37]. While patients with immune-mediated HIT were not specifically included in these two studies, they do provide evidence that argatroban might be a reasonable alternative to UFH therapy for HIT patients with acute MI that cannot be immediately managed with PCI.

Bivalirudin has not been studied in this setting, but it is reasonable to extrapolate that it may be a viable option in this situation as well.

CABG with or Without HIT

The EVOLUTION trials compared the use of heparin plus protamine reversal to bivalirudin alone in patients undergoing coronary artery bypass grafting (CABG), either on or off cardiopulmonary bypass (CPB) [38, 39]. Procedural success rates and safety were similar between the two groups in both studies, except for a higher risk of stroke in EVOLUTION-ON with the use of heparin versus bivalirudin. In the CHOOSE-ON trial, bivalirudin demonstrated good efficacy in patients with suspected or confirmed HIT requiring cardiopulmonary bypass (CPB). Bivalirudin was administered at rate of 2.5 mg/kg/h with an initial bolus of 1 mg/kg to reach a goal ACT of 2.5× baseline. Nearly all patients (94%) achieved the primary endpoint of in-hospital procedural success, defined as the absence of death, MI, repeat coronary revascularization or stroke at day 7, or hospital discharge, whichever occurred first [40].

Practical Management

Dosing

Dosing recommendations by indication for both argatroban and bivalirudin are provided in Table 4.2. As discussed previously, both bivalirudin and argatroban may require dose adjustment based on their primary method of elimination and individual patient characteristics.

Administration

Argatroban is administered by continuous intravenous infusion (with boluses if indicated) in a 1 mg/mL dilution with dextrose 5% and water, lactated Ringer's, or 0.9% sodium chloride.

Bivalirudin is administered as a continuous intravenous infusion (with boluses if indicated) in concentrations of either 5 mg/mL or 0.5 mg/mL in 5% dextrose in water or 0.9% sodium chloride.

Monitoring and Titration

HIT

Most institutions utilize a standardized, evidence-based protocol for initiation, titration, and maintenance of parenteral DTIs. In HIT, argatroban and bivalirudin are typically monitored via the aPTT, with a target of 1.5–3× and 1.5–2× baseline, respectively [5, 7]. It is important to note that the aPTT reference range will vary between labs and reagents. Individual institutions must establish their own aPTT reference range for use with parenteral DTIs and protocols that target 1.5–3× baseline values. Several underlying variables may affect the aPTT, even in the absence of anticoagulants. These may include, but are not limited to, variations in endogenous factor levels, presence of a lupus anticoagulant, liver disease, or consumptive coagulopathy [47]. If a patient's baseline aPTT is elevated to within the target range, it may preclude either the use of a DTI or use of the aPTT for monitoring. In these instances, the use of an alternative anticoagulant (e.g., fondaparinux) or an alternative assay (e.g., a DTI-specific assay) should be considered. While some institutions have developed DTI-specific assays, they are not commercially available for widespread use [47]. HIT protocols should also incorporate monitoring of other laboratory parameters (e.g., hemoglobin, hematocrit) in order to assess for bleeding.

Activated partial thromboplastin times are typically drawn 2–4 h after the start of the infusion (to allow achievement of steady-state plasma concentrations), after any dose adjustments, and every 2–4 h until therapeutic. Once the patient has two consecutive therapeutic levels, monitoring may be decreased to once or twice daily. Parenteral DTIs can be titrated either by percentage changes or by predetermined rate increments. A comparison of these two strategies showed no difference in the amount of adjustments needed but a faster time to therapeutic with the predetermined incremental rate changes [48]. Titrating in this man-

Table 4.2 Clinical utility of argatroban, bivalirudin, and fondaparinux [15, 25–28, 31, 41–46]

Agent	Indications	Dosing	Monitoring and therapy targets	Guideline recommendations
Argatroban	*Labeled* PCI	350 mcg/kg bolus, 25 mcg/kg/min infusion	ACT	AHA/ACC Mentioned as option for PCI in patients with HIT [25]
	HIT	2 mcg/kg/min infusion Hepatic impairment: 0.5 mcg/kg/min infusion Critically ill: 0.2 mcg/kg/min infusion [41]	aPTT	ACCP Preferred for treatment of HIT [15]
Bivalirudin	*Labeled* PCI	0.75 mg/kg bolus, 1.75 mg/kg/h infusion CrCl <30 mL/min: same bolus, 1 mg/kg/h infusion Hemodialysis: same bolus, 0.25 mg/kg/h infusion	ACT	AHA/ACC Bivalirudin preferred over UFH in NSTEMI PCI [25] ACCF/AHA Bivalirudin preferred over UFH in STEMI PCI [26] ESC/EACTS Bivalirudin preferred over UFH in NSTE-ACS undergoing PCI [27, 31] ESC/EACTS UFH preferred over bivalirudin in STEMI undergoing PCI [28, 31]
	Cardiac surgery	1 mg/kg bolus, 2.5 mg/kg/h infusion	ACT	
	Off-label HIT	0.15–0.2 mg/kg/h CrCl 30–60 mL/min: 0.08–0.1 mg/kg/h CrCl <30 mL/min: 0.04–0.05mg/kg/h Intermittent hemodialysis (IHD): 0.07 mg/kg/h CRRT: 0.03–0.07 mg/kg/h Sustained low-efficiency daily diafiltration (SLEDD): 0.09 mg/kg/h	aPTT	ACCP Bivalirudin not specifically discussed in HIT treatment [15]

(continued)

Table 4.2 (continued)

Agent	Indications	Dosing	Monitoring and therapy targets	Guideline recommendations
Fondaparinux	*Labeled* VTE prophylaxis VTE treatment	2.5 mg SQ daily <50 kg: 5 mg SQ daily 50–100 kg: 7.5 mg SQ daily >100 kg: 10 mg SQ daily	None May consider anti-Xa in special pops	ACCP Option for prophylaxis in medicine patients [44] Option for non-orthopedic surgery patients [43] who cannot receive other agents Option for prophylaxis in orthopedic surgery patients. However, LMWH preferred [42] Recommended over IV UFH for acute treatment of VTE [46]
	Off-label HIT	<50 kg: 5 mg SQ daily 50–100 kg: 7.5 mg SQ daily >100 kg: 10 mg SQ daily	None May consider anti-Xa in special pops	ACCP Reasonable option to bridge patients to warfarin who have a history of HIT, no acute thrombosis and normal renal function [15] AC forum guidance Fondaparinux, at treatment doses, is a reasonable option in patients with active or remote HIT [45]
	Off-label ACS	2.5 mg SQ		*STEMI with primary PCI* ACCF/AHA, ESC/EACTS Fondaparinux not recommended as sole anticoagulant in STEMI undergoing primary PCI due to risk for catheter thrombosis [26, 28, 31] *ACS* AHA/ACC, ESC/EACTS Recommend concomitant use of an anticoagulant with anti-IIa (thrombin) activity, such as unfractionated heparin, when fondaparinux is used as initial therapy in ACS to minimize risk for catheter thrombosis [25, 27, 31]

ner also decreases chances of calculation errors and thus may be a safer and more efficient option.

Coronary Reperfusion

During PCI and CABG, argatroban and bivalirudin are monitored via the ACT, as it is a more appropriate assay for measuring very high concentrations of these medications. The ACT is performed as a point-of-care test, with targets ranging from 200 to 450 s, depending on the DTI and the type of intervention (see Table 4.2).

Argatroban

The target ACT for argatroban in PCI is 300–450 s. Additional boluses of 150 mcg/kg are recommended if the ACT is less than 300 s, along with an infusion increase to 30 mcg/kg/min. If the ACT is >450 s, it is recommended to half the infusion rate. Rechecking the ACT 5–10 min after dose adjustments will provide appropriate steady-state ACTs. After the procedure is completed, and continued treatment with argatroban is required, the rate can then be adjusted based on the institutional aPTT protocol.

Bivalirudin

With bivalirudin, ACT goals of 200–250 s for PCI and >300 s for CABG have traditionally been used. ACTs are collected 5 min after the initial bolus dose of bivalirudin, and additional boluses can be given prior to starting the infusion if the ACT is not at goal. Subsequent monitoring of bivalirudin is often not required during PCI procedures (due to minimal clearance via organ systems, short half-life with no need for reversal unlike heparin, and predictable anticoagulant effects) which may be considered an advantage over other agents including argatroban and UFH [14].

Transitioning to Oral Anticoagulation

HIT

After initial therapy with a non-heparin parenteral anticoagulant, HIT patients are usually transitioned to oral anticoagulation (OAC) for longer-term treatment in the outpatient setting. Direct oral anticoagulants (DOACs), such as dabigatran, apixaban, rivaroxaban, and edoxaban, have not been extensively studied in HIT, and thus warfarin remains the preferred OAC in this setting. The ACCP guidelines recommend starting warfarin once the platelet count has recovered to $>150 \times 10^3/\mu L$ (or to patient's baseline) and to continue overlap with the chosen parenteral non-heparin anticoagulant for ≥5 days and until INR is within a target range for a period of time during the overlap. The INR should then be rechecked after discontinuation of the parenteral anticoagulant to determine an INR based solely on the warfarin [15].

Argatroban

As previously mentioned, argatroban significantly prolongs the INR which makes transitioning to warfarin a challenging process. This is an assay artifact—not a true indication of anticoagulant affect, and supratherapeutic INRs associated with argatroban have not been shown to increase bleed risk [13, 49, 50].

Argatroban labeling does not recommend a specific duration of overlap; however, it recommends to continue the overlap with a goal INR of >4 if the argatroban infusion rate is ≤2 mcg/kg/min. For rates >2 mcg/kg/min, it is recommended to temporarily reduce the rate to 2 mcg/kg/min to determine the INR at that rate [7]. However, if a patient has required infusion rates >2 mcg/k/min in order to maintain a goal INR, decreasing the rate may put the patient at risk of undertreatment. Thus, it is suggested that providers use the chromogenic factor X activity assay if available (not to be confused with an anti-FXa LMWH or UFH assays) to monitor warfarin during the transition with a goal target range of 20–40% factor X activity (corresponds to an INR of 2–3) [15]. Unfortunately, this assay is often not readily available or is a send-out lab with a prolonged turnaround time that is not conducive to acute care.

Bivalirudin

Bivalirudin also impacts the INR but much less so than argatroban. In a study of 50 patients undergoing overlap therapy with bivalirudin while transitioning to warfarin, the mean increase in INR with bivalirudin initiation was 0.6, and the mean change in INR after discontinuation of bivalirudin was 0.8 [12]. Based on this study, aiming for an INR goal of 1.0 greater than the planned warfarin target INR is likely sufficient, without need for interruption of bivalirudin therapy. For example, bivalirudin and warfarin should be overlapped ≥5 days and until the INR is >3 for at least 24 h.

Coronary Reperfusion

After PCI or CABG, parenteral DTIs are usually discontinued, and if continued antithrombotic therapy is indicated, more conventional anticoagulation or antiplatelet therapies are employed. An exception to this is patients with active or recent HIT, in whom a parenteral DTI (or fondaparinux) may be continued with transition to warfarin as described above.

Other Clinical Uses

Continuous Renal Replacement Therapy

Heparin is the most commonly utilized anticoagulant to prevent clotting of extracorporeal circuits in continuous renal replacement therapy (CRRT). However, in patients with suspected or confirmed HIT who require CRRT and therapeutic systemic anticoagulation, treatment options are limited to parenteral DTIs. Neither bivalirudin nor argatroban have been formally studied as an alternative to heparin for CRRT, and evidence comes primarily from case reports. Systemic anticoagulation with a parenteral DTI is dually utilized as anticoagulation for the circuit as well as treatment for HIT. Argatroban has been used with doses ranging from 0.5 to 2 mcg/kg/min, similar to normal treatment doses, since argatroban clearance is not affected by renal dysfunction [51]. Bivalirudin, however, is primarily excreted via the kidneys, and, thus, documented doses for treatment of HIT have been approximately 0.07 mg/kg/h, about half the normal dose, secondary to clearance via CRRT [52].

ECMO

Bivalirudin and argatroban have both been used as alternatives to heparin for anticoagulation in extracorporeal membrane oxygenation (ECMO), primarily in patients who have suspected or confirmed HIT. While not studied in a randomized fashion, bivalirudin infusions ranging from 0.03 to 0.1 mg/kg/h have shown comparable outcomes to heparin in ECMO when targeted to achieve a therapeutic aPTT with fewer aPTT variations, less titrations, and fewer bleeds compared to heparin [53, 54]. As many ECMO patients require CRRT, it is important to anticipate the need to increase bivalirudin infusion rates in order to compensate for the elimination of drug during filtration. Less information is available for argatroban as an alternative to heparin in ECMO. However, there are reports describing the successful use of argatroban in patients with suspected HIT undergoing ECMO with maintenance doses averaging 0.15 mcg/kg/min, which is an approximately one-tenth of the standard HIT dosing [41].

Adverse Effects

In clinical practice, parenteral DTIs are generally well tolerated. Bleeding is the most serious adverse effect associated with any anticoagulant, including the parenteral DTIs. In the argatroban studies for HIT, the primary safety endpoint of major bleeding occurred less frequently in the argatroban arms as compared to historical controls [17, 18]. Bivalirudin-based regimens were shown to have a lower incidence of major bleeding in several PCI studies compared to UFH-based regimens [24, 29, 30]. Additionally, in HIT studies, bivalirudin was shown to have a lower incidence of bleeding compared to other parenteral DTIs, including argatroban [20, 21].

Other non-bleeding adverse reactions that have been reported with argatroban and bivalirudin use include angina, headache, hypotension, fever, diarrhea, cardiac arrest, nausea, ventricular tachycardia, pain, vomiting, infection, coughing, and abdominal pain [5, 7].

Reversal

There are currently no specific reversal agents for argatroban or bivalirudin. Cessation of the infusion during recognition of a bleed is the most prudent intervention given their short half-lives and rapid elimination from the body. Closely monitoring the aPTT may aid in determining if persistent drug effect is present. Hemodialysis has been shown to remove approximately 20–25% of argatroban and bivalirudin, and this may be an option if bleeding persists [5, 7]. The ACCP 2012 guidelines suggest that activated recombinant factor VIIa may potentially be used to reverse the effects of argatroban and bivalirudin in urgent situations, but this has not been studied in humans [9]. General approaches to bleeding management (e.g., looking for and controlling the source of the bleed) and supportive measures, such as resuscitation and monitoring, should be employed.

Special Considerations

Pregnancy

There are no formal studies in humans evaluating the use of bivalirudin during pregnancy. Animal studies at doses exceeding the maximum human dose have not shown any harm to the fetus. However, caution is recommended, and the use of bivalirudin during pregnancy should be limited to situations that preclude the use of more conventional anticoagulants [5, 55]. The data with argatroban used during pregnancy is similarly limited, with only animal studies and case reports to support its use [7, 56]. The ACCP 2012 guidelines recommend the use of danaparoid for treatment of HIT in pregnant patients (Grade 2C) and use of lepirudin and fondaparinux only if danaparoid is unavailable (Grade 2C) [15]. Since publication of that guideline, lepirudin has been removed from the market, and danaparoid is not available in the USA. More data regarding the use of bivalirudin and argatroban in pregnancy are needed.

Breastfeeding

The extent of transfer into breast milk is unknown with either argatroban or bivalirudin, and thus the use in breastfeeding is not recommended [5, 7].

Pediatric

Recent reviews have highlighted the evidence for the use of parenteral DTIs in the pediatric population [57–59]. Studied indications include HIT, PCI, CPB, ECMO, and VTE. Bivalirudin doses have been reported as a bolus dose of 0.125–0.25 mg/kg with an infusion rate of 0.125–0.25 mg/kg/h for treatment of thrombosis. Doses for CPB or PCI are higher at 0.5–1 mg/kg bolus and infusions of 0.5–2.5 mg/kg/h, comparable to adult dosing for similar indications. The argatroban package insert recommends starting a dose of 0.75 mcg/kg/min for critically ill patients with HIT (0.2 mcg/kg/min in these same patients if they have any hepatic impairment). Reported dosages for CPB were between 7.5 and 15 mcg/kg/min with titration based on the ACT. Since little is known regarding the pharmacokinetic/pharmacodynamic profiles of DTIs in pediatric patients, it is prudent to carefully monitor coagulation parameters, such as aPTT or ACT, and adjust doses as appropriate. More studies are needed to determine the efficacy of these agents in the pediatric population compared to the more conventional agents such as heparin and LMWH.

Fondaparinux

Pharmacology

Mechanism of Action

Fondaparinux is a chemically synthesized anticoagulant specifically developed as a selective indirect factor Xa (FXa) inhibitor. Factor Xa is an attractive target for anticoagulant drug therapy given its position at the confluence of the intrinsic and extrinsic coagulation pathways (Fig. 4.1). Its inhibition significantly reduces thrombin generation irrespective of the upstream trigger that initiates the coagulation process [10]. FXa has a single function within the coagulation cascade, serving as the gatekeeper to the final common pathway of clot formation. Conversely, thrombin (FIIa) has many roles within the coagulation process, including platelet activation and mediation of endogenous anticoagulation through binding with thrombomodulin and activation of protein C (Fig. 4.1). Thus, it has been suggested FXa may be a more pure target as compared to thrombin [60].

Fondaparinux is a synthetic analog of the naturally occurring pentasaccharide sequence found within animal-derived unfractionated heparin (UFH) and low-molecular-weight heparin (LMWH) chains that binds to the plasma glycoprotein antithrombin (AT) with high affinity [61, 62]. Like UFH and LMWH, fondaparinux is an indirect anticoagulant, requiring binding to AT to exert its effect (Fig. 4.3) [61]. Because of its specific structure, fondaparinux is >95% bound to AT in the plasma, minimizing non-specific binding to other plasma proteins and cells [63]. When

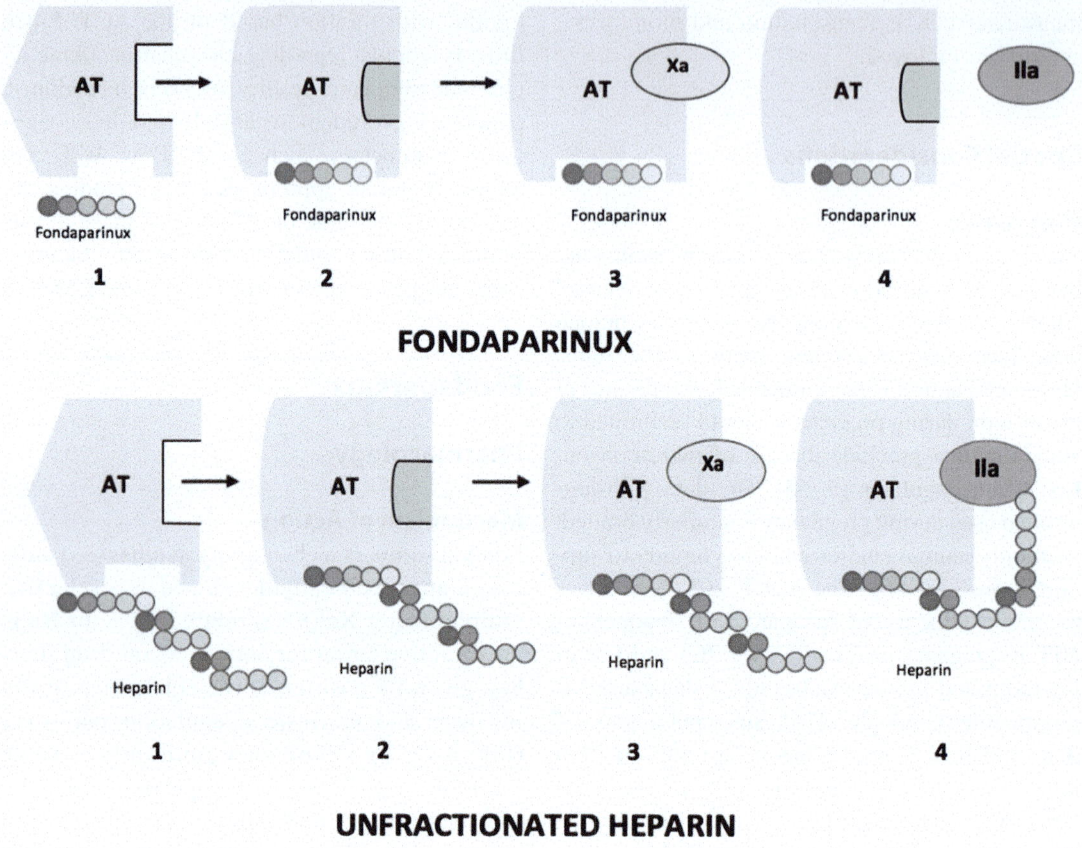

Fig. 4.3 Comparison of heparin and fondaparinux binding to antithrombin. Adapted from [70]

fondaparinux binds with AT, it induces a conformational change that catalyzes binding and inhibition of FXa. However, due to its short length compared to unfractionated heparin (≥18 saccharides), fondaparinux is unable to bind and inhibit thrombin (FIIa) [9]. Increased specificity and predictability in dose response allows fondaparinux to be administered in fixed doses without the need for routine monitoring of anticoagulant activity and reduces the potential for adverse effects [9].

Pharmacokinetics

Due to minimal binding to plasma proteins other than AT, fondaparinux exhibits linear pharmacokinetics, and thus a highly predictable dose response, across a wide range of studied doses [9]. This predictability, along with high bioavailability and a long half-life, minimizes inter- and intra-patient variability and allows fondaparinux to be given in fixed, once-daily doses without the need for routine monitoring [9].

The pharmacokinetics of fondaparinux are summarized in Table 4.1.

Absorption

Fondaparinux is not absorbed through the gastrointestinal mucosa so it must be given parenterally. Subcutaneous administration provides rapid and complete absorption of fondaparinux with 100% bioavailability. Peak plasma concentrations are achieved at approximately 2–3 h after subcutaneous administration [10]. A steady state is achieved after 3–4 doses of once-daily fondaparinux.

Distribution

Fondaparinux is highly protein bound and unable to distribute readily into tissue. Its volume of distribution is 7–11 L, which approximates the blood volume [10].

Metabolism

Fondaparinux does not undergo hepatic metabolism and is not vulnerable to pharmacokinetic drug interactions with substrates of the cytochrome P450 isoenzyme system [10].

Elimination

Decreased binding to macrophages and endothelial cells increases the plasma half-life of fondaparinux compared to UFH and LMWH. Elimination of fondaparinux is affected by multiple patient parameters, including renal function, age, and low body weight. These factors must be routinely evaluated, as they may preclude the use of fondaparinux or mandate increased monitoring for signs and symptoms of drug accumulation.

Renal Function

Fondaparinux is heavily dependent on renal elimination, with up to 77% of drug excreted unchanged in the urine. In normal renal function, the terminal half-life is 17 h in young volunteers and 21 h in elderly volunteers [10]. The half-life of fondaparinux will be prolonged, and exposure to the drug, as measured by the area under the curve (AUC), will be increased in patients with acute or chronic kidney injury (Table 4.1).

Age

In studies with prophylactic and treatment doses, the total clearance of fondaparinux was approximately 25% lower in patients >75 years old as compared to patients <65 years old. While the clinical relevance of this is unknown, close monitoring in patients of advanced age is warranted [11].

Low Body Weight

In patients weighing <50 kg, the total clearance of fondaparinux is reduced by 30%. As with advanced age, the clinical relevance of this is unknown. In clinical trials of fondaparinux for VTE prophylaxis in patients undergoing orthopedic arthroplasty or abdominal surgery, the incidence of major bleeding was higher among patients with a body weight <50 kg compared to patients ≥50 kg [11]. It is possible that reduced fondaparinux clearance along with procedural intervention cumulatively led to more bleeding. While FDA-labeling states prophylactic fondaparinux is contraindicated in these surgical populations [11], international labeling emphasizes cautious use in all patients <50 kg [64].

In patients with multiple factors that may affect fondaparinux clearance, the effect is likely to be cumulative, and use of an alternative anticoagulant may be indicated.

Pharmacodynamics

Fondaparinux binds non-covalently and reversibly to AT, increasing the innate anticoagulant activity of AT by ~300-fold. The AT-fondaparinux complex then binds and neutralizes FXa, which decreases the conversion of prothrombin (FII) to thrombin (FIIa), thereby inhibiting clot formation. Fondaparinux is then released and available to catalyze other AT molecules. When plasma AT becomes saturated, excess circulating unbound fondaparinux (which lacks anticoagulant activity) is renally excreted [65]. As it does not affect pre-existing circulating thrombin, it is theorized that fondaparinux may afford some degree of residual hemostatic function, should it be needed, at a site of injury. Fondaparinux has no known effect on platelet function fibrinogen, thrombin time, or antithrombin assays [66]. However, it can affect the PT and aPTT and may interfere with factor VIII assays. While not routinely recommended, if measurement of fondaparinux is indicated (e.g., changing renal function, extremes of weight or age), plasma concentration is most accurately assessed by use of a chromogenic anti-factor Xa activity assay. The chromogenic anti-factor Xa activity, which is reported in IU/ml, is directly proportional to the plasma concentration of fondaparinux. The result is extrapolated to a mcg/ml plasma concentration using a standard fondaparinux-calibrated curve. The assay must be calibrated to fondaparinux, as the use of assays calibrated to heparin or low-molecular-weight heparin will yield inaccurate results [67].

Concomitant use of fondaparinux and drugs that affect coagulation (e.g., antiplatelets, NSAIDs) poses a pharmacodynamic drug interaction that may potentiate bleeding risk and should be avoided whenever possible. After stopping fondaparinux, the anticoagulant effect will persist for up to 4 days and even longer in patients with reduced clearance.

Clinical Utility

Fondaparinux has been studied in numerous anticoagulation indications, including prevention and treatment of venous thromboembolism (VTE), HIT, and acute coronary syndromes (ACS).

Prevention of VTE

Orthopedic Surgery

Fondaparinux 2.5 mg SQ once daily, started 6 h postoperatively, was compared to enoxaparin at dose of either 30 mg SQ twice daily started 12–24 h postoperatively or 40 mg SQ once daily started 12 h preoperatively in four clinical trials of patients undergoing total hip (THA) or knee arthroplasty (TKA) or hip fracture surgery (HFS). In a meta-analysis of these trials [68], fondaparinux significantly reduced the incidence of asymptomatic deep vein thrombosis (DVT), symptomatic DVT, or pulmonary embolism (6.8%) compared to the gold standard enoxaparin (13.7%), with a common odds reduction of 55.2% (95% CI 46–63%; $p < 0.001$). This efficacy was consistent across several subgroups, including age, gender, weight, and duration of surgery. There was a trend toward more major bleeding with fondaparinux compared to enoxaparin (2.7 versus 1.7%; $p = 0.08$). The authors pointed out that the definitions of major bleeding varied across the studies, and the majority of events were attributable to a potentially nonclinically relevant drop in hemoglobin and need for transfusion. They further reported that clinically relevant bleeding events such as fatal bleeding, critical organ bleeding, or bleeding leading to reoperation were similar between the two groups. In a post hoc analysis, an inverse relationship was found between the timing of the first postoperative dose (ranges 3–9 h) and the occurrence of bleeding. Among fondaparinux patients who received their first injection 6–9 h postoperatively, bleeding rates were significantly reduced and similar to the enoxaparin group, with no difference in efficacy.

In the open-label randomized FLEXTRA study of 2000 patients undergoing elective hip arthroplasty, no difference in efficacy was found between fondaparinux 2.5 mg started 6 h postoperatively and delayed initiation until the first postoperative morning [69]. In response to criticism of the inclusion of asymptomatic DVT events in the fondaparinux orthopedic studies, Turpie and colleagues performed a second meta-analysis of those four trials using efficacy endpoints defined by the ACCP and considered to be more clinically relevant, including confirmed proximal DVT, symptomatic DVT, or pulmonary embolism (PE) or fatal PE [70]. The common odds reduction in favor of fondaparinux was similar to the original analysis at 49.6% ($p < 0.001$).

Extended prophylaxis with fondaparinux in hip fracture repair was investigated in the PENTHIFRA-Plus trial [71]. Fondaparinux 2.5 mg SQ once daily for up to 4 weeks compared to placebo resulted in a 89% relative risk reduction in symptomatic VTE (0.3% versus 2.7%; $p = 0.02$) with a nonsignificant increase in major bleeding ($p = 0.06$). In the most recent ACCP 2012 guidelines, fondaparinux for a minimum of 10–14 days is included as a Grade 1B option for VTE prophylaxis in patients undergoing major orthopedic surgery (THA, TKA, HFS), along with several other agents. However, the authors give a Grade 2B recommendation for the use of LMWH in preference to all other listed options, including fondaparinux. It is recommended to extend prophylaxis up to 35 days in this population [42].

Abdominal Surgery

Fondaparinux has been studied in two clinical trials among patients undergoing high-risk abdominal surgery. In the non-inferiority PEGASUS trial ($n = 2927$), fondaparinux 2.5 mg SQ which started 6 h postoperatively was compared to dalteparin initiated preoperatively [72]. The incidence of venographically detected DVT on day 10 was 4.6% in the fondaparinux arm vs. 6.1% in the dalteparin group, a relative risk reduction of 25% (95% CI −9.0–47.9%; $p = 0.144$) which achieved non-inferiority. There were no significant differences between the groups in regard to symptomatic VTE (0.4% in both groups) or major bleeding (fondaparinux 3.4% vs. 2.4% dalteparin; $p = 0.122$).

In the randomized, double-blind, placebo-controlled superiority APOLLO trial, 1309 patients undergoing major abdominal surgery were randomized to receive either prophylactic fondaparinux or subcutaneous placebo started 6–8 h postoperatively and continued for 5–9 days [73]. All patients received intermittent pneumatic compression (IPC). At day 10, the incidence of any VTE (including asymptomatic events) in the fondaparinux-treated group was 1.7% compared to 5.3% in the placebo group (odds ratio reduction 69.8%; 95% CI 27.9–87.3%; $p = 0.004$). Proximal DVT was significantly reduced with fondaparinux, as well (0.2% versus 1.7%; $p = 0.037$). Not surprisingly, major bleeding was significantly higher in the fondaparinux arm compared to placebo (1.6% versus 0.2%; $p = 0.006$). Differences in fatal bleeding and bleeding requiring reoperation could not be adequately assessed due to low event rates.

Fondaparinux is not recommended as a first-line agent for VTE prophylaxis in general surgery patients in the most recent ACCP 2012 guidelines. In a pooled analysis of the data from the orthopedic and PEGASUS trials, it was determined that fondaparinux does not significantly reduce clinically important VTE events but does increase major bleeding compared to LMWH. The ACCP recommends fondaparinux prophylaxis in general and abdominal-pelvic surgery patients at high risk for VTE only if both LMWH and UFH are contraindicated or unavailable, and the patient is not high risk for major bleeding (Grade 2C) [43].

Medically Ill Patients

The double-blind, randomized, placebo-controlled ARTEMIS trial included patients >60 years of age who were hospitalized for an acute medical illness for at least 4 days. Patients were randomized to receive fondaparinux 2.5 mg SQ once daily for 6–14 days or placebo. Fondaparinux was shown to be effective in reducing both asymptomatic and symptomatic VTE with no difference in bleeding [74]. Based on these findings, ACCP 2012 guidelines give fondaparinux a Grade 1B recommendation for prevention of VTE in at-risk hospitalized medically ill patients [44].

Treatment of VTE (DVT or PE)

In the non-inferiority MATISSE DVT ($n = 2205$) and PE ($n = 2213$) trials, fondaparinux was compared to enoxaparin and UFH, respectively. In MATISSE DVT, patients with acute symptomatic DVT were randomized to receive fondaparinux 7.5 mg SQ once daily (5 mg if weight <50 kg, 10 mg if weight >100 kg) or enoxaparin 1 mg/kg SQ BID. In MATISSE PE, the same weight-based fondaparinux regimen was compared to continuous infusion intravenous UFH titrated to an aPTT 1.5–2.5× control in patients with acute symptomatic PE. Parenteral therapies were overlapped with a vitamin K antagonist (e.g., warfarin) for ≥5 days, and until the INR was ≥2. In both trials, fondaparinux exhibited non-inferiority for the primary efficacy outcome of 3-month incidence of recurrent VTE, with similar rates of bleeding and mortality [75, 76]. A subgroup analysis of overweight patients in these two trials (11% > 100 kg, 28% BMI ≥ 30) showed that the recommended fixed dose of fondaparinux 10 mg SQ once daily in obesity provides similar protection against VTE recurrence and major bleeding as standard 7.5 mg dosing in nonobese patients [77]. This suggests that increasing the dose beyond 10 mg once daily for obese patients is not needed, which may be an advantage of fondaparinux over other parenteral agents [45]. The median body weight and BMI in the obese fondaparinux group were 110 kg and 33 kg/m^2, respectively. While some morbidly obese patients (BMI > 40) were included, their number was not sufficiently large enough to draw meaningful conclusions as to the clinical efficacy of fondaparinux in this population.

When a conventional approach to VTE is undertaken (versus the use of a direct oral anticoagulant), fondaparinux is preferred over IV UFH (Grade 2C), as is LMWH, in the acute treatment of VTE, unless there is a contraindication to its use such as significant renal impairment or potential invasive procedures [46].

Treatment of Lower Extremity Superficial Vein Thrombosis

Superficial vein thrombosis (SVT), also known as superficial thrombophlebitis, occurs most commonly in the greater saphenous vein of the leg (60–80% of cases) but can affect other superficial veins [78]. While previously considered a benign, self-limiting disease, contemporary data suggests that isolated SVT (without concomitant DVT or PE at diagnosis) may be a clinically relevant entity with the potential to progress into the deep venous system via the saphenofemoral junction (SFJ).

No consensus on optimal management of lower extremity SVT has been achieved. Recent evidence suggests that anticoagulation is the treatment of choice for those with isolated SVT of the lower extremity at increased risk for extension into the deep venous system [46, 78]. The most robust evidence for management of SVT of the lower extremity is provided by the CALISTO study [79]. In this double-blind, multicenter, prospective trial, patients with acute lower extremity SVT (≥5 cm in length on compression ultrasonography) were randomized to fondaparinux 2.5 mg subcutaneously once daily for 45 days or placebo. Fondaparinux-treated patients had an absolute risk reduction of 5% in the incidence of the composite primary outcome of all-cause mortality, symptomatic VTE or symptomatic extension, or recurrence of SVT (0.9% vs. 5.9%; RR 0.15; 95% CI 0.08–0.26; $p < 0.001$; number needed to treat = 20) compared to the placebo group, with no difference in bleeding. Based on these results, prophylactic-dose fondaparinux for 45 days may be considered for isolated lower extremity SVT of at least 5 cm in length (Grade 2B) [46]. However, fondaparinux is expensive and was found to not be cost-effective in this setting [80]. If fondaparinux is cost-prohibitive for the patient, it is reasonable to use traditional therapies of NSAIDs, compression stockings, and topical agents with close follow-up for signs and symptoms of VTE development.

HIT

Fondaparinux is not FDA-approved for treatment of suspected or confirmed HIT but is frequently used in this setting owing to similar safety and efficacy compared to approved therapies, as well as simplified management [81–83]. In the 2012 ACCP guidelines, fondaparinux is mentioned as a non-heparin anticoagulant option for acute HIT, but other therapies are preferred if available. The authors attribute this recommendation to lack of data for its use in this setting, as well as concern over a small number of case reports of fondaparinux-associated HIT [84–86]. While fondaparinux can trigger immunogenicity and generation of anti-PF4/heparin antibodies, it does not appear to promote antibody binding to PF4 complexes and subsequent HIT, possibly due to its small molecular size and/or weak PF4 affinity [87]. Importantly no cases of HIT have been reported in the thousands of patients included in clinical trials evaluating the safety and efficacy of fondaparinux in VTE treatment and prevention or in ACS. The ACCP 2012 guidelines do suggest that fondaparinux may be used in patients with normal renal function and a remote history of HIT who require anticoagulation for acute non-HIT-associated thrombosis (Grade 2C) [15]. Guidance from the Anticoagulation Forum supports its use in this setting as well but also states that it is a viable option in patients with active HIT and should be administered in therapeutic doses. The authors deem this to be reasonable based on the fact that the available data for any agent in the treatment of HIT is of low quality [45]. One often cited concern with fondaparinux in HIT patients with active thrombosis is its inability to inhibit clot-bound thrombin. As such, in unstable patients with significant HIT-associated clot burden, it is reasonable to initially utilize a parenteral DTI and then switch to fondaparinux once the patient is more stable [88].

Acute Coronary Syndrome (ACS)

UA and NSTEMI

The OASIS-5 trial (n = 20,078) compared fondaparinux to enoxaparin in patients with unstable angina (UA) or NSTEMI [89]. In this randomized, double-blind, double-dummy trial, patients received either enoxaparin 1 mg/kg SQ twice daily or fondaparinux 2.5 mg for a mean of 6 days and were followed for 6 months. The dose of fondaparinux was derived from the phase II dose-finding PENTUA study that showed a prophylactic dose of fondaparinux provided the lowest rate of outcome events (death, MI, recurrent ischemia), with similar bleeding, compared to enoxaparin 1 mg/kg BID or higher doses of fondaparinux [90]. For patients undergoing PCI (~40% of patients in each group), the study protocol called for enoxaparin patients to receive supplemental IV UFH and for fondaparinux patients to receive supplemental IV fondaparinux prior to the procedure. Early in the study, it was discovered that enoxaparin patients, but not fondaparinux patients, were receiving their supplemental anticoagulation intravenously. This was in tandem with reports from some study centers of catheter-associated thrombosis. Midway through the study, steps were taken to ensure per-protocol administration of supplemental agents, and a protocol amendment allowing for open-label use of a 200 IU heparin flush at investigator's discretion was implemented. For the primary outcome of death, MI or recurrent ischemia at day 9, there was no difference between the fondaparinux and enoxaparin groups (5.8% versus 5.7%, HR 1.01, 95% CI 0.9–1.13), which met non-inferiority criteria. There was a nonsignificant trend toward fewer of these combined events at 30 days (8% versus 8.6%, p = 0.13) and 180 days (12.3% versus 13.2%, p = 0.06) with fondaparinux compared to enoxaparin. Major bleeding at day 9 was significantly lower with fondaparinux (2.2% versus 4.1%, HR 0.52, 95% CI 0.44–0.61, $p < 0.001$), and this was sustained at all study points. When looking at the composite of the primary outcome and major bleeding at 9 days, there was a significant net benefit in favor of fondaparinux (7.3% versus 9%, HR 0.81, 95% CI 0.73–0.89, $p < 0.001$), which persisted throughout the study. Mortality was significantly reduced at 30 days (2.9% versus 3.5%, HR 0.83, 95% CI 0.71–0.97, $p = 0.02$) and 180 days (5.8% versus 6.5%, HR 0.89, 95% CI 0.8–1.0, $p = 0.05$) with fondaparinux, which was primarily driven by reductions in bleeding. Investigators reported significantly more catheter-related thrombi with fondaparinux compared to enoxaparin (0.9% versus 0.4%, RR 3.59, 95% CI 1.64–7.84, $p = 0.001$).

To avoid the complication of catheter-related thrombi, both the American College of Cardiology/American Heart Association (ACC/AHA) and European Society of Cardiology (ESC) recommend concomitant use of an anticoagulant with anti-IIa (thrombin) activity, such as unfractionated heparin, when fondaparinux is used as initial therapy in ACS [25, 27]. Based on results of the FUTURA/OASIS-8 double-blind randomized trial comparing low versus standard-dose heparin in this setting, it is recommended to administer a heparin bolus of 85 units/kg or, if patient has received concomitant GPI, a reduced dose of 60 units/kg [91].

STEMI

The OASIS-6 trial compared fondaparinux 2.5 mg with placebo (plus standard care) in 12,092 patients with STEMI [92]. Among patients undergoing primary PCI, rates of mortality, MI or severe bleeding did not differ between the groups. Additionally, as with the OASIS-5 trial, a significantly higher rate of catheter-associated thrombosis was seen with fondaparinux. Thus, both US and EU guidelines recommend against fondaparinux as initial anticoagulation for STEMI patients undergoing primary PCI, with UFH or bivalirudin being preferred therapies [26, 28]. However, in subgroup analyses of the OASIS-6 trial, fondaparinux was found to have a significant net benefit (death, MI, or severe hemorrhage at 30 days) among patients receiving fibrinolytic therapy (HR 0.77; 95% CI 0.67–0.9) or no reperfusion therapy (HR 0.81; 95% CI 0.67–0.99) [92]. When used in these setting (STEMI without primary PCI), it is recommended to give fondaparinux as a 2.5 mg IV bolus, along with a standard-dose UFH bolus as defined in the FUTURA/OASIS-8 trial mentioned above [26, 28, 91].

Practical Management

Dosing

When fondaparinux is used for VTE prophylaxis, the dose is 2.5 mg SQ once daily. Prophylactic use in patients <50 kg is contraindicated, as orthopedic studies have shown in increased risk for bleeding in low weight patients [68]. For obese patients, the same 2.5 mg prophylactic dose may be used without need for dose adjustment. When used for treatment, fondaparinux is given in fixed doses based on the patient's weight category (Table 4.2). For obese patients, a standard dose of 10 mg SQ once daily may be used without need for upward adjustment. Because it is primarily renally eliminated, it is contraindicated in patients with an estimated creatinine clearance of <30 mL/min by Cockroft-Gault equation, and caution is recommended in those with an estimated clearance of 30–50 mL/min [11].

Administration

Fondaparinux comes in pre-filled syringes of 2.5, 5, 7.5, and 10 mg strengths, which increases the feasibility and convenience of outpatient therapy. It should be administered subcutaneously in the abdomen once daily.

Monitoring

Fondaparinux has a high degree of specificity and predictability, precluding the need for routine monitoring of anticoagulant activity. An anti-Xa assay, calibrated to fondaparinux, may be considered in certain populations, such as patients with changing renal function, extremes of weight, or altered pharmacokinetics (such as pregnancy and burns) (Table 4.3).

Table 4.3 Observed plasma fondaparinux concentrations with repeat dosing [29]

Fondaparinux dose (SQ once daily)	Cmax (mcg/ml)	Cmin (mcg/ml)
Prophylaxis (2.5 mg)	0.39–0.5	0.14–0.19
Treatment (5–10 mg)	1.2–1.26	0.46–0.62

Transitioning Between Anticoagulants

Transitioning from Fondaparinux

Clinical situations that might involve transitioning from fondaparinux to an alternative anticoagulant include a desire for a shorter-acting anticoagulant (e.g., UFH, LMWH) prior to an invasive procedure or need for longer-term oral anticoagulation therapy.

- When switching from fondaparinux to an alternative anticoagulant with a rapid onset of action, such as UFH, LMWH, or a DOAC, the alternative anticoagulant should be started 24 h after the last dose of fondaparinux.
- When transitioning from fondaparinux to warfarin, such as in acute VTE using a conventional approach, fondaparinux should be overlapped with warfarin for a minimum of 5 days and until the INR is >2 for approximately 24 h. This is due to the long half-life (~40 h) and slow onset of effect of warfarin, coupled with the long half-life of pre-existing, circulating thrombin (~60 h).

Transitioning to Fondaparinux

The most common clinical situation wherein a transition to fondaparinux from another anticoagulant might occur is HIT, a potentially fatal prothrombotic condition.

- Patients with suspected or confirmed HIT who have been receiving UFH (either SQ or IV) or LMWH should have fondaparinux initiated as soon as safely possible, regardless of the timing of the previous dose of UFH or LMWH, to minimize the risk for HIT-associated thrombosis.
- This obviously may place patients at risk of excessive anticoagulation if UFH or LMWH has been recently administered and underscores the importance of using the 4T score to determine pretest probability of HIT to most accurately identify at-risk patients warranting a change in therapy.

Adverse Effects

The major side effect associated with fondaparinux, as with all anticoagulants, is bleeding. Risk may be mitigated by administering a first post-procedural prophylactic dose at least 6 h after the procedure or even the next morning, which will not compromise efficacy [68, 93]. In the MATISSE DVT and PE trials [75, 76], therapeutic fondaparinux was shown to have similar bleeding rates to therapeutic-dose enoxaparin and UFH. In ACS trials, a low, prophylactic dose significantly reduced major bleeding compared to therapeutic UFH or enoxaparin [89, 92]. This evidence collectively suggests that fondaparinux, when used at recommended doses in appropriately selected patients, has a bleeding profile similar to or better than other anticoagulants. Importantly, clinicians must ensure a patient has adequate renal function prior to and throughout fondaparinux therapy to avoid bleeding complication associated with accumulation.

Reversal

Currently there is no specific antidote for fondaparinux. It cannot be reversed with protamine, possibly due to its charge, sulfate content, molecular size, or a combination of these factors [94]. Fresh-frozen plasma (FFP) or factor concentrates such as prothrombin complex concentrate (PCC) or recombinant factor VIIa (rFVIIa) may be considered [95], but none of these have been adequately studied. Additionally, factor concentrates have been associated with a risk of thrombosis and should be reserved for clinical situations refractory to general approaches to bleeding management [96, 97].

Special Considerations

Pregnancy

In the last decade, LMWH has become preferred over UFH in pregnant women requiring anticoagulation due to reduced monitoring requirements, less osteopenia, and lower risk of HIT. However, women with confirmed or suspected HIT, or those with allergies to UFH or LMWH, require an alternative anticoagulant. There have been case reports of successful use of fondaparinux in pregnancy, but most were limited to the second or third trimester. It is a very small molecule, and anti-Xa activity has been detected in cord plasma of newborns, indicating fetal exposure, and harm is possible. Because of the low quality and paucity of existing evidence, the ACCP 2012 guidelines suggest consideration of fondaparinux only in pregnant women with a contraindication to UFH or LMWH, such as HIT or severe allergic reaction, who cannot receive an alternative agent, danaparoid (Grade 2C). It is important for clinicians to be aware that danaparoid is not available in the USA. If fondaparinux must be used, it should be avoided in the first trimester if possible [98, 99].

Breastfeeding

Warfarin, which is not excreted in breast milk due to a high degree of protein binding and low lipophilicity, and LMWHs, which are not absorbed from an infant's gut, are both acceptable anticoagulant therapies for breastfeeding women. Similar to LMWH, only miniscule amounts of fondaparinux would be expected to be absorbed from the gut of a nursing infant. However, based on the lack of evidence, ACCP suggests alternative anticoagulants rather than fondaparinux in breastfeeding women (Grade 2C) [98].

Pediatric

The evidence for use of fondaparinux in pediatric patients is limited to case reports and small pharmacokinetic studies, mostly in patients with HIT using a wide variety of doses [59, 100–102]. Until more data is available, the use in this population should be reserved for patients that are unable to receive alternative therapies.

Conclusion

While much of the recent interest in anticoagulants has focused on oral agents, such as DOACs, the need for parenteral DTIs and fondaparinux will remain, particularly in niche clinical situations where conventional therapies cannot be used. In order to promote optimized patient outcomes with these high-risk therapies, clinicians must have a good working knowledge of their pharmacology, role in therapy, as well as evidence-based recommendations for their use.

Key Points

- Parenteral DTIs may be more advantageous than heparins because they prevent both thrombus initiation and propagation.
- Bivalirudin is minimally reliant on organ elimination, being primarily cleared by plasma esterases. Thus, it is preferred in patients with diminished organ function.
- Bivalirudin monotherapy may be associated with less bleeding than UFH in PCI without HIT, but UFH in combination with a GPI may be preferred for patients at higher ischemic risk due to a potential increased risk of stent thrombosis.
- A fixed dose of fondaparinux 10 mg SQ once daily may be used in obese patients (weight ≥100 kg) with acute VTE without the need for monitoring or increased doses.
- Fondaparinux does not affect the INR or the aPTT and can be used with stable, fixed doses in HIT patients with normal renal function.
- Fondaparinux is not recommended as initial anticoagulant therapy in patients with STEMI undergoing primary PCI due to risk for catheter-associated thrombosis.

Self-Assessment Questions

1. A patient is diagnosed with HIT with active thrombosis and has been initiated on argatroban and overlapping warfarin. He has received 3 consecutive doses of warfarin 5 mg daily, and his INR this morning is 3.6. Which of the following is the most appropriate plan?
   (a) Reduce warfarin dose to 2.5 mg daily and continue overlap for another 2 days with goal INR of 2–3.
   (b) Discontinue argatroban now. Continue with the current warfarin dose and discharge the patient once INR > 4.
   (c) Disregard the elevated INR as an assay artifact and monitor the aPTT as the primary anticoagulation parameter for the warfarin during the 5 day overlap.
   (d) Continue with current warfarin dose and ensure INR > 4 prior to discontinuation of argatroban.
2. Which of the following is the most appropriate way to monitor the anticoagulant effect of bivalirudin during coronary artery bypass grafting (CABG)?
   (a) aPTT at baseline, after initial bolus, and every 30 min for the entirety of the procedure with a goal of 1.5–2.5× baseline
   (b) ACT after initial bolus and as needed throughout the procedure with a goal of >300 s
   (c) ACT at baseline, after initial bolus, and as needed throughout the procedure with a goal of 200 s
   (d) Chromogenic factor X activity assay after initial bolus and every 30 min for the entirety of the procedure with goal of 20–40%
3. A 65-year-old man has undergone a total knee arthroplasty and is to be discharged to a rehabilitation facility with postsurgical VTE prophylaxis. Which of the following would be the most reasonable regimen?
   (a) Fondaparinux 7.5 mg once daily for 2–4 weeks
   (b) Enoxaparin 1 mg/kg BID for 2–4 weeks
   (c) Fondaparinux 2.5 mg once daily indefinitely
   (d) Fondaparinux 2.5 mg once daily for 2–4 weeks
4. A 55-year-old man presents to the emergency department with left lower extremity pain, swelling, and redness. He denies any recent trauma, surgery, personal or family history of clots, or prolonged travel. His height is 157 cm, weight is 109 kg, and BMI is 44.2. His renal function and coagulation assays are normal. He is diagnosed with a right lower extremity deep vein thrombosis in the common femoral vein. He is stable and appropriate for outpatient treatment of his DVT.

(a) An anti-Xa assay should be monitored and the fondaparinux dose adjusted accordingly since he is obese.
(b) Fondaparinux should be initiated at 7.5 mg SQ once daily and overlapped with warfarin for a minimum of 3 days or until the INR is >2.
(c) Intravenous unfractionated heparin would be preferred over fondaparinux for initial VTE treatment in this patient according to the ACCP guidelines.
(d) Fondaparinux should be initiated at 10 mg SQ once daily and overlapped with warfarin for a minimum of 5 days and until the INR is >2.

5. A 68-year-old woman presents to the emergency department with a chief complaint of chest pain. She is diagnosed with an NSTEMI and is to undergo PCI. Which of the following is the most accurate statement regarding anticoagulation therapy for coronary reperfusion in this patient?
(a) Unfractionated heparin may be preferred over bivalirudin in patients at a higher risk of bleeding.
(b) Unfractionated heparin has been shown to have a higher rate of stent thrombosis compared to bivalirudin.
(c) Fondaparinux is a reasonable initial anticoagulation strategy as long as IV UFH is administered prior to PCI.
(d) Bivalirudin plus a glycoprotein inhibitor (GPI) is a reasonable alternative to IV UFH.

Self-Assessment Answers

1. (d) Continue with current warfarin dose and ensure INR > 4 prior to discontinuation of argatroban

   Argatroban is to be continued until the INR is >4 when overlapping with warfarin initiation because argatroban is known to increase the INR level.

2. (b) ACT after initial bolus and as needed throughout the procedure with a goal of >300 s

   The goal ACT level for bivalirudin administration during CABG is >300 s.

3. (d) Fondaparinux 2.5 mg once daily for 2–4 weeks

   VTE prophylaxis with fondaparinux is usually performed for 2–4 weeks at a once-daily dose of 2.5 mg.

4. (d) Fondaparinux should be initiated at 10 mg SQ once daily and overlapped with warfarin for a minimum of 5 days and until the INR is >2.

   Given that this man's weight is >100 kg, the acute VTE treatment dose for fondaparinux is 10 mg daily. This should be continued for at least 5 days and until the INR is >2 when used as overlapping therapy for warfarin initiation.

5. (d) Bivalirudin plus a glycoprotein inhibitor (GPI) is a reasonable alternative to IV UFH.

   Bivalirudin is an acceptable alternative to and may be preferred over UFH for patients undergoing PCI for NSTEMI.

References

1. Kaplan KL. Direct thrombin inhibitors. Expert Opin Pharmacother. 2003;4(5):653–66.
2. Di Nisio M, Middeldorp S, Büller HR. Direct thrombin inhibitors. N Engl J Med. 2005;353(10):1028–40.
3. Reed MD, Bell D. Clinical pharmacology of bivalirudin. Pharmacotherapy. 2002;22(6 Pt 2):105S–11S.
4. Lee CJ, Ansell JE. Direct thrombin inhibitors. Br J Clin Pharmacol. 2011;72(4):581–92.
5. Bivalirudin (Angiomax) package insert [Internet]. Available from: http://www.angiomax.com/downloads/ANG_USPI.pdf. Accessed 18 Dec 2016.
6. Swan SK, Hursting MJ. The pharmacokinetics and pharmacodynamics of argatroban: effects of age, gender, and hepatic or renal dysfunction. Pharmacotherrapy. 2000;20(3):318–29.
7. Argatroban package insert [Internet]. Available from: https://www.gsksource.com/pharma/content/dam/GlaxoSmithKline/US/en/Prescribing_Information/Argatroban/pdf/ARGATROBAN.PDF. Accessed 18 Dec 2016.
8. Robson R, White H, Aylward P, Frampton C. Bivalirudin pharmacokinetics and pharmacodynamics: effect of renal function, dose, and gender. Clin Pharmacol Ther. 2002;71(6):433–9.
9. Garcia DA, Baglin TP, Weitz JI, Samama MM. American College of Chest Physicians. Parenteral anticoagulants: antithrombotic therapy and prevention of thrombosis, 9th ed: American College of Chest Physicians Evidence-Based Clinical Practice Guidelines. Chest. 2012;141(2 Suppl):e24S–43S.
10. Donat F, Duret JP, Santoni A, Cariou R, Necciari J, Magnani H, et al. The pharmacokinetics of

fondaparinux sodium in healthy volunteers. Clin Pharmacokinet. 2002;41(Suppl 2):1–9.
11. Fondaparinux package insert [Internet]. Available from: http://www.accessdata.fda.gov/drugsatfda_docs/label/2005/021345s010lbl.pdf. Accessed 27 Nov 2016.
12. Hohlfelder B, DeiCicchi D, Sylvester KW, Connors JM. Development of a predictive nomogram for the change in PT/INR upon discontinuation of bivalirudin as a bridge to warfarin. Clin Appl Thromb Hemost. 2016;23(5):487–93.
13. Walenga JM, Drenth AF, Mayuga M, Hoppensteadt DA, Prechel M, Harder S, et al. Transition from argatroban to oral anticoagulation with phenprocoumon or acenocoumarol: effect on coagulation factor testing. Clin Appl Thromb Hemost. 2008;14(3):325–31.
14. Warkentin TE, Greinacher A, Koster A. Bivalirudin. Thromb Haemost. 2008;99(5):830–9.
15. Linkins L-A, Dans AL, Moores LK, Bona R, Davidson BL, Schulman S, et al. Treatment and prevention of heparin-induced thrombocytopenia. Chest. 2012;141(2 Suppl):e495S–530S.
16. Cuker A, Gimotty PA, Crowther MA, Warkentin TE. Predictive value of the 4Ts scoring system for heparin-induced thrombocytopenia: a systematic review and meta-analysis. Blood. 2012;120(20):4160–7.
17. Lewis BE, Wallis DE, Berkowitz SD, Matthai WH, Fareed J, Walenga JM, et al. Argatroban anticoagulant therapy in patients with heparin-induced thrombocytopenia. Circulation. 2001;103(14):1838–43.
18. Lewis BE, Wallis DE, Leya F, Hursting MJ, Kelton JG, Argatroban-915 Investigators. Argatroban anticoagulation in patients with heparin-induced thrombocytopenia. Arch Intern Med. 2003;163(15):1849–56.
19. Cuker A, Cines DB. How I treat heparin-induced thrombocytopenia. Blood. 2012;119(10):2209–18.
20. Bain J, Meyer A. Comparison of bivalirudin to lepirudin and argatroban in patients with heparin-induced thrombocytopenia. Am J Health Syst Pharm. 2015;72(17 Suppl. 2):S104–9.
21. Vo QA, Lin JK, Tong LM. Efficacy and safety of argatroban and bivalirudin in patients with suspected heparin-induced thrombocytopenia. Ann Pharmacother. 2015;49(2):178–84.
22. Zeymer U, Rao SV, Montalescot G. Anticoagulation in coronary intervention. Eur Heart J. 2016;37(45):3376–85.
23. Jang I-K, Lewis BE, Matthai WH, Kleiman NS. Argatroban anticoagulation in conjunction with glycoprotein IIb/IIIa inhibition in patients undergoing percutaneous coronary intervention: an open-label, nonrandomized pilot study. J Thromb Thrombolysis. 2004;18(1):31–7.
24. Lee MS, Liao H, Yang T, Dhoot J, Tobis J, Fonarow G, et al. Comparison of bivalirudin versus heparin plus glycoprotein IIb/IIIa inhibitors in patients undergoing an invasive strategy: a meta-analysis of randomized clinical trials. Int J Cardiol. 2011;152(3):369–74.
25. Amsterdam EA, Wenger NK, Brindis RG, Casey DE, Ganiats TG, Holmes DR, et al. 2014 AHA/ACC guideline for the management of patients with non–ST-elevation acute coronary syndromes. J Am Coll Cardiol. 2014;64(24):e139–228.
26. O'Gara PT, Kushner FG, Ascheim DD, Casey DE, Chung MK, et al. 2013 ACCF/AHA guideline for the management of ST-elevation myocardial infarction. Circulation. 2013;127(4):e362–425.
27. Roffi M, Patrono C, Collet J-P, Mueller C, Valgimigli M, Andreotti F, et al. 2015 ESC Guidelines for the management of acute coronary syndromes in patients presenting without persistent ST-segment elevation: task force for the management of acute coronary syndromes in patients presenting without persistent ST-Segment Elevation of the European Society of Cardiology (ESC). Eur Heart J. 2016;37(3):267–315.
28. Steg PG, James SK, Atar D, Badano LP, Lundqvist CB, et al. ESC Guidelines for the management of acute myocardial infarction in patients presenting with ST-segment elevation. Eur Heart J. 2012;33(20):2569–619.
29. Cavender MA, Sabatine MS. Bivalirudin versus heparin in patients planned for percutaneous coronary intervention: a meta-analysis of randomised controlled trials. Lancet. 2014;384(9943):599–606.
30. Bavry AA, Elgendy IY, Mahmoud A, Jadhav MP, Huo T. Critical appraisal of bivalirudin versus heparin for percutaneous coronary intervention: a meta-analysis of randomized trials. PLoS One. 2015;10(5):e0127832.
31. Windecker S, Kolh P, Alfonso F, Collet J-P, Cremer J, et al. ESC/EACTS Guidelines on myocardial revascularization. Eur Heart J. 2014;35(37):2541–619.
32. Lewis BE, Matthai WH, Cohen M, Moses JW, Hursting MJ, Leya F, et al. Argatroban anticoagulation during percutaneous coronary intervention in patients with heparin-induced thrombocytopenia. Catheter Cardiovasc Interv. 2002;57(2):177–84.
33. Cruz-Gonzalez I, Sanchez-Ledesma M, Baron SJ, Healy JL, Watanabe H, Osakabe M, et al. Efficacy and safety of argatroban with or without glycoprotein IIb/IIIa inhibitor in patients with heparin induced thrombocytopenia undergoing percutaneous coronary intervention for acute coronary syndrome. J Thromb Thrombolysis. 2008;25(2):214–8.
34. Mahaffey KW, Lewis BE, Wildermann NM, Berkowitz SD, Oliverio RM, Turco MA, et al. The anticoagulant therapy with bivalirudin to assist in the performance of percutaneous coronary intervention in patients with heparin-induced thrombocytopenia (ATBAT) study: main results. J Invasive Cardiol. 2003;15(11):611–6.
35. Levine GN, Bates ER, Blankenship JC, Bailey SR, Bittl JA, Cercek B, et al. 2011 ACCF/AHA/SCAI guideline for percutaneous coronary intervention:

a report of the American College of Cardiology Foundation/American Heart Association Task Force on Practice Guidelines and the Society for Cardiovascular Angiography and Interventions. J Am Coll Cardiol. 2011;58(24):e44–122.
36. Jang I-K, Brown DFM, Giugliano RP, Anderson HV, Losordo D, Nicolau JC, et al. A multicenter, randomized study of argatroban versus heparin as adjunct to tissue plasminogen activator (TPA) in acute myocardial infarction: myocardial infarction with Novastan and TPA (MINT) study. J Am Coll Cardiol. 1999;33(7):1879–85.
37. Vermeer F, Vahanian A, Fels PW, Besse P, Müller E, Van de Werf F, et al. Argatroban and alteplase in patients with acute myocardial infarction: the ARGAMI Study. J Thromb Thrombolysis. 2000;10(3):233–40.
38. Dyke CM, Smedira NG, Koster A, Aronson S, McCarthy HL, Kirshner R, et al. A comparison of bivalirudin to heparin with protamine reversal in patients undergoing cardiac surgery with cardiopulmonary bypass: the EVOLUTION-ON study. J Thorac Cardiovasc Surg. 2006;131(3):533–9.
39. Smedira NG, Dyke CM, Koster A, Jurmann M, Bhatia DS, Hu T, et al. Anticoagulation with bivalirudin for off-pump coronary artery bypass grafting: the results of the EVOLUTION-OFF study. J Thorac Cardiovasc Surg. 2006;131(3):686–92.
40. Koster A, Dyke CM, Aldea G, Smedira NG, McCarthy HL, Aronson S, et al. Bivalirudin during cardiopulmonary bypass in patients with previous or acute heparin-induced thrombocytopenia and heparin antibodies: results of the CHOOSE-ON trial. Ann Thorac Surg. 2007;83(2):572–7.
41. Beiderlinden M, Treschan T, Görlinger K, Peters J. Argatroban in extracorporeal membrane oxygenation. Artif Organs. 2007;31(6):461–5.
42. Falck-Ytter Y, Francis CW, Johanson NA, Curley C, Dahl OE, Schulman S, et al. Prevention of vte in orthopedic surgery patients: antithrombotic therapy and prevention of thrombosis, 9th ed: American College of Chest Physicians Evidence-Based Clinical Practice Guidelines. Chest. 2012 Feb 1;141(2 suppl):e278S–325S.
43. Gould MK, Garcia DA, Wren SM, Karanicolas PJ, Arcelus JI, Heit JA, et al. Prevention of VTE in nonorthopedic surgical patients: antithrombotic therapy and prevention of thrombosis, 9th ed: American College of Chest Physicians Evidence-Based Clinical Practice Guidelines. Chest. 2012;141(2 Suppl):e227S–77S.
44. Kahn SR, Lim W, Dunn AS, Cushman M, Dentali F, Akl EA, et al. Prevention of VTE in nonsurgical patients: antithrombotic therapy and prevention of thrombosis, 9th ed: American College of Chest Physicians Evidence-Based Clinical Practice Guidelines. Chest. 2012;141(2 Suppl):e195S–226S.
45. Smythe MA, Priziola J, Dobesh PP, Wirth D, Cuker A, Wittkowsky AK. Guidance for the practical management of the heparin anticoagulants in the treatment of venous thromboembolism. J Thromb Thrombolysis. 2016;41(1):165–86.
46. Kearon C, Akl EA, Comerota AJ, Prandoni P, Bounameaux H, Goldhaber SZ, et al. Antithrombotic therapy for vte disease: antithrombotic therapy and prevention of thrombosis, 9th ed: American College of Chest Physicians Evidence-Based Clinical Practice Guidelines. Chest. 2012 Feb 1;141(2 Suppl):e419S–94S.
47. Warkentin TE. HIT paradigms and paradoxes. J Thromb Haemost. 2011;9(Suppl 1):105–17.
48. Arpino PA, Goeller AJ, Fatalo A, Van Cott EM. Evaluation of 2 nomogram-based strategies for dosing argatroban in patients with known or suspected heparin induced thrombocytopenia. Clin Appl Thromb Hemost. 2015;21(3):260–5.
49. Hursting MJ, Lewis BE, Macfarlane DE. Transitioning from argatroban to warfarin therapy in patients with heparin-induced thrombocytopenia. Clin Appl Thromb Hemost. 2005;11(3):279–87.
50. Bartholomew JR, Hursting MJ. Transitioning from argatroban to warfarin in heparin-induced thrombocytopenia: an analysis of outcomes in patients with elevated international normalized ratio (INR). J Thromb Thrombolysis. 2005;19(3):183–8.
51. Tolwani AJ, Wille KM. Anticoagulation for continuous renal replacement therapy. Semin Dial. 2009;22(2):141–5.
52. Tsu LV, Dager WE. Bivalirudin dosing adjustments for reduced renal function with or without hemodialysis in the management of heparin-induced thrombocytopenia. Ann Pharmacother. 2011;45(10):1185–92.
53. Pieri M, Agracheva N, Bonaveglio E, Greco T, Bonis MD, Covello RD, et al. Bivalirudin versus heparin as an anticoagulant during extracorporeal membrane oxygenation: a case-control study. J Cardiothorac Vasc Anesth. 2013;27(1):30–4.
54. Ranucci M, Ballotta A, Kandil H, Isgrò G, Carlucci C, Baryshnikova E, et al. Bivalirudin-based versus conventional heparin anticoagulation for postcardiotomy extracorporeal membrane oxygenation. Crit Care. 2011;15:R275.
55. Angiox. European medicines agency summary of product characteristics [Internet]. Available from: http://www.angiomax.com/angiox/Angiox-PIs/Angiox%20SmPC%20en%2012.2015.pdf. Accessed 1 Jan 2017.
56. Young SK, Al-Mondhiry HA, Vaida SJ, Ambrose A, Botti JJ. Successful use of argatroban during the third trimester of pregnancy: case report and review of the literature. Pharmacotherapy. 2008; 28(12):1531–6.
57. Buck ML. Bivalirudin as an alternative to heparin for anticoagulation in infants and children. J Pediatr Pharmacol Ther. 2015;20(6):408–17.
58. Chan VHT, Monagle P, Massicotte P, Chan AK. Novel paediatric anticoagulants: a review of

the current literature. Blood Coagul Fibrinolysis. 2010;21(2):144–51.
59. Young G. Anticoagulants in children and adolescents. Hematology Am Soc Hematol Educ Program. 2015;2015:111–6.
60. Weitz JI. Factor Xa or thrombin: is thrombin a better target? J Thromb Haemost. 2007;5:65–7.
61. Olson ST, Björk I, Sheffer R, Craig PA, Shore JD, Choay J. Role of the antithrombin-binding pentasaccharide in heparin acceleration of antithrombin-proteinase reactions. Resolution of the antithrombin conformational change contribution to heparin rate enhancement. J Biol Chem. 1992;267(18):12528–38.
62. Choay J, Petitou M, Lormeau JC, Sinaÿ P, Casu B, Gatti G. Structure-activity relationship in heparin: a synthetic pentasaccharide with high affinity for antithrombin III and eliciting high anti-factor Xa activity. Biochem Biophys Res Commun. 1983;116(2):492–9.
63. Paolucci F, Claviés M-C, Donat F, Necciari J. Fondaparinux sodium mechanism of action: identification of specific binding to purified and human plasma-derived proteins. Clin Pharmacokinet. 2002;41(12):11–8.
64. Arixtra. European medicines agency summary of product characteristics [Internet]. Available from: http://www.ema.europa.eu/docs/en_GB/document_library/EPAR_-_Product_Information/human/000403/WC500027746.pdf. Accessed 27 Nov 2016.
65. Bergqvist D. Review of fondaparinux sodium injection for the prevention of venous thromboembolism in patients undergoing surgery. Vasc Health Risk Manag. 2006;2(4):365–70.
66. Koshida S, Suda Y, Sobel M, Ormsby J, Kusumoto S. Synthesis of heparin partial structures and their binding activities to platelets. Bioorg Med Chem Lett. 1999;9(21):3127–32.
67. Smogorzewska A, Brandt JT, Chandler WL, Cunningham MT, Hayes TE, Olson JD, et al. Effect of fondaparinux on coagulation assays: results of College of American Pathologists proficiency testing. Arch Pathol Lab Med. 2006;130(11):1605–11.
68. Turpie AGG, Bauer KA, Eriksson BI, Lassen MR. Fondaparinux vs enoxaparin for the prevention of venous thromboembolism in major orthopedic surgery: a meta-analysis of 4 randomized double-blind studies. Arch Intern Med. 2002;162(16):1833–40.
69. Colwell CW, Kwong LM, Turpie AGG, Davidson BL. Flexibility in administration of fondaparinux for prevention of symptomatic venous thromboembolism in orthopaedic surgery. J Arthroplast. 2006;21(1):36–45.
70. Turpie AGG, Bauer KA, Eriksson BI, Lassen MR. Superiority of fondaparinux over enoxaparin in preventing venous thromboembolism in major orthopedic surgery using different efficacy end points. Chest. 2004;126(2):501–8.
71. Eriksson BI, Lassen MR. PENTasaccharide in HIp-FRActure Surgery Plus Investigators. Duration of prophylaxis against venous thromboembolism with fondaparinux after hip fracture surgery: a multicenter, randomized, placebo-controlled, double-blind study. Arch Intern Med. 2003;163(11):1337–42.
72. Agnelli G, Bergqvist D, Cohen AT, Gallus AS, Gent M, PEGASUS investigators. Randomized clinical trial of postoperative fondaparinux versus perioperative dalteparin for prevention of venous thromboembolism in high-risk abdominal surgery. Br J Surg. 2005;92(10):1212–20.
73. Turpie AGG, Bauer KA, Caprini JA, Comp PC, Gent M, Muntz JE, et al. Fondaparinux combined with intermittent pneumatic compression vs. intermittent pneumatic compression alone for prevention of venous thromboembolism after abdominal surgery: a randomized, double-blind comparison. J Thromb Haemost. 2007;5(9):1854–61.
74. Cohen AT, Davidson BL, Gallus AS, Lassen MR, Prins MH, Tomkowski W, et al. Efficacy and safety of fondaparinux for the prevention of venous thromboembolism in older acute medical patients: randomised placebo controlled trial. BMJ. 2006;332(7537):325–9.
75. Büller HR, Davidson BL, Decousus H, Gallus A, Gent M, Piovella F, et al. Fondaparinux or enoxaparin for the initial treatment of symptomatic deep venous thrombosis: a randomized trial. Ann Intern Med. 2004;140(11):867–73.
76. Büller HR, Davidson BL, Decousus H, Gallus A, Gent M, Piovella F, et al. Subcutaneous fondaparinux versus intravenous unfractionated heparin in the initial treatment of pulmonary embolism. N Engl J Med. 2003;349(18):1695–702.
77. Davidson BL, Büller HR, Decousus H, Gallus A, Gent M, Piovella F, et al. Effect of obesity on outcomes after fondaparinux, enoxaparin, or heparin treatment for acute venous thromboembolism in the Matisse trials. J Thromb Haemost. 2007;5(6):1191–4.
78. Di Nisio M, Middeldorp S. Treatment of lower extremity superficial thrombophlebitis. JAMA. 2014;311(7):729–30.
79. Decousus H, Prandoni P, Mismetti P, Bauersachs RM, Boda Z, Brenner B, et al. Fondaparinux for the treatment of superficial-vein thrombosis in the legs. N Engl J Med. 2010;363(13):1222–32.
80. Blondon M, Righini M, Bounameaux H, Veenstra DL. Fondaparinux for isolated superficial vein thrombosis of the legs: a cost-effectiveness analysis. Chest. 2012;141(2):321–9.
81. Kang M, Alahmadi M, Sawh S, Kovacs MJ, Lazo-Langner A. Fondaparinux for the treatment of suspected heparin-induced thrombocytopenia: a propensity score-matched study. Blood. 2015;125(6):924–9.
82. Warkentin TE, Pai M, Sheppard JI, Schulman S, Spyropoulos AC, Eikelboom JW. Fondaparinux treatment of acute heparin-induced thrombocytopenia confirmed by the serotonin-release assay:

a 30-month, 16-patient case series. J Thromb Haemost. 2011;9(12):2389–96.
83. Schindewolf M, Steindl J, Beyer-Westendorf J, Schellong S, Dohmen PM, Brachmann J, et al. Frequent off-label use of fondaparinux in patients with suspected acute heparin-induced thrombocytopenia (HIT)--findings from the GerHIT multi-centre registry study. Thromb Res. 2014;134(1):29–35.
84. Warkentin TE, Maurer BT, Aster RH. Heparin-induced thrombocytopenia associated with fondaparinux. N Engl J Med. 2007;356(25):2653–5.
85. Rota E, Bazzan M, Fantino G. Fondaparinux-related thrombocytopenia in a previous low-molecular-weight heparin (LMWH)-induced heparin-induced thrombocytopenia (HIT). Thromb Haemost. 2008; 99(4):779–81.
86. Alsaleh KA, Al-Nasser SMA, Bates SM, Patel A, Warkentin TE, Arnold DM. Delayed-onset HIT caused by low-molecular-weight heparin manifesting during fondaparinux prophylaxis. Am J Hematol. 2008;83(11):876–8.
87. Warkentin TE. Fondaparinux: does it cause HIT? Can it treat HIT? Expert Rev Hematol. 2010;3(5):567–81.
88. Cuker A. Management of the multiple phases of heparin-induced thrombocytopenia. Thromb Haemost. 2016;116(5):835–42.
89. Mehta SR, Granger CB, Eikelboom JW, Bassand J-P, Wallentin L, Faxon DP, et al. Efficacy and safety of fondaparinux versus enoxaparin in patients with acute coronary syndromes undergoing percutaneous coronary intervention: results from the OASIS-5 trial. J Am Coll Cardiol. 2007;50(18):1742–51.
90. Simoons ML, Bobbink IWG, Boland J, Gardien M, Klootwijk P, Lensing AWA, et al. A dose-finding study of fondaparinux in patients with non-ST-segment elevation acute coronary syndromes: the Pentasaccharide in Unstable Angina (PENTUA) Study. J Am Coll Cardiol. 2004;43(12):2183–90.
91. Steg PG, Mehta S, Jolly S, Xavier D, Rupprecht H-J, Lopez-Sendon JL, et al. Fondaparinux with UnfracTionated heparin dUring Revascularization in Acute coronary syndromes (FUTURA/OASIS 8): a randomized trial of intravenous unfractionated heparin during percutaneous coronary intervention in patients with non-ST-segment elevation acute coronary syndromes initially treated with fondaparinux. Am Heart J. 2010;160(6):1029–34. 1034.e1.
92. Yusuf S, Mehta SR, Chrolavicius S, Afzal R, Pogue J, Granger CB, et al. Effects of fondaparinux on mortality and reinfarction in patients with acute ST-segment elevation myocardial infarction: the OASIS-6 randomized trial. JAMA. 2006;295(13):1519–30.
93. Davidson B, Turpie AGG, Colwell C, Kwong LM. Early vs delayed initiation of fondaparinux prophylaxis to prevent postoperative pulmonary embolism: a clinical endpoint study. Chest. 2004;126(4 MeetingAbstracts):783S-b–783S.
94. Crowther MA, Berry LR, Monagle PT, Chan AKC. Mechanisms responsible for the failure of protamine to inactivate low-molecular-weight heparin. Br J Haematol. 2002;116(1):178–86.
95. Bijsterveld NR, Moons AH, Boekholdt SM, van Aken BE, Fennema H, Peters RJG, et al. Ability of recombinant factor VIIa to reverse the anticoagulant effect of the pentasaccharide fondaparinux in healthy volunteers. Circulation. 2002;106(20):2550–4.
96. Dentali F, Marchesi C, Giorgi Pierfranceschi M, Crowther M, Garcia D, Hylek E, et al. Safety of prothrombin complex concentrates for rapid anticoagulation reversal of vitamin K antagonists. A meta-analysis. Thromb Haemost. 2011;106(3):429–38.
97. Levi M, Levy JH, Andersen HF, Truloff D. Safety of recombinant activated factor VII in randomized clinical trials. N Engl J Med. 2010;363(19):1791–800.
98. Bates SM, Greer IA, Middeldorp S, Veenstra DL, Prabulos A-M, Vandvik PO, et al. VTE, thrombophilia, antithrombotic therapy, and pregnancy: antithrombotic therapy and prevention of thrombosis, 9th ed: American College of Chest Physicians Evidence-Based Clinical Practice Guidelines. Chest. 2012;141(2 Suppl):e691S–736S.
99. Carolis SD, di Pasquo E, Rossi E, Sordo GD, Buonomo A, Schiavino D, et al. Fondaparinux in pregnancy: could it be a safe option? A review of the literature. Thromb Res. 2015;135(6):1049–51.
100. Young G, Yee DL, O'Brien SH, Khanna R, Barbour A, Nugent DJ. FondaKIDS: a prospective pharmacokinetic and safety study of fondaparinux in children between 1 and 18 years of age. Pediatr Blood Cancer. 2011;57(6):1049–54.
101. Ko RH, Michieli C, Lira JL, Young G. FondaKIDS II: long-term follow-up data of children receiving fondaparinux for treatment of venous thromboembolic events. Thromb Res. 2014;134(3):643–7.
102. Monagle P, Chan AKC, Goldenberg NA, Ichord RN, Journeycake JM, Nowak-Göttl U, et al. Antithrombotic therapy in neonates and children: antithrombotic therapy and prevention of thrombosis, 9th ed: American College of Chest Physicians Evidence-Based Clinical Practice Guidelines. Chest. 2012;141(2 Suppl):e737S–801S.

Direct Oral Anticoagulants

5

Natalie S. Evans

Clinical Vignettes

Case 1: *A 68-year-old woman presents to her primary physician's office with complaints of mild shortness of breath and palpitations. She has a history of hypertension, well-controlled diabetes, mild chronic kidney disease, and remote gastrointestinal bleeding related to peptic ulcer disease. Current medications are lisinopril, metformin, and omeprazole. Exam reveals irregularly irregular heartbeat. An electrocardiogram performed in the office reveals atrial fibrillation with a rate of 97 beats per minute. The physician would like to start her on a direct oral anticoagulant but has concerns about her history of bleeding.*

Case 2: *A 48-year-old man is seen in his primary physician's office a week after an emergency department visit at which he was diagnosed with a proximal deep vein thrombosis (DVT) and started on apixaban 10 mg twice daily. He has a history of well-controlled hypertension but is otherwise healthy, and no risk factor for venous thromboembolism (VTE) is identified. He is concerned because he has heard that the "new blood thinners don't have an antidote." The physician is unsure how to counsel the patient on the risks and benefits of the DOACs.*

Introduction

In 2010, the first commercially available non-vitamin K antagonist, dabigatran etexilate, was approved for stroke prevention in non-valvular atrial fibrillation, marking the advent of a new age in anticoagulation. Since then, three additional direct oral anticoagulants (DOACs) have been approved for use in patients with atrial fibrillation and venous thromboembolism. Prior to the development of dabigatran, efforts to develop a non-vitamin K antagonist (VKA) oral anticoagulant had been disappointing. The first such drug, ximelagatran, was never approved for use in the United States after completion of phase 3 trials in VTE prevention and treatment due to hepatotoxicity.

N. S. Evans (✉)
Department of Cardiovascular Medicine, Section of Vascular Medicine, Cleveland Clinic, Cleveland, OH, USA
e-mail: evansn2@ccf.org

J. F. Lau et al. (eds.), *Anticoagulation Therapy*, https://doi.org/10.1007/978-3-319-73709-6_5

Direct Thrombin Inhibitors

Pharmacology

Dabigatran is a competitive, reversible direct inhibitor of the active site of both free and clot-bound thrombin [1]. It is administered as a pro-drug (dabigatran etexilate) and rapidly converted to active drug. It reaches a peak plasma concentration within approximately 2 h of ingestion. Breaking the drug capsule may lead to increases in bioavailability, so patients must be instructed not to break, chew, or crush the capsules. It may be taken with or without food. Dabigatran interacts with the p-glycoprotein efflux transporter. Therefore, co-administration with rifampin, a strong inducer of p-GP, should be avoided, as clearance of dabigatran may be increased. Conversely, p-GP inhibitors such as dronedarone and ketoconazole can lead to increased concentrations of dabigatran, so the dose of dabigatran should be adjusted, and the medication should be avoided altogether in patients with renal insufficiency. Co-administration of other p-GP inhibitors such as verapamil and amiodarone does not require dose adjustment of dabigatran. Dabigatran is about 35% bound to plasma proteins, and about 80% of the drug is eliminated by the kidneys, with a half-life of 15–17 h [2].

Indications

Prevention of Stroke and Systemic Embolism in Non-valvular Atrial Fibrillation

Dabigatran was approved for the reduction of risk of stroke and systemic embolism in patients with non-valvular atrial fibrillation based on the results of the RE-LY trial, an unblinded non-inferiority study of more than 18,000 participants. Patients were randomly assigned to either dabigatran 150 mg or 110 mg twice daily or warfarin adjusted to maintain an INR of 2.0–3.0 [3]. The mean age of patients was 71 years, and 64% were men. Patients with Cockcroft-Gault-estimated creatinine clearance (CG-CrCl) <30 mL/min were excluded. Dabigatran at the 110 mg dose was non-inferior and at the 150 mg dose superior to warfarin in preventing stroke or systemic embolism. Rates of major bleeding—defined as a fall in hemoglobin of 2 g/dL or more, transfusion of 2 or more units of packed red blood cells, or bleeding in a critical site or with a fatal outcome—were similar (Table 5.1). Dabigatran had statistically significantly lower rates of intracranial hemorrhage but higher rates of gastrointestinal bleeding than warfarin. Patients older than 75 years taking dabigatran had higher bleeding rates than younger patients.

Although the 110 mg dose was studied in the trial, the Food and Drug Administration (FDA)-approved dose for patients with a CrCl 15–30 mL/min is 75 mg twice daily, which has not been studied in a prospective, randomized trial.

Treatment and Secondary Prevention of Deep Vein Thrombosis and Pulmonary Embolism

Dabigatran for the treatment of venous thromboembolism (VTE) was studied in the RE-COVER and RE-COVER II trials. RE-COVER randomized more than 2500 patients with acute VTE (pulmonary embolism or proximal deep vein thrombosis or both) who were initially treated with parenteral therapy for 5–10 days to dabigatran 150 mg twice daily versus warfarin adjusted to achieve an INR of 2.0–3.0 [4]. Patients with CG-CrCl <30 mL/min were excluded. RE-COVER II also randomized more than 2500 patients with VTE to the same dose of dabigatran versus warfarin [5]. Patients in both trials were relatively young, with a mean age of 56 years. The primary outcome in both trials, recurrent symptomatic VTE and related deaths over 6 months, was no different for dabigatran versus warfarin (Table 5.2). Major bleeding, which was defined similarly to that in the atrial fibrillation trial, was no different, but nonmajor clinically relevant bleeding was lower for the dabigatran group.

The RE-MEDY trial examined secondary prevention of VTE (after more than 3 months of treatment with any anticoagulant) with dabigatran versus warfarin, and the RE-SONATE trial

Table 5.1 Dabigatran versus warfarin (INR 2–3) for thromboprophylaxis in non-valvular atrial fibrillation: clinical outcomes from the RE-LY study [3]

Primary efficacy and safety outcomes for dabigatran vs. warfarin in atrial fibrillation in percent per year					
	Dabigatran 110 mg	Dabigatran 150 mg	Warfarin	110 mg vs. warfarin RR (95% CI)	150 mg vs. warfarin RR (95% CI)
Stroke or systemic embolism	1.53	1.11	1.69	0.91 (0.74–1.11)	0.66 (0.53–0.82)
Major bleeding	2.71	3.11	3.36	0.80 (0.69–0.93)	0.93 (0.81–1.07)
Intracranial hemorrhage	0.23	0.30	0.74	0.31 (0.20–0.47)	0.40 (0.27–0.60)
Gastrointestinal bleeding	1.12	1.51	1.02	1.10 (0.86–1.41)	1.50 (1.19–1.89)

Y year, *RR* relative risk, *CI* confidence interval

Table 5.2 Dabigatran versus warfarin for treatment of venous thromboembolism: results of the RE-COVER study [5]

Primary efficacy and safety outcomes			
	Dabigatran (*N* = 1273)	Warfarin (*N* = 1266)	Hazard ratio (95% confidence interval)
Recurrent symptomatic VTE and VTE-related death	30 (2.4)	27 (2.1)	1.10 (0.65–1.84)
Major bleeding	20 (1.6)	24 (1.9)	0.82 (0.45–1.48)
Intracranial hemorrhage	0	3 (0.2)	
Gastrointestinal bleeding	53 (4.2)	35 (2.8)	

compared dabigatran with placebo for secondary prevention [6]. In RE-MEDY, which randomized 2856 patients, dabigatran was non-inferior to warfarin for preventing recurrent VTE, with a similar rate of major bleeding and a lower rate of major or clinically relevant nonmajor bleeding (Table 5.3). In the RE-SONATE trial, which randomized 1343 patients, major bleeding was rare in the dabigatran arm, with just two cases compared with zero in the placebo group. However, nonmajor clinically relevant bleeding occurred more frequently, in 5.3% of patients compared with 1.8% in the placebo group [6] (Table 5.4).

In the VTE treatment and secondary prevention trials comparing dabigatran with warfarin, patients on dabigatran had significantly higher rates of myocardial infarction, 0.9% of dabigatran patients compared with 0.2% of warfarin patients.

Primary Prophylaxis After Hip Replacement Surgery

In the RE-NOVATE I and II trials [7, 8], 5549 patients were randomized to dabigatran, either 150 mg (RE-NOVATE I only) or 220 mg daily, with a half dose given within 1–4 h after surgery, or enoxaparin 40 mg started the night before surgery to prevent a composite of VTE and death after hip replacement surgery. Patients with a CG-CrCl <30 mL/min were excluded. Treatment was given for 28–35 days. Dabigatran was non-inferior to enoxaparin, with similar rates of bleeding (Table 5.5).

Dabigatran is approved by the US Food and Drug Administration (FDA) to prevent stroke in non-valvular atrial fibrillation at doses of 150 mg BID for patients with CG-CrCl >30 mL/min and 75 mg bid for CG-CrCl 15–30 mL/min. For VTE treatment, dabigatran is indicated in patients with CG-CrCl >30 mg/mL at a dose of 150 mg BID after 5–10 days of treatment with a parenteral agent. Dosing is the same for secondary prevention of recurrent VTE. For prophylaxis in knee and hip replacement surgery, the dose for patients with CrCl >30 mL/min is 110 mg on the first day post-op, followed by 220 mg daily. The drug carries black-box warnings for premature discontinuation, which can increase the risk of thrombotic events, and for spinal or epidural hematoma in patients

Table 5.3 Dabigatran versus warfarin (INR 2–3) for extended treatment of venous thromboembolism: the RE-MEDY study [6]

Primary efficacy and safety outcomes			
	Dabigatran ($N = 1430$)	Warfarin ($N = 1426$)	Hazard ratio (95% confidence interval)
Recurrent or fatal VTE	26 (1.8%)	18 (1.3%)	1.44 (0.78–2.64)
Major bleeding	13 (0.9%)	25 (1.8%)	0.52 (0.27–1.02)
Acute coronary syndrome	13 (0.9%)	3 (0.2%)	95% CI not reported $p = 0.02$

Table 5.4 Dabigatran versus placebo for extended treatment of venous thromboembolism: the RE-SONATE study [6]

Primary efficacy and safety outcomes			
	Dabigatran ($N = 681$)	Placebo ($N = 662$)	Hazard ratio (95% confidence interval)
Recurrent or fatal VTE or unexplained death	3 (0.4%)	37 (5.6%)	0.08 (0.02–0.25)
Major bleeding	2 (0.3%)	0	Not estimable
Acute coronary syndrome	1 (0.1%)	1 (0.2%)	Not reported

Table 5.5 Primary efficacy and safety outcomes for dabigatran versus enoxaparin in VTE thromboprophylaxis after hip replacement surgery [7, 8]

Primary efficacy and safety outcomes			
	Dabigatran 220 mg	Dabigatran 150 mg	Enoxaparin 40 mg
RE-NOVATE			
Total VTE and all-cause mortality	53/880 (6.0%)	75/874 (8.6%)	60/897 (6.7%)
Major bleeding	23/1146 (2.0%)	15/1163 (1.3%)	18/1154 (1.6%)
RE-NOVATE II			
Total VTE and all-cause mortality	61/792 (7.7%)		69/785 (8.8%)
Major bleeding	14/1010 (1.4%)		9/1003 (0.9%)

receiving neuraxial anesthesia or spinal puncture if the medication is not discontinued at an appropriate interval [9].

Direct Factor Xa Inhibitors

Pharmacology

The commercially available direct factor Xa inhibitors—rivaroxaban, apixaban, and edoxaban—are reversible direct inhibitors of free and clot-bound factor Xa. They all achieve rapid peak plasma concentrations within a few hours after ingestion (see Table 5.6); the non-prophylaxis dose of rivaroxaban must be taken with food for optimal absorption [10]. They have few drug-drug interactions, but because they are metabolized through the cytochrome p450 system, there are a few notable ones (Table 5.6). The direct factor Xa inhibitors also can be affected by strong inducers or inhibitors of the p-GP system. They are all eliminated to some degree by the kidneys, so decreasing renal function leads to increased drug levels [11]. The half-lives are short, from 7 to 14 h.

Rivaroxaban

Prevention of Stroke and Systemic Embolism in Non-valvular Atrial Fibrillation

Rivaroxaban is approved to prevent stroke and systemic embolism on the basis of the ROCKET AF trial, which randomized nearly 15,000 patients to treatment with rivaroxaban 20 mg daily or dose-adjusted warfarin with goal INR of 2.0–3.0 [12]. Rivaroxaban was non-inferior to warfarin, and rates of major and clinically relevant nonmajor bleeding were similar (Table 5.7). There were statistically significantly fewer intracranial hemorrhages and fatal bleeding events in patients on rivaroxaban. For patients with CrCl 15–50 mL/min, the FDA approved a 15 mg daily dose.

Table 5.6 Pharmacologic characteristics of DOAC

	Dabigatran	Rivaroxaban	Apixaban	Edoxaban
Target	Factor IIa (thrombin)	Factor Xa		
Time to peak (hours)	1.5–3	2–3	3–4	1–2
Half-life (hours)	12–17	7–11	9–14	9–11
Renal excretion (%)	>80	35	25	35–50
Antidote	Idarucizumab	Andexanet alfa (not approved)		
Significant drug-drug interactions	Dronedarone ↑, ketoconazole↑, rifampin↓	Ketoconazole↑, ritonavir↑, clarithromycin↑, rifampin↓, carbamazepine↓, phenytoin↓	Ketoconazole↑, ritonavir↑, clarithromycin↑, rifampin↓, carbamazepine↓, phenytoin↓	Rifampin↓, carbamazepine↓, phenytoin↓

↑Increases DOAC level
↓Decreases DOAC level

Table 5.7 Primary efficacy and safety outcomes for rivaroxaban versus warfarin for thromboprophylaxis in non-valvular atrial fibrillation: the ROCKET AF study [12]

Primary efficacy and safety outcomes			
	Rivaroxaban	Warfarin	Hazard ratio (95% confidence interval)
Primary outcome	269/7081 (2.1% per year)	306/7090 (2.4% per year)	0.88 (0.75–1.03)
Major bleeding	395/7111 (3.6% per year)	386/7125 (3.4% per year)	1.04 (0.90–1.20)
Intracranial hemorrhage	55/7111 (0.5% per year)	84/7125 (0.7% per year)	0.67 (0.47–0.93)
Gastrointestinal bleeding	224/7111 (3.2%)	154/7125 (2.2%)	NR; $p < 0.001$

NR not reported

Treatment and Secondary Prevention of Deep Vein Thrombosis and Pulmonary Embolism

In the EINSTEIN-DVT study, 3449 patients with acute, symptomatic proximal DVT were randomized to either rivaroxaban or dose-adjusted warfarin and followed for up to 12 months [13]. Rivaroxaban patients were given 15 mg twice daily with food for the first 21 days of treatment, followed by 20 mg daily with food. Patients with a CG-CrCl <30 mL/min were excluded. Rivaroxaban was non-inferior to warfarin in preventing recurrent symptomatic DVT, with similar major and clinically relevant nonmajor bleeding (Table 5.8). In EINSTEIN-PE, 4832 patients with acute, symptomatic PE were randomized to the same regimen as in EINSTEIN-DVT for up to 12 months, and the results were similar: non-inferior to warfarin in prevention of recurrent PE with no difference in major and clinically relevant nonmajor bleeding (Table 5.9) [14]. Comparing major bleeding alone, rivaroxaban appeared safer, with about half the rate of major bleeding compared with warfarin.

A secondary prevention study was done for patients who had been treated for 6–12 months and in whom there was equipoise with respect to need for continued anticoagulation, comparing rivaroxaban 20 mg daily with placebo [15]. As would be expected, rivaroxaban was superior to placebo in preventing recurrence. Major bleeding rates were low (<1%) in the treatment group and

Table 5.8 Primary efficacy and safety outcomes for rivaroxaban versus warfarin for treatment of DVT: the EINSTEIN-DVT study [13]

Primary efficacy and safety outcomes			
	Rivaroxaban	Warfarin	Hazard ratio (95% confidence interval)
Primary outcome	36/1731 (2.1%)	51/1718 (3.0%)	0.68 (0.44–1.04)
Major bleeding	14/1718 (0.8%)	20/1711 (1.2%)	0.65 (0.33–1.30)
Intracranial hemorrhage	NR	NR	
Gastrointestinal bleeding	3/1718 (0.2%)	0	

NR not reported

Table 5.9 Primary efficacy and safety outcomes for rivaroxaban versus warfarin for treatment of acute PE: EINSTEIN-PE study [14]

Primary efficacy and safety outcomes			
	Rivaroxaban	Warfarin	Hazard ratio (95% confidence interval)
Symptomatic recurrent VTE	50/2419 (2.1%)	44/2413 (1.8%)	1.12 (0.75–1.68)
Major bleeding	26/2412 (1.1%)	52/2405 (2.2%)	0.49 (0.31–0.79)
Intracranial hemorrhage	3 (0.1%)	12 (0.5%)	
Gastrointestinal bleeding	NR	NR	

NR not reported

Table 5.10 Primary efficacy and safety outcomes for rivaroxaban versus placebo in extended treatment of VTE: EINSTEIN-Extension [15]

Primary efficacy and safety outcomes			
	Rivaroxaban 20 mg	Placebo	Hazard ratio (95% confidence interval)
Recurrent VTE	8/602 (1.3%)	42/594 (7.1%)	0.18 (0.09–0.39)
Major bleeding	4/598 (0.7%)	0	Not reported
Major or clinically relevant nonmajor bleeding	36/598 (6.0%)	7/590 (1.2%)	5.19 (2.3–11.7)

not statistically significantly different from placebo (Table 5.10).

Prevention of VTE in Hip and Knee Replacement Surgery

Rivaroxaban was studied for VTE prevention in total hip and knee replacement in the RECORD trials, which randomized patients to rivaroxaban starting 6–8 h after wound closure versus enoxaparin started the day before surgery. RECORD-1 compared extended (35 days) rivaroxaban 10 mg daily with extended (35 days) enoxaparin 40 mg every 24 h [16]. RECORD-2 compared extended rivaroxaban 10 mg daily with enoxaparin 40 mg every 24 h for 10–14 days [17]. RECORD-3 compared 10–14 days of rivaroxaban 10 mg daily with 10–14 days of enoxaparin 40 mg every 24 h [18]. RECORD-4 compared 10–14 days of rivaroxaban 10 mg daily with 10–14 days of enoxaparin 30 mg every 12 h [19]. These studies showed rivaroxaban to be more effective than enoxaparin in preventing VTE, with relative risk reductions from 31 to 79%, and similar bleeding rates (Table 5.11).

Rivaroxaban is approved by the FDA to prevent stroke in non-valvular atrial fibrillation at doses of 20 mg daily with the evening meal for patients with CG-CrCl >50 mL/min and 15 mg daily with the evening meal for CG-CrCl 15–50 mL/min. Rivaroxaban is indicated for VTE treatment at a dose of 15 mg BID with food for 21 days, followed by 20 mg daily with food. Rivaroxaban 20 mg daily with food is indicated for secondary prevention of recurrent VTE. Rivaroxaban 10 mg daily, with or without food, is indicated for prophylaxis in knee and hip replacement surgery. The drug carries black-box warnings for premature discontinuation, which can increase the risk of thrombotic events, and for spinal or epidural hematoma in patients receiving neuraxial anesthesia or spinal puncture if the medication is not discontinued at an appropriate interval [20].

Table 5.11 Primary efficacy and safety outcomes for rivaroxaban versus enoxaparin in VTE thromboprophylaxis after hip or knee replacement [16–19]

Primary efficacy and safety outcomes				
	Rivaroxaban 10 mg daily	Enoxaparin 40 mg daily	Enoxaparin 30 mg BID	Absolute risk reduction (95% CI)
RECORD-1				
Any DVT, nonfatal PE, or death from any cause	18/1595 (1.1%)	58/1558 (3.7%)		2.6% (1.5–3.7), $p < 0.001$
Major bleeding	6/2209 (0.3%)	2/2224 (0.1%)		$P = 0.18$
RECORD-2				
Any DVT, nonfatal PE, or death from any cause	17/864 (2.0%)	81/869 (9.3%)		7.3% (5.2–9.4), $p < 0.001$
Major bleeding	1/1218 (<0.1%)	1/1229 (<0.1%)		Not reported
RECORD-3				
Any DVT, nonfatal PE, or death from any cause	79/824 (9.6%)	166/878 (18.9%)		9.2% (5.9–12.4%), $p < 0.001$
Major bleeding	7/1220 (0.6%)	6/1239 (0.5%)		$P = 0.77$
RECORD-4				
Any DVT, nonfatal PE, or death from any cause	67/965 (6.9%)		97/959 (10.1%)	3·19% (0.71–5·67), $p = 0.0362$
Major bleeding	10/1526 (0.7%)		4/1508 (0.3%)	$P = 0.1096$

Apixaban

Prevention of Stroke and Systemic Embolism in Atrial Fibrillation

Apixaban 5 mg twice daily was compared with warfarin adjusted to achieve an INR of 2.0–3.0 to prevent stroke and systemic embolism in 18,201 patients with atrial fibrillation in the ARISTOTLE trial [21]. The dose was reduced to 2.5 mg twice daily in patients with two or more of the following characteristics: age 80 or older, body weight 60 kg or less, or a serum creatinine of 1.5 mg/dL or more. The primary outcome measure was ischemic and hemorrhagic stroke and systemic embolism. Over a mean follow-up of 1.8 years, apixaban was found to be superior to warfarin in preventing stroke, with fewer major bleeds, half the rate of hemorrhagic strokes (0.24% versus 0.47%), and fewer deaths from any cause (Table 5.12). Apixaban 5 mg twice daily was also compared with low-dose aspirin in patients with atrial fibrillation who had been deemed not suitable candidates for or unwilling to take a VKA in the AVERROES trial [22]. More than 5000 patients were randomized and followed for a mean 1.1 years. The trial was stopped early because of the clear benefit of apixaban in preventing stroke or systemic embolism, with no difference in bleeding rates compared with aspirin (Table 5.13). Common reasons that patients had been deemed unsuitable for VKA therapy were patient refusal to take a VKA, concern that patients would not be able to have INR measured at requested intervals, and uncertainty about patients' ability to adhere to VKA therapy.

Table 5.12 Primary efficacy and safety outcomes for apixaban versus warfarin in non-valvular atrial fibrillation thromboprophylaxis: the ARISTOTLE study [21]

Primary efficacy and safety outcomes			
	Apixaban *n*/*N* (% per year)	Warfarin *n*/*N* (% per year)	Hazard ratio (95% confidence interval)
Stroke or systemic embolism	212/9120 (1.27)	265/9081 (1.60)	0.79 (0.66–0.95)
Major bleeding	327/9088 (2.13)	462/9052 (3.09)	0.69 (0.60–0.80)
Intracranial hemorrhage	52/9088 (0.33)	122/9052 (0.80)	0.42 (0.30–0.58)
Gastrointestinal bleeding	105/9088 (0.76)	119/9052 (0.86)	0.89 (0.70–1.15)

Table 5.13 Primary efficacy and safety outcomes for apixaban versus aspirin in non-valvular atrial fibrillation thromboprophylaxis: the AVERROES study [22]

Primary efficacy and safety outcomes			
	Apixaban *n*/*N* (% per year)	Aspirin *n*/*N* (% per year)	Hazard ratio (95% confidence interval)
Stroke or systemic embolism	51/2808 (1.6)	113/2791 (3.7)	0.45 (0.32–0.62)
Major bleeding	44/2808 (1.4)	39/2791 (1.2)	1.13 (0.74–1.75)
Intracranial hemorrhage	11/2808 (0.4)	13/2791 (0.4)	0.85 (0.38–1.90)
Gastrointestinal bleeding	12/2808 (0.4)	14/2791 (0.4)	0.86 (0.40–1.86)

Treatment of DVT and PE and Secondary Prevention of DVT and PE

The AMPLIFY study compared apixaban with warfarin in treating acute proximal DVT and PE, with the primary efficacy outcome of recurrent symptomatic venous thromboembolism or death related to venous thromboembolism [23]. More than 5000 patients were randomized to apixaban 10 mg twice daily for 7 days followed by 5 mg twice daily or subcutaneous enoxaparin overlapping with warfarin. The primary outcome in both groups was similar, with about half the rate of major bleeding in the patients taking apixaban (Table 5.14). An extension study compared apixaban 5 mg twice daily, apixaban 2.5 mg twice daily, and placebo in patients who had been anticoagulated for at least 6 months. Patients on both doses of apixaban had similar rates of recurrent VTE, with no difference in major bleeding (Table 5.15), while patients on the lower dose of apixaban had lower rates of clinically relevant nonmajor bleeding [24].

Prevention of VTE in Knee and Hip Arthroplasty

Apixaban was studied for primary VTE prevention in the ADVANCE trials. In ADVANCE-1, apixaban 2.5 mg twice daily for 10–14 days was non-inferior to enoxaparin 30 mg twice daily for 10–14 days in preventing a composite of asymptomatic and symptomatic DVT, nonfatal PE, or death from any cause during the treatment period in patients undergoing knee replacement surgery [25] (Table 5.16). There was less bleeding among apixaban patients in this trial. In ADVANCE-2 [26], which enrolled knee surgery patients, apixaban 2.5 mg twice daily for 10–14 days was more effective than enoxaparin 40 mg every 24 h for 10–14 days (Table 5.16). In ADVANCE-3 [27], enrolling hip surgery patients, apixaban 2.5 mg twice daily for 35 days was more effective than enoxaparin 40 mg every 24 h for 35 days in preventing the same composite outcome, with similar rates of bleeding (Table 5.16).

Apixaban is approved by the FDA to prevent stroke in non-valvular atrial fibrillation at doses of 5 mg twice daily and 2.5 mg twice daily if two or more of these features are present: age 80 years or older, weight 60 kg or less, or serum creatinine 1.5 mg/dL. Apixaban is indicated for VTE treatment at a dose of 10 mg twice daily for 7 days, followed by 5 mg twice daily. For extended treatment to prevent recurrent VTE, a reduced dose of 2.5 mg twice daily is recommended. Apixaban 2.5 mg twice daily for 12–35 days is indicated for prophylaxis in knee and hip replacement surgery. The drug carries black-box warnings for premature discontinuation, which can increase the risk of thrombotic events, and for spinal or epidural hematoma in patients receiving neuraxial anesthesia or spinal puncture if the medication is not discontinued at an appropriate interval [28].

Edoxaban

Prevention of Stroke and Systemic Embolism in Non-valvular Atrial Fibrillation

Edoxaban was approved to reduce rates of stroke and systemic embolism in patients with non-valvular atrial fibrillation based on results of the ENGAGE AF-TIMI study [29]. Patients were randomized to either edoxaban or warfarin adjusted to achieve an INR of 2.0–3.0; patients with normal kidney function were given edoxaban 60 mg daily and those with a CG-CrCl 30–50 mL/min, body

Table 5.14 Primary efficacy and safety outcomes for apixaban versus warfarin in the acute treatment of VTE: the AMPLIFY study [23]

Primary efficacy and safety outcomes			
	Apixaban ($N = 2691$)	Warfarin ($N = 2635$)	Hazard ratio (95% confidence interval)
Recurrent VTE or VTE-related death	59 (2.3%)	71 (2.7%)	0.84 (0.60–1.18)
Major bleeding	15 (0.6%)	49 (1.8%)	0.31 (0.17–0.55)
Intracranial hemorrhage	3 (0.1%)	6 (0.2%)	
Gastrointestinal bleeding	7 (0.3%)	18 (0.7%)	

Table 5.15 Primary efficacy and safety outcomes for apixaban versus placebo in the extended treatment of VTE: the AMPLIFY-Extension study [24]

Primary efficacy and safety outcomes						
				Relative risk (95% confidence interval)		
	Apixaban 2.5 mg BID ($N = 840$)	Apixaban 5 mg BID ($N = 813$)	Placebo ($N = 829$)	Apixaban 2.5 mg vs. placebo	Apixaban 5 mg vs. placebo	
Recurrent VTE or death from any cause	32 (3.8%)	34 (4.2%)	96 (11.6%)	0.33 (0.22–0.48)	0.36 (0.25–0.53)	Not available
Major bleeding	2 (0.2%)	1 (0.1%)	4 (0.5%)	0.49 (0.09–2.64)	0.25 (0.03–2.24)	1.93 (0.18–21.25)

weight < 60 kg, or on concomitant potent p-GP inhibitors received half the dose. Patients with CG-CrCl <30 mL/min were excluded. Over a mean follow-up of 2.8 years, edoxaban was non-inferior in preventing stroke or systemic embolism, with lower rates of bleeding—about half the rate for warfarin in the low-dose edoxaban group (Table 5.17).

Treatment of DVT and PE

Edoxaban for symptomatic proximal DVT or PE was studied in the HOKUSAI-VTE trial, which randomized patients to either high- or low-dose edoxaban versus warfarin after 5–10 days of parenteral therapy [30]. The same criteria as in ENGAGE AF-TIMI 48 were used to determine who got high- versus low-dose edoxaban. The primary efficacy outcome was recurrent symptomatic VTE; the primary safety outcome was major or clinically relevant non-major bleeding. Rates of recurrence were similar for edoxaban and warfarin, with statistically significantly lower rates of major or clinically relevant nonmajor bleeding in the edoxaban group. This study also examined more than 900 patients with right ventricular dysfunction as measured by elevated N-terminal pro-brain natriuretic peptide. Patients on edoxaban had about half the rate of recurrent VTE as patients on warfarin (Table 5.18).

Edoxaban is approved by the FDA to prevent stroke in non-valvular atrial fibrillation at doses of 60 mg daily for patients with CG-CrCl >50 mL/min and ≤95 mL/min and 30 mg daily for those with CG-CrCl 15–50 mL/min or weight ≤60 kg. Edoxaban is indicated for VTE treatment at doses of 60 mg daily for patients with CG-CrCl >50 mL/min and ≤95 mL/min and 30 mg daily for those with CG-CrCl 15–50 mL/min or weight ≤60 kg. The drug carries black-box warnings for decreased efficacy in preventing stroke in patients with CG-CrCl >95 mL/min; premature discontinuation, which can increase the risk of thrombotic events; and for spinal or epidural hematoma in patients receiving neuraxial anesthesia or spinal puncture if the medication is not discontinued at an appropriate interval [31].

Table 5.16 Primary efficacy and safety outcomes for apixaban versus enoxaparin for VTE thromboprophylaxis after hip or knee replacement [25–27]

Primary efficacy and safety outcomes				
	Apixaban 2.5 mg BID	Enoxaparin 30 mg every 12 h	Enoxaparin 40 mg every 24 h	Relative risk (95% CI)
ADVANCE-1				
All VTE and death from any cause	104/1157 (9.0%)	100/1130 (8.8%)		1.02 (0.78–1.32)
Major bleeding	11/1596 (0.7%)	22/1588 (1.4%)		NR
ADVANCE-2				
All VTE and all-cause death	147/976 (15.1%)		243/997 (24.4%)	0.62 (0.51–0.74)
Major bleeding	9/1501 (0.6%)		14/1508 (0.9%)	
ADVANCE-3				
All VTE and death from any cause	29/1949 (1.4%)		74/1917 (3.9%)	0.36 (0.22–0.54)
Major bleeding	22/2673 (0.8%)		18/2659 (0.7%)	

Table 5.17 Primary efficacy and safety outcomes for edoxaban versus warfarin in non-valvular atrial fibrillation thromboprophylaxis: the ENGAGE AF-TIMI48 study [29]

Primary efficacy and safety outcomes					
	Edoxaban 30 mg *n*/*N* (% per year)	Edoxaban 60 mg *n*/*N* (% per year)	Warfarin *n*/*N* (% per year)	30 mg vs. warfarin HR (95% CI)	60 mg vs. warfarin HR (95% CI)
Stroke and systemic embolism	253/7034 (1.61)	182/7035 (1.18)	232/7036 (1.50)	1.07 (0.87–1.31)	0.79 (0.63–0.99)
Major bleed	254/7002 (1.61)	418/7012 (2.75)	524/7012 (3.43)	0.80 (0.71–0.91)	0.47 (0.41–0.55)
Intracranial hemorrhage	41/7002 (0.26)	61/7012 (0.39)	132/7012 (0.85)	0.30 (0.21–0.43)	0.47 (0.34–0.63)
GI bleed	129/7002 (0.82)	232/7012 (1.51)	190/7012 (1.23)	0.67 (0.53–0.83)	1.23 (1.02–1.50)

Real-World Experience

As real-world experience with the DOACs accumulates, results tend to mirror those seen in the trials. In a Danish cohort of more than 60,000 patients started on a DOAC for atrial fibrillation, no outcomes were worse on DOACs than with warfarin [32]. A US Medicare population study showed reduced rates of intracranial hemorrhage and increased rates of GI bleeding for dabigatran [33]. Another group looked at more than 60,000 patients on DOACs and found more bleeding with rivaroxaban and similar rates for dabigatran and apixaban [34].

Perioperative Management

Because of the DOACs' relatively short half-life compared with warfarin, generally they can be stopped prior to invasive procedures without the need for "bridging" therapy with a parenteral anticoagulant. The timing of preoperative cessation depends upon renal function; for patients with CG-CrCl >50 mL/min undergoing procedures with low bleeding risk, the DOACs should be held for approximately 2–3 half-lives, or 24–48 h, and for procedures with high bleeding risk, 4–5 half-lives, or 48–72 h [35] (Table 5.19). In patients with renal insufficiency, these times should be increased, since drug clearance will be

Table 5.18 Primary efficacy and safety outcomes for edoxaban versus warfarin for treatment of VTE: the HOKUSAI-VTE study [30]

Primary efficacy and safety outcomes			
	Edoxaban ($N = 4118$)	Warfarin ($N = 4122$)	Hazard ratio (95% confidence interval)
Recurrent VTE or VTE-related death	130 (3.2%)	146 (3.5%)	0.89 (0.70–1.13)
Major bleeding	56 (1.4%)	66 (1.6%)	0.84 (0.59–1.21)
Intracranial hemorrhage	5 (0.1%)	12 (0.3%)	
Gastrointestinal bleeding	1 (<0.1%)	2 (<0.1%)	

Table 5.19 Suggested perioperative interruption of DOACs [35]

Drug	Renal function	Low bleeding risk	High bleeding risk
Dabigatran			
	CG-CrCl >50 mL/min	Skip two doses	Skip four doses
	CG-CrCl 15–50 mL	Skip four doses	Skip six to eight doses
Rivaroxaban			
	CG-CrCl >30 mL/min	Skip one dose	Skip two doses
	CG-CrCl 15–29 mL/min	Skip two doses	Skip three doses
Apixaban			
	CG-CrCl >50 mL/min	Skip two doses	Skip four doses
	CG-CrCl 15–50 mL	Skip four doses	Skip six doses
Edoxaban			
	CG-CrCl >50 mL/min	Skip one doses	Skip two doses
	CG-CrCl 15–29 mL/min	Skip one doses	Skip three doses

delayed. For low-bleeding-risk procedures such as tooth cleaning and skin biopsy, the DOACs can be continued. The timing of drug resumption depends on factors such as the bleeding risk of the surgery, how difficult it was to achieve hemostasis, and the patient's individual risk for bleeding. Because of the DOACs' short time to peak action, resumption should be delayed at least 48–72 h postoperatively for high-bleeding-risk procedures. Clinicians may wish to start patients who are immobilized on a prophylaxis dose of anticoagulation in the interim. Please refer to Chap. 9 for a more in-depth discussion on this topic.

Management of the Bleeding Patient/ Drug Reversal

Certain basic measures should be taken for all patients who have severe bleeding on anticoagulation, including stopping the medication, controlling bleeding mechanically as possible, and supporting circulation with fluids and blood products as needed. The short half-life of the DOACs means that the majority of the drug is cleared within 24 h in patients with normal renal function. For patients on dabigatran with life-threatening bleeding and in case of need for urgent or emergent surgery, a reversal agent, idarucizumab, is available. It was studied in 90 patients on dabigatran with either serious bleeding or in need of an urgent invasive procedure. The primary outcome was the maximum percentage reversal of the anticoagulant effect of the drug, which was achieved within minutes for the majority of patients [36]. Dabigatran can be cleared via hemodialysis, but the role of this approach in cases of life-threatening bleeding is not clear. For more information, please refer to Chap. 6.

The factor Xa inhibitors cannot be removed with hemodialysis, and there is no FDA-approved antidote. A reversal agent, andexanet alfa, is being studied in patients with major bleeding who had taken one of the direct Xa inhibitors or the low-molecular-weight heparin (enoxaparin) within the preceding 18 h. Of note, patients with major thrombosis within 2 weeks were excluded from the trial. Patients were given one of two doses depending on timing of last dose of factor Xa inhibitor aimed at rapid reversal of 80% of factor Xa activity. The primary outcomes were anti-factor Xa activity and hemostatic efficacy 12 h after the infusion. After completion of the 2-h infusion, factor Xa activity was reduced approximately 90% for both rivaroxaban and apixaban (no patients taking edoxaban had been enrolled at the time the initial results were published), but anti-Xa activity returned toward pre-treatment baseline by 4.5 h post-infusion. Nevertheless, 79% of patients had good or excellent hemostatic efficacy at 12 h.

There are several important steps in the approach to the patient who has bleeding in the context of DOAC administration. One should learn the patient's dosing regimen and time of last dose, as well as other medications that could potentially influence the concentration of the DOACs and drugs that could influence hemostasis. Obtain serum creatinine levels as well as hemoglobin and platelet count. If necessary, give blood volume replacement and transfuse platelets if there is significant thrombocytopenia. Prothrombin complex concentrates and activated prothrombin complex concentrates may also be administered [37].

Monitoring

Because of their predictable pharmacokinetics, routine monitoring of DOACs is unnecessary. Dabigatran has an unpredictable effect on both the prothrombin time and the activated partial thromboplastin time (aPTT). A normal aPTT indicates negligible circulating drug. The thrombin time can also detect the presence of dabigatran, and because of this test's high sensitivity, a normal result indicates no circulating dabigatran. The dilute thrombin time, available commercially as the Hemoclot® thrombin inhibitor test, used with the appropriate reagent, can be used to monitor plasma concentrations of dabigatran [38].

As with dabigatran, routine monitoring of the anticoagulant effect of the direct factor Xa inhibitors is unnecessary. The Xa inhibitors have an unpredictable effect on the PT and aPTT [39, 40]. Nevertheless, a normal PT excludes significant anticoagulation activity with the Xa inhibitors [31]. The ecarin clotting time and thrombin time tests are not significantly affected by the Xa inhibitors. Chromogenic anti-Xa activity, with testing calibrated specifically to the Xa inhibitors, has been shown to reliably predict drug concentration [41].

Special Populations

Valvular Atrial Fibrillation, Bioprosthetic Heart Valves, and Mechanical Heart Valves

All of the DOACs carry black-box warnings against use in patients with mechanical heart valves. The RE-ALIGN study of dabigatran versus warfarin for patients with bileaflet mechanical valves was terminated early because of excess thrombosis in the dabigatran group [42]. They also are not indicated for patients with atrial fibrillation associated with rheumatic mitral stenosis, bioprosthetic valve, or mitral valve repair. Sub-analyses of patients with aortic stenosis, aortic regurgitation, and mitral regurgitation showed no safety or efficacy differences, but more study is needed before routinely prescribing the DOACs to these patients [43].

Cancer

Incident VTE is common among cancer patients, who also have a high risk of recurrent VTE. Patients with active cancer were excluded from the large randomized controlled trials of the DOACs, but more post-marketing data are being acquired regarding the use of DOACs in cancer patients. Current practice guidelines recommend LMWH for initial treatment of VTE in patients with active malignancy, but suggest that either a VKA or a DOAC may be used after that time, if transitioning therapy, based on weak evidence. A meta-analysis of cancer patients in the DOAC trials showed that rates of recurrence were comparable to those of warfarin [44]. Please refer to Chap. 20 for a more in-depth discussion on this topic.

Thrombophilia

Data on the use of the DOACs for VTE treatment and secondary prevention in patients with inherited thrombophilia—deficiencies of antithrombin and proteins C and S and factor V Leiden and prothrombin gene mutations—and the acquired antiphospholipid syndrome are sparse, as thrombophilia was not expressly studied in the major DOAC trials. Patients with primary thrombophilia made up less than 5% of the total patients studied. A post hoc subset analysis of the RE-COVER and RE-MEDY trials including 933 patients with thrombophilia (mostly factor V Leiden mutation) showed no difference in rates of recurrent VTE or VTE death among those patients randomized to dabigatran [45]. To date, there are only case series of patients with thrombophilia on the factor Xa inhibitors [46] (please refer to Chaps. 14 and 15 for more in-depth discussions on this topic).

Obese Patients

The randomized controlled trials for DOACs for all indications did not exclude obese patients, but few very obese patients were enrolled. This could be of particular concern with respect to VTE, because obesity increases the risk of VTE. In the EINSTEIN and EINSTEIN-PE studies of rivaroxaban, about 14% of patients weighed more than 100 kg [13, 14]; in the AMPLIFY study of apixaban, about 19% of patients weighed more than 100 kg [23]; and in the HOKUSAI-VTE study of edoxaban, about 15% of patients weighed more than 100 kg [30]. There was no difference in outcomes among the subsets of weight [44, 47]. Nevertheless, because of limited data on outcomes among obese patients, the International Society on Thrombosis and Haemostasis recommends against using these drugs in patients with BMI > 40 kg/m^2 or weight > 120 kg [48].

Prophylaxis of High-Risk Medical Patients

In the recent randomized, double-blind, placebo-controlled APEX trial, patients older than 40 hospitalized for acute medical illness and deemed high risk for VTE were randomized to betrixaban 80 mg daily for 35–42 days versus enoxaparin 40 mg every 24 h for 10 ± 4 days. The primary outcome, a composite of asymptomatic proximal DVT and symptomatic VTE, occurred in 5.3% of the total population on betrixaban versus 7.0% of patients on enoxaparin (relative risk 0.76, 95% confidence interval 0.63–0.92). The primary safety outcome, major bleeding, was not significantly different for either group [49]. Inclusion criteria were complex, so patients who may benefit must be carefully selected.

Atherosclerotic Vascular Disease

The COMPASS trial (ClinicalTrials.gov NCT01776424) focused on the role of rivaroxaban in patients with stable atherosclerotic vascular disease, with the goal of identifying whether its use can affect the primary outcome comprising a composite of cardiovascular death, stroke, or myocardial infarction. Specifically, the COMPASS trial was a double-blind randomized controlled trial that evaluated 27,395 patients in three arms receiving either rivaroxaban 2.5 mg twice daily plus aspirin 100 mg/day (n = 9152), rivaroxaban 5 mg daily (n = 9117), or aspirin 100 mg/day (n = 9126) [50]. Inclusion criteria included patients with atherosclerosis in two or more vascular beds, or two additional risk factors that include smoking, diabetes, heart failure, renal insufficiency, or nonlacunar ischemic stroke ≥1 month. What initially generated great interest was that the study was stopped early after a mean follow-up period of only 23 months, as the primary endpoint for major adverse cardiovascular events met its prespecified criteria for superiority in the rivaroxaban-plus-aspirin group, in which the primary outcome occurred in 4.1%. The primary outcome occurred in 4.9% in the rivaroxaban alone group and in 5.4% in the aspirin alone group ($p < 0.001$ for rivaroxaban-plus-aspirin versus aspirin alone; $p = 0.12$ for rivaroxaban alone versus aspirin alone). However, for the rivaroxaban-plus-aspirin group, the significant decrease in primary outcomes came at the expense of an increase in major bleeding: 3.1% for rivaroxaban-plus-aspirin, 2.8% for rivaroxaban alone, and 1.9% for aspirin alone ($p < 0.001$ for both rivaroxaban-plus-aspirin versus aspirin alone and rivaroxaban alone versus aspirin alone cohorts).

Findings were similar among those with peripheral artery disease in the parallel COMPASS PAD study. While those who received both rivaroxaban-plus-aspirin sustained significantly fewer major adverse cardiac events (MACE), including limb-threatening ischemia and amputations, compared to those within the rivaroxaban alone and aspirin alone cohorts, there also were increased major bleeding events. It is worthy to highlight that although major bleeding events were significantly higher for the rivaroxaban-plus-aspirin arms in both COMPASS and COMPASS PAD, the risk of more catastrophic events such as fatal or critical organ bleeding was not higher.

Additional longer-term studies will likely be needed before findings from COMPASS and COMPASS PAD change practice guidelines. However, these results certainly refocus the role of anticoagulants in atherosclerotic vascular disease therapy.

Summary

The DOACs, which require no monitoring or dose adjustment, have simplified anticoagulation for many patients. They have been shown to be non-inferior or superior to warfarin for a number of different indications, including prevention of stroke in non-valvular atrial fibrillation, prevention of VTE after joint surgery, and treatment of VTE. The utility of DOACs in atherosclerotic vascular disease is certainly noteworthy but still requires further investigation.

A reversal agent is available for dabigatran only, and certain basic supportive measures should be applied to all anticoagulated patients who develop bleeding. Caution should be used in prescribing these medications to patients with thrombophilia and morbid obesity, given lack of data in these populations.

Key Points

- DOACs target a single clotting factor and provide predictable anticoagulant effect for the majority of patients.
- DOACs have been shown to be non-inferior and often with better safety profile than VKA therapy for the prevention of stroke in non-valvular atrial fibrillation and the treatment of VTE.
- Specific reversal agents are available for dabigatran and in development for the factor Xa inhibitors.
- DOACs should be avoided or used with caution in patients with advanced renal dysfunction, thrombophilia, and morbid obesity.

Self-Assessment Questions

1. Which of the following clotting factors is the target for one or more of the direct oral anticoagulants (DOACs)?
   (a) Factor VII
   (b) Factor Xa
   (c) Factor XII
   (d) Protein C
   (e) Protein S
2. In the large randomized trials, which of the DOAC medications has been shown to be superior to aspirin for the prevention of stroke or systemic embolism in patient with non-valvular atrial fibrillation?
   (a) Apixaban
   (b) Betrixaban
   (c) Dabigatran
   (d) Edoxaban
   (e) Rivaroxaban

3. Which of the following DOAC medications requires 5–10 days of parenteral heparin treatment prior to DOAC initiation in patients with acute venous thromboembolism?
   (a) Apixaban
   (b) Betrixaban
   (c) Dabigatran
   (d) Rivaroxaban
4. Which of the following DOAC medications will not be specifically reversed by andexanet alpha?
   (a) Apixaban
   (b) Betrixaban
   (c) Dabigatran
   (d) Edoxaban
   (e) Rivaroxaban
5. Which of the following laboratory tests is necessary to ensure accurate dosing of the DOAC medications?
   (a) Hemoglobin
   (b) White blood count
   (c) Serum protein
   (d) Serum creatinine
   (e) Total cholesterol

Self-Assessment Answers

1. (b) Factor Xa.

   Factor Xa is the target for the DOACs apixaban, betrixaban, edoxaban, and rivaroxaban. Dabigatran inhibits thrombin (factor II), while warfarin inhibits the production of vitamin K-dependent clotting factors (II, VII, IX, X, protein C, and protein S).
2. (a) Apixaban.

   In the AVERROES study, patients who were deemed not suitable candidates for warfarin were randomized to apixaban or aspirin. Patient treated with apixaban had a lower rate of stroke or systemic embolism (HR 0.45, 95% CI 0.32–0.62) than patient randomized to aspirin therapy.
3. (c) Dabigatran.

   Dabigatran requires 5–10 days of parenteral therapy prior to starting dabigatran for treatment of acute venous thromboembolism. Apixaban and rivaroxaban can be used without parenteral lead-in therapy, and betrixaban has not been studied for treatment of acute venous thromboembolism.
4. (c) Dabigatran.

   Dabigatran, as a direct thrombin inhibitor, is not affected directly by andexanet alpha (a factor Xa decoy). Andexanet will specifically reverse all of the factor Xa inhibitors, including apixaban, betrixaban, edoxaban, and rivaroxaban.
5. (d) Serum creatinine.

   Since nearly all of the DOAC medications are cleared renally (at least in part), proper dosing is based on serum creatinine (for apixaban) or calculated creatinine clearance level (for dabigatran, edoxaban, and rivaroxaban).

References

1. Ganetsky M, Babu KM, Salhanick SD, Brown RS, Boyer EW. Dabigatran: review of pharmacology and management of bleeding complications of this novel oral anticoagulant. J Med Toxicol. 2011;7(4):281–7.
2. Stangier J, Clemens A. Pharmacology, pharmacokinetics, and pharmacodynamics of dabigatran etexilate, an oral direct thrombin inhibitor. Clin Appl Thromb Hemost. 2009;15(Suppl 1):9s–16s.
3. Connolly SJ, Ezekowitz MD, Yusuf S, Eikelboom J, Oldgren J, Parekh A, et al. Dabigatran versus warfarin in patients with atrial fibrillation. N Engl J Med. 2009;361(12):1139–51.
4. Schulman S, Kearon C, Kakkar AK, Mismetti P, Schellong S, Eriksson H, et al. Dabigatran versus warfarin in the treatment of acute venous thromboembolism. N Engl J Med. 2009;361(24):2342–52.
5. Schulman S, Kakkar AK, Goldhaber SZ, Schellong S, Eriksson H, Mismetti P, et al. Treatment of acute venous thromboembolism with dabigatran or warfarin and pooled analysis. Circulation. 2014;129(7):764–72.
6. Schulman S, Kearon C, Kakkar AK, Schellong S, Eriksson H, Baanstra D, et al. Extended use of dabigatran, warfarin, or placebo in venous thromboembolism. N Engl J Med. 2013;368(8):709–18.
7. Eriksson BI, Dahl OE, Huo MH, Kurth AA, Hantel S, Hermansson K, et al. Oral dabigatran versus enoxaparin for thromboprophylaxis after primary total hip arthroplasty (RE-NOVATE II*). A randomised, double-blind, non-inferiority trial. Thromb Haemost. 2011;105(4):721–9.
8. Eriksson BI, Dahl OE, Rosencher N, Kurth AA, van Dijk CN, Frostick SP, et al. Dabigatran etexilate versus enoxaparin for prevention of venous thromboembolism after total hip replacement: a ran-

domised, double-blind, non-inferiority trial. Lancet. 2007;370(9591):949–56.
9. Pradaxa. Package insert, Boehringer Ingelheim Pharmaceuticals. 2015.
10. Kreutz R. Pharmacokinetics and pharmacodynamics of rivaroxaban—an oral, direct factor Xa inhibitor. Curr Clin Pharmacol. 2014;9(1):75–83.
11. Kubitza D, Becka M, Mueck W, Halabi A, Maatouk H, Klause N, et al. Effects of renal impairment on the pharmacokinetics, pharmacodynamics and safety of rivaroxaban, an oral, direct Factor Xa inhibitor. Br J Clin Pharmacol. 2010;70(5):703–12.
12. Patel MR, Mahaffey KW, Garg J, Pan G, Singer DE, Hacke W, et al. Rivaroxaban versus warfarin in nonvalvular atrial fibrillation. N Engl J Med. 2011;365(10):883–91.
13. Bauersachs R, Berkowitz SD, Brenner B, Buller HR, Decousus H, Gallus AS, et al. Oral rivaroxaban for symptomatic venous thromboembolism. N Engl J Med. 2010;363(26):2499–510.
14. Buller HR, Prins MH, Lensin AW, Decousus H, Jacobson BF, Minar E, et al. Oral rivaroxaban for the treatment of symptomatic pulmonary embolism. N Engl J Med. 2012;366(14):1287–97.
15. Romualdi E, Donadini MP, Ageno W. Oral rivaroxaban after symptomatic venous thromboembolism: the continued treatment study (EINSTEIN-extension study). Expert Rev Cardiovasc Ther. 2011;9(7):841–4.
16. Eriksson BI, Borris LC, Friedman RJ, Haas S, Huisman MV, Kakkar AK, et al. Rivaroxaban versus enoxaparin for thromboprophylaxis after hip arthroplasty. N Engl J Med. 2008;358(26):2765–75.
17. Kakkar AK, Brenner B, Dahl OE, Eriksson BI, Mouret P, Muntz J, et al. Extended duration rivaroxaban versus short-term enoxaparin for the prevention of venous thromboembolism after total hip arthroplasty: a double-blind, randomised controlled trial. Lancet. 2008;372(9632):31–9.
18. Lassen MR, Ageno W, Borris LC, Lieberman JR, Rosencher N, Bandel TJ, et al. Rivaroxaban versus enoxaparin for thromboprophylaxis after total knee arthroplasty. N Engl J Med. 2008;358(26):2776–86.
19. Turpie AG, Lassen MR, Davidson BL, Bauer KA, Gent M, Kwong LM, et al. Rivaroxaban versus enoxaparin for thromboprophylaxis after total knee arthroplasty (RECORD4): a randomised trial. Lancet. 2009;373(9676):1673–80.
20. Xarelto. Package insert, Janssen Pharmaceuticals.
21. Granger CB, Alexander JH, McMurray JJ, Lopes RD, Hylek EM, Hanna M, et al. Apixaban versus warfarin in patients with atrial fibrillation. N Engl J Med. 2011;365(11):981–92.
22. Connolly SJ, Eikelboom J, Joyner C, Diener HC, Hart R, Golitsyn S, et al. Apixaban in patients with atrial fibrillation. N Engl J Med. 2011;364(9):806–17.
23. Agnelli G, Buller HR, Cohen A, Curto M, Gallus AS, Johnson M, et al. Oral apixaban for the treatment of acute venous thromboembolism. N Engl J Med. 2013;369(9):799–808.
24. Agnelli G, Buller HR, Cohen A, Curto M, Gallus AS, Johnson M, et al. Apixaban for extended treatment of venous thromboembolism. N Engl J Med. 2013;368(8):699–708.
25. Lassen MR, Raskob GE, Gallus A, Pineo G, Chen D, Portman RJ. Apixaban or enoxaparin for thromboprophylaxis after knee replacement. N Engl J Med. 2009;361(6):594–604.
26. Lassen MR, Raskob GE, Gallus A, Pineo G, Chen D, Hornick P. Apixaban versus enoxaparin for thromboprophylaxis after knee replacement (ADVANCE-2): a randomised double-blind trial. Lancet. 2010;375(9717):807–15.
27. Lassen MR, Gallus A, Raskob GE, Pineo G, Chen D, Ramirez LM. Apixaban versus enoxaparin for thromboprophylaxis after hip replacement. N Engl J Med. 2010;363(26):2487–98.
28. Eliquis. Package insert, Bristol Myers Squibb and Pfizer.
29. Giugliano RP, Ruff CT, Braunwald E, Murphy SA, Wiviott SD, Halperin JL, et al. Edoxaban versus warfarin in patients with atrial fibrillation. N Engl J Med. 2013;369(22):2093–104.
30. Buller HR, Decousus H, Grosso MA, Mercuri M, Middeldorp S, Prins MH, et al. Edoxaban versus warfarin for the treatment of symptomatic venous thromboembolism. N Engl J Med. 2013;369(15):1406–15.
31. Savaysa. Package insert, Daiichi Sankyo.
32. Larsen TB, Skjoth F, Nielsen PB, Kjaeldgaard JN, Lip GY. Comparative effectiveness and safety of non-vitamin K antagonist oral anticoagulants and warfarin in patients with atrial fibrillation: propensity weighted nationwide cohort study. BMJ. 2016;353:i3189.
33. Graham DJ, Reichman ME, Wernecke M, Hsueh YH, Izem R, Southworth MR, et al. Stroke, bleeding, and mortality risks in elderly medicare beneficiaries treated with dabigatran or rivaroxaban for nonvalvular atrial fibrillation. JAMA Int Med. 2016;176(11):1662–71.
34. Villines TC, Peacock WF. Safety of direct oral anticoagulants: insights from postmarketing studies. Am J Med. 2016;129(11s):S41–s6.
35. Spyropoulos AC, Douketis JD. How I treat anticoagulated patients undergoing an elective procedure or surgery. Blood. 2012;120(15):2954–62.
36. Pollack CV Jr, Reilly PA, Eikelboom J, Glund S, Verhamme P, Bernstein RA, et al. Idarucizumab for dabigatran reversal. N Engl J Med. 2015;373(6):511–20.
37. Heidbuchel H, Verhamme P, Alings M, Antz M, Diener HC, Hacke W, et al. Updated European Heart Rhythm Association practical guide on the use of non-vitamin-K antagonist anticoagulants in patients with non-valvular atrial fibrillation: Executive summary. Eur Heart J. 2017;38(27):2137–49.
38. Stangier J, Feuring M. Using the HEMOCLOT direct thrombin inhibitor assay to determine plasma concentrations of dabigatran. Blood Coagul Fibrinolysis. 2012;23(2):138–43.
39. Cuker A, Siegal D. Monitoring and reversal of direct oral anticoagulants. Hematology Am Soc Hematol Educ Program. 2015;2015:117–24.
40. Douxfils J, Mani H, Minet V, Devalet B, Chatelain B, Dogne JM, et al. Non-VKA oral anticoagulants:

accurate measurement of plasma drug concentrations. Biomed Res Int. 2015;2015:345138.

41. Barrett YC, Wang Z, Frost C, Shenker A. Clinical laboratory measurement of direct factor Xa inhibitors: anti-Xa assay is preferable to prothrombin time assay. Thromb Haemost. 2010;104(6):1263–71.
42. Eikelboom JW, Connolly SJ, Brueckmann M, Granger CB, Kappetein AP, Mack MJ, et al. Dabigatran versus warfarin in patients with mechanical heart valves. N Engl J Med. 2013;369(13):1206–14.
43. Owens RE, Kabra R, Oliphant CS. Direct oral anticoagulant use in nonvalvular atrial fibrillation with valvular heart disease: a systematic review. Clin Cardiol. 2017;40(6):407–12.
44. van Es N, Buller HR. Using direct oral anticoagulants (DOACs) in cancer and other high-risk populations. Hematology Am Soc Hematol Educ Program. 2015;2015:125–31.
45. Goldhaber SZ, Eriksson H, Kakkar A, Schellong S, Feuring M, Fraessdorf M, et al. Efficacy of dabigatran versus warfarin in patients with acute venous thromboembolism in the presence of thrombophilia: findings from RE-COVER(R), RE-COVER II, and RE-MEDY. Vasc Med. 2016;21(6):506–14.
46. Skelley JW, White CW, Thomason AR. The use of direct oral anticoagulants in inherited thrombophilia. J Thromb Thrombolysis. 2017;43(1):24–30.
47. Di Minno MN, Lupoli R, Di Minno A, Ambrosino P, Scalera A, Dentali F. Effect of body weight on efficacy and safety of direct oral anticoagulants in the treatment of patients with acute venous thromboembolism: a meta-analysis of randomized controlled trials. Ann Med. 2015;47(1):61–8.
48. Martin K, Beyer-Westendorf J, Davidson BL, Huisman MV, Sandset PM, Moll S. Use of the direct oral anticoagulants in obese patients: guidance from the SSC of the ISTH. J Thromb Haemost. 2016;14(6):1308–13.
49. Cohen AT, Harrington RA, Goldhaber SZ, Hull RD, Wiens BL, Gold A, et al. Extended thromboprophylaxis with betrixaban in acutely Ill medical patients. N Engl J Med. 2016;375(6):534–44.
50. Eikelboom JW, Connolly SJ, Bosch J, Dagenais GR, Hart RG, Shestakovska O, et al. COMPASS investigators. Rivaroxaban with or without aspirin in stable cardiovascular disease. N Engl J Med. 2017;377(14):1319–30. https://doi.org/10.1056/NEJMoa1709118.

6 Anticoagulation Reversal

Deborah Hornacek and Marcelo P. V. Gomes

Clinical Vignettes

Case 1: *An 82-year-old woman with atrial fibrillation on long-term anticoagulation with warfarin is placed on sulfamethoxazole/trimethoprim for urinary tract infection. Her INR has been stable within the therapeutic target range (2.0–3.0) for several months without warfarin dose changes, but 5 days after starting antibiotic therapy, her INR is >8.0. She denies any bleeding.*

Case 2: *A 53-year-old man is seen in the emergency department after a fall from a ladder with head injury. He is anticoagulated on warfarin for history of recurrent deep vein thrombosis, and his INR is currently 2.8. Brain CT confirms intracranial hemorrhage with midline shift; he is being prepared to go for decompressive hemicraniotomy.*

Introduction

Antithrombotic therapy is commonly prescribed for the prevention and treatment of venous and arterial thromboembolism. Contemporary antithrombotic therapy can be achieved by the prescription of several different anticoagulants that are now available for clinical use. These anticoagulants include unfractionated heparin (UFH), low-molecular-weight heparins (LMWHs), pentasaccharides, parenteral and oral direct thrombin inhibitors (DTIs), vitamin K antagonists (VKAs), as well as direct oral factor Xa inhibitors. These classes of drugs have been approved for clinical use because large-scale randomized clinical trials (RCTs) have demonstrated a net clinical benefit in which their efficacy (generally evaluated in terms of prevention of thrombus propagation, embolization, and recurrence) outweighs their adverse effects. The most common and feared adverse event associated with the various antithrombotic drugs is bleeding, with the rates of minor bleeding, clinically relevant

D. Hornacek
Department of Cardiovascular Medicine, Section of Vascular Medicine, Cleveland Clinic, Cleveland, OH, USA
e-mail: hornacd@ccf.org

M. P. V. Gomes (✉)
Department of Cardiovascular Medicine, Section of Vascular Medicine, Cleveland Clinic, Cleveland, OH, USA
e-mail: gomesm3@ccf.org

J. F. Lau et al. (eds.), *Anticoagulation Therapy*, https://doi.org/10.1007/978-3-319-73709-6_6

nonmajor bleeding, and/or major bleeding being the safety outcomes typically reported in clinical trials of antithrombotics old and new. The annual risk of bleeding associated with anticoagulation varies according to individual patient-specific risk factors and drug-specific characteristics, as well as the underlying indication(s) [1]. In addition, the specific rates of hemorrhagic complications will vary depending upon the anatomical site involved. In a pooled analysis derived from clinical trials enrolling patients treated with vitamin K antagonists for prevention of cardioembolic stroke in the setting of atrial fibrillation, the annual risk of major bleeding was 1.3%, and the specific risk of intracranial hemorrhage was 0.3% [2]. A meta-analysis of clinical trials of patients treated with vitamin K antagonists for acute venous thromboembolic events (VTE) reported an annual risk of major bleeding of 1.1% [3]. Higher annual rates of major bleeding ranging from 1.7% to 3.4% have been reported in patients treated with vitamin K antagonists in "real-world" clinical practice [4, 5]. Analyses of data from trials of direct oral anticoagulants (DOACs) for prevention of cardioembolic stroke in patients with nonvalvular atrial fibrillation reveal less intracranial hemorrhage (ICH) compared to VKA [6], but patients receiving DOACs for VTE and acute coronary syndromes (ACS) may have an increased risk of gastrointestinal (GI) bleeding [7].

Despite the fact that the efficacy and safety outcomes of antithrombotic drugs have been extensively evaluated in multiple clinical trials, there is a paucity of prospective data evaluating methods to reverse the effects of different anticoagulant drugs and to guide management of anticoagulant-related hemorrhage. While correction of minor bleeding may not require specific therapy beyond a brief interruption (one or two doses) of an anticoagulant drug, the use of reversal strategies or specific antidotes is required to treat anticoagulation-related major or life-threatening bleeding, as well as for reversal of anticoagulation prior to emergent invasive procedures.

This chapter will review available data pertaining to reversal strategies for the different classes of anticoagulant drugs that are either currently available for clinical use or have completed advanced stages of clinical development.

Vitamin K Antagonists

Vitamin K antagonists exert their anticoagulant properties by inhibiting vitamin K epoxide reductase and interfering with the cyclic interconversion of vitamin K and its epoxide, thus preventing the γ-carboxylation of glutamic acid residues on the N-terminal regions of vitamin K-dependent coagulation factors II, VII, IX, and X [8–10]. Because γ-carboxylation is required for the enzymatic activity of those vitamin K-dependent proteins, VKA therapy results in hepatic synthesis of proteins with reduced coagulation factor activity [11–14]. Warfarin, acenocoumarol, phenprocoumon, and fluindione are the different VKAs available in various countries around the world. Because warfarin is the most widely available VKA, most studies have focused on management of warfarin-associated coagulopathy (i.e., elevated INRs) or warfarin-induced major bleeding. This section will focus on relevant aspects to be taken into consideration for reversal of warfarin, although the general principles and strategies likely apply to all VKAs.

The strategy for reversal of the anticoagulant effect of warfarin is dependent on the indication and urgency of the situation. Frequently encountered reasons for warfarin reversal include the following:

- Supratherapeutic INR without bleeding
- Major bleeding with a therapeutic INR
- Supratherapeutic INR values with serious or major bleeding
- Need for urgent surgery or other invasive procedures with increased bleeding risk while the INR is within therapeutic range

The presence of life-threatening bleeding or bleeding within a critical area of the body, such as

ICH, is a major determinant of the urgency with which VKA anticoagulation must be reversed.

Additional consideration must be given to the risks associated with anticoagulation reversal. These include the risk of thromboembolism associated with the patient's original indication for anticoagulation, as well as potential adverse effects related to specific reversal strategies.

Overview of Anticoagulation with Warfarin

Warfarin is rapidly absorbed by the gastrointestinal tract, reaching peak plasma levels within 90 min after oral administration [15, 16]. It has high bioavailability and a plasma half-life of 36–42 h [14, 15]. Its antithrombotic effect is achieved predominantly by the reduction of prothrombin (factor II) levels [17–19], and can be measured by the prolongation of the prothrombin time (PT) and increase in the international normalized ratio (INR). Because factor II has a plasma half-life of 60–72 h, warfarin will achieve its desired antithrombotic effect only after at least 4 or 5 days of therapy, hence the need for simultaneous administration of a parenteral anticoagulant drug when initiating warfarin for a patient with acute arterial or venous thromboembolism [14]. Typically, a minimum 5-day overlap is necessary until the PT/INR increases to the desired therapeutic target range.

Patient education and regular INR monitoring are important to provide high-quality anticoagulation with warfarin and to prevent thromboembolic events while minimizing potential bleeding complications. A patient's risk of bleeding with warfarin is highest when anticoagulation is initially started. The level of anticoagulation, comorbidities, and specific patient factors contribute to the associated bleeding risk. Specific patient characteristics associated with an increased risk for bleeding independent of INR include increasing age, heart failure, chronic kidney or liver disease, chronic pulmonary disease, diabetes, alcohol abuse, anemia, hypertension, prior history of major bleeding, prior stroke, fall risk, malignancy, thrombocytopenia, and concomitant use of antiplatelet drugs [20–23].

Variability of the INR is also associated with an increased risk for bleeding [24]. Commonly encountered risk factors for INR instability include a need for frequent dose adjustments [25], dietary variation in vitamin K intake, addition or discontinuation of other medications, and temporary interruption and restarting of warfarin. Acute illness can affect the INR in previously stable patients; over-anticoagulation is most commonly reported with fever and especially diarrheal illness [26]. Thus the frequency of INR monitoring should be increased during any of these time periods. Clinicians should also be aware that there may be no documented supratherapeutic INR or only a brief period of INR instability heralding a bleeding event [27] and that the risk of bleeding approximately doubles for each point of increase in the INR between 3.0 and 6.0 to 6.5 [28, 29]. Indeed, in a retrospective review of patients anticoagulated with VKAs for mechanical heart valves, the risk of major hemorrhage increased in a logarithmic fashion: patients with INRs between 3.0 and 4.5 had the lowest risk (~2 events per 100 patient-years), while patients with INR > 6.5 had the highest risk (75 events per 100 patient-years) [29]. Episodes of extreme over-anticoagulation, defined as INR ≥ 8.0, have been found to be associated with later under-anticoagulation with inadequate time in therapeutic range, placing these patients both at increased risk of bleeding and also increased risk of thrombosis within a short period of time [30].

Vitamin K

Vitamin K_1, or phytonadione, is a fat-soluble, plant-derived form of vitamin K administered to help restore the hepatic synthesis of functional vitamin K-dependent factors II, VII, IX, and X, as well as the natural anticoagulant proteins C and S [31, 32]. The vitamin K antagonist effect of warfarin can be overcome by relatively low doses of vitamin K_1. Other forms include vitamin K_2 (menaquinone) and K_3 (menadione) which are neither widely available for clinical use nor have they been well-studied for reversal of warfarin-associated coagulopathy [31]. For the purpose of this chapter, use of the term vitamin K will refer to phytonadione.

Vitamin K is available in oral tablets or a solution that is administered via intravenous (IV) or subcutaneous (SC) route. Low-dose vitamin K oral tablets can be administered in addition to withholding warfarin doses in patients who do not require urgent reversal of the INR. Alternatively, in countries where vitamin K tablets are not available, low-dose vitamin K dose can be administered safely and effectively by adding 1–2 mg of the intravenous solution to a cup of orange juice [33]. While vitamin K could also be administered via intramuscular (IM) injection, this should be avoided due to high risk of hematoma and bleeding in a patient with a supratherapeutic INR.

Because the risk of bleeding associated with VKAs increases exponentially when the INR is greater than 4.5 [34], studies evaluating the effectiveness of INR reversal with vitamin K have typically included patients with moderately elevated INR values (between 4.5 and 10.0 or between 6.0 and 10.0), or with extremely elevated INR values (>10.0), as well as with or without active bleeding. Some studies measured magnitude and timing of INR reversal (laboratory endpoint), whereas other studies attempted to determine whether vitamin K supplementation was in fact associated with a lower risk of bleeding in follow-up (clinical endpoint). Laboratory reversal of the INR with adequate correction of VKA-related coagulopathy does not necessarily translate into more effective clinical outcomes such as lower bleeding rates.

In a RCT which included patients with INR values between 6.0 and 10.0 without bleeding, a strategy of low-dose oral vitamin K combined with temporary interruption of warfarin was associated with INR < 4.0 in less than 2 days [35]. However, four randomized controlled trials (RCTs) showed that the rates of both major bleeding and thromboembolic events were similar during follow-up periods of 1–3 months in patients who were treated with oral vitamin K versus placebo for moderately elevated INR values (between 4.5 and 10.0) without bleeding [33, 36–38].

In patients with INRs greater than 10.0 without active bleeding, one retrospective study showed that low-dose oral vitamin K (2 mg) was associated with a lower frequency of INR > 5.0 after 72 h compared to placebo (11.1% versus 46.7%) [39], whereas a prospective cohort study reported a low rate (3.9%) of major bleeding after 90 days of administration of low-dose (2.5 mg) vitamin K [40].

Based on available data, current guidelines suggest against routine use of vitamin K for patients with INRs between 4.5 and 10.0 without active bleeding. But the use of low-dose oral vitamin K is suggested for patients with INR > 10.0 without active bleeding because of their exceptionally high risk of hemorrhagic complications (Table 6.1) [41].

Subcutaneous vitamin K has been shown to be less effective than oral administration, likely due to inconsistent absorption. Clinical trials have demonstrated that less than 50% of patients achieve an INR < 4.0 at 24 h after SC dosing [42, 43]. Similarly, SC administration is not as effective as IV dosing. In one RCT, low-dose (0.5 mg) intravenous administration of vitamin K was shown to correct supratherapeutic INRs more rapidly than a SC dose of 3 mg, with 95% and 45% of patients having INR values <5.0 measured 24 h after IV and SC dosing, respectively [44]. Therefore, the best available evidence suggests that the SC route of administration of vitamin K should not be used.

In patients with elevated INRs between 6.0 and 10.0 without active bleeding, low-dose oral (2.5–5 mg) and low-dose IV (0.5–1 mg) vitamin

Table 6.1 Warfarin reversal prior to invasive procedures

Day of surgery = day 0 • Hold warfarin 5 days before major surgeries or interventions with high risk of bleeding • Recheck PT/INR the day before the procedure – If INR still between 1.4 and 1.9, give vitamin K 1 mg PO
Warfarin may not have to be held prior to minor procedures (such as single tooth extractions) or may be withheld 3–4 days prior to procedures which can be performed with an INR of 1.5–1.8

K yield similar reductions in INR values 24 h after dosing [45, 46]. However, IV vitamin K has a more rapid onset of action than oral administration. In a RCT trial of patients with INRs between 6.0 and 10.0 without bleeding, low-dose IV vitamin K was successful at correcting the warfarin-related coagulopathy and bringing the INR down to the therapeutic range in 11 of 24 patients 6 h after dosing (versus 0 of 23 patients who received low-dose oral vitamin K) [45]. When administered at higher doses, IV vitamin K has even more rapid onset of action with reduction of the INR beginning within 2 h, and normalization of the INR within 12–16 h (assuming normal hepatic function), compared to normalization of the INR in up to 24 h after oral vitamin K administration [31, 44, 45, 47].

Therefore, even though there are no prospective trials comparing IV vitamin K with no IV vitamin K for treatment of VKA-associated bleeding events, extrapolation from those studies in patients with elevated INR but without bleeding indicates that IV is the preferred route of vitamin K administration in patients with VKA-related major bleeding. The optimal IV dose is unknown; most reports used a dose ranging from 5 to 10 mg (Table 6.1). In these situations, the INR should be repeated every 6–12 h [47, 48], and repeat dose(s) of vitamin K may be necessary 12 h after the initial dose. It is important to note that higher doses of vitamin K (single or cumulative, regardless of route of administration) are associated with a greater risk of resistance to VKA therapy once it is resumed [49].

Anaphylactoid reactions have been reported with intravenous administration of vitamin K, with an estimated incidence of 3 cases per 10,000 administered doses; one case was reported after IM administration, and a review did not identify any reports after oral or SC administration [50]. Most documented cases occurred with rapid administration of large intravenous doses of vitamin K containing polyethoxylated castor oil (PEO-CO) as the solubilizing vehicle [31, 50]. As a pharmaceutical grade inactive excipient, PEO-CO is commonly used to emulsify and solubilize oils and other water-insoluble substances; PEO is common to many formulations available in the United States. Anaphylaxis has also been reported after the administration of other drugs solubilized in polyethylene oxide (PEO)-based formulations, including cyclosporine and cisplatin [51–54]. Pretreatment with antihistamines or corticosteroids is not routinely recommended before the administration of vitamin K; however, patients should be closely monitored during the infusion, and pretreatment could be considered in patients with prior reactions [50]. To reduce the risk of reactions, it is recommended that vitamin K be mixed with at least 50 mL of intravenous fluid and be administered over a minimum of 20–30 min or not exceeding 1 mg per minute [31, 55]. Current vitamin K formulations with mixed micelles of lecithin and glycol appear to be safer than the previous preparations containing PEO-CO [56, 57]. The oral form of vitamin K does not contain PEO-CO. There are no reports of reactions following oral administration of the intravenous solution.

Warfarin Reversal Prior to Surgery

It is recommended that patients stop warfarin 5 days before elective surgery and certain invasive procedures [56, 58, 59]. This recommendation is based on an expected warfarin half-life of 36–42 h and usually allows for regeneration of vitamin K-dependent coagulation factors, normalization of the INR, and achievement of normal hemostasis. However, due to variation between patients, it is recommended that the PT/INR be checked on the day before surgery to ensure normalization [59]. If a patient on warfarin has an INR between 1.4 and 1.9 the day before surgery, administration of 1 mg of oral vitamin K reduces the INR to less than 1.5 in 91% of patients by the next day (i.e., the day of surgery) [59]. However, similar strategies will have a much higher failure rate if patients hold their VKA only 2 days before surgery, especially if taking VKAs with a longer plasma half-life than warfarin (such as acenocoumarol or fluindione) [60]. Certain procedures with a lower bleeding risk may be performed safely when the INR is lowered to a range of 1.5–1.8; thus a shorter interval of withholding warfarin may be appropriate in these instances. It is important to discuss the perioperative anticoagulation plan with the surgeon/proceduralist to ensure adequate hemostasis can be achieved with partial reversal of the INR (Table 6.1).

Stopping warfarin and allowing the INR to fall are the most frequently used strategies for warfarin-associated coagulopathy in the absence of bleeding or the urgent need for an invasive procedure [61]. While an elevated INR is a marker for increased bleeding risk, there are no data to support that a rapidly corrected supratherapeutic INR is associated with a reduction in bleeding risk [31, 36]. An in-depth review of perioperative management of warfarin and other anticoagulants is discussed in Chap. 9.

Plasma

Transfusions of plasma remain one of the most commonly used strategies to reverse the anticoagulant effect of warfarin in patients with major bleeding. In large part, this is due to clinician familiarity with the product which contains all vitamin K-dependent coagulation factors as well as other plasma proteins [55]. Unfortunately, plasma contains relatively low concentrations of these proteins (1 unit/mL); thus large volumes are required to significantly reduce the INR.

A major pitfall of plasma transfusions for VKA reversal is the potential for rebound coagulopathy if a patient with active bleeding receives plasma without concomitant vitamin K replacement. The elevated PT/INR may correct soon after the transfusion is completed, but a rebound increase in the INR (with the potential for recurrent bleeding) may occur within 36–72 h if the patient does not receive vitamin K initially. This occurs because the plasma half-life of some of the infused coagulation factors is shorter than the plasma half-life of warfarin. Therefore, supplemental vitamin K is required to adequately restore hepatic production of functionally normal vitamin K-dependent coagulation factors [55].

There are a number of other potential risks and limitations associated with plasma transfusions, including (1) delays in availability and administration that may occur because of the need for cross-matching for ABO group specificity and thawing (such delays may be 30 min or longer), (2) risk of transmission of blood-borne pathogens because most plasma products are not virally inactivated, (3) risk of allergic reactions including urticaria (quite common) and anaphylaxis (estimated incidence of 1 in 20,000 transfusions), and (4) risk of transfusion-related acute lung injury (TRALI) which is estimated to occur in approximately 1 in 5000 FFP transfusions [56, 62–67]. Moreover, as previously mentioned, plasma requires large transfusion volumes, leading to prolonged transfusion times of up to several hours and, most importantly, risk of intravascular volume overload [56, 62]. The recommended dose of fresh frozen plasma (FFP) in the setting of major bleeding is typically 15 mL/kg (10–20 mL/kg), which for an adult weighing 100 kg would correspond to 1500 mL (4–6 units) of FFP [62, 67]. In a small RCT comparing transfusion of FFP alone or in combination with a factor IX complex concentrate, five of eight patients receiving FFP alone developed fluid overload despite intensive monitoring of central venous pressure and furosemide use [66]. Lower transfusion volumes of FFP may be required as a supplemental source of factor VII concomitant to 3-factor prothrombin complex concentrate (PCC) infusion [56].

Given the available data on PCCs, the use of plasma transfusions for management of acute major bleeding associated with VKA therapy should only be considered in circumstances and/or locations when PCCs are not available (Table 6.2) [56, 62, 71, 72].

Prothrombin Complex Concentrates

Prothrombin complex concentrates were originally developed for the treatment of patients with hemophilia B [65, 73], but currently they are primarily used for prevention and treatment of bleeding associated with VKA therapy [73]. Compared to FFP, PCCs do not require cross-matching, can be infused within less than 30 min, and are not associated with the risk of volume overload [55, 56, 73]. Indeed, the typical doses of PCC required to achieve 50–100% of vitamin K-dependent coagulation factor levels in plasma can be administered in volumes as little as 1–2 mL/kg [73]. In a recent prospective trial, the median volume of PCC infused was 90 mL over 12 min [74]. These products also undergo one or two steps of viral inactivation or elimination techniques, such as pasteurization, nanofiltration, vapor heat treatment, and/or addition of solvent detergent [56, 73].

Prothrombin complex concentrates are produced by ion-exchange chromatography from pooled human plasma after removal of antithrombin and factor XI [75]. Different processing techniques enable production of 3- or 4-factor concentrates, with a final coagulation factor concentration approximately 25 times higher than in normal plasma [67]. There are three types of PCC products with variable availability in different countries:

1. 4-factor PCCs contain adequate levels of all vitamin K-dependent coagulation factors (II, VII, IX, X) as well as protein C and protein S. The 4-factor PCCs also contain heparin;

Table 6.2 Strategies for reversal of anticoagulant drugs [68–70]

Anticoagulant class	Specific drug	Reversal agent	Dose (comments)
Vitamin K antagonist	Warfarin	Oral vitamin K (no bleeding) Intravenous vitamin K (with bleeding) PCCs FFP	• 1 mg–5 mg PO (complete effect in 24 h) • 5 mg–10 mg IV (complete effect in 6–12 h) KCentra® [68] • If INR 2–3.9 = >25 IU/kg • If INR 4.0–6.0 = >35 IU/kg • If INR >6.0 = >50 IU/kg (concomitant IV vitamin K replacement recommended) Profilnine® SD, Bebulin® [69, 70] • 1.0 IU/kg multiplied by desired % increase in factor IX (plasma levels of factor IX should be monitored during replacement therapy) • 10–15 mL/kg (if PCCs not available); concomitant vit. K replacement recommended
Heparins	Unfractionated heparin (UFH)	Protamine sulfate	• 1 mg per 100 anti-Xa units of UFH administered within previous 3–4 h; complete immediate reversal • Total dose not to exceed 50 mg
	Low-molecular-weight heparins (LMWHs)	Protamine sulfate	• 1 mg per 100 anti-Xa units (administered within the last 8 h) • 0.5 mg per 100 anti-Xa units (if bleeding not controlled after initial dose or if last dose more than 8 h prior to bleeding) • Total dose not to exceed 50 mg (provides incomplete reversal)
Pentasaccharides	Fondaparinux	Recombinant factor VIIa	• 90 µg/kg IV (reports in healthy volunteers; no clinical studies in patients with bleeding)
	Idrabiotaparinux[a]	Avidin	• 75–100 mg IV (experimental therapy)
Direct thrombin inhibitors	Parenteral	Argatroban, bivalirudin Lepirudin[b]	• rFVIIa (no studies or recommended doses in clinical bleeding, typical doses range 80–90 mcg/kg); hemodialysis • rFVIIa and hemodialysis with high-flux capillary membranes

(continued)

Table 6.2 (continued)

Anticoagulant class	Specific drug	Reversal agent	Dose (comments)
	Oral (dabigatran)	Idarucizumab	• Two 2.5 g doses (50 mL each) administered as IV bolus, 15 min apart
Oral direct factor Xa inhibitors[c]	Apixaban Rivaroxaban	Andexanet alfa[d]	• Apixaban-treated patients: 400 mg bolus during a period of 15–30 min, followed by 480 mg infusion over 2 h • Rivaroxaban-treated patients – If last dose >7 h prior to bleeding: 400 mg bolus during a period of 15–30 min, followed by 480 mg infusion over 2 h – If last dose ≤7 h prior to bleeding: 800 mg bolus during a period of 15–30 min, followed by 960 mg infusion over 2 h

PO per os (per oral), *IV* intravenous, *PCCs* prothrombin complex concentrates, *IU* international units, *kg* kilograms, *FFP* fresh frozen plasma, *rFVIIa* recombinant factor VIIa
[a]Not FDA-approved
[b]No longer available in the United States
[c]No edoxaban-treated patients were included in the ANNEXA-4 study data that have been published to this date
[d]Not yet approved by the FDA

thus they should be avoided in patients with heparin-induced thrombocytopenia [56].

2. 3-factor PCC products contain factors II, IX, and X but only low levels of factor VII. Failure to restore factor VII activity may result in suboptimal reversal of VKA-induced coagulopathy due to persistently low levels of factor VII [56, 62, 76]. Despite this concern, there have been reports of successful reversal of warfarin coagulopathy without concomitant transfusion of FFP [56, 77–79].
3. Activated PCC products contain therapeutic levels of activated factors VIIa and Xa and nonactivated factor II and IX levels. In the United States, they are labeled for control of bleeding and periprocedural bleeding management in patients with hemophilia A and B who have factor inhibitors, but they have been used "off-label" for warfarin reversal as well.

Despite the fact that optimal doses for the different PCC products have not been determined, PCCs are clearly more effective in correcting the INR than FFP [55, 56, 62, 66, 80–90]. The only RCT which compared PPCs with FFP alone (i.e., without concomitant use of vitamin K) showed that a 3-factor PCC was more effective in reducing the INR compared to FFP in patients anticoagulated with warfarin for mechanical heart valves who required interventional procedures [90]. In this study, INRs were measured serially between 15 min and 48 h after infusion of either PCC or FFP. A target INR (defined as INR < 2.5) was achieved in 76% and 20% of patients in the PCC and FFP groups, respectively, 48 h after infusion [90]. A recent meta-analysis, which included five RCTs and eight observational studies comparing use of PCCs with FFP, revealed that PCC was more likely associated with INR correction and that INR normalization was achieved in a shorter time than after FFP transfusions [89].

Earlier studies with either 3-factor or 4-factor PCCs demonstrated more rapid correction of the INR, but not until a few h post-PCC infusion. In a small case series of 17 patients with VKA-associated intracranial hemorrhage, the use of a 3-factor PCC led to complete correction of the INR from 2.8 to 1.2 within 4.8 h, compared to INR reduction from ~3.0 to 1.7 within 7.3 h in patients who received only FFP transfusions [81]. Similarly, a small RCT comparing a factor IX complex concentrate combined with FFP versus FFP transfusions alone demonstrated much more rapid normalization of the INR in the group of patients receiving factor IX concentrate plus FFP compared with FFP alone (2.95 h versus 8.9 h, respectively) [66].

While the use of individualized dosing of a 4-factor PCC was not more effective than fixed dosing in achieving a target INR in one study [83], there is increasing evidence to support different doses of 4-factor PCCs according to initial INR, with higher doses resulting in more effective INR reversal in patients with higher baseline INR values [56, 74, 84, 85]. In a prospective trial, the use of a 4-factor PCC resulted in INR ≤ 1.3 in 93% of patients [74]. This study used higher doses of PCC according to the initial INR on presentation: 25, 35, and 50 international units (IU)/kg for INR values of <4.0, 4.0–6.0, and >6.0, respectively [74]. Time to INR correction post-infusion of a 4-factor PCC has been reported to be as rapid as within 10–30 min [74, 84, 86]. Moreover, it is recommended that patients receiving PCCs also be treated with vitamin K supplementation [56, 62, 81].

The potential risk of suboptimal INR correction with the use of a 3-factor PCC was observed in a prospective study with historical controls, in which 40 consecutive patients with INR > 5 were treated with a 3-factor PCC at either a low-dose (25 units/kg) or a high-dose (50 units/kg) [76]. Only 50% and 43% of patients achieved the target INR < 3.0 in the low- and high-dose groups, respectively, compared with 63% of patients with INR < 3.0 in the historical group that had received FFP transfusions alone [76]. Additional transfusion of FFP (mean, 2 units) increased the rate of achieving an INR < 3.0 to 89% and 88% in the low- and high-dose groups, respectively [76]. Furthermore, a retrospective cohort study showed that only 58% of patients had adequate INR correction after receiving a 3-factor PCC [91]. Among the 42% who had inadequate control of the INR, the initial INR was significantly higher than in the group of individuals with adequate reversal but only moderately so (3.5 versus 2.5) [91]. Another study using a 3-factor PCC also demonstrated that the lowest rate of INR correction was seen in patients with the highest initial INR values [92]. In this small prospective cohort study, the use of 3-factor PCC was associated with adequate INR reversal in 89%, 33%, and 0% of patients who had initial INR values between 2.0 to 4.0, 4.0 to 6.0, and >6.0, respectively [92].

Thus, despite the fact that 3-factor PCCs are more effective than FFP transfusions alone in reversing VKA-associated coagulopathy, these products may not be the PCC of choice for reversal of VKA-induced bleeding unless they are administered with concomitant plasma transfusion [62]. While this recommendation has been disputed by recent reports of successful reversal of warfarin coagulopathy without concomitant transfusion of FFP [56, 77–79], definitive recommendations are not possible due to the lack of prospective RCTs comparing the different PCC products with or without concomitant FFP. Therefore, given the best available evidence to date, and until prospective randomized data comparing 4-factor and 3-factor PCCs become available, 4-factor PCCs (if available) are preferred over 3-factor PCCs for reversal of VKA-induced coagulopathy [62].

Even though it is clear that PCCs lead to a more effective laboratory correction of VKA-associated coagulopathy (laboratory endpoint), data are much more limited in terms of cessation of bleeding (clinical endpoint). Nevertheless, in one prospective study of patients presenting with VKA-associated major bleeding (n = 17) or requiring immediate INR reversal for emergent invasive procedures (n = 26), administration of 4-factor PCC resulted in a clinical hemostatic efficacy deemed "good or very good" in 98% (n = 42) [74]. In addition, PCCs have also been associated with reduced progression of intracranial hemorrhage as defined by clinical and imaging criteria in one small series [81].

Data on the safety of PCCs are limited. While thromboembolic events have rarely been reported, accurate rates of thromboembolic complications are not known. In a prospective study, there was one fatal pulmonary embolism out of 43 patients who received a 4-factor PCC [74]. One review of the literature reported a rate of thromboembolic events of 1.5% (n = 7) among 460 patients who received PCCs for reversal of VKA [88]. In a meta-analysis of 27 studies using PCCs for rapid reversal of VKAs, the rate of thromboembolic events was 1.8% [93]. A meta-analysis of five RCTs and eight observational studies showed that PCC use was associated with lower all-cause mortality (odds ratio, 0.56; p = 0.006) without any statistically significant difference in the risk of thromboembolic events after administration of PCC or FFP (odds ratio, 0.91) [89].

Recombinant Factor VIIa

Recombinant factor VIIa (rFVIIa) is a prohemostatic agent first reported as a treatment for bleeding in patients with hemophilia A in 1983 [94]. Based on a modern understanding of normal hemostasis in vivo, rFVIIa likely exerts its prohemostatic effect by initially binding to exposed tissue factor at the sites of vascular injury, resulting in an increase in thrombin generation. But rFVIIa is also likely capable of generating a "thrombin burst" via tissue factor-independent pathways, by interacting with activated platelets even in the presence of significant underlying platelet dysfunction [55, 95, 96]. Data on the use of rFVIIa for the reversal of VKA-associated coagulopathy and bleeding are limited; thus rFVIIa is not approved specifically for reversal of VKA. Nevertheless, rFVIIa administration led to complete correction of INRs >2.0 in healthy volunteers who received acenocoumarol [97]. The duration of INR correction was >24 h in those who received higher doses (i.e., > 120 μg/kg) [97]. In two small case series, which included patients with major bleeding or who required rapid reversal of the INR for emergent interventions, rFVIIa infusion resulted in variable reductions in the INR within 2 h after infusion [98, 99]. Complete correction of the mean INR from 2.7 to <1.2 was seen following rFVIIa administration in another small case series of seven patients presenting with intracranial hemorrhage associated with warfarin use, but some patients also received vitamin K and FFP transfusions [100].

It is important to note, however, that correction of a laboratory endpoint does not necessarily translate into an adequate hemostatic response with clinical cessation of bleeding. Indeed, rFVIIa failed to provide a clinically adequate hemostatic effect despite correction of the INR in animal models of VKA-induced bleeding [101]. But a small case series of patients with VKA-associated intracranial hemorrhage reported not only adequate reversal of VKA-associated coagulopathy but also adequate control of bleeding as defined by clinical criteria [102]. Moreover, several case reports and a small case series have reported that the use of rFVIIa resulted in effective control and/or cessation of bleeding in VKA-treated patients [103, 104]. Other reports indicated that administration of rFVIIa was also successful for prevention of bleeding in patients receiving VKAs who required invasive procedures [98, 103].

The dose of rFVIIa used to treat bleeding in hemophiliacs with inhibitors is typically 90 μg/kg administered as an IV bolus over 2–5 min. When such patients present with major bleeding, this dose results in the successful arrest of bleeding within 2–3 h in >80–93% of patients [104]. In contrast, there are no prospective trials of rFVIIa for the treatment of VKA-associated major bleeding, so there are no specific dosing recommendations for this indication. Case reports and small case series have used widely different rFVIIa doses for VKA-related coagulopathy and/or bleeding, varying from 5 to 320 μg/kg [97, 98, 102–104]. It is important to note that the plasma half-life of rFVIIa is much shorter (~2 h) than that of PCCs (~8 h) which also contain other vitamin K-dependent factors with longer half-lives than factor VII [104]. Thus there is a potential concern for a rebound in the INR as well as recurrent clinical bleeding.

Furthermore, the safety of rFVIIa administration for correction of VKA-associated coagulopathy with or without bleeding is not well defined. Because these patients are presumably prothrombotic (as opposed to hemophiliacs) given their need for anticoagulation, the risk of thromboembolic complications is an issue of concern. Although precise data on thromboembolic complications following administration of rFVIIa are not available in the setting of VKA reversal, rFVIIa administration has been associated with both arterial and venous thromboembolism in patients with hemophilia and in patients presenting with intracranial hemorrhage not related to anticoagulation [104–107]. Thromboembolic events were reported in 1% of hemophilic patients who received rFVIIa [105], and there are also reports of acute myocardial infarction [104, 106]. In one randomized, double-blind, placebo-controlled trial of rFVIIa for treatment of intracranial hemorrhage in patients not receiving any anticoagulation, the rate of thromboembolic events was 7% ($n = 21$) in patients who received doses of rFVIIa ranging from 40, 80, to 160 μg/kg [107]. In all, 76% of the events were arterial (acute coronary syndromes and acute ischemic stroke), and 24% were venous (acute deep vein thrombosis and pulmonary embolism); all but 4 events occurred within 72 h of rFVIIa administration [107]. While there are no prospective RCTs comparing the use of rFVIIa with PCCs, it has been estimated that the incidence of thromboembolic events following rFVIIa administration may be three times higher than that of PCCs (24.6 per 10,000 infusions versus 8.2 per 10,000 infusions of rFVIIa and PCCs, respectively) [108].

In 1999, the US Food and Drug Administration (FDA) approved rFVIIa for treatment of bleeding episodes in patients with hemophilia A or B and inhibitors to factor VIII or factor IX. In 2005, the FDA extended the label of rFVIIa to include surgical procedures in patients with hemophilia A or B (and inhibitors) and treatment of bleeding episodes in patients with factor VII deficiency. A review of the FDA's Adverse Event Reporting System (AERS) database showed that the estimated number of hospitalized patients treated with rFVIIa increased 13-fold between 2000 and 2004 [109]. During that period, there were 185 adverse events which were due to thromboembolic complications, 52% of which occurred within 24 h of rFVIIa dosing. Off-label use of rFVIIa accounted for the majority ($n = 151$) of the reports [109]. Arterial thromboembolic events (54.1%) included acute ischemic stroke (21.3%), acute myocardial infarction (18.6%), and peripheral embolism (14.2%) including hepatic, renal, splenic, femoral, and iliac arterial embolism. Venous thromboembolic events included acute pulmonary embolism (17.5%) and acute deep vein thrombosis (22.9%) involving the lower extremity, internal jugular, superior mesenteric, portal, renal, and retinal veins. There were also device-related thromboses (5%) involving extracorporeal membrane oxygenation (ECMO) lines, hemodialysis catheters, and grafts. Of 50 reported deaths, the probable cause of death was thromboembolism in 36 (72%) [109]. These findings raise the concern that rFVIIa may be more thrombogenic in non-hemophiliac patients.

Recombinant factor VIIa is not FDA-approved for reversal of VKA-associated coagulopathy or bleeding. Based on available data, and given the existence of more appropriate and targeted therapies for VKA reversal, the use of rFVIIa for this indication should only be considered in extreme circumstances, such as treatment of life-threatening bleeding when PCCs are not available and FFP would require long transfusion times and thus not provide rapid INR reversal [55, 62, 110]. The use of rFVIIa has also been suggested as a "rescue" therapy if PCCs and FFP transfusions fail to stop bleeding and/or completely reverse a supratherapeutic INR [55, 62, 110].

Heparins

Unfractionated heparin (UFH) and low-molecular-weight heparins (LMWHs) are antithrombotic drugs approved for prevention and treatment of venous and arterial thromboembolic events. Heparin was originally discovered in 1916 by McLean and Howell [111], whereas LMWHs were originally described in 1976 [112–114]. Heparins are negatively charged polysaccharides which exert their anticoagulant properties by binding to and activating antithrombin [115–118]. Heparins bind to the lysine site of the antithrombin molecule through a glucosamine unit contained within a high-affinity pentasaccharide sequence [117–120]. Such binding induces a conformational change in the arginine-reactive site on antithrombin that converts it into a rapid inhibitor of a number of coagulation serine proteases, including factors IIa (thrombin), IXa, Xa, XIa, and XIIa [116–118]. Of these, factors IIa and Xa are the most sensitive to inhibition. The conformational change induced by heparin-binding accelerates the antithrombin's reaction kinetics by several 1000-fold [118].

In order to inhibit thrombin (factor IIa), heparin must simultaneously bind to antithrombin and thrombin [121]. Heparin molecules bind to antithrombin through their unique pentasaccharide sequence, and a minimum of 13 additional saccharide units are necessary to simultaneously bind to thrombin. Unfractionated heparin molecules with chain lengths less than 18 saccharide units are incapable of binding simultaneously to antithrombin and thrombin [121]. The inhibition of factor Xa by heparins is also dependent on heparin-antithrombin binding through the unique pentasaccharide sequence, but it does not require simultaneous binding to the factor Xa molecule [119, 121]. At clinically administered doses, only one-third of unfractionated heparin molecules bind to antithrombin and have anticoagulant function [121].

The LMWHs result from chemical or enzymatic depolymerization of the larger UFH molecules, resulting in smaller fragments. Those with chain lengths containing less than 18 saccharide units are incapable of binding to both antithrombin and thrombin and hence cannot catalyze thrombin inhibition. While some clinically available LMWHs are still capable of generating anti-IIa activity, the predominant anticoagulant effect of LMWHs is exerted via anti-Xa activity. This is because LMWHs are still capable of binding to antithrombin through the unique pentasaccharide sequence, thus catalyzing the inhibition of factor Xa by antithrombin [121–124]. Therefore, LMWHs are indirect factor Xa inhibitors because such inhibition is mediated by their binding to antithrombin.

Even though UFH inhibits factors IIa and Xa in a 1:1 ratio, its anticoagulant effect is primarily driven by its inhibition of factor IIa because human thrombin is tenfold more sensitive to inactivation by the heparin-antithrombin complex than human factor Xa [118–121]. Conversely, LMWHs have much less anti-factor IIa activity than UFH but maintain its antithrombotic and anticoagulant properties by predominantly inhibiting factor Xa [121]. While the anti-factor IIa activity of UFH is expressed by its prolongation of the activated partial thromboplastin time (aPTT), the anticoagulant effect of LMWHs cannot be measured by the aPTT as the anti-Xa/anti-IIa ratios of LMWHs range between 2:1 and 4:1 [121, 125–129].

Compared to UFH, LMWHs have a reduced IIa to Xa ratio [125], more predictable anticoagulant response, less nonspecific binding to positively charged plasma and cellular proteins, lower immunogenicity, and lower activation of osteoclasts. These differences result in a longer plasma half-life (allowing for once- or twice-daily subcutaneous administration), lower incidence of heparin-induced thrombocytopenia (HIT), and lower incidence of osteoporosis compared to UFH. Moreover, LMWHs do not require laboratory monitoring due to more predictable pharmacokinetics and pharmacodynamics in individuals with normal renal function [121].

Protamine Sulfate

The plasma half-life of UFH is approximately 60–90 min after intravenous administration of a typical clinical dose; as a result, most of the anticoagulant effect of UFH will disappear within 4 h of discontinuation of an intravenous infusion [130]. If a major bleeding event occurs and immediate reversal is required, the anticoagulant effect of UFH can be rapidly neutralized by protamine sulfate. Protamine is a cationic protein derived from fish sperm which binds to the anionic UFH molecule forming a stable salt with a neutralization ratio of 1 mg of protamine sulfate per 100 units of heparin [130]. Due to the short plasma half-life of UFH, the dose of protamine sulfate required to reverse the effect of UFH should be calculated taking into consideration only the proportion of the total units of UFH administered over the previous 3–4 h (bolus included) (Table 6.2). A fall in the aPTT can be used to confirm heparin neutralization [131]. The thrombin time also normalizes after heparin neutralization by protamine, which has a plasma half-life of approximately 7 min [130].

Protamine can only partially reverse the anticoagulant effect of LMWHs because it only neutralizes the larger molecular weight moieties that preferentially inhibit factor IIa activity while incompletely neutralizing their predominant anti-Xa activity [121, 132–136]. As a result, protamine sulfate only neutralizes approximately 60% and 80% of the anticoagulant effect of enoxaparin and dalteparin, respectively. The degree of neutralization of anti-Xa activity by protamine is strongly correlated with the total sulfate content of the LMWHs; thus theoretically protamine would be more effective at neutralizing dalteparin than enoxaparin [136]. However, there are no clinical data to confirm or refute this hypothesis. In animal models, protamine has been reported to be effective in controlling microvascular bleeding despite persistent anti-Xa activity [137–139]. However, the clinical efficacy of such incomplete anti-Xa neutralization in controlling bleeding complications in humans is unknown. In a small case series of patients undergoing cardiac surgery with extracorporeal circulation, protamine failed to control bleeding in two of three patients who had developed excessive bleeding [140].

Protamine dosing recommendations for reversal of bleeding related to LMWHs are not based on clinical studies but recommendations by the manufacturer and consist of a dose of protamine of 1 mg per 100 anti-Xa units if the last dose of LMWHs was administered within 8 h, with smaller doses required if bleeding persists or if the last dose of LMWHs was more than 8 h ago (0.5 mg protamine per 100 anti-Xa units) [130] (Table 6.1).

Serious adverse reactions such as hypotension, bradycardia, and anaphylaxis have been reported in individuals receiving intravenous bolus doses of protamine. Individuals felt to be at higher risk of developing such severe allergic reactions include those with previous exposure to protamine or to protamine-containing insulin, as well as those who have undergone vasectomy or have hypersensitivity to fish. Pretreatment with antihistamines or steroids may be considered in those individuals who might be at increased risk of having preformed antibodies against protamine [130].

Experimental Therapies

There is one case report of successful use of rFVIIa to control bleeding in a patient with acute renal failure who was receiving LMWH and aspirin [141]. Synthetic variants of protamine appear to be very effective at neutralizing the anticoagulant effect of LMWH, including anti-Xa activity, in animal models, but there are no reports of their use in humans [130, 142, 143].

Andexanet alfa is a modified factor Xa decoy that is devoid of enzymatic activity but possesses high-affinity binding sites capable of binding and inhibiting direct and indirect factor Xa inhibitors [144]. ANNEXA-4 is an ongoing prospective open-label study evaluating the efficacy of andexanet alfa in patients with acute major bleeding while on anticoagulation with apixaban, rivaroxaban, or enoxaparin [145]. A total of 67 patients were evaluated in the published interim report, but only four patients had major bleeding while on enoxaparin at doses of 90–200 mg daily. Those patients had baseline anti-Xa activity levels ranging from 0.4 to 0.6 anti-Xa units/mL; thus only one patient was included in the efficacy analysis (those with <0.5 units/mL were excluded from the efficacy analysis but included in the safety analysis). In that one patient, anti-factor Xa activity of enoxaparin was reduced from 0.61 anti-Xa units/mL to 0.15 anti-Xa units/mL at the end of the bolus administration and to 0.19 anti-Xa units/mL after the 2-h infusion. The anti-Xa activity increased to 0.46 anti-Xa units/mL 4 h after the end of the infusion. Therefore, andexanet alfa is considered a potential reversal agent for enoxaparin pending additional data on enoxaparin-treated patients being included in the ongoing, active ANNEXA-4 study [145].

Ciraparantag is a synthetic, water-soluble molecule that is capable of binding directly to anionic molecules. Thus, it is potentially capable of neutralizing the effects of several anticoagulants including UFH and LMWH. In a Phase 1/2 trial, four cohorts of ten healthy subjects received escalating doses of ciraparantag (100–300 mg) IV or placebo approximately 4 h after a single SC 1.5 mg/kg dose of enoxaparin [146]. The study demonstrated a complete and rapid reversal of enoxaparin as measured by the whole blood clotting time in the treated group, compared to placebo. Such differences were no longer present at 12 and 24 h after the IV dose, and there was no increase in the plasma levels of procoagulant markers (D-dimer, fragment F1.2) [146].

Pentasaccharides

The synthetic pentasaccharide fondaparinux is an indirect factor Xa inhibitor that binds to antithrombin and accelerates its inactivation of factor Xa. Due to its very short chain length consisting solely of the unique pentasaccharide sequence which binds with high affinity to the lysine site of the antithrombin molecule, fondaparinux enhances antithrombin-mediated factor Xa inhibition without any factor IIa inhibition given the lack of the additional glycosaminoglycan saccharide residues necessary to bind to thrombin [120, 121, 147–149].

Fondaparinux is a synthetic analog of that unique pentasaccharide sequence with a structural modification that increases its affinity for antithrombin and plasma half-life (~17–21 h). Its specific anti-Xa activity is approximately seven times higher than LMWHs [130]. Idraparinux and idrabiotaparinux are other synthetic pentasaccharides that have completed Phase 3 trials for treatment of venous thromboembolic disease. Idraparinux has a much longer plasma half-life (~130 h) than fondaparinux, and its elimination half-life prolongs to approximately 600 h after once-weekly dosing for >12 weeks [150]. In Phase 3 clinical trials, the termination half-life (*t* 1/2) during steady state (35 days) of idraparinux prolonged to 60 days [151, 152].

There are no specific antidotes for reversal of the anticoagulant effects of pentasaccharides. Fondaparinux does not bind to protamine sulfate [130]. The use of rFVIIa has been evaluated for reversal of fondaparinux and idraparinux in randomized, placebo-controlled studies with healthy volunteers [153, 154]. Laboratory endpoints were used to demonstrate that a single IV dose of rFVIIa (90 μg/kg) was effective in normalizing the aPTT and PT while simultaneously normalizing the thrombin generation time (TGT) and endogenous thrombin potential (ETP) within 6 h after injection [153, 154]. A small case series was published on the use of rFVIIa in eight patients who were being treated with fondaparinux and developed major bleeding [155]. The dose of rFVIIa was 90 μg/kg IV once, but FFP was also given to some patients. Adequate control of bleeding within 6 h after rFVIIa dosing was observed in 4 patients, but 3 other patients were deemed to have had inadequate clinical control of bleeding following rFVIIa [155].

Idrabiotaparinux consists of the idraparinux molecule with an added biotin moiety introduced at position 2 of the nonreducing end glucose of idraparinux [150]. Biotin was added in a position that does not interact with antithrombin and does modify the anti-Xa activity of the pentasaccharide [156, 157]. The biotinylated idraparinux molecule was developed specifically so that the drug could be completely reversed by avidin [150]. Avidin is a tetrameric protein derived from the egg whites of many species; it has low antigenicity and a plasma half-life of 2 min in animal models [158]. Because of its high affinity for biotin, avidin is used as a reagent for in vitro detection of biotinylated proteins [159]. In animal models, avidin completely neutralized the anti-Xa activity of idrabiotaparinux at a molar ratio of 1:1 without any observed rebound phenomenon 5 days after dosing [157]. In a placebo-controlled, double-blind Phase 1 study, healthy volunteers who received idrabiotaparinux were randomized to receive a single 30-min intravenous infusion of avidin or placebo [160]. In this study, the primary outcome was defined as the change in factor Xa activity measured immediately before and after avidin infusions at doses of 25 mg, 75 mg, and 100 mg. Avidin rapidly reversed the anti-Xa activity of idrabiotaparinux by 66% at the 25 mg dose and 84–90% at the 75 mg and 100 mg doses [160]. In addition, in a prospective sub-study of the EQUINOX trial, 55 patients who were receiving weekly idrabiotaparinux injections for 6 months were randomized to receive avidin ($n = 33$) or placebo ($n = 22$). In the EQUINOX sub-study, the degree of anti-Xa activity reversal was similar to that observed in the healthy volunteer study. There was no evidence of rebound anti-Xa activity at the end of the study period in healthy volunteers (follow-up 14 days) or DVT patients (follow-up 5 days) and no evidence of VTE recurrence 3 months after avidin infusion [160]. Idrabiotaparinux is not approved for prevention or treatment of VTE in the United States.

Parenteral Direct Thrombin Inhibitors (DTIs)

The recombinant hirudins (desirudin and lepirudin), the synthetic polypeptide, bivalirudin, and the L-arginine derivative argatroban exert their anticoagulant effects by directly binding to the active site of thrombin. Because of exclusive factor IIa inhibition, they prolong the thrombin time, and their anticoagulant effects can be measured by the aPTT [130].

There are no specific reversal agents for the DTIs. Experimental therapies that have been reported include rFVIIa and desmopressin acetate (DDAVP). Recombinant factor VIIa has been shown to reduce DTI-related bleeding in animal models. One report demonstrated restoration of thrombin generation after ex vivo addition of recombinant FVIIa to whole blood (harvested from healthy volunteers) that had been spiked with the DTI melagatran [161]. However, it remains unclear whether laboratory demonstration of restored thrombin generation will translate into clinical benefit in reversing DTI-associated bleeding in patients. The use of DDAVP—a synthetic analogue of vasopressin—has been shown to reduce the anticoagulant effect of recombinant hirudin in vitro in a study using blood from patients treated with r-hirudin [162] and reduced the duration of spontaneous rebleeding in animal models of continuous DTI infusion [163]. Large-volume transfusion of cryoprecipitate (>10 units) has also been described [164].

Hemodialysis can remove argatroban and bivalirudin from plasma, whereas hemodialysis using high-flux capillary membranes with a cut point of 50,000 daltons appears to efficiently remove lepirudin from plasma [130].

Oral Direct Thrombin Inhibitor

Dabigatran etexilate is a reversible, oral direct thrombin (factor IIa) inhibitor (DTI) that binds directly to the active site on the thrombin molecule. Dabigatran etexilate is a prodrug, which is rapidly converted to the active drug dabigatran after oral administration and absorption. Peak plasma levels occur within 1–3 h after oral administration, and its plasma half-life is approximately 14–17 h [165]. It is approved for prevention of cardioembolic stroke in patients with nonvalvular atrial fibrillation and for prevention and treatment of acute venous thromboembolic disease.

There is limited ex vivo data supporting the use of activated charcoal to decrease dabigatran absorption from the gastrointestinal tract if given within 2–3 h after dabigatran ingestion. Thus, activated charcoal may be useful for cases of overdose or major bleeding that happen soon after ingestion of dabigatran [166]. Hemodialysis may also be considered for dabigatran-associated bleeding, given dabigatran's limited binding to plasma proteins and lipophilic profile [167, 168].

Unfortunately, PCCs failed to correct coagulation assays (aPTT, thrombin time, and ecarin clotting time) and did not restore thrombin generation potential in a randomized, controlled, crossover study in which 12 healthy volunteers on dabigatran 150 mg twice daily for 2.5 days received a single infusion of a 4-factor PCC (50 IU/kg) [169]. Likewise, rFVIIa failed to show in vitro reversal of the anticoagulant effects of the DTI melagatran when administered to healthy subjects [170].

Idarucizumab is a monoclonal antibody fragment specifically directed against dabigatran. Idarucizumab binds to both free and thrombin-bound dabigatran with an affinity 350 times higher than thrombin, resulting in immediate reversal of dabigatran's anticoagulant effects [171, 172]. Because it does not exhibit thrombin-like enzymatic activity, idarucizumab does not bind to thrombin-like substrates and is devoid of procoagulant effects in vitro. In preclinical studies, idarucizumab was associated with immediate reversal of dabigatran-associated anticoagulant effects and reduction in blood loss in a porcine trauma model [173], as well as clinical bleeding in a rat animal model [174]. In Phase 1 trials in healthy male volunteers aged 18–45 years, peak plasma concentrations of idarucizumab were achieved at or shortly after the end of 5-min or 1-h infusions [175].

The RE-VERSE AD study is an ongoing prospective cohort study examining the efficacy and safety of idarucizumab in dabigatran-treated patients who either present with serious bleeding (Group 1) or require urgent surgery or invasive procedures that require normal hemostasis and cannot be delayed for more than 8 h (Group 2) [176]. An interim analysis of the first 90 patients enrolled a subject population with a median age of 76 years; only one patient was on dabigatran for treatment of acute venous thromboembolic disease. Idarucizumab was administered intravenously as two 50 mL bolus doses containing 2.5 g each, no more than 15 min apart, for a total idarucizumab dose of 5 g. The primary endpoint of RE-VERSE AD was the maximal percentage reversal of the anticoagulant effect of dabigatran as determined by the dilute thrombin time (dTT) or ecarin clotting time (ECT) performed from the end of the first infusion up to 4 h after the second infusion. Secondary endpoints included the percentage of patients with complete reversal of the anticoagulant effect of dabigatran, reduction in the plasma concentration of dabigatran, and clinical outcomes consisting of the time to cessation of bleeding (Group 1) and achievement of hemostasis (Group 2) as assessed by treating clinicians. Approximately two-thirds of patients in this interim cohort analysis were on the 110 mg twice-daily dose of dabigatran, with the remainder taking 150 mg twice-daily (27%) or 75 mg twice-daily (2%). The most common types of serious bleeding in Group 1 were gastrointestinal (39%), intracranial (35%), and trauma-related bleeding (20%) [176].

Eighty-eight percent and 98% of patients demonstrated rapid (within minutes) and complete reversal of the anticoagulant effect of dabigatran as measured by the dTT and ECT, respectively. Plasma levels of dabigatran were <20 ng/mL in all but one patient, confirming the presence of little to no residual anticoagulant effect. Such low levels of unbound dabigatran were present in 79% of patients at 24 h post-infusion. In Group 1, the median investigator-reported time to cessation of bleeding was 11.4 h, and in Group 2, normal intraoperative hemostasis was reported in 92% of the cohort [176].

There were a total of five thrombotic events, with some of the patients having one or more of the following events: acute deep vein thrombosis (DVT), pulmonary embolism, left atrial thrombus, non-ST segment elevation myocardial infarction, and acute ischemic stroke. Only one patient had acute DVT and PE within 72 h after idarucizumab administration [176].

Idarucizumab is now FDA-approved for reversal of dabigatran-associated major bleeding (Table 6.2).

Direct Oral Factor Xa Inhibitors

Unlike UFH, LMWHs, and the synthetic pentasaccharides, which are indirect factor Xa inhibitors because Xa inhibition is dependent on their binding to antithrombin, the direct oral factor Xa inhibitors apixaban, edoxaban, and rivaroxaban directly inhibit factor Xa. Peak plasma levels are achieved within 1–3 h after oral administration, and plasma half-lives range from 5 to 9 h (rivaroxaban), 8 to 15 h (apixaban), and 9 to 11 h (edoxaban), assuming normal renal function [165].

In an animal model, rFVIIa failed to control bleeding induced by rivaroxaban overdose [177]. In contrast, the use of a 4-factor PCC (50 IU/kg) in a randomized, controlled, crossover study of 12 healthy volunteers who received therapeutic doses of rivaroxaban for 2.5 days did result in almost immediate normalization of the PT and near-complete restoration of endogenous thrombin potential immediately following the infusion [169].

Activated charcoal has been shown to reduce plasma levels of apixaban in healthy subjects if given up to 6 h after ingestion of apixaban, with best effects when given within 2 h of the last apixaban dose [178]. Because rivaroxaban and apixaban are more highly protein-bound, it is unlikely that they can be removed from plasma by hemodialysis [167].

Andexanet alfa is a specific reversal agent designed to neutralize the anticoagulant effects of both direct and indirect factor Xa inhibitors [144]. Andexanet alfa is a recombinant, modified factor Xa decoy that binds to both direct and indirect factor Xa inhibitors with very high affinity at a 1:1 stoichiometric ratio, thus neutralizing their anticoagulant effects [144]. Despite the fact that andexanet alfa is structurally similar to native human factor Xa, it is devoid of enzymatic activity due to a substitution of a serine residue with an alanine at the active site. However, the molecule retains the ability to bind and sequester factor Xa inhibitors within the vascular space, thus restoring endogenous factor Xa activity. Preclinical animal and human blood in vitro studies demonstrated that andexanet alfa rapidly and completely reversed the anticoagulant effects of direct factor Xa inhibitors as demonstrated by restored hemostasis and reduced bleeding. The plasma half-life of andexanet alfa is approximately 1 h [144, 179].

The ANNEXA-A and ANNEXA-R trials were double-blind, placebo-controlled studies designed to evaluate the ability of andexanet alfa to reverse the anticoagulant effects of apixaban and rivaroxaban, respectively, as well as its safety in healthy volunteers [180]. Andexanet alfa was administered either as an intravenous bolus dose of 400 mg or a bolus dose (400 mg) followed by a 2-h infusion (4 mg/min for 120 min). There were 24 and 27 volunteers in the ANNEXA-A (apixaban) and ANNEXA-R (rivaroxaban) trials, respectively. The primary endpoint was the mean percentage change in anti-factor Xa activity as measured by a specific chromogenic factor Xa activity assay. Secondary endpoints included the proportion of participants with 80% or greater reduction in anti-factor Xa activity, percentage change in unbound plasma Xa inhibitor, and change in thrombin generation as measured by endogenous thrombin potential (ETP) from baseline to the nadir after administration of andexanet alfa or placebo. In participants treated with apixaban, administration of a 400 mg bolus of andexanet alfa was associated with a 94% reduction in anti-factor Xa activity, a reduction in the unbound apixaban concentration by 9.3 ng/mL, and restoration of thrombin generation in 100% of participants. In contrast, in placebo recipients, anti-factor Xa only declined by 21% and unbound apixaban concentrations by only 1.9 ng/mL, and only 11% demonstrated restoration of thrombin generation. In rivaroxaban-treated participants, administration of a 400 mg andexanet alfa bolus was associated with a 92% reduction in anti-factor Xa activity, a 23.4 ng/mL reduction in unbound rivaroxaban concentration, and restoration of thrombin generation in 96% of participants versus 18%, 4.2 ng/mL, and 7% in placebo-treated participants, respectively [180].

The ANNEXA-4 study is an ongoing, multicenter, prospective, open-label single-group study evaluating the use of andexanet alfa for treatment of acute major bleeds in patients taking apixaban, rivaroxaban, or enoxaparin [145]. A total of 67 patients were included in the interim report. Based on data from the aforementioned studies in healthy subjects, all 67 patients received a bolus dose (over a 15- to 30-min period) followed by a 2-h infusion. For patients who had taken the last dose of apixaban or rivaroxaban >7 h (but less than 18 h) prior to developing acute bleeding, the dose of andexanet alfa was 400 mg bolus followed by 480 mg infusion. For those who had taken rivaroxaban ≤7 h prior to development of acute bleeding, the dose of andexanet alfa was 800 mg bolus followed by 960 mg infusion in rivaroxaban-treated patients and 400 mg bolus followed by 480 mg infusion in apixaban-treated patients. Study patients were evaluated for reversal of anti-Xa activity as well as for clinical hemostatic efficacy at 12 h after administration of the study drug. In total, there were 32 patients receiving rivaroxaban (median daily dose, 20 mg) and 31 patients receiving apixaban (median daily dose, 5 mg). Of those, 33 and 28 presented with gastrointestinal and intracranial bleeding, respectively. Among the patients included in the efficacy analysis (those with anti-Xa activity levels >75 ng/mL), andexanet alfa significantly reversed the anti-Xa activity of the oral Xa inhibitors. At the end of the bolus administration, there was an observed relative decrease in anti-factor Xa activity by 89% (from 277 ng/mL to 16.8 ng/mL) and by 93% (from 149.7 ng/mL to 10.3 ng/mL) from baseline in rivaroxaban- and apixaban-treated patients, respectively. A similar relative decrease in anti-Xa activity from baseline was observed after the 2-h infusion, whereas the observed relative decrease from baseline was 39% and 30% for rivaroxaban- and apixaban-treated patients, respectively. Of the 47 patients included in the clinical efficacy analysis, 37 (79%) were adjudicated as having achieved excellent (n = 31) or good (n = 6) hemostatic control 12 h after completion of the andexanet infusion, with 9 reporting poor or no hemostatic control. The rates of excellent or good hemostatic control were 84% for gastrointestinal bleeding and 80% for intracranial bleeding. This preliminary analysis of the ANNEXA-4 study suggests that andexanet alfa is a potentially effective reversal agent for the oral factor Xa inhibitors, apixaban and rivaroxaban. This interim analysis did not include any patients receiving edoxaban [145]. Of the 67 patients included in the safety analysis, 12 (18%) were diagnosed with a thromboembolic event during the 30-day follow-up period; four of those 12 patients had a thromboembolic event within 3 days after receiving andexanet alfa [145].

Ciraparantag is a synthetic, water-soluble molecule that is capable of binding directly to anionic molecules. Thus, it is potentially capable of neutralizing the effects of several anticoagulants including UFH, LMWHs, fondaparinux, oral direct factor Xa inhibitors, and dabigatran [181]. In a Phase 1 study, ciraparantag safely and completely reversed the anticoagulant effects of the direct factor Xa inhibitor edoxaban [182]. In this study, escalating single IV doses of ciraparantag (100–300 mg) were administered alone and following a 60 mg oral dose of edoxaban in a double-blind, placebo-controlled fashion to 80 healthy subjects. Full reversal of the anticoagulant effect of edoxaban was observed within 10 min and sustained for 24 h after IV dose administration. This effect was not associated with increases in the levels of prothrombotic markers [182]. Ciraparantag does not bind to warfarin or argatroban [181].

As of Fall 2017, andexanet alfa is still being evaluated by regulatory agencies for its role in the reversal of anticoagulant effects of direct oral factor Xa inhibitors and is therefore not available for commercial use. Nonspecific hemostatic agents that have been suggested for off-label use in reversing excessive bleeding in patients taking the direct oral factor Xa inhibitors such as rivaroxaban and apixaban include recombinant factor VIIa, 3-factor and 4-factor PCC, and activated PCC.

Conclusion

The occurrence of major or life-threatening bleeding is the most feared complication of anticoagulation therapy. Although UFH and VKA have been available for decades and have reasonably specific strategies for reversal, the same is not true for other classes of anticoagulants, including LMWHs, pentasaccharides, and parenteral DTIs. Bleeding associated with these drugs has to be managed by carefully balancing the risks and benefits of experimental reversal therapies which may have preliminary evidence of efficacy but are neither validated nor specific reversal strategies. Recent data from studies of specific reversal agents for the direct oral anticoagulants (DOACs) have shown promising results in interim analyses of ongoing prospective studies. New and emerging reversal agents are in initial stages of clinical development and may provide safer, more targeted reversal therapy for anticoagulant-related hemorrhagic events (see Table 6.2).

Key Points

- Reversal strategies are important both for the treatment of major hemorrhagic complications and also for minimizing the risk of major bleeding in patients who require emergent invasive procedures while on anticoagulation.
- Most common reversal strategies for the treatment and prevention of bleeding caused by older anticoagulants such as UFH and VKAs are based on the use of

drugs and/or blood products that replace and/or boost the synthesis of coagulation proteins inhibited by those anticoagulants.

- The latest generation of anticoagulant drugs such as the DOACs has a target-specific mechanism of action with predominant or exclusive inhibition of one coagulation protein. More target-specific reversing agents are therefore being developed to neutralize the anticoagulant effect of these new anticoagulants.
- Frequently encountered reasons for warfarin reversal include the following: (1) supratherapeutic INR without bleeding, (2) major bleeding with a therapeutic INR, (3) supratherapeutic INR values with serious or major bleeding, and (4) need for urgent surgery or other invasive procedures with increased bleeding risk while the INR is within therapeutic range.
- Idarucizumab binds to both free and thrombin-bound dabigatran with an affinity 350 times higher than thrombin, resulting in immediate reversal of dabigatran's anticoagulant effects.
- Andexanet alfa is a specific reversal agent designed to neutralize the anticoagulant effects of both direct and indirect factor Xa inhibitors. Preliminary analysis of the ANNEXA-4 study suggests that andexanet alfa is a potentially effective reversal agent for the oral factor Xa inhibitors, apixaban and rivaroxaban. Of note, a small number of trial participants (18%) were diagnosed with a thromboembolic event during the 30-day follow-up period. Ongoing studies will need to evaluate this finding.

Self-Assessment Questions

1. An 82-year-old woman with chronic atrial fibrillation on long-term anticoagulation with warfarin is placed on sulfamethoxazole/trimethoprim for a recurrent urinary tract infection. Her INR has been stable within the therapeutic target range (2.0–3.0) for several months without warfarin dose changes, but 5 days after starting antibiotic therapy, her INR is >8.0. She denies any bleeding. You recommend, based on current guidelines, that the best option at this time is to:
   (a) Stop the antibiotic, and hold warfarin. Monitor INR, allowing it to drift down. No reversal agents are necessary at this time.
   (b) Stop the antibiotic and give oral vitamin K to reverse the anticoagulant effects of warfarin. The patient is at higher risk of bleeding.
   (c) Stop the antibiotic and give intravenous vitamin K to reverse the anticoagulant effects of warfarin. The patient is at higher risk of bleeding.
   (d) Continue sulfamethoxazole/trimethoprim, but give half of her usual daily dose of warfarin. The INR will eventually decrease.
   (e) None of the above options are recommended.
2. A 53-year-old man is seen in the emergency department after a fall from a ladder with head injury. He is anticoagulated on warfarin for history of recurrent deep vein thrombosis, and his INR is currently 2.8. Brain CT confirms intracranial hemorrhage with midline shift; he is being prepared to go for decompressive hemicraniotomy. At this time, you recommend that the following is the next best option:
   (a) This is an emergency, and there is no time to consider the use of reversal agents. The patient should proceed with surgery without need for reversal agents. Reversal of anticoagulant effects will also place patient at great risk of recurrent VTE.
   (b) Give oral vitamin K immediately prior to surgery, because the INR is within the therapeutic range.
   (c) Give intravenous vitamin K immediately prior to surgery, because the INR is within the therapeutic range.
   (d) Give fresh frozen plasma (FFP) during the peri- and intraoperative periods.

(e) Give prothrombin complex concentrates (PCC) during the peri- and intraoperative periods

3. *The* difference between 3-factor and 4-factor prothrombin complex concentrates (PCCs) is that 3-factor PCC has very low levels of:
   (a) Factor II
   (b) Factor VII
   (c) Factor IX
   (d) Factor X
   (e) Proteins C and S
4. A 65-year-old man is seen in the emergency department after a fall from a ladder with head injury. He is anticoagulated on dabigatran for history of paroxysmal atrial fibrillation. He had taken his last dose approximately 4 h ago prior to presentation. Brain CT confirms intracranial hemorrhage with midline shift; he is being prepared to go for decompressive hemicraniotomy. At this time, you recommend that the following is the next best option:
   (a) This is an emergency, and there is no time to consider the use of reversal agents. The patient should proceed with surgery without need for reversal agents. Reversal of anticoagulant effects will also place patient at greater risk of embolic stroke.
   (b) Give fresh frozen plasma (FFP) during the peri- and intraoperative periods.
   (c) Give prothrombin complex concentrates (PCC) during the peri- and intraoperative periods
   (d) Give 2 boluses of idarucizumab 2.5 mg, separated by no more than 15 min apart.
   (e) Start a bolus of andexanet alfa 800 mg, followed by an infusion of 960 mg.
5. A 76-year-old man is seen in the emergency department after a fall from a ladder with head injury. He is anticoagulated on rivaroxaban for chronic atrial fibrillation. He had taken his last dose approximately 3 h prior to presentation. Brain CT confirms intracranial hemorrhage with midline shift; he is being prepared to go for decompressive hemicraniotomy. At this time, you recommend that the following is the next best option:
   (a) This is an emergency, and there is no time to consider the use of reversal agents. The patient should proceed with surgery without need for reversal agents. Reversal of anticoagulant effects will also place patient at greater risk of embolic stroke.
   (b) Give fresh frozen plasma (FFP) during the peri- and intraoperative periods.
   (c) Give prothrombin complex concentrates (PCC) during the peri- and intraoperative periods.
   (d) Give 2 boluses of idarucizumab 2.5 mg, separated by no more than 15 min apart.
   (e) Start a bolus of andexanet alfa 800 mg, followed by an infusion of 960 mg.

Self-Assessment Answers

1. (a) Stop the antibiotic, and hold warfarin. Monitor INR, allowing it to drift down. No reversal agents are necessary at this time.

   Choice A represents the best option at this time, as per current guideline recommendations. Although she is at increased risk of bleeding with an elevated INR, she is currently not bleeding and not about to undergo an invasive procedure.
2. (e) Give prothrombin complex concentrates (PCC) during the peri- and intraoperative periods.

   Choice E represents the best choice in this clinical scenario. Compared to FFP, PCCs do not require cross-matching, can be infused within 30 min, and are not associated with the risk of volume overload. If PCCs are not available, FFP (Choice D) may be used.
3. (b) Factor VII

   3-factor PCC has very low levels of factor VII. Please note that failure to restore factor VII activity may result in suboptimal reversal of VKA-induced coagulopathy.
4. (d) Give 2 boluses of idarucizumab 2.5 mg, separated by no more than 15 min apart.

   Choice D represents the best option for this patient. Idarucizumab is a monoclonal antibody fragment specifically directed against dabigatran. In the United States, idarucizumab is FDA-approved for reversal of dabigatran-associated major bleeding.

5. (c) Give prothrombin complex concentrates (PCC) during the peri- and intraoperative periods.
   As of Fall 2017, andexanet alfa is still being evaluated by regulatory agencies for its role in the reversal of anticoagulant effects of direct oral factor Xa inhibitors and is therefore not available for commercial use. Nonspecific hemostatic agents that have been suggested for off-label use in reversing excessive bleeding in patients taking the direct oral factor Xa inhibitors such as rivaroxaban include recombinant factor VIIa, 3 factor and 4-factor PCC, and activated PCC.

References

1. Schulman S, Beyth RJ, Kearon C, Levine MN. Hemorrhagic complications of anticoagulant and thrombolytic treatment. American College of Chest Physicians Evidence-Based Clinical Practice Guidelines (8th Edition). Chest. 2008;133:257S–98S.
2. Atrial Fibrillation Investigators. Risk factors for stroke and efficacy of antithrombotic therapy in atrial fibrillation: analysis of pooled data from five randomized controlled trials. Arch Intern Med. 1994;154:1449–57.
3. Ost D, Tepper J, Mihara H, et al. Duration of anticoagulation following venous thromboembolism: a meta-analysis. JAMA. 2005;294:706–15.
4. Abdelhafiz AH, Wheeldon NM. Results of an open-label, prospective study of anticoagulant therapy for atrial fibrillation in an outpatient anticoagulation clinic. Clin Ther. 2004;26:1470–8.
5. Jackson SL, Peterson GM, Vial JH, et al. Outcomes in the management of atrial fibrillation: clinical trial results can apply in practice. Intern Med J. 2001;31:329–36.
6. Miller CS, Grandi SM, Shimony A, et al. Meta-analysis of efficacy and safety of new oral anticoagulants (Dabigatran, Rivaroxaban, Apixaban) versus warfarin in patients with atrial fibrillation. Am J Cardiol. 2012;110:453–60.
7. Holster IL, Valkhoff VE, Kuipers EJ, Tjwa ETTL. New oral anticoagulants increase risk for gastrointestinal bleeding: a systematic review and meta-analysis. Gastroenterology. 2013;145:105–12.
8. Stenflo J, Fernlund P, Egan W, Roepstorff P. Vitamin K dependent modifications of glutamic acid residues in prothrombin. Proc Natl Acad Sci U S A. 1974;71:2730–3.
9. Nelsestuen GL, Zytkovicz TH, Howard JB. The mode of action of vitamin K. Identification of gamma-carboxyglutamic acid as a component of prothrombin. J Biol Chem. 1974;249:6347–50.
10. Whitlon DS, Sadowski JA, Suttie JW. Mechanism of coumarin action: significance of vitamin K epoxide reductase inhibition. Biochemistry. 1978;17:1371–7.
11. Friedman PA, Rosenberg RD, Hauschka PV, Fitz-James A. A spectrum of partially carboxylated prothrombins in the plasmas of coumarin-treated patients. Biochim Biophys Acta. 1977;494:271–6.
12. Malhotra OP, Nesheim ME, Mann KG. The kinetics of activation of normal and gamma-carboxyglutamic acid-deficient prothrombins. J Biol Chem. 1985;260:279–87.
13. Choonara IA, Malia RG, Haynes BP, et al. The relationship between inhibition of vitamin K1 2,3-epoxide reductase and reduction of clotting factor activity with warfarin. Br J Clin Pharmacol. 1988;25:1–7.
14. Hirsh J, Dalen JE, Anderson DR, et al. Oral anticoagulants: mechanism of action, clinical effectiveness, and optimal therapeutic range. American College of Chest Physicians Evidence-Based Clinical Practice Guidelines (6th Edition). Chest. 2001;119:8S–21S.
15. Breckenridge A. Oral anticoagulant drugs: pharmacokinetic aspects. Semin Hematol. 1978;15:19–26.
16. Kelly JG, O'Malley K. Clinical pharmacokinetics of oral anticoagulants. Clin Pharmacokinet. 1979; 4:1–15.
17. Wessler S, Gitel SN. Warfarin. From bedside to bench. N Engl J Med. 1984;311:645–52.
18. Zivelin A, Rao LV, Rapaport SI. Mechanism of the anticoagulant effect of warfarin as evaluated in rabbits by selective depression of individual procoagulant vitamin K-dependent clotting factors. J Clin Invest. 1993;92:2131–40.
19. Patel P, Weitz J, Brooker LA, Paes B, Mitchell L, Andrew M. Decreased thrombin activity of fibrin clots prepared in cord plasma compared with adult plasma. Pediatr Res. 1996;39:826–30.
20. Sanden P, Renlund H, Svensson PJ, Själander A. Bleeding complications in venous thrombosis patients on well-managed warfarin. J Thromb Thrombolysis. 2016;41:351–8.
21. Goodman SG, Wojdyla DM, Piccini JP, et al. Factors associated with major bleeding events: insights from the ROCKET-AF trial (rivaroxaban once-daily oral direct factor Xa inhibition compared with vitamin K antagonism for prevention of stroke and embolism trial in atrial fibrillation). J Am Coll Cardiol. 2014;63:891–900.
22. DiMarco JP, Flaker G, Waldo AL, et al. Factors affecting bleeding risk during anticoagulant therapy in patients with atrial fibrillation: observations from the Atrial Fibrillation Follow-up Investigation of Rhythm Management (AFFIRM) study. Am Heart J. 2005;149:650–6.
23. Gage BF, Yan Y, Milligan PE, et al. Clinical classification schemes for predicting hemorrhage: results

from the National Registry of Atrial Fibrillation (NRAF). Am Heart J. 2006;151:713–9.
24. Sandén P, Renlund H, Svensson PJ, Själander A. Bleeding complications and mortality in warfarin-treated VTE patients, dependence of INR variability and iTTR. Thromb Haemost. 2017;117:27–32.
25. Rose AJ, Ozonoff A, Berlowitz DR, et al. Warfarin dose management affects INR control. J Thromb Haemost. 2009;7:94–101.
26. Penning-van Beest FJ, van Meegen E, Rosendaal FR, Stricker BH. Characteristics of anticoagulant therapy and comorbidity related to overanticoagulation. Thromb Haemost. 2001;86:569–74.
27. Kucher N, Connolly S, Beckman JA, et al. International normalized ratio increase before warfarin-associated hemorrhage: brief and subtle. Arch Intern Med. 2004;164:2176–9.
28. Odén A, Fahlén M. Oral anticoagulation and risk of death: a medical record linkage study. BMJ. 2002;325:1073–5.
29. Cannegieter SC, Rosendaal FR, Wintzen AR, et al. Optimal oral anticoagulant therapy in patients with mechanical heart valves. N Engl J Med. 1995; 333:11–7.
30. Kooistra HA, Veeger NJGM, Khorsand N, et al. Long-term quality of VKA treatment and clinical outcome after extreme overanticoagulation in 14,777 AF and VTE patients. Thromb Haemost. 2015;113:881–90.
31. Dentali F, Ageno W, Crowther MA. Treatment of coumarin-associated coagulopathy: a systematic review and proposed treatment algorithms. J Thromb Haemost. 2006;4:1853–63.
32. Fondevila CG, Grosso SH, Santarelli MT, Pinto MD. Reversal of excessive oral anticoagulation with a low oral dose of vitamin K1 compared with acenocoumarine discontinuation. A prospective, randomized, open study. Blood Coagul Fibrinolysis. 2001;12:9–16.
33. Crowther MA, Julian J, McCarty D, et al. Treatment of warfarin-associated coagulopathy with oral vitamin K: a randomized clinical trial. Lancet. 2000;356:1551–3.
34. Hylek EM, Chang YC, Skates SJ, et al. Prospective study of the outcomes of ambulatory patients with excessive warfarin anticoagulation. Arch Intern Med. 2000;160:1612–7.
35. Patel RJ, Witt DM, Saseen JJ, et al. Randomized, placebo-controlled trial of oral phytonadione for excessive anticoagulation. Pharmacotherapy. 2000;20: 1159–66.
36. Crowther MA, Ageno W, Garcia D, et al. Oral vitamin K versus placebo to correct excessive anticoagulation in patients receiving warfarin: a randomized trial. Ann Intern Med. 2009;150:293–300.
37. Ageno W, Crowther M, Steidl L, et al. Low dose oral vitamin K to reverse acenocoumarol-induced coagulopathy: a randomized controlled trial. Thromb Haemost. 2002;88:48–51.
38. Ageno W, Garcia D, Silingardi M, et al. A randomized trial comparing 1 mg of oral vitamin K with no treatment in the management of warfarin-associated coagulopathy in patients with mechanical heart valves. J Am Coll Cardiol. 2005; 46:730–42.
39. Gunther KE, Conway G, Leibach L, Crowther MA. Low-dose oral vitamin K is safe and effective for outpatient management of patients with an INR>10. Thromb Res. 2004;113:205–9.
40. Crowther MA, Garcia D, Ageno W, et al. Oral vitamin K effectively treats international normalised ratio (INR) values in excess of 10. Results of a prospective cohort study. Thromb Haemost. 2010;104:118–21.
41. Holbrook A, Schulman S, Witt DM, et al. Evidence-based management of anticoagulation therapy. American College of Chest Physicians Evidence-Based Clinical Practice Guidelines (8^{9h} Edition). Chest. 2012;141:e152S–84S.
42. Crowther MA, Douketis JD, Schnurr T, et al. Oral vitamin K lowers the international normalized ratio more rapidly than subcutaneous vitamin K in the treatment of warfarin-associated coagulopathy. A randomized, controlled trial. Ann Intern Med. 2002; 137:251–4.
43. Dezee KJ, Shimeall WT, Douglas KM, et al. Treatment of excessive anticoagulation with phytonadione (vitamin K): a meta-analysis. Arch Intern Med. 2006;166:391–7.
44. Nee R, Doppenschmidt D, Donovan DJ, Andrews TC. Intravenous versus subcutaneous vitamin K1 in reversing excessive oral anticoagulation. Am J Cardiol. 1999;83:286–8.
45. Lubetsky A, Yonath H, Olchovsky D, et al. Comparison of oral vs intravenous phytonadione (vitamin K1) in patients with excessive anticoagulation: a prospective randomized controlled study. Arch Intern Med. 2003;163:2469–73.
46. Watson HG, Baglin T, Laidlaw SL, et al. A comparison of the efficacy and rate of response to oral and intravenous vitamin K in reversal of over-anticoagulation with warfarin. Br J Haematol. 2001; 115:145–9.
47. Raj G, Kumar R, McKinney WP. Time course of reversal of anticoagulant effect of warfarin by intravenous and subcutaneous phytonadione. Arch Intern Med. 1999;159:2721–4.
48. Lubetsky A, Shasha Y, Olchovsky D, et al. Impact of pre-treatment INR level on the effect of intravenous low dose vitamin K in patients with excessive anticoagulation. Thromb Haemost. 2003;90:71–6.
49. Denas G, Marzot F, Offelli P, et al. Effectiveness and safety of a management protocol to correct over-anticoagulation with oral vitamin K: a retrospective study of 1,043 cases. J Thromb Thrombolysis. 2009;27:340–7.
50. Riegert-Johnson DL, Volcheck GW. The incidence of anaphylaxis following intravenous phytonadione

(vitamin K1): a 5-year retrospective review. Ann Allergy Asthma Immunol. 2002;89:400–6.
51. Riegert-Johnson DL, Kumar S, Volcheck GW. A patient with anaphylactoid hypersensitivity to intravenous cyclosporine and subcutaneous phytonadione (vitamin K1). Bone Marrow Transplant. 2001;28:1176–7.
52. Rich EC, Drage CW. Severe complications of intravenous phytonadione therapy. Two cases with one fatality. Postgrad Med. 1982;72:303–6.
53. Ciesielski-Carlucci C, Leong P, Jacobs C. Case report of anaphylaxis from cisplatin/paclitaxel and review of their hypersensitivity reaction profiles. Am J Clin Oncol. 1997;20:373–5.
54. Volcheck GW, Van Dellen RG. Anaphylaxis to intravenous cyclosporin and tolerance to oral cyclosporin: case report and review of the literature. Ann Allergy Asthma Immunol. 1998;80:159–63.
55. Ageno W, Gallus AS, Wittkowsky A, et al. Oral anticoagulant therapy. Antithrombotic Therapy and Prevention of Thrombosis (9th edition): American College of Chest Physicians Evidence-Based Clinical Practice Guidelines. Chest. 2012;141(Suppl):e44S–88S.
56. Tran HA, Chunilal SD, Harper PL, et al. An update of consensus guidelines for warfarin reversal. Med J Aust. 2013;198:1–7.
57. Fiore LD, Scola MA, Cantillon CE, Brophy MT. Anaphylactoid reactions to vitamin K. J Thromb Thrombolysis. 2001;11:175–83.
58. Douketis JD, Spyropoulos AC, Spencer FA, et al. Perioperative management of antithrombotic therapy. Antithrombotic Therapy and Prevention of Thrombosis (9th edition). American College of Chest Physicians Evidence-Based Clinical Practice Guidelines. Chest. 2012;141(Suppl):e326S–50S.
59. Woods K, Douketis JD, Kathirgamanathan K, et al. Low-dose oral vitamin k to normalize the international normalized ratio prior to surgery in patients who require temporary interruption of warfarin. J Thromb Thrombolysis. 2007;24:93–7.
60. Steib A, Barre J, Mertes M, et al. Can oral vitamin K before elective surgery substitute for preoperative heparin bridging in patients on vitamin K antagonists? J Thromb Haemost. 2010;8:499–503.
61. Glover JJ, Morrill GB. Conservative treatment of overanticoagulated patients. Chest. 1995;108:987–90.
62. Ageno W, Garcia D, Aguilar MI, et al. Prevention and treatment of bleeding complications in patients receiving vitamin K antagonists, part 2: treatment. Am J Hematol. 2009;84:584–8.
63. Contreras M, Ala FA, Greaves M, et al. Guidelines for the use of fresh frozen plasma. British Committee for Standards in Haematology, Working Party of the Blood Transfusion Task Force. Transfus Med. 1992;2:57–63.
64. Popovsky MA. Transfusion-related acute lung injury: incidence, pathogenesis and the role of multicomponent apheresis in its prevention. Transfus Med Hemother. 2008;35:76–9.
65. Chapman SA, Irwin ED, Beal AL, et al. Prothrombin complex concentrate versus standard therapies for INR reversal in trauma patients receiving warfarin. Ann Pharmacother. 2011;45:869–75.
66. Boulis NM, Bobek MP, Schmaier A, Hoff JT. Use of factor IX complex in warfarin-related intracranial hemorrhage. Neurosurgery. 1999;45:1113–9.
67. Schulman S, Bijsterveld NR. Anticoagulants and their reversal. Transfus Med Rev. 2007;21:37–48.
68. KCentra. Highlights of prescribing information. Revised 02/2017. http://labeling.cslbehring.com/PI/US/Kcentra/EN/Kcentra-Prescribing-Information.pdf.
69. Profilnine SD. Prescribing information. Revised 08/2010. https://www.fda.gov/ucm/groups/fdagov-public/@fdagov-bio-gen/documents/document/ucm261964.pdf.
70. Bebulin. Prescribing information. Revised 09/2015. http://www.shirecontent.com/PI/PDFs/BEBULIN_USA_ENG.pdf.
71. Baglin TP, Keeling DM, Watson HG. Guidelines on oral anticoagulation (warfarin): third edition–2005 update. Br J Haematol. 2006;132:277–85.
72. Palareti GA. Guide to oral anticoagulant therapy. Italian federation of anticoagulation clinics. Haemostasis. 1998;28(Suppl 1):1–46.
73. Franchini M, Lippi G. Prothrombin complex concentrates: an update. Blood Transfus. 2010;8:149–54.
74. Pabinger I, Brenner B, Kalina U, et al. Prothrombin complex concentrate (Beriplex® P/N) for emergency anticoagulation reversal: a prospective multinational clinical trial. J Thromb Haemost. 2008;6:622–31.
75. Hellstern P. Production and composition of prothrombin complex concentrates correlation between composition and therapeutic efficiency. Thromb Res. 1999;95:S7–S12.
76. Holland L, Warkentin TE, Refaai M, et al. Suboptimal effect of a three-factor prothrombin complex concentrate (Profilnine-SD) in correcting supratherapeutic international normalized ratio due to warfarin overdose. Transfusion. 2009;49:1171–7.
77. Tran H, Collecutt M, Whitehead S, Salem HH. Prothrombin complex concentrates used alone in urgent reversal of warfarin anticoagulation. Intern Med J. 2011;41:337–43.
78. Chiu D, Grigg M, Levi E. Operating on patients with warfarin: simpler alternative approach [letter]. ANZ J Surg. 2009;79:409–10.
79. Crawford JH, Augustson BM. Prothrombinex use for the reversal of warfarin: is fresh frozen plasma needed [letter]? Med J Aust. 2006;184:365–6.
80. Makris M, Greaves M, Phillips WS, et al. Emergency oral anticoagulant reversal: the relative efficacy of infusions of fresh frozen plasma and clotting factor concentrate on correction of the coagulopathy. Thromb Haemost. 1997;77:477–80.
81. Fredriksson K, Norrving B, Strömblad LG. Emergency reversal of anticoagulation after intracerebral hemorrhage. Stroke. 1992;23:972–7.

82. Cartmill M, Dolan G, Byrne JL, Byrne PO. Prothrombin complex concentrate for oral anticoagulant reversal in neurosurgical emergencies. Br J Neurosurg. 2000;14:458–61.
83. Khorsand N, Veeger NJ, Muller M, et al. Fixed versus variable dose of prothrombin complex concentrate for counteracting vitamin K antagonist therapy. Transfus Med. 2011;21:116–23.
84. Preston FE, Laidlaw ST, Sampson B, Kitchen S. Rapid reversal of oral anticoagulation with warfarin by a prothrombin complex concentrate (Beriplex®): efficacy and safety in 42 patients. Br J Haematol. 2002;116:619–24.
85. van Aart L, Eijkhout HW, Kamphuis JS, et al. Individualized dosing regimen for prothrombin complex concentrate more effective than standard treatment in the reversal of oral anticoagulant therapy: an open, prospective randomized controlled trial. Thromb Res. 2006;118:313–20.
86. Lorenz R, Kienast J, Otto U, et al. Successful emergency reversal of phenprocoumon anticoagulation with prothrombin complex concentrate: a prospective clinical study. Blood Coagul Fibrinolysis. 2007;18:565–70.
87. Imberti D, Barillari G, Biasioli C, et al. Prothrombin complex concentrates for urgent anticoagulation reversal in patients with intracranial hemorrhage. Pathophysiol Haemost Thromb. 2009;36:259–65.
88. Leissinger CA, Blatt PM, Hoots WK, Ewenstein B. Role of prothrombin complex concentrates in reversing warfarin anticoagulation: a review of the literature. Am J Hematol. 2008;83:137–43.
89. Chai-Adisaksopha C, Hillis C, Siegal DM, et al. Prothrombin complex concentrates versus fresh frozen plasma for warfarin reversal. A systematic review and meta-analysis. Thromb Haemost. 2016;116:879–90.
90. Farsad BF, Golpira R, Najafi H, et al. Comparison between prothrombin complex concentrate (PCC) and fresh frozen plasma (FFP) for the urgent reversal of warfarin in patients with mechanical heart valves in a tertiary care cardiac center. Iran J Pharm Res. 2015;14:877–85.
91. Baggs JH, Patanwala AE, Williams EM, Erstad BL. Dosing of 3-factor prothrombin complex concentrate for international normalized ratio reversal. Ann Pharmacother. 2012;46:51–6.
92. Imberti D, Barillari G, Biasioli C, et al. Emergency reversal of anticoagulation with a three-factor prothrombin complex concentrate in patients with intracranial haemorrhage. Blood Transfus. 2011;9:148–55.
93. Dentali F, Marchesi C, Pierfranceschi MG, et al. Safety of prothrombin complex concentrates for rapid anticoagulation reversal of vitamin K antagonists: a meta-analysis. Thromb Haemost. 2011;106:429–38.
94. Hedner U, Kisiel W. Use of human factor VIIa in the treatment of two hemophilia a patients with high-titer inhibitors. J Clin Invest. 1983;71:1836–41.
95. ten Cate H, Bauer KA, Levi M, et al. The activation of factor X and prothrombin by recombinant factor VIIa in vivo is mediated by tissue factor. J Clin Invest. 1993;92:1207–12.
96. Butenas S, Brummel KE, Branda RF, et al. Mechanism of factor VIIa-dependent coagulation in hemophilia blood. Blood. 2002;99:923–30.
97. Erhardtsen E, Nony P, Dechavanne M, et al. The effect of recombinant factor VIIa (NovoSeven) in healthy volunteers receiving acenocoumarol to an International Normalized Ratio above 2.0. Blood Coagul Fibrinolysis. 1998;9:741–8.
98. Deveras RAE, Kessler CM. Reversal of warfarin-induced excessive anticoagulation with recombinant human factor VIIa concentrate. Ann Intern Med. 2002;137:884–8.
99. Lin J, Hanigan WC, Tarantino M, Wang J. The use of recombinant activated factor VII to reverse warfarin-induced anticoagulation in patients with hemorrhages in the central nervous system: preliminary findings. J Neurosurg. 2003;98:737–40.
100. Freeman WD, Brott TG, Barrett KM, et al. Recombinant factor VIIa for rapid reversal of warfarin anticoagulation in acute intracranial hemorrhage. Mayo Clin Proc. 2004;79:1495–500.
101. Tanaka KA, Szlam F, Dickneite G, Levy JH. Effects of prothrombin complex concentrate and recombinant activated factor VII on vitamin K antagonist induced anticoagulation. Thromb Res. 2008;122:117–23.
102. Sorensen B, Johansen P, Nielsen GL, et al. Reversal of the International Normalized Ratio with recombinant activated factor VII in central nervous system bleeding during warfarin thromboprophylaxis: clinical and biochemical aspects. Blood Coagul Fibrinolysis. 2003;14:469–77.
103. Berntorp E, Stigendal L, Lethagen S, et al. NovoSeven in warfarin-treated patients. Blood Coagul Fibrinolysis. 2000;11(Suppl 1):S113–5.
104. Levi M, Peters M, Büller HR. Efficacy and safety of recombinant factor VIIa for treatment of severe bleeding: a systematic review. Crit Care Med. 2005; 33:883–90.
105. Roberts HR. Clinical experience with activated factor VII: focus on safety aspects. Blood Coagul Fibrinolysis. 1998;9(Suppl 1):S115–8.
106. Peerlinck K, Vermylen J. Acute myocardial infarction following administration of recombinant activated factor VII (NovoSeven) in a patient with haemophilia A and inhibitor. Thromb Haemost. 1999;82:1775–6.
107. Mayer SA, Brun NC, Vegtrup K, et al. Recombinant activated factor VIIa for acute intracerebral hemorrhage. N Engl J Med. 2005;352:777–85.
108. Aledort LM. Comparative thrombotic event incidence after infusion of recombinant factor VIIa versus factor VIII inhibitor bypass activity. J Thromb Haemost. 2004;2:1700–8.
109. O'Connell KA, Wood JJ, Wise RP, et al. Thromboembolic adverse events after use of recom-

binant human coagulation factor VIIa. JAMA. 2006;295:293–8.
110. Rosovsky RP, Crowther MA. What is the evidence for the off-label use of recombinant factor VIIa (rFVIIa) in the acute reversal of warfarin? ASH evidence-based review 2008. Hematology Am Soc Hematol Educ Program. 2008;2008:36–8.
111. McLean J. The thromboplastic action of cephalin. Am J Phys. 1916;41:250–7.
112. Johnson E, Mulloy B. The molecular weight range of commercial heparin preparations. Carbohydr Res. 1976;51:119–27.
113. Johnson E, Kirkwood T, Stirling Y, et al. Four heparin preparations: anti-Xa potentiating effect of heparin after subcutaneous injection. Thromb Hamost. 1976;35:586–91.
114. Andersson L, Barrowcliffe T, Holmer E, et al. Anticoagulant properties of heparin fractionated by affinity chromatography chromatography on matrix-bound antithrombin III and by gel filtration. Thromb Res. 1976;9:575–83.
115. Abildgaard U. Highly purified antithrombin III with heparin cofactor activity prepared by disc electrophoresis. Scand J Clin Lab Invest. 1968;21:89–91.
116. Rosenberg R, Lam L. Correlation between structure and function of heparin. Proc Natl Acad Sci U S A. 1979;76:1218–22.
117. Lindahl U, Backstrom G, Hook M, et al. Structure of the antithrombin-binding site of heparin. Proc Natl Acad Sci U S A. 1979;76:3198–202.
118. Rosenberg R, Bauer K. The heparin-antithrombin system: a natural anticoagulant mechanism. 3rd ed. Philadelphia, PA: Lippincott; 1994.
119. Casu B, Oreste P, Torri G, et al. The structure of heparin oligosaccharide fragments with high anti-(factor Xa) activity containing the minimal antithrombin III-binding sequence. Biochem J. 1981;97:599–609.
120. Choay J, Lormeau J, Petitou M, et al. Structural studies on a biologically active hexasaccharide obtained from heparin. Ann N Y Acad Sci. 1981;370:644–9.
121. Hirsh J, Warkentin TE, Shaughnessy SG, et al. Heparin and low-molecular-weight heparin: mechanisms of action, pharmacokinetics, dosing, monitoring, efficacy, and safety. American College of Chest Physicians Evidence-Based Clinical Practice Guidelines (6th Edition). Chest. 2001;119:64S–94S.
122. Andersson L-O, Barrowcliffe T, Holmer E, et al. Molecular weight dependency of the heparin potentiated inhibition of thrombin and activated factor X: effect of heparin neutralization in plasma. Thromb Res. 1979;5:531–41.
123. Rosenberg RD, Jordon RE, Favreau LV, et al. Highly active heparin species with multiple binding sites for antithrombin. Biochem Biophys Res Commun. 1979;86:1319–24.
124. Danielsson A, Raub E, Lindahl U, et al. Role of ternary complexes in which heparin binds both antithrombin and proteinase, in the acceleration of the reactions between antithrombin and thrombin or factor Xa. J Biol Chem. 1986;261:15467–73.
125. Lane D, Denton J, Flynn A, et al. Anticoagulant activities of heparin oligosaccharides and their neutralization by platelet factor 4. Biochem J. 1984; 218:725–32.
126. Oosta G, Gardner W, Beeler D, et al. Multiple functional domains of the heparin molecule. Proc Natl Acad Sci U S A. 1981;78:829–33.
127. Jordan R, Oosta G, Gardner W, et al. The kinetics of hemostatic enzyme-antithrombin interactions in the presence of low molecular weight heparin. J Biol Chem. 1980;255:10081–90.
128. Holmer E, Kurachi K, Soderstrom G. The molecular-weight dependence of the rate-enhancing effect of heparin on the inhibition of thrombin, factor Xa, factor IXa, factor XIa, factor XIIa and kallikrein by antithrombin. Biochem J. 1981;193:395–400.
129. Holmer E, Soderberg K, Bergqvist D, et al. Heparin and its low molecular weight derivatives: anticoagulant and antithrombotic properties. Haemostasis. 1986;16:1–7.
130. Garcia DA, Baglin TP, Weitz JI, et al. Parenteral anticoagulants. Antithrombotic Therapy and Prevention of Thrombosis (9th edition). American College of Chest Physicians Evidence-Based Clinical Practice Guidelines. Chest. 2012;141(Suppl):e24S–43S.
131. Protamine sulfate heparin agents 20:12.08. In: McEvoy GK, Litvak K, Welsh OH, et al, editors. AHFS drug information 1999. Bethesda, MD: American Society of Health-System Pharmacists; 1999. p. 1265–7.
132. Lindblad B, Borgström A, Wakefield TW, et al. Protamine reversal of anticoagulation achieved with a low molecular weight heparin. The effects on eicosanoids, clotting and complement factors. Thromb Res. 1987;48:31–40.
133. Racanelli A, Fareed J, Walenga JM, Coyne E. Biochemical and pharmacologic studies on the protamine interactions with heparin, its fractions and fragments. Semin Thromb Hemost. 1985;11:176–89.
134. Wolzt M, Weltermann A, Nieszpaur-Los M, et al. Studies on the neutralizing effects of protamine on unfractionated and low molecular weight heparin (Fragmin) at the site of activation of the coagulation system in man. Thromb Haemost. 1995;73:439–43.
135. Hirsh J, Levine MN. Low molecular weight heparin. Blood. 1992;79:1–17.
136. Crowther MA, Berry LR, Monagle PT, Chan AK. Mechanisms responsible for the failure of protamine to inactivate low-molecular-weight heparin. Br J Haematol. 2002;116:178–86.
137. Doutremepuich C, Bonini F, Toulemonde F, et al. In vivo neutralization of low-molecular weight heparin fraction CY 216 by protamine. Semin Thromb Hemost. 1985;11:318–22.

138. Racanelli A, Fareed J, Huan XQ. Low molecular weight heparin induced bleeding can be neutralized by protamine. Haemostasis. 1988;18(Suppl 2):163–4.
139. Van Ryn-McKenna J, Cai L, Ofosu FA, et al. Neutralization of enoxaparine-induced bleeding by protamine sulfate. Thromb Haemost. 1990;63:271–4.
140. Massonnet-Castel S, Pelissier E, Bara L, et al. Partial reversal of low molecular weight heparin (PK 10169) anti-Xa activity by protamine sulfate: in vitro and in vivo study during cardiac surgery with extracorporeal circulation. Haemostasis. 1986;16:139–46.
141. Ng HJ, Koh LP, Lee LH. Successful control of postsurgical bleeding by recombinant factor VIIa in a renal failure patient given low molecular weight heparin and aspirin. Ann Hematol. 2003;82:257–8.
142. Wakefield TW, Andrews PC, Wrobleski SK, et al. Effective and less toxic reversal of low-molecular weight heparin anticoagulation by a designer variant of protamine. J Vasc Surg. 1995;21:839–50.
143. Wakefield TW, Andrews PC, Wrobleski SK, et al. A [+18RGD] protamine variant for nontoxic and effective reversal of conventional heparin and low-molecular-weight heparin anticoagulation. J Surg Res. 1996;63:280–6.
144. Lu G, DeGuzman FR, Hollenbach SJ, et al. A specific antidote for reversal of anticoagulation by direct and indirect inhibitors of coagulation factor Xa. Nat Med. 2013;19:446–51.
145. Connolly SJ, Milling TJ Jr, Eikelboom JW, et al. Andexanet alfa for acute major bleeding associated with factor Xa inhibitors. N Engl J Med. 2016;375:1131–41.
146. Ansell JE, Laulicht BE, Bakhru SH, et al. Ciraparantag safely and completely reverses the anticoagulant effects of low-molecular weight heparin. Thromb Res. 2016;146:113–8.
147. Choay J, Petitou M, Lormeau JC, et al. Structure-activity relationship in heparin: a synthetic pentasaccharide with high affi nity for antithrombin III and eliciting high anti-factor Xa activity. Biochem Biophys Res Commun. 1983;116:492–9.
148. Thunberg L, Bäckström G, Lindahl U. Further characterization of the antithrombin-binding sequence in heparin. Carbohydr Res. 1982;100:393–410.
149. Choay J. Biologic studies on chemically synthesized pentasaccharide and tetrasaccharide fragments. Semin Thromb Hemost. 1985;11:81–5.
150. Harenberg J. Development of idraparinux and idrabiotaparinux for anticoagulant therapy. Thromb Haemost. 2009;102:811–5.
151. Harenberg J, Jörg I, Vukojevic Y, et al. Anticoagulant effects of idraparinux after termination of therapy for prevention of recurrent venous thromboembolism: observations from the van Gogh trials. Eur J Clin Pharmacol. 2008;64:555–63.
152. Veyrat-Follet C, Vivier N, Trellu M, et al. The pharmacokinetics of idraparinux, a long-acting indirect factor Xa inhibitor: population pharmacokinetic analysis from Phase III clinical trials. J Thromb Haemost. 2009;7:559–65.
153. Bijsterveld NR, Moons AH, Boekholdt SM, et al. Ability of recombinant factor VIIa to reverse the anticoagulant effect of the pentasaccharide fondaparinux in healthy volunteers. Circulation. 2002;106:2550–4.
154. Bijsterveld NR, Vink R, van Aken BE, et al. Recombinant factor VIIa reverses the anticoagulant effect of the long-acting pentasaccharide idraparinux in healthy volunteers. Br J Haematol. 2004;124:653–8.
155. Luporsi P, Chopard R, Janin S, et al. Use of recombinant factor VIIa (NovoSeven®) in 8 patients with ongoing life-threatening bleeding treated with fondaparinux. Acute Card Care. 2011;13:93–8.
156. Huntington JA, McCoy A, Belzar KJ, et al. The conformational activation of antithrombin. A 2.85-A structure of a fluorescein derivative reveals an electrostatic link between the hinge and heparin binding regions. J Biol Chem. 2000;275:15377–83.
157. Savi P, Herault JP, Duchaussoy P, et al. Reversible biotinylated oligosaccharides: a new approach for a better management of anticoagulant therapy. J Thromb Haemost. 2008;6:1697–706.
158. Kang YS, Saito Y, Pardridge WM. Pharmacokinetics of [3H] biotin bound to different avidin analogues. J Drug Target. 1995;3:159–65.
159. Wilchek M, Bayer EA. The avidin–biotin complex in bioanalytical applications. Anal Biochem. 1988;171:1–32.
160. Paty I, Trellu M, Destors J-M, et al. Reversibility of the anti-FXa activity of idrabiotaparinux (biotinylated idraparinux) by intravenous avidin infusion. J Thromb Haemost. 2010;8:722–9.
161. Sørensen B, Ingerslev JA. Direct thrombin inhibitor studied by dynamic whole blood clot formation. Haemostatic response to ex-vivo addition of recombinant factor VIIa or activated prothrombin complex concentrate. Thromb Haemost. 2006;96:446–53.
162. Ibbotson SH, Grant PJ, Kerry R, et al. The influence of infusions of 1-desamino-8-D-arginine vasopressin (DDAVP) in vivo on the anticoagulant effect of recombinant hirudin (CGP39393) in vitro. Thromb Haemost. 1991;65:64–6.
163. Bove CM, Casey B, Marder VJDDAVP. Reduces bleeding during continued hirudin administration in the rabbit. Thromb Haemost. 1996;75:471–5.
164. Warkentin TE, Crowther MA. Reversing anticoagulants both old and new. Can J Anaesth. 2002;49:S11–25.
165. Nutescu E, Chuatrisom I, Hellenbart E. Drug and dietary interactions of warfarin and novel oral anticoagulants: an update. J Thromb Thrombolysis. 2011; 31:326–43.
166. van Ryn J, Sieger P, Kink-Eiband M, Gansser D, Clemens A. Adsorption of dabigatran etexilate in water or dabigatran in pooled human plasma by activated charcoal in vitro. Blood. 2009;114:440.

167. Crowther M, Crowther MA. Antidotes for novel oral anticoagulants: current status and future potential. Arterioscler Thromb Vasc Biol. 2015;35:1736–45.
168. Chai-Adisaksopha C, Hillis C, Lim W, Boonyawat K, Moffat K, Crowther M. Hemodialysis for the treatment of dabigatran-associated bleeding: a case report and systematic review. J Thromb Haemost. 2015;13:1790–8.
169. Eerenberg ES, Kamphuisen PW, Sijpkens MK, et al. Reversal of rivaroxaban and dabigatran by prothrombin complex concentrate: a randomized, placebo-controlled, crossover study in healthy subjects. Circulation. 2011;124:1573–9.
170. Woltz M, Levi M, Sarich TC, et al. Effect of recombinant factor VIIa on melagatran-induced inhibition of thrombin generation and platelet activation in healthy volunteers. Thromb Haemost. 2004;91:1090–6.
171. van Ryn J, Stangier J, Haertter S, et al. Dabigatran etexilate — a novel, reversible, oral direct thrombin inhibitor: interpretation of coagulation assays and reversal of anticoagulant activity. Thromb Haemost. 2010;103:1116–27.
172. Schiele F, van Ryn J, Canada K, et al. A specific antidote for dabigatran: functional and structural characterization. Blood. 2013;121:3554–62.
173. van Ryn J, Spronk HM, Rossaint R, Grottke O. Ex vivo prothrombin complex concentrates and a specific antidote are effective in reversing dabigatran-induced coagulopathy in pigs. Blood. 2013;122(21):A2387. (Abstract).
174. van Ryn J, Litzenburger T, Gan G, Coble K, Schurer J. In vitro characterization, pharmacokinetics and reversal of supratherapeutic doses of dabigatran-induced bleeding in rats by a specific antibody fragment antidote to dabigatran. ASH Ann Meet Abstr. 2012;120(21):3418.
175. Glund S, Stangier J, Schmohl M, et al. A specific antidote for dabigatran: immediate, complete and sustained reversal of dabigatran induced anticoagulation in healthy male volunteers. Circulation. 2013;128(22):A17765. (Abstract).
176. Pollack CV Jr, Reilly PA, Eikelboom J, et al. Idarucizumab for dabigatran reversal. N Engl J Med. 2015;373:511–20.
177. Godier A, Miclot A, Le Bonniec B, et al. Evaluation of prothrombin complex concentrate and recombinant activated factor VII to reverse rivaroxaban in a rabbit model. Anesthesiology. 2012;116:94–102.
178. Wang X, Mondal S, Wang J, et al. Effect of activated charcoal on apixaban pharmacokinetics in healthy subjects. Am J Cardiovasc Drugs. 2014;14:147–54.
179. Crowther M, Lu G, Conley PB, et al. Reversal of factor Xa inhibitors-induced anticoagulation in healthy subjects by andexanet alfa. Crit Care Med. 2014;42(12):A1469.
180. Siegal DM, Curnutte JT, Connolly SJ, et al. Andexanet alfa for the reversal of factor Xa inhibitor activity. N Engl J Med. 2015;373:2413–24.
181. Laulicht B, Bakhru S, Lee C, et al. Small molecule antidote for anticoagulants. Circulation. 2012;126:Abstract #11395.
182. Ansell JE, Bakhru SH, Laulicht BE, et al. Single-dose ciraparantag safely and completely reverses anticoagulant effects of edoxaban. Thromb Haemost. 2017;117:238–45.

Transitioning Between Anticoagulants

7

Maya Serhal and Marcelo P. V. Gomes

Case Vignettes

Case 1: *A 45-year-old man is admitted with a hemodynamically stable acute pulmonary embolism. He is also found to have a right lower extremity femoropopliteal DVT. He is started on anticoagulation in the form of intravenous unfractionated heparin, and after 48 h of a stable course during his hospitalization, he is informed of different options for outpatient anticoagulation, including warfarin, parenteral (subcutaneous) anticoagulants, and direct oral anticoagulants. Because he has no contraindications to any of the available anticoagulant drugs, and he has good prescription drug coverage, he asks for any treatment options that would allow him to be discharged within 24 h.*

Case 2: *A 54-year-old woman undergoes aortic valve replacement with a mechanical valve. She is started on anticoagulation with intravenous unfractionated heparin postoperatively but develops heparin-induced thrombocytopenia which prompts discontinuation of heparin infusion and initiation of an intravenous direct thrombin inhibitor. She remains stable and without arterial or venous thromboembolic events, and her platelet count recovers within a few days. She asks about her options for oral anticoagulant therapy when she leaves the hospital and wants to know how long she will have to remain hospitalized.*

Introduction

Anticoagulation is one of the most rapidly evolving areas of medicine. While unfractionated heparin (UFH) and vitamin K antagonists (VKAs) were the only anticoagulants available for several decades until the early 1990s, the following 25 years have witnessed a surge in the clinical development of different classes of anticoagulants. Initially, drug development was focused on parenteral drugs with more specific mechanism of action and reliable pharmacokinetics (PK) and pharmacodynamics (PD), such as low-molecular-weight heparins (LMWHs) and pentasaccharides, which did away with the need for continuous intravenous (IV) infusion and can be

M. Serhal · M. P. V. Gomes (✉)
Department of Cardiovascular Medicine, Section of Vascular Medicine, Cleveland Clinic, Cleveland, OH, USA
e-mail: serhalm@ccf.org; gomesm3@ccf.org

J. F. Lau et al. (eds.), *Anticoagulation Therapy*, https://doi.org/10.1007/978-3-319-73709-6_7

administered in the outpatient setting via subcutaneous (SC) injections at fixed and/or weight-based doses [1–11]. Then the parenteral direct thrombin inhibitors (DTIs) became available as alternative anticoagulants for patients with heparin-induced thrombocytopenia or during percutaneous coronary interventions [12, 13]. Although administered by continuous IV infusion and requiring monitoring by the activated partial thromboplastin time (aPTT), the DTIs proved to be more reliable than UFH in terms of more stable levels of anticoagulation, less fluctuation of the aPTT during infusion, and much shorter plasma half-lives. More recently, research efforts to develop new, direct oral anticoagulants (DOACs) to replace VKAs have come to fruition, with the approval of an oral DTI and three oral direct factor Xa inhibitors [14–24]. These new oral anticoagulants have brought the field of anticoagulation and antithrombotic therapy one step closer to the "ideal anticoagulant," i.e., one that is rapid-acting, is fully reversible, does not require monitoring, and can be used in patients with end-stage renal disease and moderate-severe liver dysfunction. Other anticoagulants in advanced stages of clinical development may become available in a not so distant future [25].

All of these classes of anticoagulant drugs have been approved following the results of several large-scale, multicenter, prospective clinical trials which compared them against UFH, LMWHs, and VKAs for different indications. Each new drug has specific benefits while posing different challenges and risks as compared to traditional anticoagulants. In addition, the new parenteral and oral anticoagulants also have contraindications of their own; thus, UFH and VKA may still remain the only option to deliver safe and efficacious anticoagulation therapy to patients with certain comorbidities. Therefore, depending on the clinical indication and patient-specific characteristics, some anticoagulants may be more or less appropriate for a given clinical scenario.

With the advent of so many options for anticoagulation, the need to transition from one anticoagulant to another has become increasingly common in routine clinical practice. However, prospective data on the safest and most appropriate strategies for transition are lacking. Therefore, guidance for transitioning between anticoagulants is in part derived from the vast experience acquired from transition recommendations between UFH and LMWHs to VKAs and in part extrapolated from pharmacokinetic data of the DOACs. This chapter will provide a brief overview of PK/PD of the different anticoagulants and outline potential strategies to be adopted when transitioning between different anticoagulants.

Heparins

Unfractionated heparin and LMWHs exert their anticoagulant effects by inhibiting factors IIa (thrombin) and Xa. Their mechanism of action depends upon its unique high-affinity pentasaccharide sequence through which UFH and LMWHs are capable of binding to the lysine site of the antithrombin molecule [26–32]. Such binding converts antithrombin into a rapid inhibitor of factors IIa and Xa [27–29]. Therefore, UFH and LMWHs are indirect factor Xa inhibitors because such inhibition is mediated by their binding to antithrombin.

Heparins are appealing due to their rapid onset of activity. While UFH can be administered via IV or subcutaneous (SC) routes, an immediate anticoagulant effect requires IV administration, with a plasma half-life ranging from 30 to 90 min following weight-based IV bolus at clinically recommended doses [33]. The LMWHs reach peak plasma anti-Xa activity within 3–4 h after SC injection, with plasma half-life ranging from 4 to 8 h depending on the specific LMWH preparation [33]. The effect of UFH can be monitored by the aPTT, which provides guidance with regard to the intensity of anticoagulation, whereas LMWH preparations offer the advantage of fixed, weight-based SC dosing without the need for close monitoring or titration (Table 7.1). Because

Table 7.1 Selected PK/PD features of different anticoagulants

	UFH	Argatroban	Bivalirudin	LMWH[a]	Fondaparinux	Warfarin	Dabigatran	Apixaban	Edoxaban	Rivaroxaban
Mechanism of action	Indirect factors Xa/IIa inhibitors (1:1 ratio)	Direct factor IIa (thrombin) inhibitor	Direct factor IIa (thrombin) inhibitor	Indirect factors Xa/IIa inhibition (2–4:1 ratio)	Indirect factor Xa inhibitor	Inhibitor of vitamin K-dependent factors II,VII, IX, X	Direct factor IIa (thrombin) inhibitor	Direct factor Xa inhibitor	Direct factor Xa inhibitor	Direct factor Xa inhibitor
Route of administration	IV or SC	IV	IV	SC	SC	PO or IV[a]	PO	PO	PO	PO
Peak plasma level	6 h[b]	2 h[b]	2 h[b]	3–4 h	3–4 h	90 min[c]	1–2 h	~3 h	1–2 h	2–3 h
Plasma half-life (steady state)	30–90 min	35–45 min	25 min	4–8 h	17–21 h	36–42 h	12–17 h	8–14 h	8–10 h	7–11 h
Renal metabolism	No	No	20%	Yes	Yes	No	~80%	~25%	~35%	~66%

PK pharmacokinetics, *PD* pharmacodynamics, *UFH* unfractionated heparin, *LMWH* low-molecular-weight heparin, *IV* intravenous, *SC* subcutaneous, *PO* per oral, *min* minutes

[a]Data for enoxaparin, dalteparin

[b]Immediate onset of anticoagulant action; time (in hours) for therapeutic aPTT with weight-based IV administration

[c]Maximum antithrombotic effect achieved after 5–6 days of therapy (with adequate reduction of factors II and X)

they have less anti-factor IIa activity compared to UFH, LMWHs may not prolong the aPTT [32].

While UFH is the most common IV anticoagulant used in the intraoperative period for endovascular procedures in general, cardiopulmonary bypass, and vascular surgeries, as well as during hemodialysis, the LMWHs allow for outpatient treatment of acute venous thromboembolism (VTE) and have been shown to be superior to VKAs in the setting of cancer-related VTE [4, 5, 34–36]. However, therapeutic-intensity doses of LMWHs are contraindicated in patients with calculated creatinine clearance <30 mL/min.

Pentasaccharides

Fondaparinux is a synthetic analog of the unique pentasaccharide unit contained in the molecules of UFH and LMWHs. The fondaparinux molecule has a structural modification that increases its affinity for antithrombin; its specific anti-Xa activity is approximately seven times higher than LMWHs [33]. But because it contains only the pentasaccharide sequence, the fondaparinux-antithrombin complex is capable of binding to factor Xa but not to factor IIa (thrombin) [31, 32, 37–39]. Thus, fondaparinux is also an indirect factor Xa inhibitor in that its anti-factor Xa activity is dependent upon its binding to antithrombin.

Fondaparinux is administered via SC injections, with a peak plasma anti-Xa activity similar to LMWHs at 3–4 h after SC injection (Table 7.1). Its terminal half-life is approximately 17–18 h in young individuals and up to 21 h in elderly volunteers with normal renal function. The elimination of fondaparinux is also dependent on renal function, and the drug is contraindicated in individuals with chronic kidney disease and a creatinine clearance < 30 mL/min [33].

Direct Thrombin Inhibitors

Hirudin is a 65-amino acid polypeptide originally isolated from the salivary glands of leech saliva (*Hirudo medicinalis*) [40, 41]. Recombinant hirudins (desirudin and lepirudin) and bivalirudin (a 20-amino acid synthetic peptide that is an analog of hirudin) are parenteral direct thrombin inhibitors. These drugs bind to the thrombin molecule in a bivalent fashion: their amino terminal domains interact with the active site of thrombin, while their carboxy-terminal peptides bind to the exosite 1 (substrate-binding site) of the thrombin molecule [33]. Recombinant hirudins are irreversible DTIs with a plasma half-life of 60–90 min (lepirudin) with IV administration and ~120 min (desirudin) after SC administration, whereas bivalirudin has a very short plasma half-life of 25 min with IV continuous infusion (Table 7.1) [33, 42]. Unlike recombinant hirudins which are dependent on renal function and accumulate in the plasma of patients with advanced renal insufficiency, bivalirudin is eliminated mostly via cell-based mechanisms with only 20% renal clearance [43].

Argatroban is an L-arginine derivative that binds non-covalently to the active site of thrombin in a competitive and reversible fashion. It has a plasma half-life of 35–45 min which may be prolonged in patients with liver dysfunction but is not dependent on renal function (Table 7.1) [44, 45].

As with IV UFH, therapy with parenteral DTIs is typically monitored by the aPTT even though this is not an ideal or specific assay for parenteral DTIs because of variable dose responses and sensitivities of different aPTT reagents [33]. While the ecarin clotting time appears to be a more accurate assay for parenteral DTI monitoring, this assay is not widely available for clinical use [33].

Vitamin K Antagonists

Vitamin K antagonists inhibit the vitamin K epoxide reductase enzyme and interfere with the cyclic interconversion of vitamin K and its epoxide, ultimately resulting in reduced hepatic synthesis of vitamin K-dependent coagulation factors II, VII, IX, and X [1, 46–51]. Warfarin is the most widely available and best-studied VKA and exerts its antithrombotic effect predominantly by the reduction of prothrombin (factor II) levels [52, 53]. The plasma half-life of warfarin after oral dosing is 36–42 h, which is not dependent on renal function (Table 7.1) [1, 54, 55].

Despite the fact that warfarin is widely used, there are many challenges and practical limitations associated with warfarin therapy, including a number of significant drug–drug and dietary interactions. Commonly interacting drug classes include antibiotics, chemotherapy, and antiepileptic agents (including phenytoin) [56]. In addition, the efficacy of warfarin is greatly affected by diet, particularly by the consumption of vitamin K-containing foods and vitamin K-containing supplements [56]. Given these practical considerations with regard to prolonged warfarin therapy, it is no surprise that patients often present for follow-up care with questions about fluctuating INR values, the difficulty and inconvenience of regular laboratory monitoring, and the various dietary restrictions.

Direct Oral Anticoagulants

Dabigatran is a reversible, oral DTI that binds directly to the active site on the thrombin molecule [57]. Dabigatran is administered as a prodrug, dabigatran etexilate, which is rapidly converted to the active metabolite upon absorption. Such conversion begins in the gut and is completed in the liver [58]. Dabigatran etexilate is administered in capsules containing hundreds of pellets with a tartaric acid core in order to improve dissolution and absorption of the prodrug independent of gastric pH [56]. Peak plasma concentrations are achieved within 1–2 h following oral administration, and the plasma half-life at steady state is 12–17 h (Table 7.1) [58–61]. Elimination of dabigatran is 80% dependent on renal clearance, and the terminal half-life can be prolonged to 28–35 h in patients with creatinine clearance <30 mL/min [61]. It is noteworthy that, in the prospective randomized clinical trial (RCT) of dabigatran for acute VTE treatment (RE-COVER trial), all patients had to receive a parenteral anticoagulant (UFH, LMWH, or fondaparinux) for at least 5 days prior to initiation of study drugs [18]. The mean total duration of parenteral anticoagulation before starting dabigatran was 9 days in the RE-COVER trial [18].

Apixaban, edoxaban, and rivaroxaban are oral direct Xa inhibitors which selectively and competitively bind to the active site of factor Xa [25]. As with dabigatran, the oral factor Xa inhibitors have also been studied for prevention of cardioembolic stroke in patients with non-valvular atrial fibrillation and for acute treatment of VTE [15–17, 19–24]. Peak plasma levels are achieved within 1–3 h after oral administration, and plasma half-lives range from 8 to 14 h (apixaban), 8 to 10 h (edoxaban), and 7 to 11 h (rivaroxaban) in patients with normal renal function. Approximately 60% of rivaroxaban is eliminated by the kidneys, whereas apixaban (25%) and edoxaban (35%) are less dependent on renal clearance [25, 56, 62–66].

It is important to note that, in the prospective RCT of edoxaban for acute VTE treatment, all patients had to receive at least 5–10 days of a parenteral anticoagulant prior to initiation of edoxaban [23]. Conversely, prospective RCTs of apixaban and rivaroxaban for acute VTE treatment did not require a parenteral anticoagulant prior to initiation of study drug. While apixaban and rivaroxaban have been approved for treatment of acute VTE as the sole anticoagulant therapy, i.e., without the need for a parenteral anticoagulant prior to initiation of the oral drug, the percentage of patients receiving a parenteral anticoagulant for 24–48 h in the rivaroxaban-DVT, rivaroxaban-PE, and apixaban-VTE trials was 73%, 92%, and 86%, respectively [19, 20, 22].

Transitioning Between Different Anticoagulants

Background and General Concepts

Because anticoagulation therapy consisted solely of parenteral UFH and oral VKAs for many decades until the 1990s, the early concept of transition between anticoagulants in patients with acute venous or arterial thromboembolic events became almost synonymous with anticoagulant therapy itself. In those settings, an overlap between UFH and VKA is necessary because a complete antithrombotic effect is not achieved until at least 5 days into VKA therapy. Therefore, a transition period is required in order to achieve immediate antithrombotic effect. The rationale behind such requirement is based on experiments performed decades ago in animal models of warfarin anticoagulation, which demonstrated that the antithrombotic effect of warfarin is achieved predominantly by the reduction of prothrombin (factor II) levels [52, 53]. Because factor II has a plasma half-life of 60–72 h, warfarin will achieve its desired antithrombotic effect only after at least 5–6 days of therapy [59]. Hence the need for simultaneous administration of a parenteral anticoagulant when initiating warfarin (or any VKA) in a patient with acute arterial or venous thromboembolism [14].

The need to transition from a parenteral anticoagulant (UFH, LMWH, fondaparinux, or parenteral DTI) to warfarin has become widely referred to as "bridging therapy" because both drugs—the parenteral anticoagulant and warfarin—are administered simultaneously for a period of at least 5 days.

While the term "bridging" therapy is appropriate for clinical scenarios when an oral VKA will be used as the maintenance anticoagulant drug in the outpatient setting, "bridging" is not an appropriate term when other oral anticoagulants are used. This is because DOACs have a target-specific mechanism of action and a short plasma half-life. As a result, when a patient's anticoagulant therapy will be transitioned from a parenteral anticoagulant to a DOAC, the general recommendation is that the DOAC be started either at the time of the next scheduled or expected dose of the SC anticoagulant or within 1–4 h after discontinuation of the IV anticoagulant (Table 7.2).

Transition between different anticoagulants may be either necessary or considered for various reasons, including:

- Hospital discharge planning
- Specific indications (for instance, LMWHs best recommended for cancer-related VTE; DOACs not recommended for mechanical heart valves)
- Prior to elective invasive procedure or major surgery
- Change in clinical status (such as acute kidney injury, acute malabsorption states, inability to take oral drugs, hospitalization in intensive care unit where IV anticoagulants are more appropriate, heparin-induced thrombocytopenia)
- Drug-specific, nonhemorrhagic side effects
- Anticoagulant "failure" (for instance, recurrent thromboembolism despite adequate and compliant anticoagulant therapy with a given anticoagulant drug)
- To minimize or avoid drug–drug interactions (e.g., DOACs not recommended with concomitant antiretroviral therapy, rifampin)
- Prohibitive drug cost
- When lack of need for INR monitoring becomes important, such as in patients living in remote areas and/or without ease of access to anticoagulation clinics for INR monitoring
- Poor or non-compliance with oral anticoagulant therapy, when INR monitoring is desirable in order to minimize the risk of recurrent thromboembolism (due to missing frequent doses of short-acting DOACs), the risk of major bleeding (due to wrong, excessive doses), and/or to avoid mislabeling recurrent thromboembolic events as "anticoagulant failures"
- Patient preference (including preference for once-daily versus twice-daily dosing schedules)

Compared to warfarin, the DOACs bring several potential advantages, including (1) rapid onset of action which may eliminate the need for parenteral anticoagulation altogether, (2) lack of need for laboratory monitoring, (3) minimal to no dietary restrictions, and (4) less drug–drug interactions. Conversely, VKAs may be preferred over DOACs because:

Table 7.2 Suggested strategies for transition between the different anticoagulant drugs currently available for clinical use

To From	Unfractionated heparin (UFH)	Low-molecular-weight heparin (LMWH)	Fondaparinux	Warfarin	Apixaban	Rivaroxaban	Dabigatran	Edoxaban
Unfractionated heparin (UFH)		Discontinue UFH 1–2 h after first dose of LMWH	Discontinue UFH 1–2 h after first dose of fondaparinux	Overlap for at least 5 days and until INR is within therapeutic range for 2 consecutive days	Take first dose at the same time UFH is discontinued[a]			Take first dose 4 h after UFH is discontinued
Low-molecular-weight heparin (LMWH)	Begin infusion (without initial bolus) within 6 h prior to the next expected dose of LMWH		Discontinue LMWH, and start fondaparinux at time of next scheduled dose	Overlap for at least 5 days and until INR is within therapeutic range for 2 consecutive days	Discontinue LMWH, and begin oral anticoagulant at the time of next expected dose of LMWH[a]			
Fondaparinux	Begin UFH infusion (without initial bolus) or SC LMWH at the time of the next expected dose of fondaparinux			Overlap for at least 5 days and until INR is within therapeutic range for 2 consecutive days	Discontinue LMWH, and begin oral anticoagulant at the time of next expected dose of fondaparinux[a]			
Warfarin	Stop warfarin, and begin parenteral agent 36 h after warfarin has been discontinued If daily INRs are available, begin parenteral agent when INR ≤ 2.0				Take first dose when INR < 2.0[a]	Take first dose when INR < 3.0[a]	Take first dose when INR < 2.0	Take first dose when INR < 2.0

(continued)

Table 7.2 (continued)

To From	Unfractionated heparin (UFH)	Low-molecular-weight heparin (LMWH)	Fondaparinux	Warfarin	Apixaban	Rivaroxaban	Dabigatran	Edoxaban
Apixaban	Discontinue apixaban, and initiate parenteral agent at the time of next expected dose of apixaban			Discontinue apixaban, and initiate overlap to warfarin using a parenteral anticoagulant		Discontinue apixaban, and take first dose of rivaroxaban or dabigatran at the time of next expected dose of apixaban		Discontinue the other oral anticoagulant, and take first dose of edoxaban at the time of next expected dose of the other anticoagulant
Rivaroxaban	Discontinue rivaroxaban, and initiate parenteral agent at the time of next expected dose of rivaroxaban			Discontinue rivaroxaban, and initiate overlap to warfarin using a parenteral anticoagulant	Discontinue rivaroxaban, and take first dose at the time of next expected dose of rivaroxaban		Discontinue rivaroxaban, and take first dose at the time of next expected dose of rivaroxaban	
Dabigatran	If CrCl ≥30 ml/min, stop dabigatran, and begin parenteral agent at the time of next expected dose of dabigatran If CrCl <30 ml/min, stop dabigatran, and wait 24 h prior to initiation of parenteral agent			Discontinue dabigatran, and initiate overlap to warfarin using a parenteral anticoagulant	Discontinue dabigatran, and take first dose of apixaban or rivaroxaban at the time of next expected dose of dabigatran			
Edoxaban	Discontinue edoxaban, and begin parenteral anticoagulant at the time of next expected dose of edoxaban			Discontinue edoxaban, and initiate overlap to warfarin using a parenteral anticoagulant	Stop edoxaban, and take first dose of other oral anticoagulant at time of next expected dose of edoxaban			

[a]In the setting of acute venous thrombosis, a higher ("loading") dose of apixaban and rivaroxaban should be used initially

1. Warfarin has been available for several decades, and information on the efficacy and safety of long-term therapy (>10 years) with DOACs is lacking.
2. VKAs are fully reversible, whereas not all DOACs have approved strategies for reversal at this time.
3. DOACs may not be indicated or may not be the preferred anticoagulant regimen (due to lack of specific data) in several clinical settings and specific patient populations, including patients with mechanical heart valves, active malignancy, and antiphospholipid syndrome; those who are pregnant and breastfeeding or who take chronic medications which have significant drug–drug interactions with DOACs (such as antiretroviral drugs); as well as the pediatric population and patients in extremes of body weight (<50 kg or >150 kg).

Because therapy with DOACs can make anticoagulation therapy overall more convenient than VKA therapy, some guidelines have suggested that DOACs be considered over VKAs for patients who are being started on anticoagulation and do not have a contraindication to the new anticoagulants [36]. However, in patients who have been on warfarin for some time and have had no complications from such therapy, yet for whom any of the oral anticoagulants available—either VKAs or DOACs—could be appropriate options, the decision to switch from VKA to DOAC may at times be made by taking into consideration specific evidence-based information.

The RE-LY trial was a prospective, double-blind, open-label RCT of dabigatran versus warfarin for prevention of cardioembolic stroke in patients with non-valvular atrial fibrillation [14]. In that trial, dabigatran met the statistical criteria for non-inferiority compared to warfarin. When the analysis was broken down according to the dabigatran doses used in the trial (either 150 mg or 110 mg twice daily), pre-specified subgroup analyses for superiority showed that dabigatran 150 mg twice daily was superior to warfarin in preventing cardioembolic stroke, but the 110 mg twice-daily dose was not superior to warfarin [14]. Opposite findings were seen in the analysis of safety outcomes: dabigatran at a dose of 110 mg twice daily was associated with statistically significant less major bleeding than warfarin, whereas the rates of major bleeding were identical between the dabigatran 150 mg twice-daily and warfarin groups. Overall, rates of intracranial hemorrhage (ICH) were lower with dabigatran, but the rates of gastrointestinal bleeding were higher with dabigatran, compared to warfarin [14]. During the RE-LY trial, patients randomized to the warfarin group had a time in therapeutic range (TTR) of 64% on average (i.e., had a therapeutic target INR of 2.0–3.0 for 64% of the study time). Further analysis of the RE-LY trial data taking into consideration different levels of INR control during the study demonstrated that in patients randomized to the warfarin group who had a TTR > 65.5%, dabigatran 150 mg twice daily was not superior to warfarin in preventing cardioembolic events [67]. However, compared to the RE-LY overall data, safety outcome analysis was unchanged irrespective of the TTR. Therefore, patients with atrial fibrillation who have been on long-term warfarin therapy and are deemed to have very good to excellent INR control (defined as TTR > 65%) may have no benefit in terms of prevention of cardioembolic stroke by transitioning from warfarin to dabigatran. Similar analyses are lacking for the oral direct Xa inhibitors, as well as for patients enrolled in the VTE trials comparing DOACs with warfarin (see Chap. 11).

It is important to emphasize the fact that any guidance or suggestions regarding strategies for transition between classes of anticoagulants or between specific anticoagulant drugs are not derived from RCTs or prospective studies. Rather, suggested strategies are based either on published guidelines or on our expert opinion, combined with information derived from drug-specific PK/PD data and approved prescribing information outlined by different manufacturers.

Transitioning Between Different Anticoagulants

Specific Recommendations for Transition

Transition from Parenteral Anticoagulants to Oral VKAs (and Vice Versa)

Current guidelines for acute VTE treatment recommend overlapping a parenteral anticoagulant with warfarin for a minimum of 5 days and until two consecutive therapeutic range INRs (between 2.0 and 3.0) are achieved [59]. As previously discussed, this recommendation is based on available evidence suggesting that the achievement of an adequate antithrombotic effect with warfarin requires at least 5 days of treatment and a reduction in the plasma levels of factor II (and to a lesser extent, factor X). Therefore, the term "bridging" implies the need for ongoing parenteral anticoagulation, while the plasma levels of warfarin increase progressively with daily doses, which in turn results in progressive reduction in the plasma levels of factors II and X. This recommendation applies to transition from IV UFH, SC LMWHs, SC fondaparinux, or IV DTIs to warfarin.

But transition from parenteral DTIs to warfarin poses a greater challenge due to the fact that argatroban (and to a lesser extent, bivalirudin) interferes with the INR in vitro in a way that patients on therapeutic IV argatroban therapy oftentimes have high INR values despite no doses of warfarin being administered [33, 68]. In one study of patients who were being transitioned from argatroban to warfarin, 21% of those who had INR of 3.0 while on concomitant argatroban-warfarin therapy had subtherapeutic INRs checked after a 4-h interruption of argatroban infusion [69]. In these patients, one suggested strategy (which is not based on prospective data) is to follow the INR daily until it is >5.0 (or ≥4.0 for 2 consecutive days) on argatroban-warfarin "bridging" for at least 5 days, at which time argatroban infusion should be interrupted for approximately 4 h and INR repeated [70, 71]. If the INR off argatroban is <2.0, DTI infusion should be resumed for another 24 h, and the same strategy should be followed daily until a therapeutic INR of 2.5 (acceptable range 2.0–3.0) is achieved while off DTI therapy. But because patients with heparin-induced thrombocytopenia are exquisitely hypercoagulable, there is a risk of thrombosis when holding argatroban if the patient has a subtherapeutic INR [33, 69]. Thus, some have suggested that monitoring VKA therapy with chromogenic factor X levels may be safer because it will minimize the risk that argatroban infusion is held for a few hours in a patient who may still potentially have a subtherapeutic INR [33, 72–74]. Regardless of the strategy used during the "bridging" period between the parenteral DTI and VKA, it is imperative that the DTI not be discontinued until after a minimum of 5 days of overlap with a VKA [71, 75].

When transitioning from warfarin to parenteral anticoagulants, therapy with the parenteral drug (UFH, DTI, LMWH, or fondaparinux) should be started as soon as the INR is <2.0.

Transition from IV UFH to LMWHs or Fondaparinux (and Vice Versa)

Based on the plasma half-life of IV UFH and the time to peak plasma levels of LMWHs and fondaparinux (Table 7.1), the suggested strategy is to discontinue IV UFH infusion 1–2 h after the first SC injection of LMWH or fondaparinux is administered.

If transition from LMWH or fondaparinux to IV UFH is necessary, the SC anticoagulant should be discontinued and IV UFH infusion initiated approximately 6 h prior to the next scheduled dose of the SC drug.

Transition from IV UFH to DOACs

Based on the plasma half-life of IV UFH and the time to peak plasma levels of all currently available DOACs (which achieve peak plasma concentrations faster than LMWHs—Table 7.1), the suggested strategy is to administer the first oral dose of the DOAC at the same time that infusion of UFH is discontinued [76–78]. But the prescribing information of edoxaban differs from the other DOACs in that the recommendation is to give the first dose of edoxaban 4 h after discontinuation of UFH infusion [79].

If dabigatran or edoxaban is prescribed for acute VTE therapy, it is important to note that a 5–10 day period of therapy with IV UFH or SC LMWH is necessary prior to initiation of the DOAC, as per clinical trial protocols [18, 23].

If apixaban or rivaroxaban is prescribed for acute VTE therapy, it is important to follow the dosing protocols used in the RCTs, which consist of a "loading" initial dose of apixaban 10 mg twice daily for 7 days and rivaroxaban 15 mg twice daily for 21 days, prior to reducing the doses to apixaban 5 mg twice daily and rivaroxaban 20 mg once daily for the remainder of the acute VTE therapy [19, 20, 22]. In the clinical trials that compared apixaban or rivaroxaban with warfarin for prevention of cardioembolic stroke in patients with non-valvular atrial fibrillation, the dose of apixaban was 5 mg twice daily and rivaroxaban 20 mg once daily [15, 16].

Despite the fact that there have been an increasing number of case reports on the use of DOACs in patients with heparin-induced thrombocytopenia (HIT) [80], the efficacy and safety of DOACs in the setting of HIT are unknown. But if transition from IV DTI to DOACs was desired, it would be appropriate to initiate the DOAC at the same time of discontinuation of DTI infusion.

Transition from LMWHs or Fondaparinux to DOACs (or Vice Versa)

Taking into account the peak plasma levels and plasma half-lives of LMWHs, fondaparinux, and DOACs (Table 7.1), it is reasonable to recommend that, after LMWH or fondaparinux has been discontinued, the first dose of a DOAC be administered at the time of the next scheduled dose of LMWH or fondaparinux. This strategy is listed as a recommendation in the package inserts of DOACs in the United States [76–79].

Likewise, when transitioning from a DOAC to LMWH or fondaparinux, the first dose of the SC anticoagulant should be administered at the time of the next scheduled dose of the DOAC that was discontinued [76–79].

If dabigatran or edoxaban is chosen for acute VTE therapy, it is important to note that a 5- to 10-day period of therapy with the SC anticoagulant is necessary prior to initiation of the DOAC, as per clinical trial protocols [18, 23].

If apixaban or rivaroxaban is chosen for acute VTE therapy, it is important to follow the dosing protocols used in the RCTs, which consist of a "loading" initial dose of apixaban 10 mg twice daily for 7 days and rivaroxaban 15 mg twice daily for 21 days, prior to reducing the doses to apixaban 5 mg twice daily and rivaroxaban 20 mg once daily for the remainder of the acute VTE therapy [19, 20, 22]. In the clinical trials that compared apixaban or rivaroxaban with warfarin for prevention of cardioembolic stroke in patients with non-valvular atrial fibrillation, the dose of apixaban was 5 mg twice daily and rivaroxaban 20 mg once daily [15, 16].

Transition from Warfarin to DOACs

The most common reasons why clinicians and/or patients may prefer to transition from warfarin to a DOAC include added convenience (lack of need for laboratory monitoring), more favorable pharmacologic properties of DOACs over warfarin (lack of dietary interactions, fewer drug–drug interactions), and some data suggesting lower rates of ICH with DOACs compared to warfarin in some of the clinical trials.

When transitioning from warfarin to dabigatran, the strategy adopted in the RE-LY trial was to give the first dose of dabigatran when the INR was ≤2.3 [14]. While that trial did not report increased risk of bleeding with this strategy, the prescribing information recommends beginning dabigatran only when the INR declines to <2.0 after discontinuation of warfarin [76].

When transitioning from warfarin to apixaban, it is recommended that the first dose of apixaban be taken when the INR declines to <2.0 after discontinuation of warfarin [77].

When transitioning from warfarin to edoxaban, the manufacturer's prescribing information recommends starting edoxaban when the INR declines to <2.5 after discontinuation of warfarin [79].

When transitioning from warfarin to rivaroxaban, the strategy used in the ROCKET AF trial was to give the first dose of rivaroxaban as soon as the INR was ≤3.0 after discontinuation of warfarin in order to avoid periods of inadequate anticoagulation [16]. This recommendation is included in the approved prescribing information for rivaroxaban [78].

It is important to note that point-of-care (POC) INR devices should not be used to assess the INR during transitions between warfarin and DOACs because there are data suggesting that dabigatran and rivaroxaban can interfere with POC-INR values and cause variable INR increases due to differences in the sensitivity of coagulometers and reagents [64, 81, 82]. While no such data exists specifically for apixaban and edoxaban, the same recommendation should apply for all DOACs.

Transition from DOACs to Warfarin

The most common reasons why clinicians and/or patients may prefer to transition from a DOAC to warfarin include prohibitive cost of the new anticoagulants compared to warfarin, patients' preferences (which may be related to the lack of long-term data [>10 years] on DOACs or lack of an approved specific antidote for the oral Xa inhibitors), and some data suggesting higher rates of gastrointestinal bleeding with DOACs compared to warfarin in some of the clinical trials.

Taking into consideration the plasma half-life of dabigatran, as well as the fact that the maximum effect of warfarin will not be achieved before a minimum of 5 days (when reduction of factor II levels may finally be adequate), the suggested transition strategy described in the manufacturer package insert is to discontinue dabigatran after 3 days (doses) of warfarin therapy for patients with creatinine clearance >50 mL/min and after 2 days (doses) of warfarin therapy for those with creatinine clearance of 30–50 mL/min [76]. However, not only has this recommendation not been tested in prospective trials, but there are also data suggesting that dabigatran may prolong the INR in some patients [81]; thus, the INR may not be a reliable surrogate marker of the coagulant effect of warfarin until 48 h after the last dose of dabigatran. Thus, the safety of this strategy is unknown.

The strategy recommended by the manufacturer of edoxaban is to reduce the dose of edoxaban by half (thus, patients who were on 60 mg once daily would have their dose reduced to 30 mg once daily) and to overlap edoxaban and warfarin until the INR is >2.0 [79]. However, this strategy has not been validated in prospective trials. Moreover, data on another oral factor Xa inhibitor (rivaroxaban) suggest that the INR may not be reliable because of the Xa inhibitors' potential interference with the INR [64, 82]. In an open-label study that evaluated pharmacodynamic changes during transition from rivaroxaban to warfarin in healthy volunteers, co-administration of rivaroxaban with warfarin for 2–4 days led to higher INR values (2.79–4.15) than with similar doses of warfarin alone without rivaroxaban overlap (INR values of 1.41–1.74) [83]. In subjects taking both rivaroxaban and warfarin, the smallest effect on the INR was seen at trough rivaroxaban concentrations. Thus, while the safety of such transition strategy is still uncertain, the study suggested that INR should be performed at the trough rivaroxaban concentration (i.e., just before the next dose of rivaroxaban) if such "bridging" strategy from rivaroxaban to warfarin is chosen [83].

The 2015 European Heart Rhythm Association Practical Guide on DOACs in patients with nonvalvular atrial fibrillation has suggested a strategy of transitioning from DOACs to warfarin in which the INR should be performed at the expected trough level of the DOAC, beginning after the third day of overlap; the DOAC should be continued until the INR is greater than 2.0, but the INR should then be repeated within 24 h to ensure a therapeutic VKA level [84]. While this strategy has been reported as successful [17, 85], incorrect transitioning from DOAC to a VKA without a parenteral anticoagulant as a "bridging" agent has been associated with increased risk of cardioembolic stroke in patients with atrial fibrillation [16, 86, 87].

Given the lack of high-grade evidence derived from prospective trials comparing different strategies for transition from DOAC to warfarin, the safest recommendation in 2017 is to adopt the well-known, evidence-based strategy that would consist of (1) discontinuation of the DOAC and (2) initiation of a parenteral anticoagulant (UFH, LMWH, or fondaparinux) at the time the next dose of the DOAC would have been taken, and (3) proceed with the typical overlap ("bridging" therapy) from parenteral anticoagulants to warfarin for a minimum of 5 days and until a therapeutic INR value is achieved for 2 consecutive days [59]. Such strategy should be preferred both for patients with non-valvular atrial fibrillation and VTE, until evidence from prospective controlled trials demonstrating the safety of alternative strategies becomes available.

Transition Between DOACs

Given the similar peak plasma levels and plasma half-lives of dabigatran, rivaroxaban, apixaban, and edoxaban, if a patient should be transitioned from one DOAC to another, the new drug should be started at the time when the next dose of the previous discontinued DOAC would have been administered.

Conclusion

Recommendations for transitioning patients from one anticoagulant to another have been summarized in Table 7.2. Because there are no prospective randomized data comparing different strategies of transition, management recommendations should focus on strategies that are most likely to be safe and will minimize the risk of thromboembolic and hemorrhagic complications during periods of transition. These strategies are based on limited data extrapolated from RCTs, on available PK/PD data for each individual drug, and on approved prescribing information for selected drugs. It is also important to tailor the treatment plan to the individual patient and to bear in mind the fact that different anticoagulants may interfere with clot-based assays (aPTT, INR) in variable and sometimes unpredictable ways. Ultimately, given the lack of properly validated strategies for transitioning between different anticoagulant drugs, the choice of anticoagulant regimen will have to take into consideration multiple variables including the underlying indication, patient-specific comorbidities, and the prescribing clinicians' familiarity with the different options available for clinical use.

Key Points

- For a variety of reasons, patients may require switching between various oral anticoagulants during their treatment course.
- Strategies to transition between DOAC medications and warfarin should balance bleeding and thromboembolic risk while adjusting for individual patient factors.
- Transitions between individual DOAC medications and warfarin differ and should be followed according to the package insert.

Self-Assessment Questions

1. Your 72-year-old patient who is currently taking warfarin for chronic atrial fibrillation wants to start taking one of the direct oral anticoagulants (DOACs). He wants to start taking rivaroxaban because his friend is also taking it and has had no issues because he felt inconvenienced by the dietary restrictions and the frequent INR checks. He has no other medical concerns. His INR today was 2.5. You instruct him to:
   (a) Stop warfarin, and start a loading dose of rivaroxaban 15 mg to be taken twice daily for 21 days, starting tonight.
   (b) Stop warfarin, and start rivaroxaban 20 mg tonight.
   (c) Stop warfarin, and recheck INR tomorrow. If INR is <2.0, start a loading dose of

rivaroxaban 15 mg to be taken twice daily for 21 days and then take 20 mg daily.
(d) Stop warfarin, and recheck INR tomorrow. If INR is <2.0, then start rivaroxaban 20 mg daily.
(e) Continue taking warfarin because his bleeding risks are excessively high, and he should therefore avoid taking rivaroxaban.

2. Your 78-year-old patient with a previous history of two embolic strokes and chronic atrial fibrillation currently on apixaban 5 mg twice daily was noted to have acute worsening renal function on a recent routine blood test. His serum creatinine (Cr) was 3.2 mg/dL, and his GFR was 26. Of note, he has no other medical concerns. You instruct him that the best option is to:
(a) Decrease the dose of apixaban to 2.5 mg twice daily.
(b) Stop apixaban, and start warfarin tomorrow without bridging therapy.
(c) Start warfarin and stop apixaban 3 days later.
(d) Stop apixaban, begin enoxaparin and warfarin at the same time apixaban would have been due, and then stop enoxaparin when INR becomes therapeutic.
(e) Stop apixaban, begin unfractionated heparin (UFH) and warfarin at the same time apixaban would have been due, and then stop UFH when INR becomes therapeutic.

3. A 56-year-old man with unprovoked bilateral segmental pulmonary emboli has been admitted onto your service. He is currently receiving unfractionated heparin intravenously. He has chosen to start anticoagulation with warfarin. Current guidelines recommend:
(a) Stopping heparin immediately so you can initiate therapy with warfarin to achieve therapeutic INR
(b) Overlapping heparin with warfarin and stopping heparin immediately once the INR is therapeutic
(c) Overlapping heparin with warfarin for at least 3 days and stopping heparin once the INR is therapeutic
(d) Overlapping heparin with warfarin for at least 5 days and stopping heparin once the INR is therapeutic
(e) Overlapping heparin with warfarin for at least 5 days and stopping heparin once the INR has been therapeutic for 2 consecutive days

4. A 77-year-old woman who was in the MICU for respiratory failure related to pneumonia was diagnosed with a provoked right lower extremity deep vein thrombosis (DVT) and was started on intravenous unfractionated heparin. Over the next several days, her platelet count was noted to drop, and she was started on argatroban in the setting of suspected heparin-induced thrombocytopenia (HIT). During her recovery on the medical wards, you initiate discussion with the patient about her transition to oral anticoagulation with warfarin, and she agrees. The following is an acceptable strategy to transition the patient to warfarin:
(a) Overlap argatroban with warfarin at least 3 days, and if INR is therapeutic, can stop argatroban.
(b) Stop argatroban, and start warfarin. Discharge patient when INR is therapeutic.
(c) Overlap argatroban with warfarin for at least 5 days until INR is greater than 5, and then stop argatroban and reassess INR immediately. If INR is therapeutic, no need to resume argatroban.
(d) Overlap argatroban with warfarin for at least 5 days until INR is greater than 5, and then stop argatroban and re-assess INR 4 h after. If INR is therapeutic, no need to resume argatroban.
(e) Overlap argatroban with warfarin until INR is between 2 and 3; then stop argatroban and reassess 4 h after. If INR is still therapeutic, you need to bridge 1 more day; resume argatroban for another 24 h before stopping completely.

5. A 50-year-old man was diagnosed with provoked pulmonary embolism after a recent 10 h nonstop flight. The ER physician started him on enoxaparin. The patient has requested that he be started on dabigatran because there

is currently an FDA-approved reversal agent available. You advise the patient that:

(a) He can stop enoxaparin and start dabigatran immediately.
(b) He can stop enoxaparin. He will need to take a loading dose of dabigatran in the first 7 days before he transitions to a maintenance dose.
(c) He needs to overlap enoxaparin with dabigatran for 5 days.
(d) He needs to take enoxaparin for 5–10 days first, before starting dabigatran.
(e) Dabigatran is not currently recommended for treatment of venous thromboembolism (VTE).

Self-Assessment Answers

1. (d) Stop warfarin, and recheck INR tomorrow. If INR is <2.0, then start rivaroxaban 20 mg daily.

   The patient's CHA_2DS_2VASc score is at least 2, and he should remain on anticoagulation. He can start taking rivaroxaban 20 mg daily once the INR falls below 2.0.
2. (e) Stop apixaban, begin unfractionated heparin (UFH) and warfarin at the same time apixaban would have been due, and then stop UFH when INR becomes therapeutic.

   The patient's CHA_2DS_2VASc score is at least 3, and he has already demonstrated a high thromboembolic risk because of his history of two prior strokes. Because of his elevated risk of stroke, choice B is therefore not the best option. He should be started on warfarin with bridging therapy. Because of renal dysfunction, UFH should be considered over enoxaparin. He can start taking rivaroxaban 20 mg daily once the INR falls below 2.0. Choice C may be the next best alternative, although apixaban should be stopped with acute renal dysfunction.
3. (e) Overlapping heparin with warfarin for at least 5 days and stopping heparin once the INR have been therapeutic for 2 consecutive days.

   The recommendation is based on available evidence suggesting that the achievement of an adequate antithrombotic effect with warfarin requires at least 5 days of treatment with a parenteral anticoagulant such as heparin.
4. (d) Overlap argatroban with warfarin for at least 5 days until INR is greater than 5, and then stop argatroban and reassess INR 4 h after. If INR is therapeutic, no need to resume argatroban.

   Choice D provides the best strategy when transitioning a patient from argatroban to warfarin. If the INR is subtherapeutic upon reassessment following cessation of argatroban for 4 h, resume argatroban, and reassess in similar fashion the next day and until the INR is therapeutic while off argatroban.
5. (d) He needs to take enoxaparin for 5–10 days first, before starting dabigatran.

   There is no loading dose for dabigatran. As per clinical trial protocols, if dabigatran is chosen for treatment of acute VTE, a 5–10-day period of therapy with a subcutaneous anticoagulant such as enoxaparin is necessary before initiating therapy with dabigatran.

References

1. Hirsh J, Raschke R. Heparin and low-molecular-weight heparin. The seventh ACCP conference on antithrombotic and thrombolytic therapy. Chest. 2004;126:188S–203S.
2. Lensing AW, Prins MH, Davidson BL, Hirsh J. Treatment of deep venous thrombosis with low-molecular-weight heparins: a meta-analysis. Arch Intern Med. 1995;155:601–7.
3. Siragusa S, Cosmi B, Piovella F, et al. Low-molecular-weight heparins and unfractionated heparin in the treatment of patients with acute venous thromboembolism: results of a meta-analysis. Am J Med. 1996;100:269–77.
4. Levine M, Gent M, Hirsh J, et al. A comparison of low-molecular-weight heparin administered primarily at home with unfractionated heparin administered in the hospital for proximal deep-vein thrombosis. N Engl J Med. 1996;334:677–81.
5. Koopman MM, Prandoni P, Piovella F, et al. Treatment of venous thrombosis with intravenous unfractionated heparin administered in the hospital as compared with

subcutaneous low-molecular-weight heparin administered at home. The Tasma Study Group. N Engl J Med. 1996;334:682–7.
6. Weitz JI, Hirsh J, Samama MM. New anticoagulant drugs. The seventh ACCP conference on antithrombotic and thrombolytic therapy. Chest. 2004;126:265S–86S.
7. Buller HR, Davidson BL, Decousus H, et al. Fondaparinux or enoxaparin for the initial treatment of symptomatic deep venous thrombosis: a randomized trial. Ann Intern Med. 2004;140:867–73.
8. The MATISSE Investigators. Subcutaneous fondaparinux versus intravenous unfractionated heparin in the initial treatment of pulmonary embolism. N Engl J Med. 2003;349:1695–702.
9. Harenberg J. Development of idraparinux and idrabiotaparinux for anticoagulant therapy. Thromb Haemost. 2009;102:811–5.
10. Büller HR, Gallus AS, Zpillion G, et al. Enoxaparin followed by once-weekly idrabiotaparinux versus enoxaparin plus warfarin for patients with acute symptomatic pulmonary embolism: a randomised, double-blind, double-dummy, non-inferiority trial. Lancet. 2012;379:123–9.
11. The EQUINOX Investigators. Efficacy and safety of once weekly idrabiotaparinux in the treatment of patient with symptomatic deep venous thrombosis. J Thromb Haemost. 2011;9:92–9.
12. Hirsh J, Heddle N, Kelton JG. Treatment of heparin-induced thrombocytopenia: a critical review. Arch Intern Med. 2004;164:361–9.
13. Joseph L, Casanegra AI, Dhariwal M, et al. Bivalirudin for the treatment of patients with confirmed or suspected heparin-induced thrombocytopenia. J Thromb Haemost. 2014;12:1044–55.
14. Connolly SJ, Ezekowitz MD, Yusuf S, et al. Dabigatran versus warfarin in patients with atrial fibrillation. N Engl J Med. 2009;361:1139–51.
15. Granger CB, Alexander JH, McMurray JJV, et al. Apixaban versus warfarin in patients with atrial fibrillation. N Engl J Med. 2011;365:981–92.
16. Patel MR, Mahaffey KW, Garg J, et al. Rivaroxaban versus warfarin in nonvalvular atrial fibrillation. N Engl J Med. 2011;365:883–91.
17. Giugliano RP, Ruff CT, Braunwald E, et al. Edoxaban versus warfarin in patients with atrial fibrillation. N Engl J Med. 2013;369:2093–104.
18. Schulman S, Kearon K, Kakkar AJ, et al. Dabigatran versus warfarin in the treatment of acute venous thromboembolism. N Engl J Med. 2009;361:2342–52.
19. The EINSTEIN Investigators. Oral rivaroxaban for symptomatic venous thromboembolism. N Engl J Med. 2010;363:2499–510.
20. The EINSTEIN-PE Investigators. Oral rivaroxaban for the treatment of symptomatic pulmonary embolism. N Engl J Med. 2012;366:1287–97.
21. Agnelli G, Büller HR, Cohen A, et al. Apixaban for extended treatment of venous thromboembolism. N Engl J Med. 2013;368:699–708.
22. Agnelli G, Büller HR, Cohen A, et al. Oral apixaban for the treatment of acute venous thromboembolism. N Engl J Med. 2013;369:799–808.
23. The Hokusai-VTE Investigators. Edoxaban versus warfarin for the treatment of symptomatic venous thromboembolism. N Engl J Med. 2013;369:1406–15.
24. Weitz JI, Lensing AWA, Prins MH, et al. Rivaroxaban or aspirin for extended treatment of venous thromboembolism. N Engl J Med. 2017;376(13):1211–22. https://doi.org/10.1056/NEJMoa1700518.
25. Weitz JI, Eikelboom JW, Samama MM. New antithrombotic drugs: antithrombotic therapy and prevention of thrombosis, 9th ed: American College of Chest Physicians Evidence-Based Clinical Practice Guidelines. Chest. 2012;141:e120S–51S.
26. Abildgaard U. Highly purified antithrombin III with heparin cofactor activity prepared by disc electrophoresis. Scand J Clin Lab Invest. 1968;21:89–91.
27. Rosenberg R, Lam L. Correlation between structure and function of heparin. Proc Natl Acad Sci U S A. 1979;76:1218–22.
28. Lindahl U, Backstrom G, Hook M, et al. Structure of the antithrombin-binding site of heparin. Proc Natl Acad Sci U S A. 1979;76:3198–202.
29. Rosenberg R, Bauer K. The heparin-antithrombin system: a natural anticoagulant mechanism. 3rd ed. Philadelphia, PA: Lippincott; 1994.
30. Casu B, Oreste P, Torri G, et al. The structure of heparin oligosaccharide fragments with high anti-(factor Xa) activity containing the minimal antithrombin III-binding sequence. Biochem J. 1981;97:599–609.
31. Choay J, Lormeau J, Petitou M, et al. Structural studies on a biologically active hexasaccharide obtained from heparin. Ann N Y Acad Sci. 1981;370:644–9.
32. Hirsh J, Warkentin TE, Shaughnessy SG, et al. Heparin and low-molecular-weight heparin: mechanisms of action, pharmacokinetics, dosing, monitoring, efficacy, and safety. American College of Chest Physicians Evidence-Based Clinical Practice Guidelines (6th Edition). Chest. 2001;119:64S–94S.
33. Garcia DA, Baglin TP, Weitz JI, et al. Parenteral anticoagulants. Antithrombotic therapy and prevention of thrombosis, 9th ed: American College of Chest Physicians Evidence-Based Clinical Practice Guidelines. Chest. 2012;141(Suppl):e24S–43S.
34. Lyman GH, Khorana AA, Kuderer NM, et al. Venous thromboembolism prophylaxis and treatment in patients with cancer: American Society of Clinical Oncology Clinical Practice Guideline. J Clin Oncologia. 2013;31:2189–204.
35. Carrier M, Cameron C, Delluc A, et al. Efficacy and safety of anticoagulant therapy for the treatment of acute cancer-associated thrombosis: a systematic review and meta-analysis. Thromb Res. 2014;134:1214–9.
36. Kearon C, Akl EA, Ornelas J, et al. Antithrombotic therapy for VTE disease: chest guideline and expert panel report. Chest. 2016;149:315–52.

37. Choay J, Petitou M, Lormeau JC, et al. Structure-activity relationship in heparin: a synthetic pentasaccharide with high affinity for antithrombin III and eliciting high anti-factor Xa activity. Biochem Biophys Res Commun. 1983;116:492–9.
38. Thunberg L, Bäckström G, Lindahl U. Further characterization of the antithrombin-binding sequence in heparin. Carbohydr Res. 1982;100:393–410.
39. Choay J. Biologic studies on chemically synthesized pentasaccharide and tetrasaccharide fragments. Semin Thromb Hemost. 1985;11:81–5.
40. Toschi V, Lettino M, Gallo R, et al. Biochemistry and biology of hirudin. Coron Artery Dis. 1996;7:420–8.
41. Wallis RB. Hirudins: from leeches to man. Semin Thromb Hemost. 1996;22:185–96.
42. Fox I, Dawson A, Loynds P, et al. Anticoagulant activity of Hirulog, a direct thrombin inhibitor, in humans. Thromb Haemost. 1993;69:157–63.
43. Robson R. The use of bivalirudin in patients with renal impairment. J Invasive Cardiol. 2000;12(Suppl F):33F–6F.
44. Hursting MJ, Alford KL, Becker JC, et al. Novastan (brand of argatroban): a small-molecule, direct thrombin inhibitor. Semin Thromb Hemost. 1997;23:503–16.
45. Swan SK, Hursting MJ. The pharmacokinetics and pharmacodynamics of argatroban: effects of age, gender, and hepatic or renal dysfunction. Pharmacotherapy. 2000;20:318–29.
46. Stenflo J, Fernlund P, Egan W, Roepstorff P. Vitamin K dependent modifications of glutamic acid residues in prothrombin. Proc Natl Acad Sci U S A. 1974;71:2730–3.
47. Nelsestuen GL, Zytkovicz TH, Howard JB. The mode of action of vitamin K. Identification of gamma-carboxyglutamic acid as a component of prothrombin. J Biol Chem. 1974;249:6347–50.
48. Whitlon DS, Sadowski JA, Suttie JW. Mechanism of coumarin action: significance of vitamin K epoxide reductase inhibition. Biochemistry. 1978;17:1371–7.
49. Friedman PA, Rosenberg RD, Hauschka PV, Fitz-James A. A spectrum of partially carboxylated prothrombins in the plasmas of coumarin-treated patients. Biochim Biophys Acta. 1977;494:271–6.
50. Malhotra OP, Nesheim ME, Mann KG. The kinetics of activation of normal and gamma-carboxyglutamic acid-deficient prothrombins. J Biol Chem. 1985;260:279–87.
51. Choonara IA, Malia RG, Haynes BP, et al. The relationship between inhibition of vitamin K1 2,3-epoxide reductase and reduction of clotting factor activity with warfarin. Br J Clin Pharmacol. 1988;25:1–7.
52. Wessler S, Gitel SN. Warfarin. From bedside to bench. N Engl J Med. 1984;311:645–52.
53. Zivelin A, Rao LV, Rapaport SI. Mechanism of the anticoagulant effect of warfarin as evaluated in rabbits by selective depression of individual procoagulant vitamin K-dependent clotting factors. J Clin Invest. 1993;92:2131–40.
54. Breckenridge AM. Oral anticoagulant drugs: pharmacokinetic aspects. Semin Hematol. 1978;15:19–26.
55. Kelly JG, O'Malley K. Clinical pharmacokinetics of oral anticoagulants. Clin Pharmacokinet. 1979;4:1–15.
56. Nutescu EA, Chuatrisom I, Hellenbart E. Drug and dietary interactions of warfarin and novel oral anticoagulants: an update. J Thromb Thrombolysis. 2011;31:326–43.
57. Nutescu EA, Shapiro NL, Chevalier A. New anticoagulant agents: direct thrombin inhibitors. Cardiol Clin. 2008;26:169–87. v–vi.
58. Stangier J, Rathgen K, Stahle H, et al. The pharmacokinetics, pharmacodynamics and tolerability of dabigatran etexilate, a new oral direct thrombin inhibitor, in healthy male subjects. Br J Clin Pharmacol. 2007;64:292–303.
59. Ageno W, Gallus AS, Wittkowsky A, et al. Oral anticoagulant therapy: antithrombotic therapy and prevention of thrombosis, 9th ed: American College of Chest Physicians Evidence-Based Clinical Practice Guidelines. Chest. 2012;141(Suppl):e44S–88S.
60. Stangier J. Clinical pharmacokinetics and pharmacodynamics of the oral direct thrombin inhibitor dabigatran etexilate. Clin Pharmacokinet. 2008;47:285–95.
61. Stangier J, et al. Influence of renal impairment on the pharmacokinetics and pharmacodynamics of oral dabigatran etexilate: an open-label, parallel-group, single-centre study. Clin Pharmacokinet. 2010;49:259–68.
62. Jiang X, Crain EJ, Luettgen JM, et al. Apixaban, an oral direct factor Xa inhibitor, inhibits human clot-bound factor Xa activity in vitro. Thromb Haemost. 2009;101:780–2.
63. Raghavan N, Frost CE, Yu Z, et al. Apixaban metabolism and pharmacokinetics after oral administration to humans. Drug Metab Dispos. 2009; 37:74–81.
64. Kubitza D, Becka M, Wensing G, et al. Safety, pharmacodynamics, and pharmacokinetics of BAY59-7939—an oral, direct Factor Xa inhibitor—after multiple dosing in healthy male subjects. Eur J Clin Pharmacol. 2005;61:873–80.
65. Mueck W, Becka M, Kubitza D, et al. Population model of the pharmacokinetics and pharmacodynamics of rivaroxaban—an oral, direct factor Xa inhibitor—in healthy subjects. Int J Clin Pharmacol Ther. 2007;45:335–44.
66. Ogata K, Mendell-Harary J, Tachibana M, et al. Clinical safety, tolerability, pharmacokinetics, and pharmacodynamics of the novel factor Xa inhibitor edoxaban in healthy volunteers. J Clin Pharmacol. 2010;50:743–53.
67. Wallentin L, Yusuf S, Ezekowitz MD, et al. Efficacy and safety of dabigatran compared with warfarin at different levels of international normalized ratio control for stroke prevention in atrial fibrillation: an analysis of the RE-LY trial. Lancet. 2010;376:975–83.
68. Warkentin TE, Greinacher A, Craven S, et al. Differences in the clinically effective molar concentrations of four direct thrombin inhibitors explain

their variable prothrombin time prolongation. Thromb Haemost. 2005;94:958–64.
69. Bartholomew JR, Hursting MJ. Transitioning from argatroban to warfarin in heparin-induced thrombocytopenia: an analysis of outcomes in patients with elevated international normalized ratio (INR). J Thromb Thrombolysis. 2005;19:183–8.
70. Argatroban. Highlights of prescribing information. Revised 05/2016. https://www.accessdata.fda.gov/drugsatfda_docs/label/2016/022485s009lbl.pdf.
71. Watson H, Davidson S, Keeling D. Haemostasis and Thrombosis Task Force of the British Committee for Standards in Haematology Guidelines on the diagnosis and management of heparin-induced thrombocytopenia: second edition. Br J Haematol. 2012;159:528–40.
72. Arpino PA, Demirjian Z, Van Cott EM. Use of the chromogenic factor X assay to predict the international normalized ratio in patients transitioning from argatroban to warfarin. Pharmacotherapy. 2005;25:157–64.
73. Bartholomew J. Transition to an oral anticoagulant in patients with heparin-induced thrombocytopenia. Chest. 2005;127:27S–34S.
74. Hursting MJ, Lewis BE, Macfarlane DE. Transitioning from argatroban to warfarin therapy in patients with heparin-induced thrombocytopenia. Clin Appl Thromb Hemost. 2005;11:279–87.
75. Kinkins L-A, Dans AL, Moores LK, et al. Treatment and prevention of heparin-induced thrombocytopenia: antithrombotic therapy and prevention of thrombosis, 9th ed: American College of Chest Physicians Evidence-Based Clinical Practice Guidelines. Chest. 2012;141(Suppl):e495S–530S.
76. Pradaxa. Highlights of prescribing information. Revised 11/2015. http://docs.boehringer-ingelheim.com/Prescribing%20Information/PIs/Pradaxa/Pradaxa.pdf.
77. Eliquis. Highlights of prescribing information. Revised 07/2016. https://www.accessdata.fda.gov/drugsatfda_docs/label/2016/202155s012lbl.pdf.
78. Xarelto. Highlights of prescribing information. Revised 05/2016. https://www.accessdata.fda.gov/drugsatfda_docs/label/2016/202439s017lbl.pdf.
79. Savaysa. Highlights of prescribing information. Revised 09/2016. https://hemonc.org/w/images/9/96/Edoxaban.pdf.
80. Shatzel JJ, Crapster-Pregont M, Seloughery TG. Non-vitamin K antagonist oral anticoagulants for heparin-induced thrombocytopenia. A systematic review of 54 reported cases. Thromb Haemost. 2016;116:397–400.
81. Baruch L, Sherman O. Potential inaccuracy of point-of-care INR in dabigatran-treated patients. Ann Pharmacother. 2011;45(7–8):e40.
82. Samama MM, Martinoli JL, LeFlem L, et al. Assessment of laboratory assays to measure rivaroxaban: an oral, direct factor Xa inhibitor. Thromb Haemost. 2010;103:815–25.
83. Moore KT, Byra W, Vaidyanathan S, et al. Switching from rivaroxaban to warfarin: an open-label pharmacodynamic study in healthy subjects. Br J Clin Pharmacol. 2014;79:907–17.
84. Heidbuchel H, Verhamme P, Alings M, Antz M, Diener HC, Hacke W, et al. Updated European Heart Rhythm Association Practical Guide on the use of non-vitamin antagonist anticoagulants in patients with non-valvular atrial fibrillation. Europace. 2015;17:1467–507.
85. Ruff CT, Giugliano RP, Braunwald E, Mercuri M, Curt V, Betcher J, et al. Transition of patients from blinded study drug to open-label anticoagulation: the ENGAGE AF-TIMI 48 trial. J Am Coll Cardiol. 2014;64:576–84.
86. Granger C, Alexander JH, Hanna M, Wang J, Mohan P, Lawrence J, et al. Events after discontinuation of randomized treatment at the end of the ARISTOTLE trial. Eur Heart J. 2012;33(Suppl):685–6. (Abstract).
87. Granger CB, Lopes RD, Hanna M, Ansell J, Hylek EM, Alexander JH, et al. Clinical events after transitioning from apixaban versus warfarin to warfarin at the end of the Apixaban for Reduction in Stroke and Other Thromboembolic Events in Atrial Fibrillation (ARISTOTLE) trial. Am Heart J. 2015;169:25–30.

Part II

Clinical Applications of Anticoagulant Therapy

The Anticoagulation Clinic

8

Nathan P. Clark and Daniel M. Witt

Clinical Vignettes

Case 1: *An internal medicine physician begins a new practice joining a family health clinic in rural Colorado. She is surprised to learn that despite its modest size, the practice cares for several hundred patients anticoagulated with warfarin and a few dozen more taking DOACs. There currently is no formal system for tracking anticoagulated patients or managing labs, which has generated safety concerns from the provider team. The quality of warfarin management is not currently being measured, and it is not clear if there is room for improved INR control. The group agrees that establishing a formal process for anticoagulation management is overdue but is not quite sure where to start. What staffing model should they pursue for the AMS? What drug therapy policy and procedures should be developed?*

Case 2: *The AMS has been up and running for 6 months and includes a pharmacist, 2 nurses, and 2 clerks to manage the 630 anticoagulated patients. Most of the patients are seen during visits in the office using a point-of-care INR instrument. However, a few patients have complained about a long commute from rural areas into the clinic. What other options might be available for these patients? The AMS team has been doing well but is requesting more education regarding the coagulation cascade and pharmacology of the DOACs. What opportunities are available for them?*

Background and Introduction

Warfarin management is a labor-intensive endeavor involving thorough patient education, frequent patient-provider interactions, fastidious laboratory monitoring, and careful data management [1]. A major obstacle to the safety and effectiveness of warfarin therapy is the poor quality of dose management in real-world clinical practice. Poorly managed anticoagulation ther-

N. P. Clark (✉)
Clinical Pharmacy Anticoagulation and Anemia Service, Kaiser Permanente Colorado, Aurora, CO, USA
e-mail: nathan.clark@kp.org

D. M. Witt
University of Utah College of Pharmacy, Salt Lake City, UT, USA
e-mail: dan.witt@pharm.utah.edu

J. F. Lau et al. (eds.), *Anticoagulation Therapy*, https://doi.org/10.1007/978-3-319-73709-6_8

apy can result in life-threatening complications, and warfarin remains among the medications commonly implicated in emergency hospitalizations for adverse drug events in older adults [2]. In the late 1960s, when it became apparent that a systematic approach was needed to realize the therapeutic benefits of warfarin therapy while ensuring patient safety, anticoagulation management services (AMS) began to emerge [1]. The initial objective of these services was to relieve busy primary care physicians of the complex task of coordinating warfarin therapy [3]. Veterans Administration and academic medical centers were among early adopters of AMS models [4, 5]. Over time additional reports describing various AMS models and associated outcomes have appeared in the literature as summarized in a recent meta-analysis [6]. Although the American College of Chest Physicians Consensus Conference on Antithrombotic Therapy endorsed the advantage of systematic elements associated with an AMS, the superiority of AMS compared with other models needs to be confirmed in future research [6, 7]. This chapter will review various AMS models, training of AMS staff, services provided by AMS, quality improvement activities, and the future of AMS as available oral anticoagulants expand beyond warfarin.

Anticoagulation Management Service Structure

Required structural elements of an AMS have not been set forth by guidelines or formally endorsed within expert panels [8]. Their assembly over time has largely occurred according to available resources at the source of care delivery, such as nurses within a cardiology clinic or pharmacists within a hospital pharmacy. Smaller practices (e.g., less than 200 anticoagulated patients) often coordinate duties by designating one or more staff as the anticoagulation provider. Larger AMS centers benefit from common structural elements, which include clerical staff, management, clinical leadership, and patient care delivery by frontline staff. An example of AMS structure is provided in Fig. 8.1.

Clerical staff may include clerks, medical assistants, and pharmacy technicians. It is important to maximize the utility of support staff to minimize the amount of time spent by frontline providers on nonclinical duties. Examples of clerical duties include:

- Triaging incoming telephone calls and faxes
- Managing the electronic medical record in-basket
- Coordinating labs and updating standing orders
- Intake of new patient referrals and coordinating annual referral updates
- Drug interaction documentation and coordination of follow-up labs
- Scheduling patient appointments
- Updating and maintaining patient demographics and contact information
- Reminder calls and letters to patients overdue for lab monitoring
- Acquiring lab and anticoagulant dose history from hospital records or other healthcare settings
- Patient notification of stable, in-range lab results (may require prior review by trained medical personnel)

Leadership within the anticoagulation clinic takes two primary forms: clinical leadership and operational management, although there is often overlap and much needed partnership within these roles. Managers are responsible for the day-to-day administration of the AMS, including developing staff schedules, training, performance management, clinic infrastructure, and ensuring compliance with state and federal regulations, as well as establishing performance metrics and quality assurance process and successfully developing business cases for additional staff in the event of clinical growth. In many settings, ensuring financial success of the AMS is dependent upon appropriate coding for services. An in-depth description of AMS coding

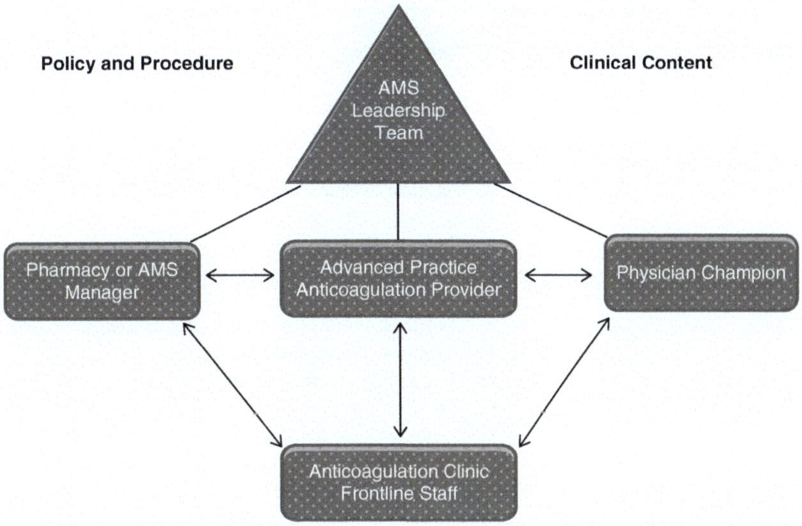

Fig. 8.1 Example structure of an outpatient anticoagulation management service. *AMS* Anticoagulation management service

practices can be found in work published by Wirth and Moore [9].

Clinical leadership of the AMS is derived from several sources, including from within the AMS. In addition, a physician champion is integral in developing AMS staff and coordinating with stakeholders from medical and surgical specialties throughout the healthcare system in the development of evidence-based clinical practices. Clinical leadership is responsible for the development and maintenance of AMS policy and procedures, training materials, best practices, and continuously evaluating for quality improvement opportunities. Potential areas of coordination between the AMS and other specialties are described in Table 8.1.

Frontline AMS providers require specialized training in thrombosis and hemostasis concepts, prothrombotic disease state pathophysiology, anticoagulant pharmacology, and practical knowledge of anticoagulant drug therapy management [8]. Providers of anticoagulant care should be a licensed healthcare provider, such as:

- Licensed practical nurse
- Registered nurse
- Advanced practice nurse/nurse practitioners
- Pharmacist
- Clinical pharmacy specialist
- Trainees
  - Interns
  - Residents

One or more of these healthcare professionals may be included in the AMS team. Successful AMS models have established divisions of responsibility according to staff training background and patient acuity. There are several ways to organize AMS care delivery, and no one method, structure, or discipline has proven definitively superior to any other. Standards of care for outpatient anticoagulant structure, personnel, and care delivery have been published by the Anticoagulation Forum (ACF) and are highlighted in Table 8.2.

Pharmacist Versus Nurse Anticoagulation Management Service

Pharmacy and nursing are the two most common disciplines found within AMS. Each discipline brings unique and valuable expertise to AMS

Table 8.1 Example areas of coordination between AMS and specialties

Specialty	Example topics
Cardiology/electrophysiology	• Evidence-based management of AF • Protocols for cardioversion and AF ablation • Periprocedural anticoagulation management
Cardiovascular surgery	• Protocols for prosthetic heart valve replacement
Hematology	• Duration of therapy guidelines for VTE • Bleeding management • Thrombophilia testing policy and procedures
Family practice/internal medicine	• Definition of roles and responsibilities in long-term anticoagulation management • Coordination of laboratory and medication ordering • Communication around referrals • Management of non-adherence
Hospital medicine	• Transitions of care • Periprocedural anticoagulation management • Use of formulary and preferred agents
Hospital pharmacy	• Coordination of anticoagulation care • Warfarin dose/INR history communication
Gastroenterology	• Procedure planning for colonoscopy/EGD
Obstetrics/gynecology	• Anticoagulation management during preconception planning • Contraceptive recommendations and management in VTE
Anesthesiology	• Anticoagulation management around neuraxial anesthesia and epidural steroid injections
General surgery	• Perioperative anticoagulation management • VTE prophylaxis guidelines

AF atrial fibrillation, *VTE* venous thromboembolism, *INR* international normalized ratio, *EGD* esophagogastro-duodenoscopy

care delivery. Observational studies supporting AMS benefit have evaluated both nurse- and pharmacy-led approaches in the outpatient AMS setting [10–16]. Greater autonomy in drug therapy management and prescribing are often available to those AMS with advance practitioners, such as nurse practitioners or clinical pharmacists with advanced training.

Traditional Laboratory Versus Point-of-Care INR Testing

Point-of-care (POC) testing utilizes a drop of capillary whole blood from a finger stick which is then rapidly analyzed by the POC device to determine the INR [17]. The POC device may be located within the AMS or the patients' home to facilitate patient self-testing (PST) or patient self-management (PSM). The use of POC testing is less invasive than traditional laboratory venipuncture and is particularly well suited to face-to-face AMS models as INR results are rapidly available.

There are a few barriers to consider with POC testing. The clinician or patient must receive adequate training to use the POC device properly to provide accurate INR results. The POC device requires an initial capital investment, takes up storage space, and must be regularly maintained and calibrated to ensure accuracy. Both traditional lab and POC INR testing are viable options, and each can have a role within the AMS [8]. However, there is potential for lack of agreement between two methods, and it is advisable for patients to stick to one methodology [18].

Patient Self-Testing and Patient Self-Management

Patient self-testing (PST) refers to INR monitoring at home with a POC device used by the patient. In many cases, PST INR results are

Table 8.2 Summary of ACF recommendations for optimized outpatient anticoagulant therapy [8]

Section	Recommendation
Qualifications of personnel	Licensed healthcare providers in pharmacy, nursing, or medicine engaged in anticoagulant care delivery should possess core competency in anticoagulant management
Leadership and reporting	If day-to-day management of anticoagulant therapy has been delegated to an AMS, CDTM practice agreements should be in place with the healthcare provider ultimately responsible for the patient care. The CDTM should be as descriptive and explicit as possible in the description of AMS responsibilities, job description, and accountability
Care management and coordination	Policies and procedures for anticoagulant care delivery should be established and approved by AMS leadership and the provider or provider group responsible for patient care
	These policy and procedures should enable communication regarding anticoagulation care delivery between healthcare providers accountable for high-quality anticoagulation care delivery
	A patient scheduling and tracking system should be utilized to facilitate efficient anticoagulant care delivery
Documentation	The AMS documentation should be accurate and readily available to members of the healthcare team
	Documentation should include relevant anticoagulant therapy details with current and historical information
Patient education	The AMS should provide thorough patient education which is tailored according to the educational needs of patients and their caregivers
	Provision of patient education should be documented in the medical record and/or the AMS program
Patient selection	Anticoagulant therapy should be initiated only after careful consideration of the risk and benefit for an individual patient
	The goals of anticoagulant therapy should be periodically reassessed to ensure the risk/benefit profile and patient preferences favor ongoing therapy
Laboratory monitoring	Optimal anticoagulation should include regular laboratory monitoring of warfarin with use of the prothrombin time test and reported as an INR
	Warfarin monitoring using the prothrombin time should be performed on either plasma samples in a clinical laboratory or on whole blood capillary (finger stick) samples utilizing point-of-care devices
	Routine monitoring of the anticoagulant effect of DOACs is not necessary
	Routine coagulation monitoring for long-term LMWH is rarely indicated. Anti-factor Xa concentration is the appropriate test to assess LMWH if necessary
Anticoagulation initiation	Anticoagulation should be initiated using a systematic, evidence-based approach
	A reminder mechanism to support timely anticoagulation drug therapy transitions for acute DVT/PE should be established
Anticoagulation maintenance	Anticoagulant care delivery should employ a systematic process for ongoing patient assessment, anticoagulant dose adjustment, and scheduling of follow-up laboratory monitoring
	Renal function should be periodically assessed for patients receiving long-term (e.g., greater than 45 days) DOAC or LMWH therapy
	A systematic approach should be established for management of anticoagulant therapy around elective invasive procedures
	Unexpected events such as bleeding and thrombosis should be systematically assessed and documented by the AMS
Anticoagulation cessation	A systematic approach should be established for determining appropriate patient-specific duration of anticoagulant therapy
	Anticoagulation discontinuation date and reason should be clearly documented by the AMS

AMS anticoagulation management service, *CDTM* collaborative drug therapy management, *DOAC* direct oral anticoagulant, *DVT* deep vein thrombosis, *LMWH* low-molecular-weight heparin

reported to an AMS or physician for warfarin dose adjustment. Patients endeavoring to perform PST typically require 30–60 min of training on the POC instrument prior to initiating PST [17].

Patient self-management occurs when a patient interprets their PST INR result and independently adjusts their warfarin dose and determines an appropriate recheck INR interval [7, 19]. PSM requires an additional training requirement where patients learn basic warfarin pharmacology and dose titration [20, 21]. Although a large, randomized controlled trial comparing PST to high quality AMS care did not identify important differences, meta-analysis suggests a decreased rate of thrombotic events among patients taking warfarin and using PST/PSM [22, 23]. The patient or family member performing PST/PSM will need good vision and hand-eye coordination to perform the POC test and read the results reliably. Patient characteristics that may be particularly amenable to PST/PSM include:

- Engaged and educated regarding their disease state and medications
- Difficulty getting into the AMS or a laboratory
- Frequent travel
- Poor venous access
- Not a suitable candidate for an alternative anticoagulant (i.e., direct oral anticoagulant)

Although the literature describing PST/PSM outcomes is generally favorable, there are barriers to implementing PST/PSM into a structured AMS. The first consideration is whether the AMS will provide the POC instrument, supplies, and training or outsource this to a third party. If the AMS elects to manage the instrument supply chain, planning is required to determine the up-front capital investment, storage, and staffing required for patient training. A vendor can manage the logistics surrounding POC instrument but may require weekly INR testing in order to recoup the up-front investment. Although weekly INR testing was often employed during PST trials [22], weekly or biweekly INR testing is unnecessary in otherwise stable patients and can overwhelm an AMS depending on patient volume. PST/PSM may also erode billable visits by an in-office AMS model.

In-Office Versus Telephonic Anticoagulation Management Service Care Delivery

Telephone and in-office visits are the two predominant AMS care delivery options. In-office AMS care delivery usually occurs within a single center, where patients are scheduled into 10- or 15-min appointment slots. The INR is done either immediately preceding or at the time of the appointment, often via POC, and the results are discussed and medications adjusted during the visit.

Telephonic AMS generally can accept INR results from many different laboratories and receives results electronically through the medical record, by fax or by phone. Electronic results from laboratories within the health system or network are preferred to optimize the timeliness of patient follow-up and efficiency with AMS processes. Frontline staff at the telephonic AMS reviews results as they are received and relays the INR result and warfarin dose information and rechecks INR interval to the patient via phone, letter, or secure messaging through the electronic medical record.

A study comparing telephonic management to in-office visits found similar anticoagulation outcomes between the two care models [24]. The optimal AMS model depends on the needs of the healthcare system, patient access, and whether the AMS is able to bill for services. The respective advantages of these two modes of anticoagulation care delivery are presented in Table 8.3.

Table 8.3 Telephone versus in-office AMS model

Characteristic	Telephone	In-office
Facilitate "show-and-tell" education and nonverbal communication		✓
Revenue generation from billable visits		✓
Refer patients for immediate physical assessment where indicated		✓
Managing patients with cognitive, hearing, or technical limitations		✓
No appointments (non-adherence is less disruptive to AMS)	✓	
High volume AMS without revenue incentive (e.g., veterans administration)	✓	
Patient convenience (use of their local laboratory, no appointments)	✓	
Management of homebound patients, assisted or skilled nursing facilities	✓	
Wide geographic service area	✓	

AMS anticoagulation management service

Panel-Based AMS Structure

The panel-based AMS bonds individual patients to an individual AMS provider. The same AMS provider is generally responsible for all aspects of anticoagulant care delivery, from patient education and invasive procedure planning to management of stable, in-range INRs. Although the clerical staff still works to support frontline providers, there are no distinct divisions of labor among the nurses or pharmacists providing anticoagulant care in a panel-based AMS.

The panel-based approach facilitates formation of a relationship between the patient and provider, which can be mutually rewarding. In addition, the AMS provider becomes familiar with the clinical picture of the patients in their panel. Historical challenges with patient memory, adherence, or previous adverse events are readily recalled by the AMS provider and do not require extensive chart review with each new laboratory result. Vacation and sick day coverage can be a challenge in a panel-based AMS to ensure all provider panels are covered each day. However, continuity in the AMS provider has been associated with improved INR control compared to a team-based approach [25].

Team-Based AMS Structure

Daily assignments in a team-based AMS may be made according to volume, by rotating assignment, or by acuity. Breaking up the work according to volume tends to focus initially on INR management, whereby the work is assigned in equal proportions to frontline staff. Assigning the work according to acuity is a particularly good option for a multidisciplinary AMS where assignments can be made to leverage the strengths of an individual provider or discipline. For example:

- New referrals and invasive procedure planning (pharmacist)
- Stable patients and in-range INRs (licensed practical nurse)
- Physical assessments during point-of-care (POC) testing (registered nurse A)
- Out-of-range INRs and incoming patient/provider calls (registered nurse B)
- Non-adherence reminders and drug interaction documentation (pharmacy intern or technician)

Patients managed in an AMS with a team-based approach may interact with any number of different providers throughout their anticoagulation care. Advantages to team-based structure include facilitating AMS staff working to their maximal scope of practice. The AMS workload can be assigned according to escalating acuity to providers with advanced degrees or greater training and development. There is also potential for an assembly-line approach when managing large volumes of patients and laboratory results with a team-based approach. Consistency in documentation is required in all AMS settings, but it is particularly crucial in a team-based structure where AMS providers may be less familiar with patients and rely on timely retrieval of relevant information during day-to-day activities.

Decision Support and Technology

Early anticoagulation management often occurred on paper flow sheets that tracked warfarin dosing and INR trends over time. Although effective, technologic advance facilitated AMS transition from paper systems to computer programs in the 1990s. Early AMS and warfarin monitoring was dominated by CoumaCare®, a widely used program provided for free by Bristol-Myers Squibb (formerly DuPont), Princeton, New Jersey. The program was widely used in many AMS settings for documenting INR results, warfarin doses, and tracking patients [26]. Many AMS locations leveraged local computer programmers to develop their own anticoagulation management systems. It is likely some of these programs continue today, although increased federal regulation regarding privacy safeguards has made it difficult for these programs to maintain compliance.

Several specialized anticoagulation management programs currently available are listed in Table 8.4. The data to support improved warfarin outcomes with these programs over use of a traditional nomogram is mixed [27, 28]; however the efficiency and utility gained in the AMS by using specialized software are undeniable. Programs can import INR results, provide warfarin dose and recheck INR interval decision support, prepopulate form letters, retain drug interaction and adverse event data, as well as interface patient data back into existing EMRs which eliminates double documentation and copy/paste errors. Productivity, safety, and quality reports can be generated easily and made available for clinical feedback. Functionality also exists to support tracking of patients on DOACs.

Training

Anticoagulation providers staffing AMS should receive training and demonstrate proficiency in core elements of anticoagulation therapy delivery (Table 8.5). Each AMS should determine minimum competencies for staff members operating in various roles. Minimum competencies should ensure that AMS staff operates within applicable scope-of-practice rules and regulations. Documentation that each AMS staff member has successfully completed designated training programs and meets minimum competencies should be available for inspection by state regulatory agencies. Continuing education should also be facilitated to ensure anticoagulation providers stay abreast of the latest consensus guideline recommendations and new additions to available anticoagulant medications.

Several resources are available to assist with training program development and continuing education (Table 8.6). The National Certification Board for Anticoagulation Providers (NCBAP) has developed a certification process for anticoagulation providers and is currently the only

Table 8.4 Available software packages for anticoagulation management

Name and company	Web address
Alere CoagClinic by standing stone	http://www.standingstoneinc.com/
CoagTrak by Medimatics	http://www.coagtrak.com/coumacare.html
Dawn AC by 4S information systems	http://www.4s-dawn.com/products/anticoagulation/dawnac/
Dose response by keystone therapeutics	http://www.doseresponse.com/
Anticoagulation CSO by IntraMed	http://www.intramed.dk/index.php/en/products
Posologic by Pharmafile solutions	http://en.posologic.com/
Web INR by Abington memorial hospital	http://www.webinr.com/

Table 8.5 Core competencies for anticoagulation providers [8]

Understand the role of coagulation and thrombogenesis in the pathophysiology of disease states requiring anticoagulation therapy
Describe how the pharmacokinetic and pharmacodynamic properties of anticoagulant medications may affect therapeutic decision-making
Identify medications, disease states, and dietary and lifestyle changes that may alter the response to anticoagulation therapy
Determine when a patient is experiencing a thromboembolic or bleeding complication and when a physician referral is warranted
Identify, triage, and refer medical problems not related to anticoagulation therapy to the appropriate healthcare provider
Understand the effects of socioeconomic, behavioral, psychological, and environmental factors on patient adherence to anticoagulation therapy instructions
Describe the meaning of laboratory tests used to measure the effect of anticoagulant medications on the hemostatic system, their limitations, and reasons for variability within and between laboratories
Interpret INR, aPTT, anti-Xa, and other laboratory values and adjust anticoagulant medication doses accordingly
Determine the optimal intensity and duration of anticoagulation therapy for individual patients based on evidence in the medical literature
Communicate effectively with patients, caregivers, and other healthcare providers
Coordinate ongoing anticoagulation therapy follow-up with patients, caregivers, and other healthcare providers

INR international normalized ratio, *aPTT* activated partial thromboplastin time; *anti-Xa* anti-factor Xa activity

available multidisciplinary credentialing opportunity [29] (see https://www.ncbap.org/index.aspx). The Anticoagulation Forum Centers of Excellence is an online tool which includes an assessment that can be taken by AMS leadership to identify gaps in AMS care. Anticoagulation services achieving a passing grade on the survey receive a 3-year certification from the Anticoagulation Forum as a "Center of Excellence." In addition, Anticoagulation Forum Centers of Excellence facilitates peer-to-peer sharing of AMS policy and procedures, best practices, and critical references which are maintained online and available free of charge (see http://excellence.acforum.org/) [30].

Medication Management

Table 8.7 highlights demographic and clinical factors to be assessed during patient intake and drug therapy and monitoring parameters relating to AMS activities [8]. Review of these parameters along with a discussion with the patient to ensure shared decision-making should guide (1) whether to initiate anticoagulation and (2), if starting anticoagulation, what agent and starting dose are most appropriate.

Warfarin and INR Monitoring

Warfarin dosing nomograms are beneficial and should be employed wherever possible, as described later [7]. Frequent INR monitoring is necessary during warfarin initiation or after a dose change or in the setting of dietary changes or new drug interactions [7]. The ACF recommends INR checks at least two to three times per week in the first 7–10 days or until a stable warfarin dose is achieved [8]. The maximum interval between INR tests in very stable warfarin patients is between 4 and 12 weeks [31, 32]. Once a stable warfarin dose is established, future dose adjustments should target ±5 to 20% of the weekly warfarin dose.

Heparin and Low-Molecular-Weight Heparin

Unfractionated heparin (UFH) is monitored by either the aPTT or anti-factor Xa (anti-Xa) concentration and low-molecular-weight heparin (LMWH) by anti-Xa concentration. UFH is only given by subcutaneous injection when used in the ambulatory setting. Monitoring and dose adjustment of these agents are rarely indicated for short-term outpatient use, and evidence supporting a therapeutic anti-Xa range has not been established for LMWH.

The dose of LMWH should be determined according to indication, actual body weight, and renal function. Anti-Xa monitoring has been suggested for patients at extremes of body

Table 8.6 Training program resources

Program	Description	Information
Anticoagulation therapy management program—University of Southern Indiana	Six-week, 40-h interactive internet certificate program	https://www.usi.edu/health/certificate-programs/anticoagulation-therapy-management-program/
Anticoagulation therapy Management for Pharmacists—University of Florida	12-week interactive internet certificate program	http://cpe.pharmacy.ufl.edu/courses/certificate/anticoagulation/
Anticoagulation traineeship—University of Connecticut Health Center	Two-day practice-based traineeship for registered pharmacists	http://pharmacy.uconn.edu/academics/ce/anticoagulation/
Stop the clot®—What every healthcare professional should know	Self-paced interactive internet continuing education program	https://www.stoptheclot.org/learn_more/curriculum.htm
Anticoagulation Forum Bootcamp	Two-day in-person continuing education program	http://acforum.org/

weight, CrCL <30, and during pregnancy [33]. Protocols for dose adjustment of these agents should be considered for patients with unpredictable pharmacokinetic parameters requiring long-term UFH or LMWH therapy, such as during pregnancy or malignancy-associated VTE treatment with variable renal function or extremes of body weight.

The use of UFH in the ambulatory setting is not common outside of pregnancy. If UFH is needed for acute DVT or PE management, an initial subcutaneous dose of 333 units/kg followed 12 h later by 250 units/kg subcutaneously twice daily without aPTT or anti-Xa monitoring was found to be as safe and effective as LMWH [34].

Excessive Anticoagulation

Patients presenting with excessive anticoagulation in the absence of bleeding should usually be managed in the outpatient setting according to established AMS policy and procedure. The AMS provider should review signs and symptoms of bleeding and attempt to identify factors contributing to excessive anticoagulation. Vitamin K should be reserved for patients presenting with an INR above 10 or if patient exposure to excessive anticoagulation is expected to be prolonged (e.g., INR > 5.0 for more than 72 h) [7]. The lowest effective vitamin K dose should be given orally, typically 1–2.5 mg. Intramuscular vitamin K administration should be avoided.

Monitoring for Adverse Events

The AMS provider is often the first point of contact for an anticoagulated patient in crisis. Often, the timely notification of healthcare providers of a problem relies on successful patient education. Anticoagulated patients need to know what symptoms are serious and which are life-threatening. Table 8.8 is provided for example only; AMS providers in collaboration with their physician champion and stakeholders should identify appropriate venue recommendations for patients according to their complaint or symptom.

Managing Patient Non-adherence

An AMS should have explicit procedures for managing patient non-adherence including documentation requirements and a communication plan for the patient and referring provider. Patients may be non-adherent with warfarin dosing, follow-up INR recheck, and/or dietary recommendations. Non-adherence with pill taking can result

Table 8.7 Baseline assessment and anticoagulant guidelines

Baseline assessment	
Accurate patient height, weight, and age	
Assessment for active bleeding and bleeding risk factors	
Identify potential drug interactions prior to anticoagulant selection	
Assessment of renal function prior to anticoagulant initiation	
Assessment of CBC prior to anticoagulant initiation	
Anticoagulant dosing guidelines	
Oral anticoagulant dosing guidelines and/or nomograms	
Direct thrombin inhibitor	Dabigatran
Factor Xa inhibitors	Rivaroxaban
	Apixaban
	Edoxaban
Vitamin K antagonist	Warfarin
Parenteral anticoagulant dosing guidelines	
Factor Xa inhibitors	Fondaparinux
Low-molecular-weight heparins	Dalteparin
	Enoxaparin
Unfractionated heparin	Heparin
Use of LMWHs, factor Xa inhibitors, and DTIs in renal failure and dialysis	
Use of warfarin, UFH, LMWHs, factor Xa inhibitors, and DTIs in pregnancy	
Use of warfarin, UFH, LMWHs, factor Xa inhibitors, and DTIs in pediatric patients	
Drug interaction recognition and management	
Selection of dosing and reversal therapies according to anticoagulant exposure	
Anticoagulant monitoring	
Target INR and INR goal range for various indications	
Frequency of INR monitoring	
Target aPTT or anti-factor Xa assay and goal range for various indications	
Frequency of aPTT or anti-factor Xa monitoring	
Patient monitoring for signs and symptoms of bleeding and thrombosis	

aPTT activated partial thromboplastin time, *CBC* complete blood count, *DTI* direct thrombin inhibitor, *LMWH* low-molecular-weight heparin, *UFH* unfractionated heparin, *VTE* venous thromboembolism

Table 8.8 Examples of bleeding and thromboembolic symptoms with recommended follow-up

Symptom	Concern	Action
Chest pain, shortness of breath, dizziness	Pulmonary embolism/acute coronary syndrome	Call 911 or go to emergency department
Slurred speech, one-sided weakness, drooping face, confusion, difficulty finding words	Stroke	Call 911 or go to emergency department
Debilitating headache like "bolt out of the blue" with nausea or vision impairment	Intracranial hemorrhage	Call 911 or go to emergency department
Fall with impact of the head		
Sudden onset of painful, cold extremity (e.g., hand or foot)	Arterial embolism	Call 911 or go to emergency department
Coffee ground emesis or black, tarry stools or blood in stool or filling the toilet ± fatigue/ light-headedness	Gastrointestinal hemorrhage	Call 911 or go to emergency department
Unexplained somnolence or decreased level of consciousness	Unknown	Call 911 or go to emergency department
One-sided leg pain, swelling, redness, and/or warm to touch	DVT	Urgent follow-up within 24 h
Blood on tissue paper or small amount in stool	Hemorrhoid bleeding	Urgent follow-up within 24 h
Extensive painful bruising that is raised or warm to the touch	Hematoma	Urgent follow-up within 24 h
Spontaneous nosebleed controlled with pressure after 15 min	Epistaxis	Follow up with AMS provider
		Recheck INR

(continued)

Table 8.8 (continued)

Symptom	Concern	Action
Unexplained, abnormal bruising	Elevated INR	Follow up with AMS provider
		Recheck INR
Blood on toothbrush	Elevated INR	Follow up with AMS provider
		Recheck INR

INR international normalized ratio, *AMS* anticoagulation management service, *DVT* deep vein thrombosis

from patient fear of being "too thin" or "too thick." It is important to have clear communication regarding roles and responsibilities and to set appropriate expectations with anticoagulated patients up-front as non-adherence during warfarin therapy can degrade time in therapeutic range (TTR) and increase the risk of adverse events [35, 36]. Referring providers are important allies, and the AMS should leverage physician support in managing patient non-adherence. For patients prescribed direct oral anticoagulants (DOACs), there is no summary statistic of anticoagulation control, but adherence is likely an important surrogate marker for quality care. The proportion of days covered, or PDC, has been evaluated as a marker of adherence in patients with atrial fibrillation prescribed dabigatran [37, 38]. A 10% reduction in PDC among patients with atrial fibrillation treated with dabigatran was associated with a 13% increased hazard of the combined outcome of stroke and all-cause mortality [37].

Invasive Procedure Management

The American College of Cardiology (ACC) recently published a guidance document for the management of anticoagulation around invasive procedures for patients with atrial fibrillation [39]. Low-molecular-weight heparin bridge therapy is suggested for patients with low bleeding risk and high risk of thromboembolism, including those with stroke or transient ischemic attack within the previous 3 months or a CHA_2DS_2-VASc score ≥7. These recommendations are controversial since the only randomized, placebo-controlled trial found low-molecular-weight heparin bridge therapy resulted in excess major bleeding without a corresponding reduction in stroke in patients with atrial fibrillation [40]. Guidelines for the perioperative management of warfarin for patients with DVT/PE or mechanical heart valves have not been updated since the American College of Chest Physicians (ACCP) guideline in 2012 [41]. In general, protocols should limit the application of bridge therapy to those patients thought to be at greatest risk for thromboembolism given we are without direct evidence as to the benefits of low-molecular-weight heparin bridging, whereas the bleeding risks are well known. Standardized practice guidelines should be implemented in the AMS to identify:

- Procedures that can be performed without warfarin or DOAC interruption
- Timing and goal pre-procedure INR values according to procedure bleeding risk
- Thromboembolic risk factors warranting the use of LMWH bridging:
  - Recommended LMWH dosing for eligible patients
  - Timing of perioperative LMWH dosing:
    - Last preoperative LMWH dose:
      Once-daily dosing versus twice-daily dosing
      Resumption of therapeutic LMWH 24 h after standard bleeding risk procedures
      Resumption of therapeutic LMWH 48–72 h after high bleeding risk procedures
- Exclusions to receiving LMWH bridging

Recommendations for warfarin reintroduction and the timing of post-procedure INRs with and without bridge therapy.

Patient Education

Patient education is an essential element of high-quality anticoagulation care [7]. Informed patients are more likely to be engaged in their care, and knowledge of anticoagulation therapy has been associated with improved TTR among anticoagulated outpatients [42]. Printed and published materials should be written at the eight grade reading level, but there is evidence that teaching materials frequently exceed the level of patient comprehension [43]. Additional methods of education may include group sessions, audiovisual presentations, web-based training, and printed materials [44]. Tools to assess knowledge and retention, including teach-back and validated anticoagulation knowledge tests, can assist AMS providers in verifying patient comprehension [21, 44]. Elements to be included in patient education checklist are presented in Table 8.9.

Table 8.9 Anticoagulant therapy patient education checklist [8]

Reason for anticoagulation
Name of the anticoagulant medication (trade and generic)
How the medication works
Onset and duration of activity
Dosing, frequency, storage, and duration of therapy
Common signs/symptoms of bleeding and instructions for follow-up when they occur
Common signs/symptoms of thrombosis and instructions for follow-up when they occur
Implications for pregnancy and the need for effective birth control
Reinforce appropriate use of safety equipment for recreation and motor vehicle operation
Avoidance of high-risk behavior for traumatic injury
Common side effects other than bleeding
Recommendations to notify other healthcare providers of anticoagulant therapy
When to notify AMS provider (e.g., invasive procedures, new dietary habits, recent hospitalization)
Options for anticoagulation identification (e.g., bracelet or medication card)
Use one pharmacy for all prescription drugs to facilitate drug interaction screening
The risk of non-adherence or taking too much anticoagulant medication
Limit or avoid alcohol
Instructions for timing of administration and missed dose
The reason for and timing of laboratory monitoring
The meaning of the INR, target INR range, and the rationale for timely testing (warfarin only)
The influence of vitamin K and the rationale for dietary consistency (warfarin only)

AMS anticoagulation management service, *INR* international normalized ratio

Anticoagulation Metrics and Quality Improvement

Providing quality anticoagulation therapy involves balancing decreasing the risk of pathologic clot formation with increasing the risk of bleeding. In order to ensure patient safety and address the needs of patients and their caregivers, anticoagulation therapy outcomes and care processes should be continually measured, evaluated, and improved [45]. Measurements help identify potential improvement targets and provide ongoing feedback as to whether quality improvement initiatives are having the intended effect. Table 8.10 provides an overview of various measurement types that can support quality improvement activities.

The most definitive measure of anticoagulation therapy quality, the proportion of patients who suffer bleeding or thromboembolic adverse events directly attributable to anticoagulation therapy, may not be the optimal care quality measure. This is because bleeding and thromboembolic complications occur infrequently, and occurrence rates may be difficult to quantify with accuracy. Perhaps, more importantly, bleeding and thromboembolism can occur despite therapeutic anticoagulation and therefore may not directly correlate with high-quality anticoagulation therapy management. Therefore, warfarin therapy quality is most often assessed indirectly using various measures of the ability to keep INRs within the targeted therapeutic range [45].

Maintaining therapeutic INR control during warfarin therapy has been shown to correlate strongly with reducing the risk of therapeutic failure and bleeding [46]. The most widely accepted method for assessing warfarin ther-

Table 8.10 Types of quality improvement measures

Measure	Used to assess	Examples
Process	System components and whether they are performing as intended	• Percentage of INR encounters documented according to specified guidelines • Percentage of patients who miss INR appointments that are contacted within 10 days
Outcome	The end care result	• Bleeding or thromboembolism • TTR • Patient satisfaction • Percentage of INRs >5 or <1.5
Balancing	The effect of changes on one system aspect on other parts of the system	• Does reducing INR recall interval following out-of-range INR increase TTR • Does change of laboratory thromboplastin impact TTR

AMS anticoagulation management service, *INR* international normalized ratio, *TTR* time in therapeutic INR range

apy quality over time is TTR. A variety of methods for measuring TTR are available but no consensus exists as to which is preferred [47]. Even in AMS where warfarin management may be better than average, efforts to drive TTR higher will likely result in improved patient outcomes. A brief description of strategies used by AMS to improve TTR follows (see also Table 8.11).

In addition to TTR, several estimates of INR variability or variance growth rate have been associated with bleeding and thromboembolism during anticoagulant therapy [48–50]. Variability in INR can be calculated as the difference between the measured INR and the target INR (e.g., 2.5) or the difference between successive INRs [48, 49]. Unstable INRs have been more closely associated with bleeding risk than TTR in one analysis; however the lack of a benchmark value and the complexity in calculating INR variability or variance growth rate over time limit its utility as an AMS quality indicator.

Table 8.11 Suggestions to improve time in therapeutic INR range

Clinical scenario	Recommendation
Patient with previously stable therapeutic INRs presenting with single out-of-range INR within 0.2 below or above target range	Continue the current warfarin dose, and test the next INR within 1–2 weeks
Patient with INRs in the target range consistently over 3 months with no need for warfarin dose changes presents with another in-range INR	Test next INR at increasing intervals as long as INR remains in target range, up to a maximum of 12 weeks
Patient with target INR 2–3 presents with an out-of-range INR needs to know when to return for next test	For INR ≥4.0 or ≤1.5, return within 7 days; for INR 3.1–3.9 or 1.6–1.9, return within 14 days
Patient needs instruction regarding what warfarin dose to take and when to return for next INR based on current INR results	Use a validated dosing nomograms (paper or computerized) rather than an ad hoc approach

INR international normalized ratio

Warfarin Dosing Algorithms

There is evidence indicating that most warfarin dosing decisions are made in an ad hoc manner [51]. Adherence to warfarin dosing algorithms (manual or computerized) has been convincingly shown to predict improved TTR [27, 46, 52]. In one study, each 10% increase in algorithm-consistent dosing independently predicted a 6% increase in TTR and an 8% decrease in rate of adverse clinical outcomes [46]. Evidence-based guidelines suggest using validated decision support tools (paper-based nomograms or computer-assisted dosing programs) is preferable to no decision support during maintenance warfarin therapy [7].

INR Recall Interval

A systematic approach to determining the interval between INR tests (INR recall interval) should optimize clinical outcomes as well as the combination of TTR, patient convenience, and healthcare resource utilization [53]. The promptness of repeat testing after an out-of-range INR value has been shown to correlate with TTR [54]. Research suggests that TTR is improved considerably by rechecking INRs within 7 days after a high (≥4.0) or low (≤1.5) INR result and within 14 days after a mildly high (3.1–3.9) or mildly low (1.6–1.9) result. Investigation of the impact of INR recall interval on TTR following in-range INRs indicates that after the first or second in-range INR value, a maximum recall interval of 28 days is optimal, but after the third or greater consecutive in-range INR, longer recall intervals do not worsen TTR [55]. Consensus panel guidelines citing evidence from both observational and randomized controlled trials suggest that INR recall intervals of up to 12 weeks are acceptable for warfarin patients with consistently stable INRs [7].

Non-adherence with INR Monitoring

Non-adherence with INR monitoring has been shown to increase the risk of thromboembolic complications during warfarin therapy [36]. Centers with more gaps greater than 56 days between INRs per patient-year have been shown to have worse anticoagulation control [56]. Strategies to identify and reduce INR monitoring non-adherence may therefore improve anticoagulation control and reduce thromboembolic risk [36, 56]. However, strategies to durably improve long-term adherence with INR monitoring have yet to be identified. A recent report of patient-specific factors influencing adherence with INR monitoring suggested the following [57]:

- Assign anticoagulation providers to work with the same patients consistently.
- Provide formal INR reminders.
- Avoid harsh language or lecturing patients following missed INR tests.
- Reinforce the clinical and psychological utility of INR results.
- Facilitate access to INR testing.

Providing formal INR reminders can be a burden on AMS providers. Interactive voice response telephone reminders have yielded mixed results due to their complexity, but text messaging may offer a reliable and less intrusive option for delivery of mass patient reminders [58].

No Tamper Zone

For patients demonstrating INR stability, warfarin dose changes in response to slightly out-of-range INR values may serve merely to perturb the INR, setting up a cycle of adjustment and readjustment [59]. The single mildly out-of-range INR in this scenario often represents random variation and does not warrant a change in VKA dose. Adjusting warfarin doses every time the INR is out-of-range without regard to prior INR stability patterns can be considered "tampering." There is evidence suggesting that instituting a "no tamper zone" wherein the INR is simply rechecked a week later without any particular intervention is likely to improve TTR for patients with otherwise stable INR control [7, 59]. For patients with targeted INR ranges of 2.0–3.0, a no tamper zone of 1.8–3.2 has been suggested [59].

Standard INR Targets

Narrower target ranges have been suggested in certain situations (e.g., INR 2.0–2.5 has been recommended in patients requiring warfarin, aspirin, and clopidogrel following percutaneous coronary intervention) [60]. Such narrow ranges are not supported by good evidence and make maintaining therapeutic INR control more difficult and usually result in the need for more frequent INR testing. The AMS should mandate using standardized "full point" INR target ranges as a precondition for assuming responsibility for warfarin therapy monitoring [7]. The proportion of patients with a mean INR value between 2.3 and 2.7 has been shown to measure the extent to which a given site is pursuing a guideline-concordant target range of 2–3 for most patients, as opposed to another target [61].

Dashboard to Support Efforts to Improve TTR

Efforts to improve TTR within a given AMS or health system can be supported by targeted audit and feedback [62]. Some health systems have developed online reporting systems (so-called dashboards), which provide real-time performance measurement data to clinicians. Dashboards can report TTR at both the patient and the site level [63]. Performance on processes of care that have been linked to TTR, including those outlined above, can also be included in dashboard reports. Dashboards have been used successfully to improve TTR in AMS in large health systems such as the Veterans Administration [54–56, 59, 61, 63].

Quality Reporting

In order to ensure patient safety, outcomes and processes associated with core elements of anticoagulation therapy delivery should be continually measured, evaluated, and improved. Therefore, each AMS should have a formal system in place to measure TTR performance (or a similar measure for assessing the quality of INR control among patients receiving warfarin therapy) and endeavor to improve performance over time [64]. Comparing TTR across different healthcare settings and to values reported in the literature allows benchmarking of performance provided the same TTR measuring methodology is used. It may also be worthwhile to track definitive outcomes of anticoagulation therapy using consistent methodology over time to identify trends within a given health system that might indicate need for further investigation and intervention.

The Future of Anticoagulation Management Services

The DOACs do not require routine coagulation monitoring, have a wider therapeutic index than warfarin, and rarely require dose adjustment. This has led some to speculate the eventual end to AMS. However, the AMS can play a vital role in ensuring patients initiating DOACs receive the same high-quality anticoagulation care as patients on warfarin [65]. A Veterans Administration study found that pharmacist-led monitoring of patients taking dabigatran was associated with better medication adherence compared to patients taking dabigatran without such support [37]. Despite the relatively straightforward prescribing of DOACs, dosing errors, off-label use, and duplicate errors are common [66]. Increasing use of rivaroxaban and dabigatran has been observed in patients with atrial fibrillation on dialysis, despite being contraindicated in this setting (Fig. 8.2) [67]. Even more worrisome, many of these patients received therapeutic doses without any adjustment to account for the decreased elimination and extended half-life expected for these drugs in the setting of severe renal insufficiency. Unsurprisingly, patients requiring dialysis and receiving rivaroxaban and dabigatran were exposed to increased risk for hospitalization and death related to bleeding than those receiving warfarin [67]. These data underscore just one of the many important interventions an AMS can make in a DOAC population; other activities include:

- Verifying the appropriateness of anticoagulant therapy
- Checking for DOAC contraindications
- Patient education:
  - Discuss financial implications of oral anticoagulant options.
- Dose adjustment:
  - DVT/PE treatment:

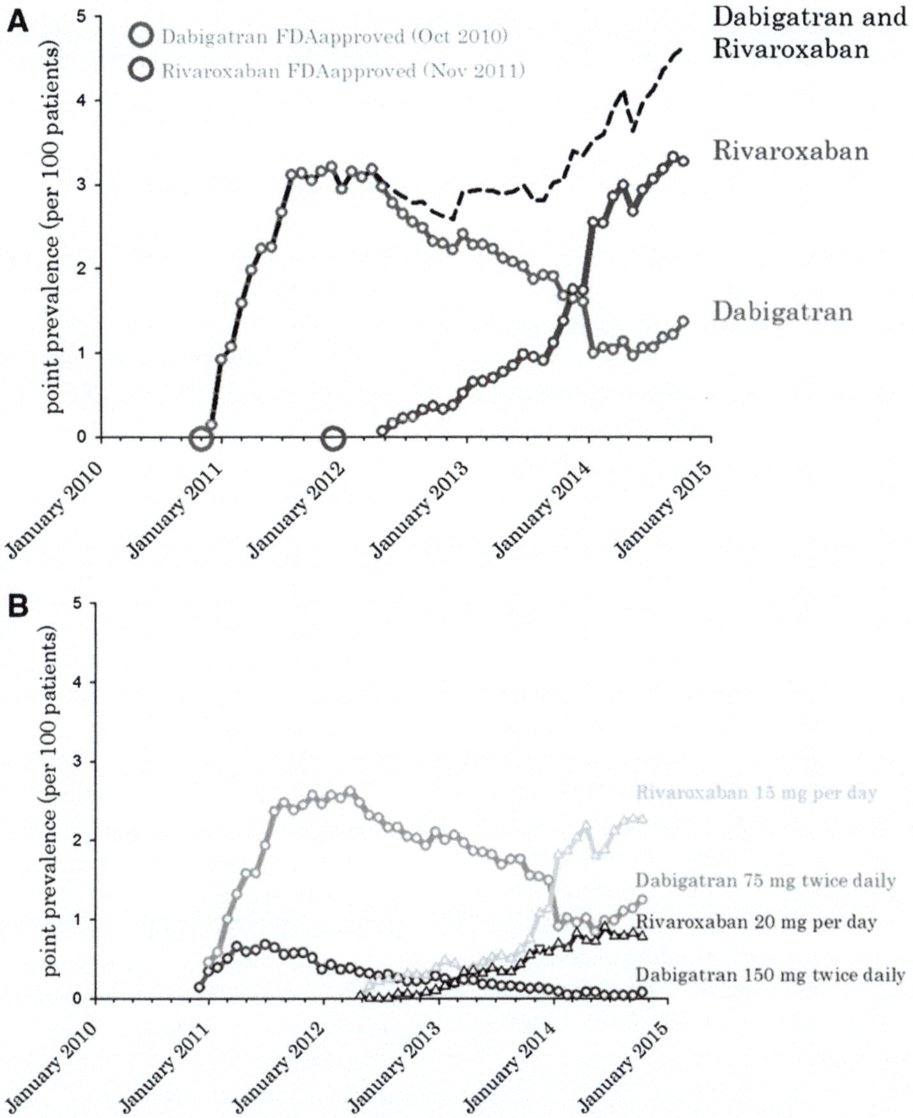

Fig. 8.2 (**a**) Point prevalence of dabigatran and rivaroxaban among anticoagulated chronic hemodialysis patients with atrial fibrillation. (**b**) Point prevalence of dabigatran and rivaroxaban among anticoagulated chronic hemodialysis patients with atrial fibrillation, by drug dose. FDA indicates Food and Drug Administration [67]. (Reprinted with permission from Chan KE, Edelman ER, Wenger JB, Thadhani RI, Maddux FW. Dabigatran and rivaroxaban use in atrial fibrillation patients on hemodialysis. Circulation, Vol. 131, No. 11, pages 972–979, © 2015, http://circ.ahajournals.org/content/131/11/972.long, with permission from Wolters Kluwer Health, Inc)

- Acute management:
  - Parenteral anticoagulants:
    - Yes (dabigatran, edoxaban)
    - No (rivaroxaban, apixaban)
  - Duration of intensified oral therapy
    - 7 days (apixaban)
    - 21 days (rivaroxaban)
    - Not applicable (dabigatran, edoxaban)
- Intermediate management
- Duration of therapy
- Long-term secondary management:
  - Dose reduction (apixaban, rivaroxaban)

  - Renal function
  - Clinical factors (body weight, serum creatinine, age, and drug interactions)
- Perioperative management
- Adherence monitoring
- Drug interaction screening
- Annual or ongoing assessment of dose requirement according to clinical factors
- Bleeding management
- Transitions between anticoagulant therapies

Ensuring these areas are effectively managed is essential for optimal anticoagulant therapy during DOAC administration, and the outpatient AMS is particularly well-suited to facilitate these processes.

Conclusion

A successful AMS must leverage available resources to optimally manage anticoagulated patients and effectively interface within the healthcare system it serves. High-quality anticoagulant care delivery is a continuous process, and efforts to measure and improve anticoagulation therapy outcomes are warranted. We have entered a new era in anticoagulant therapy, but the addition of DOACs has introduced another layer of complexity in anticoagulant care delivery and presents yet another opportunity for the AMS to establish its value.

Key Points

- A large, randomized trial comparing PST to high-quality AMS warfarin management found no difference in bleeding or thromboembolic outcomes, but patients performing PST reported improved satisfaction with their anticoagulation care and quality of life.
- Effective education can improve patient adherence and the quality of anticoagulation care; however, printed materials provided by the AMS are often written at levels beyond patient comprehension.
- Following a warfarin dosing algorithm or decision support programs improves TTR and anticoagulation outcomes.
- AMS quality improvement efforts to optimize INR recall intervals can simultaneously target shorter intervals (i.e., 7 days) for very out-of-range INRs while allowing longer intervals (i.e., up to 12 weeks) for very stable patients.

Self-Assessment Questions

1. Which of the following statements regarding the structure of an AMS *is most correct*?
   (a) An AMS utilizing pharmacists provides the best patient outcomes due to their in-depth understanding of anticoagulant pharmacology.
   (b) An AMS utilizing nurses provides the best patient outcomes due to their ability to perform a complete physical assessment.
   (c) Only physicians should manage anticoagulant therapy.
   (d) Successful AMS examples have employed a variety of medical professionals.
2. Which of the following *is the most commonly* reported quality indicator during warfarin management?
   (a) Time in therapeutic range
   (b) Fihn INR variability
   (c) Cross section of the files
   (d) Duration of low-molecular-weight heparin bridge therapy
3. Which of the following systematic changes *is most likely* to result in improved INR control during warfarin therapy?
   (a) In-office AMS visits rather than telephone follow-up
   (b) 7-day recheck intervals after significantly out-of-range INR values
   (c) Daily vitamin K supplementation
   (d) Transition from paper-based warfarin nomograms to computerized decision support

4. Which of the following is not an important element of anticoagulant therapy education?
   (a) Trade and generic medication names
   (b) Expected duration of anticoagulation
   (c) Avoidance of vitamin K-containing foods
   (d) The importance of adherence with medication dosing and laboratory monitoring
5. Which of the following *are key characteristics* of a successful AMS?
   (a) Frontline staff made up of licensed healthcare professionals.
   (b) Descriptive policy and procedures detail roles and responsibilities of AMS team members.
   (c) AMS documentation is accurate and readily available to members of the healthcare team.
   (d) All of the above.

Self-Assessment Answers

1. (d) Successful AMS examples have employed a variety of medical professionals.

   Many different models for AMS have been employed, including nurses and pharmacist in key patient management roles.
2. (a) Time in therapeutic range

   Time in therapeutic range is the most widely validated measure of warfarin quality. This is best estimated using the Rosendaal method of linear interpolation.
3. (b) 7-day recheck intervals after significantly out-of-range INR values

   AMS have shown excellent efficacy in both phone-based and in-person management as well as with paper nomogram or computer-based dosing. Short recheck intervals for significantly out-of-range INR values are most likely to improve INR control.
4. (c) Avoidance of vitamin K-containing foods

   Patients should not be told to avoid vitamin K-containing foods. Rather, they should be educated to consume a consistent daily amount of vitamin K in their diet.
5. (d) All of the above

   Successful AMS will include licensed and trained healthcare professionals that follow policies and standardized documentation for the management of anticoagulated patients.

References

1. Ansell JE, Buttaro ML, Thomas OV, Knowlton CH. Consensus guidelines for coordinated outpatient oral anticoagulation therapy management. Anticoagulation Guidelines Task Force. Ann Pharmacother. 1997;31:604–15.
2. Budnitz DS, Lovegrove MC, Shehab N, Richards CL. Emergency hospitalizations for adverse drug events in older Americans. N Engl J Med. 2011;365:2002–12.
3. Davis FB, Estruch MT, Samson-Corvera EB, Voigt GC, Tobin JD. Management of anticoagulation in outpatients: experience with an anticoagulation service in a municipal hospital setting. Arch Intern Med. 1977;137:197–202.
4. Reinders TP, Steinke WE. Pharmacist management of anticoagulant therapy in ambulant patients. Am J Hosp Pharm. 1979;36:645–8.
5. Witte K, Gurwich EL, Anzalone R, Campagna MA. Audit of an oral anticoagulant teaching program. Am J Hosp Pharm. 1980;37:89–91.
6. Zhou S, Sheng XY, Xiang Q, Wang ZN, Zhou Y, Cui YM. Comparing the effectiveness of pharmacist-managed warfarin anticoagulation with other models: a systematic review and meta-analysis. J Clin Pharm Ther. 2016;41:602–11.
7. Holbrook A, Schulman S, Witt DM, et al. Evidence-based management of anticoagulant therapy: Antithrombotic Therapy and Prevention of Thrombosis, 9th ed: American College of Chest Physicians Evidence-Based Clinical Practice Guidelines. Chest. 2012;141:e152S–84S.
8. Garcia DA, Witt DM, Hylek E, et al. Delivery of optimized anticoagulant therapy: consensus statement from the Anticoagulation Forum. Ann Pharmacother. 2008;42:979–88.
9. Wirth D, Moore J. Developing a business plan for an anticoagulation management service. In: Ansell J, Oertel L, Wittkowsky A, editors. Managing oral anticoagulation therapy: clinical and operational guidelines. 3rd ed. Philadelphia: Lippincott Williams & Wilkins; 2009.
10. Vadher BD, Patterson DL, Leaning M. Comparison of oral anticoagulant control by a nurse-practitioner using a computer decision-support system with that by clinicians. Clin Lab Haematol. 1997;19:203–7.
11. Fitzmaurice DA, Murray ET, Allan TF, Holder RL, Rose PE, Hobbs FD. A comparison of international normalised ratio (INR) measurement in hospital and general practice settings: evidence for lack of standardisation. J Clin Pathol. 2000;53:803-4.
12. Donovan JL, Drake JA, Whittaker P, Tran MT. Pharmacy-managed anticoagulation: assessment of in-hospital efficacy and evaluation of financial impact and community acceptance. J Thromb Thrombolysis. 2006;22:23–30.
13. Locke C, Ravnan SL, Patel R, Uchizono JA. Reduction in warfarin adverse events requiring patient hospitalization after implementation of a pharmacist-

managed anticoagulation service. Pharmacotherapy. 2005;25:685–9.
14. Schillig J, Kaatz S, Hudson M, Krol GD, Szandzik EG, Kalus JS. Clinical and safety impact of an inpatient pharmacist-directed anticoagulation service. J Hosp Med. 2011;6:322–8.
15. Witt DM, Sadler MA, Shanahan RL, Mazzoli G, Tillman DJ. Effect of a centralized clinical pharmacy anticoagulation service on the outcomes of anticoagulation therapy. Chest. 2005;127:1515–22.
16. Rudd KM, Dier JG. Comparison of two different models of anticoagulation management services with usual medical care. Pharmacotherapy. 2010;30:330–8.
17. Nutescu EA, Bathija S, Sharp LK, Gerber BS, Schumock GT, Fitzgibbon ML. Anticoagulation patient self-monitoring in the United States: considerations for clinical practice adoption. Pharmacotherapy. 2011;31:1161–74.
18. Dorfman DM, Goonan EM, Boutilier MK, Jarolim P, Tanasijevica M, Goldhaber SZ. Point-of-care (POC) versus central laboratory instrumentation for monitoring oral anticoagulation. Vasc Med. 2005;10:23–7.
19. McCahon D, Murray ET, Jowett S, et al. Patient self management of oral anticoagulation in routine care in the UK. J Clin Pathol. 2007;60:1263–7.
20. Simmons BJ, Jenner KM, Delate T, Clark NP, Kurz D, Witt DM. Pilot study of a novel patient self-management program for warfarin therapy using venipuncture-acquired international normalized ratio monitoring. Pharmacotherapy. 2012;32:1078–84.
21. Jenner KM, Simmons BJ, Delate T, Clark NP, Kurz D, Witt DM. An education program for patient self-management of Warfarin. Perm J. 2015;19:33–8.
22. Matchar DB, Jacobson A, Dolor R, et al. Effect of home testing of international normalized ratio on clinical events. N Engl J Med. 2010;363:1608–20.
23. Heneghan CJ, Garcia-Alamino JM, Spencer EA, et al. Self-monitoring and self-management of oral anticoagulation. Cochrane Database Syst Rev. 2016;7:CD003839.
24. Wittkowsky AK, Nutescu EA, Blackburn J, et al. Outcomes of oral anticoagulant therapy managed by telephone vs in-office visits in an anticoagulation clinic setting. Chest. 2006;130:1385–9.
25. Bishop MA, Streiff MB. Effects of anticoagulation provider continuity on time in therapeutic range for warfarin patients. J Thromb Thrombolysis. 2016;42:283–7.
26. Garcia DA, Regan S, Crowther M, Hylek EM. The risk of hemorrhage among patients with warfarin-associated coagulopathy. J Am Coll Cardiol. 2006;47:804–8.
27. Poller L, Keown M, Ibrahim S, et al. A multicentre randomised assessment of the DAWN AC computer-assisted oral anticoagulant dosage program. Thromb Haemost. 2009;101:487–94.
28. Nieuwlaat R, Hubers LM, Spyropoulos AC, et al. Randomised comparison of a simple warfarin dosing algorithm versus a computerised anticoagulation management system for control of warfarin maintenance therapy. Thromb Haemost. 2012;108:1228–35.
29. National Certification Board for Anticoagulation Providers (NCBAP). https://www.ncbap.org/index.aspx.
30. Anticoagulation Forum Centers of Excellence. http://excellence.acforum.org/.
31. Schulman S, Parpia S, Stewart C, Rudd-Scott L, Julian JA, Levine M. Warfarin dose assessment every 4 weeks versus every 12 weeks in patients with stable international normalized ratios: a randomized trial. Ann Intern Med. 2011;155:653–9. W201-3.
32. Witt DM, Delate T, Clark NP, et al. Twelve-month outcomes and predictors of very stable INR control in prevalent warfarin users. J Thromb Haemost. 2010;8:744–9.
33. Clark NP. Low-molecular-weight heparin use in the obese, elderly, and in renal insufficiency. Thromb Res. 2008;123(Suppl 1):S58–61.
34. Kearon C, Ginsberg JS, Julian JA, et al. Comparison of fixed-dose weight-adjusted unfractionated heparin and low-molecular-weight heparin for acute treatment of venous thromboembolism. JAMA. 2006;296:935–42.
35. Parker CS, Chen Z, Price M, et al. Adherence to warfarin assessed by electronic pill caps, clinician assessment, and patient reports: results from the IN-RANGE study. J Gen Intern Med. 2007;22(9):1254.
36. Witt DM, Delate T, Clark NP, et al. Nonadherence with INR monitoring and anticoagulant complications. Thromb Res. 2013;132:e124–30.
37. Shore S, Carey EP, Turakhia MP, et al. Adherence to dabigatran therapy and longitudinal patient outcomes: insights from the veterans health administration. Am Heart J. 2014;167:810–7.
38. Gorst-Rasmussen A, Skjoth F, Larsen TB, Rasmussen LH, Lip GY, Lane DA. Dabigatran adherence in atrial fibrillation patients during the first year after diagnosis: a nationwide cohort study. J Thromb Haemost. 2015;13:495–504.
39. Doherty JU, Gluckman TJ, Hucker WJ, et al. 2017 ACC expert consensus decision pathway for periprocedural management of anticoagulation in patients with nonvalvular atrial fibrillation: a report of the American College of Cardiology Clinical Expert Consensus Document Task Force. J Am Coll Cardiol. 2017;69:871–98.
40. Douketis JD, Spyropoulos AC, Kaatz S, et al. Perioperative bridging anticoagulation in patients with atrial fibrillation. N Engl J Med. 2015;373:823–33.
41. Douketis JD, Spyropoulos AC, Spencer FA, et al. Perioperative management of antithrombotic therapy: Antithrombotic Therapy and Prevention of Thrombosis, 9th ed: American College of Chest Physicians Evidence-Based Clinical Practice Guidelines. Chest. 2012;141:e326S–50S.
42. Barcellona D, Contu P, Marongiu F. Patient education and oral anticoagulant therapy. Haematologica. 2002;87:1081–6.

43. Estrada CA, Hryniewicz MM, Higgs VB, Collins C, Byrd JC. Anticoagulant patient information material is written at high readability levels. Stroke. 2000;31:2966–70.
44. Moore SJ, Blair EA, Steeb DR, Reed BN, Hull JH, Rodgers JE. Impact of video technology on efficiency of pharmacist-provided anticoagulation counseling and patient comprehension. Ann Pharmacother. 2015;49:631–8.
45. Witt DM. Quality measures and benchmarking for warfarin therapy. J Thromb Thrombolysis. 2011;31:242–8.
46. Van Spall HG, Wallentin L, Yusuf S, et al. Variation in warfarin dose adjustment practice is responsible for differences in the quality of anticoagulation control between centers and countries: an analysis of patients receiving warfarin in the randomized evaluation of long-term anticoagulation therapy (RE-LY) trial. Circulation. 2012;126:2309–16.
47. Schmitt L, Speckman J, Ansell J. Quality assessment of anticoagulation dose management: comparative evaluation of measures of time-in-therapeutic range. J Thromb Thrombolysis. 2003;15:213–6.
48. Ibrahim S, Jespersen J, Poller L, European Action on Anticoagulation. The clinical evaluation of international normalized ratio variability and control in conventional oral anticoagulant administration by use of the variance growth rate. J Thromb Haemost. 2013;11:1540–6.
49. Fihn SD, McDonell M, Martin D, et al. Risk factors for complications of chronic anticoagulation. A multicenter study. Warfarin Optimized Outpatient Follow-up Study Group. Ann Intern Med. 1993;118:511–20.
50. van Leeuwen Y, Rosendaal FR, Cannegieter SC. Prediction of hemorrhagic and thrombotic events in patients with mechanical heart valve prostheses treated with oral anticoagulants. J Thromb Haemost. 2008;6:451–6.
51. Nieuwlaat R, Barker L, Kim YK, et al. Underuse of evidence-based warfarin dosing methods for atrial fibrillation patients. Thromb Res. 2010;125:e128–31.
52. Kim YK, Nieuwlaat R, Connolly SJ, et al. Effect of a simple two-step warfarin dosing algorithm on anticoagulant control as measured by time in therapeutic range: a pilot study. J Thromb Haemost. 2010;8:101–6.
53. Fihn SD, McDonell MB, Vermes D, et al. A computerized intervention to improve timing of outpatient follow-up: a multicenter randomized trial in patients treated with warfarin. National Consortium of Anticoagulation Clinics. J Gen Intern Med. 1994;9:131–9.
54. Rose AJ, Hylek EM, Berlowitz DR, Ash AS, Reisman JI, Ozonoff A. Prompt repeat testing after out-of-range INR values: a quality indicator for anticoagulation care. Circ Cardiovasc Qual Outcomes. 2011;4:276–82.
55. Rose AJ, Ozonoff A, Berlowitz DR, Ash AS, Reisman JI, Hylek EM. Reexamining the recommended follow-up interval after obtaining an in-range international normalized ratio value: results from the veterans Affairs study to improve anticoagulation. Chest. 2011;140:359–65.
56. Rose AJ, Miller DR, Ozonoff A, et al. Gaps in monitoring during oral anticoagulation: insights into care transitions, monitoring barriers, and medication nonadherence. Chest. 2013;143:751–7.
57. Kauffman YS, Schroeder AE, Witt DM. Patient specific factors influencing adherence to INR monitoring. Pharmacotherapy. 2015;35:740–7.
58. Zallman L, Bearse A, West C, Bor D, McCormick D. Patient preferences and access to text messaging for health care reminders in a safety-net setting. Inform Health Soc Care. 2017;42:32–42.
59. Rose AJ, Ozonoff A, Berlowitz DR, Henault LE, Hylek EM. Warfarin dose management affects INR control. J Thromb Haemost. 2009;7:94–101.
60. King SB 3rd, Smith SC Jr, Hirshfeld JW Jr, et al. 2007 focused update of the ACC/AHA/SCAI 2005 guideline update for percutaneous coronary intervention: a report of the American College of Cardiology/ American Heart Association Task Force on Practice Guidelines: 2007 Writing Group to Review New Evidence and Update the ACC/AHA/SCAI 2005 Guideline Update for Percutaneous Coronary Intervention, Writing on Behalf of the 2005 Writing Committee. Circulation. 2008;117:261–95.
61. Rose AJ, Berlowitz DR, Miller DR, et al. INR targets and site-level anticoagulation control: results from the Veterans AffaiRs Study to Improve Anticoagulation (VARIA). J Thromb Haemost. 2012;10:590–5.
62. Hysong SJ, Sawhney MK, Wilson L, et al. Improving outpatient safety through effective electronic communication: a study protocol. Implement Sci. 2009;4:62.
63. Rose AJ, Hylek EM, Ozonoff A, Ash AS, Reisman JI, Berlowitz DR. Risk-adjusted percent time in therapeutic range as a quality indicator for outpatient oral anticoagulation: results of the Veterans Affairs Study to Improve Anticoagulation (VARIA). Circ Cardiovasc Qual Outcomes. 2011;4:22–9.
64. Rose AJ, Delate T, Ozonoff A, Witt DM. Comparison of the abilities of summary measures of international normalized ratio control to predict clinically relevant bleeding. Circ Cardiovasc Qual Outcomes. 2015;8:524–31.
65. Barnes GD, Nallamothu BK, Sales AE, Froehlich JB. Reimagining anticoagulation clinics in the era of direct oral anticoagulants. Circ Cardiovasc Qual Outcomes. 2016;9:182–5.
66. Chowdhry U, Jacques A, Karovitch A, Giguere P, Nguyen ML. Appropriateness of dabigatran and rivaroxaban prescribing for hospital inpatients. Can J Hosp Pharm. 2016;69:194–201.
67. Chan KE, Edelman ER, Wenger JB, Thadhani RI, Maddux FW. Dabigatran and rivaroxaban use in atrial fibrillation patients on hemodialysis. Circulation. 2015;131:972–9.

Perioperative Management of Anticoagulants

9

Ibrahim M. Ali, Alexander Volodarskiy, and Joe F. Lau

Clinical Vignettes

Case 1: *A 62-year-old woman with a history of coronary artery disease who underwent percutaneous coronary intervention with a drug-eluting stent to her proximal left anterior descending (LAD) artery 2 weeks prior presents to the emergency room with right upper quadrant abdominal pain. Her history is also significant for chronic atrial fibrillation. Her medications include warfarin 5 mg daily, aspirin 81 mg daily, clopidogrel 75 mg daily, and metoprolol 25 mg twice a day. Her surgical history is significant for cesarean section at the age of 25. She has never smoked and does not drink alcohol.*

On physical exam, she is noted to be tachycardic at a rate of 115 beats/min. She is in mild distress due to pain. Palpation of her right upper quadrant of her abdomen elicits tenderness and guarding, with a positive Murphy's sign.

Labs are significant for an INR of 2.3, alkaline phosphatase of 220 U/L, and total bilirubin of 2.2 mg/dL. A right upper quadrant ultrasound shows choledocholithiasis.

The patient is evaluated by the gastroenterology and general surgery consultation services with a recommendation to perform endoscopic retrograde cholangiopancreatography (ERCP) followed by an elective outpatient laparoscopic cholecystectomy.

How would you manage her perioperative antiplatelet and anticoagulation medications in the periprocedural period?

I. M. Ali
Department of Cardiology, Northwell Health, Zucker School of Medicine at Hofstra/Northwell, Manhasset, NY, USA
e-mail: iali@northwell.edu

A. Volodarskiy
Department of Cardiology, New York-Presbyterian/Queens, Flushing, NY, USA
e-mail: alv9062@nyp.org

J. F. Lau (✉)
Department of Cardiology, Zucker School of Medicine at Hofstra/Northwell, Northwell Health, Manhasset, NY, USA
e-mail: JLau@northwell.edu

J. F. Lau et al. (eds.), *Anticoagulation Therapy*, https://doi.org/10.1007/978-3-319-73709-6_9

Case 2: *A 58-year-old man with a history of hypertension, hyperlipidemia, and recent unprovoked bilateral pulmonary embolism and right lower extremity deep vein thrombosis diagnosed just 2 months ago presents to the hospital with sudden onset epigastric abdominal pain. He was found to have acute appendicitis on CT scan. The surgeon recommends a laparoscopic appendectomy and is requesting your recommendation on perioperative management of his anticoagulation. His current medications include apixaban 5 mg twice daily, metoprolol 25 mg twice daily, lisinopril 10 mg daily, and atorvastatin 40 mg daily.*

How would you manage his perioperative and postoperative anticoagulation, particularly in the setting of a recent unprovoked venous thromboembolic event?

Introduction

More than two million people in North America are treated with oral anticoagulation [1, 2]. Of these, approximately 250,000 patients on anticoagulation undergo surgical or invasive procedures annually [3]. Moreover, approximately 1 in 10 people on a vitamin K antagonist will have to undergo a surgical procedure [3, 4]. Quite often, patients on anticoagulant therapy are also taking antiplatelet agents, thus potentially complicating perioperative management strategies. When caring for patients on anticoagulant and antiplatelet therapies undergoing surgical and invasive procedures, it is important to formulate a plan that will place the patient at the lowest possible risk of bleeding, while at the same time maintaining a low risk of thromboembolic events. Depending on the clinical scenario at hand, anticoagulant and antiplatelet regimens may be continued, stopped, or replaced with short-term parenteral ("bridge") therapy. Temporary interruption, or the cessation of one or more dose of an oral anticoagulant in advance of surgery, may be necessary in order to decrease bleeding risk associated with the procedure. Determining the safest course of action can therefore be a daunting task for any clinician.

The initial step in perioperative management is to consider the timing and need for surgery. Is the surgical procedure urgent, or can it be delayed until the patient is no longer on anticoagulation? If possible, avoiding or delaying the surgery until anticoagulation is no longer needed is always preferable.

If the surgical procedure is deemed necessary, the clinician will need to evaluate both the periprocedural thromboembolic and bleeding risks (Fig. 9.1).

Step 1: Assess Periprocedural Thromboembolic Risk

The periprocedural thromboembolic risk for patients with venous thromboembolism and atrial fibrillation will be evaluated.

Thrombotic Risk Stratification for Patients with Venous Thromboembolism

When untreated, venous thromboembolism (VTE), which encompasses both deep vein thrombosis (DVT) and pulmonary embolism (PE), can lead to substantial morbidity and mortality. In the United States, more than 100,000 deaths per year are attributed to PE. For patients with a history of both provoked and unprovoked VTE, the risk of recurrent thromboembolism is substantially higher during the perioperative period. Perioperative management of anticoagulant therapy must therefore be determined carefully. Further, management strategies can vary depending on whether the patient is taking warfarin or one of the direct oral anticoagulants (DOACs) [5].

The thrombotic risk of all patients with VTE must be weighed. Every patient should be stratified as high, moderate, or low thrombotic risk using the criterion outlined in Table 9.1.

High Thrombotic Risk

Patients at a high thrombotic risk include patients with episodes of VTE within the last 3 months or with profound thrombophilic conditions such as protein C and S deficiency, antithrombin (III) deficiency, and/or antiphos-

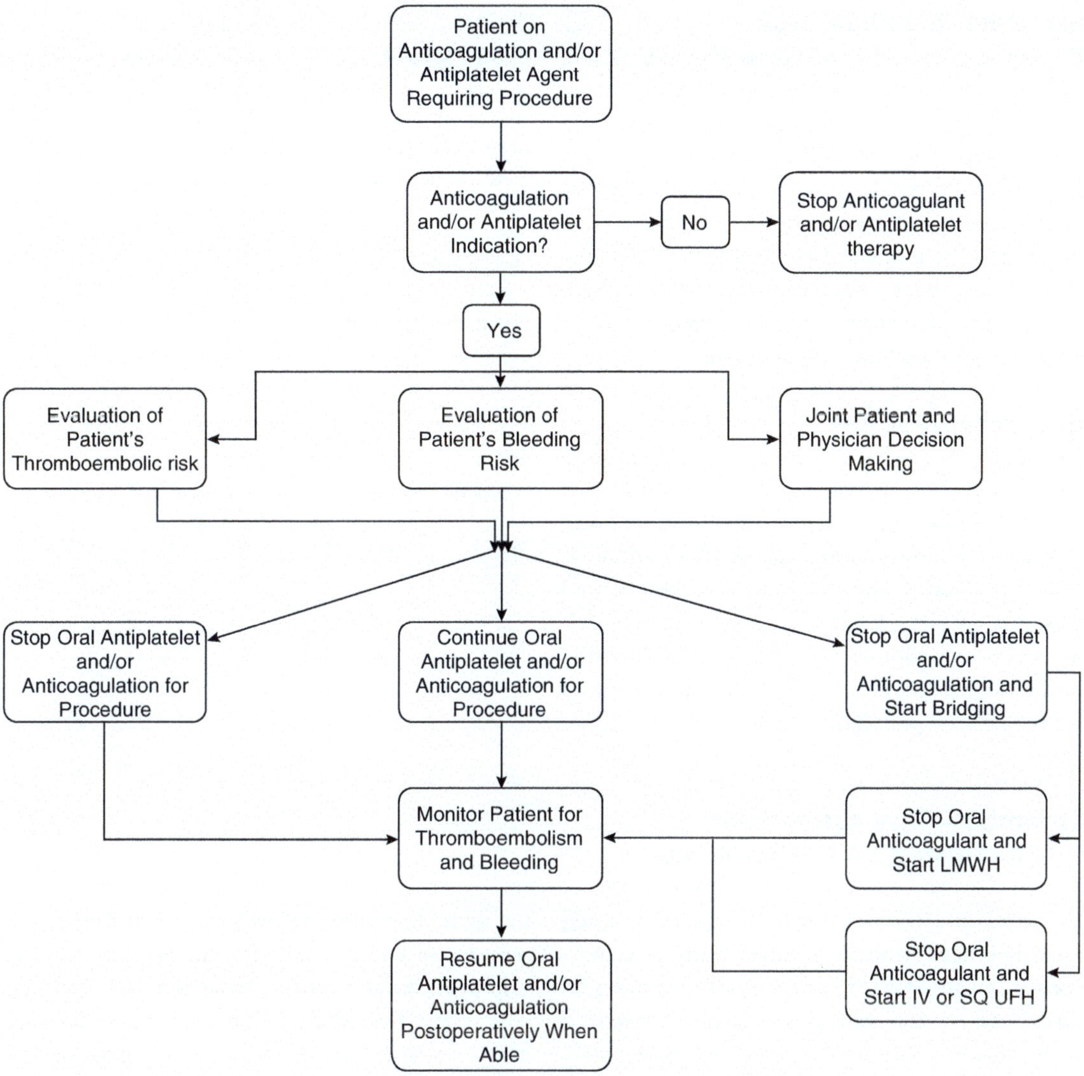

Fig. 9.1 Decision-making process in the periprocedural management of anticoagulation and antiplatelet therapies

Table 9.1 Thrombotic risk stratification for patients with VTE [6]

High risk	• VTE within the past 3 months • Severe thrombophilia
Moderate risk	• VTE within the past 3–12 months • Non-severe thrombophilia • Recurrent VTEs • Active cancer
Low risk	• VTE more than 12 months ago with no other risk factors

pholipid antibody syndrome [6] (Table 9.1). If anticoagulation therapy is discontinued or interrupted in these patients, the chance of propagation of existing DVT or the formation of a new VTE is high. Although much of the data is extrapolated from non-procedural situations, one can perceive that the approach would be similar. Kearon and colleagues found that the risk of reoccurrence of VTE within 3 months of a proximal DVT was estimated at 50% in the absence of anticoagulation therapy. Short-term periprocedural VTE risk when withholding anticoagulation in these patients has not been extensively studied.

Moderate Thrombotic Risk

Patients that are considered to be at moderate risk for VTE include those who have had VTE within the past 3–12 months, had multiple reoccurring VTE events, have active malignancy, or have thrombophilic traits such as heterozygosity or homozygosity for the factor V Leiden and prothrombin gene mutations [6] (Table 9.1). Patients in this group have a 15% per year incidence rate of VTE [7], which has to be weighed carefully against periprocedural bleeding risk.

Low Thrombotic Risk

Patients are considered to be at a low thrombotic risk if they had an episode of VTE more than 12 months prior to the surgery and have no other risk factors for thrombotic disease [6] (Table 9.1). These patients completed anticoagulation, and their risk of VTE is considered to be low enough not to warrant anticoagulation [7]. Therefore, the precautions to prevent VTE are the same as those for the general population [3, 6].

Table 9.2 CHA_2D_2-VASc score [8]

CHA_2DS_2-VASc	Points
Congestive heart failure	1
Hypertension	1
Age ≥75	2
Diabetes mellitus	1
Stroke/TIA	2
Vascular disease	1
Age 65–74	1
Sex	1
Total possible score	9

Table 9.3 CHA_2D_2-VASc stroke risk [8]

CHA_2DS_2-VASc score	Yearly stroke risk without anticoagulation
0	0%
1	1.3%
2	2.2%
3	3.2%
4	4.0%
5	6.7%
6	9.8%
7	9.6%
8	6.7%
9	15.20%

Thrombotic Risk Assessment for Patients with Atrial Fibrillation

In atrial fibrillation, there is uncoordinated electrical activation of the atria leading to ineffective contraction [8]. Lack of coordinated atrial contraction causes stasis and increased rates of atrial thrombus formation particularly in the left atrial appendage. Left atrial appendage thrombi may result in arterial thromboembolism (ATE) and stroke. It is estimated that non-valvular atrial fibrillation (NVAF) causes a fivefold increase in the risk of stroke. In the setting of mitral stenosis, the stroke risk may be as high as 20-fold [9]. Strokes due to atrial fibrillation have also been associated with higher mortality [10]. Anticoagulation has been shown to reduce the risk of stroke and other ATE in atrial fibrillation patients [8].

Risk stratification has been more intensely studied in patients with atrial fibrillation than those with VTE. Commonly used risk assessment tools such as the CHA_2DS_2-VASc score (Table 9.2) have been validated to help predict the annualized risk of stroke in atrial fibrillation patients in the absence of anticoagulation in the non-procedural setting (Table 9.3) [8, 11, 12]. The CHA_2DS_2-VASc score covers a broader array of risk factors when compared to the $CHADS_2$ score and is better in discriminating patients that benefit from anticoagulation for stroke prevention, particularly those with a lower risk score (e.g., 0–1) [13].

The 2014 AHA/ACC/HRS guidelines recommend the use of CHA_2DS_2-VASc score when risk stratifying atrial fibrillation patients [8]. Patients with a CHA_2DS_2-VASc score of 2 or greater benefit from long-term anticoagulation. On the other hand, the European Society of Cardiology (ESC) guidelines recommend that men with a risk score of 1 or greater and women with a risk score of 2 or greater receive full-dose anticoagulation [14]. The difference in recommendation stems from a controversy over the relative importance of the several risk factors considered in calculating the

Table 9.4 Thrombotic risk stratification in patients with atrial fibrillation [6]

High risk	• Elevated CHA_2DS_2-VASc ≥7+ (annualized stroke risk >10%) • Prior thromboembolic event within the past 3 months • Rheumatic valvular heart disease
Moderate risk	• CHA_2DS_2-VASc 5–6 (annualized stroke risk 5–10%) • Prior thromboembolic event >3 months
Low risk	• CHA_2DS_2-VASc 1–4 (annualized risk <5%) • No prior thromboembolic event

CHA_2DS_2-VASc score and determining the best treatment strategy (aspirin versus anticoagulation) for patients with a CHA_2DS_2-VASc score of 1, especially if the only risk factor is female gender [8, 15–17]. In fact, a recent retrospective analysis of Swedish national registries involving 140,420 patients with atrial fibrillation noted that the annual incidence of ischemic stroke in patients with a CHA_2DS_2-VASc score of 1 was lower than previously thought (i.e., 0.1–0.2% in women and 0.5–0.7% in men) [18]. Lower CHA_2DS_2-VASc scores have worse predictive accuracy of embolic events, and the true risk of bleeding in the patients is contentious. Of particular concern is the risk of intracranial hemorrhage, which may be greater in those taking vitamin K antagonists compared to DOACs. Accordingly, DOACs may be a reasonable alternative to aspirin for patients with a CHA_2DS_2-VASc score of 1. Patients with a score of 0 should not receive antiplatelet or anticoagulant therapy.

Although the CHA_2DS_2-VASc may be useful for thromboembolic risk stratification when considering the appropriateness of long-term anticoagulation, the scoring system has not been well studied as a perioperative risk stratification tool (Table 9.4).

High Thrombotic Risk

Patients who have atrial fibrillation along with an elevated CHA_2DS_2-VASc score ≥7 (or $CHADS_2$ score of 5 or greater), a history of a recent stroke or TIA within the prior 3 months, or a history of rheumatic valvular heart disease are at high thrombotic risk [6]. The risk of stroke or systemic embolism within this cohort is >10% per year. However, there is substantial debate concerning which risk factors fulfill criteria for high thrombotic risk as even the BRIDGE (Bridging Anticoagulation in Patients who Require Temporary Interruption of Warfarin Therapy for an Elective Invasive Procedure or Surgery) investigators used CVA as the only criteria for high thrombotic risk [19]. As a prothrombotic state, surgery may increase the risk of thromboembolism further. Therefore, the time off anticoagulation should be minimized. *The utilization of short-term parenteral or "bridge" therapy after cessation of oral anticoagulants is recommended in these patients.*

Moderate Thrombotic Risk

Patients with an intermediate CHA_2DS_2-VASc score of 5 or 6 (or $CHADS_2$ of 3 or 4) are considered to be at moderate risk for thromboembolism, with an annualized risk of 5–10% per year [8]. For these patients, the clinician must counterbalance the individual's thromboembolic risk with bleeding risk. A meta-analysis performed by Siegal and colleagues showed that periprocedural bridging therapy can increase the risk of major bleeding (defined as fatal bleeding, bleeding at a critical site, need for transfusion, a decrease in hemoglobin by greater than 2 g/L, need for hospitalization due to bleeding, or requirement of surgical hemostasis), from 0.9% to 3.4% [20].

However, recent data published by Douketis and the BRIDGE investigators demonstrated that in patients with atrial fibrillation or atrial flutter who require periprocedural interruption of anticoagulation, a strategy of discontinuing treatment without the use of a bridge was not inferior to the use of bridging anticoagulation [19]. BRIDGE was a randomized, double-blind, placebo-controlled study of 1884 patients on warfarin for chronic atrial fibrillation or atrial flutter who were scheduled for an elective procedure requiring interruption of anticoagulation therapy. Most enrolled subjects underwent elective cardiothoracic, gastrointestinal, or orthopedic procedures. All patients discontinued anticoagulation 5 days before the procedure and resumed therapy a day after surgery. Patients were randomized to receive either subcutaneous dalteparin or placebo from 3 days to 24 h before the procedure and for 5–10 days afterward. Either dalteparin or placebo was resumed 12–24 h after a minor procedure and 48–72 h after a major procedure. The primary efficacy outcome was arterial thromboembolism—either stroke, transient ischemic attack, or systemic embolism—within 30 days after surgery. The study also evaluated safety outcome measures including major bleeding.

The BRIDGE investigators noted no difference in the incidence of arterial thromboembolism between the bridging and the placebo groups (0.3% *versus* 0.4%; $p = 0.73$). Of note, major bleeding was significantly greater in the cohort that received bridging therapy with LMWH (low-molecular-weight heparin) (3.2% versus 1.3%; $p = 0.005$), as was minor bleeding (20.9% *versus* 12.0%; $p < 0.001$). There was no significant difference between the two groups with regard to myocardial infarction, thromboembolic events, or death [19]. Thus, findings from BRIDGE suggest that in patients with atrial fibrillation or flutter, who require perioperative interruption of warfarin for an elective procedure, the use of bridging anticoagulation may increase risk of bleeding without reducing the risk of thromboembolism.

What are the recommendations for the cohort deemed to possess moderate risk for thromboembolism? The overall recommendation for the moderate-risk cohort is to avoid bridging for those with increased risk of bleeding. If the patient has no significant risk of bleeding, one can consider utilizing bridging, particularly in those who have had previous stroke, TIA, or other thromboembolic events.

Low Thrombotic Risk

Patients on warfarin for atrial fibrillation and at a low risk for ATE are those who have a calculated CHA_2DS_2-VASc scores ≤4. The annualized risk of stroke in these patients with atrial fibrillation, when not on anticoagulant therapy, is less than 5% [8]. The BRIDGE trial included a high percentage of low-risk patients with atrial fibrillation and demonstrated non-inferiority between those who received short-term parenteral bridging therapy and those who did not. As expected, there was also decreased bleeding in the group that did not receive bridging therapy [19].

Therefore, patients considered to possess low thrombotic risk can stop anticoagulant therapy several days prior to the procedure. The timing to hold therapy depends upon which anticoagulant the patient is taking. *Bridging therapy is not necessary in this cohort.* Anticoagulant therapy should be resumed as soon as feasible following the surgical procedure. Although considerably lower, the risk of thromboembolism or stroke while not on anticoagulant therapy should still be addressed with the patient during the planning stages prior to surgery.

Thrombotic Risk Assessment in Patients with Mechanical Heart Valves

Mechanical prosthetic heart valves are durable replacement choices for dysfunctional native heart valves but come at a cost of higher arterial thromboembolic risk. Increased thrombogenicity is in part due to turbulent nature of prosthetic valve flow and the resultant shear stress that lead to increased platelet activation [21]. Patients with mechanical heart valves who are not on anticoagulant therapy can have up to a 1.8% annual incidence of valve thrombosis, although the rate has been as high as 5.2% in smaller studies. Furthermore, the incidence of major embolic events (stroke, peripheral ischemia, and death) is as high as 4% per year [22, 23]. Anticoagulation for patients with mechanical valves is associated with a 75% risk reduction for embolic events [7].

Additional factors to consider in managing patients with mechanical heart valves perioperatively are the location and type of the valve. Mechanical mitral valves have a 1.5-fold increase in the risk for major embolism compared to mechanic aortic prosthesis [22]. Ball-and-cage valves have almost twice the risk for embolism when compared to bileaflet valves [24]. Table 9.5 shows the thrombogenicity of the different types of valves.

Moderate and High Thrombotic Risk

High-risk patients include those with mechanical mitral valve replacements, ball-and-cage valves, tilting disc aortic valves, and prior thromboembolic events such as TIA or stroke within the past

6 months [6]. Moderate-risk patients include patients with bileaflet aortic valves or those with atrial fibrillation, prior stroke or TIA (more than 6 months old), hypertension, diabetes, or congestive heart failure [6]. All patients possessing moderate to high thromboembolic risk should receive short-term parenteral anticoagulant. The utility of this approach is currently under trial in the PERIOP 2 study [21].

Low Thrombotic Risk

Patients with bileaflet aortic valves with no other thrombotic risk factors arc considered to possess low risk for thromboembolic events in the perioperative period. These patients have less than a 4% chance of developing thrombotic disease annually [6, 25]. The risk of bleeding from bridging therapy in these patients outweighs the risk of thromboembolism, and these patients should not be routinely bridged perioperatively.

Table 9.5 Thrombotic risk stratification for patients with mechanical valves [6]

High risk	• Prosthetic mitral valve • Cage and ball valve • Aortic tilting disc valve • Thrombotic event in last 6 months
Moderate risk	• Bileaflet aortic valve and one or more thrombotic risk factors: - Atrial fibrillation - Stroke - TIA - Hypertension - Diabetes mellitus - Heart failure - Age >75
Low risk	• Bileaflet aortic valve and no thrombotic risk factors

Step 2: Assess Periprocedural Bleeding Risk

Assessment of periprocedural bleeding risk must focus on (1) the bleed risk of the procedure itself and (2) patient-related bleed risk.

Assessing Procedural Bleed Risk

The incidence and risk of bleeding will depend upon the type of surgery. In fact, while intraoperative bleeding risk is obviously a concern, up to two-thirds of bleeding events occur in the immediate postoperative period.

It is important to note that various professional societies have published their own consensus documents delineating recommendations for periprocedural management of anticoagulation therapy that are specific to their procedures [6, 26–35]. In general, most procedures are classified to possess either low or high bleeding risk, with infrequent classification of intermediate risk for certain procedures in several guidelines. In contrast, the recently published 2017 ACC expert consensus document on periprocedural anticoagulation management in patients with NVAF classified commonly performed procedures into four procedural bleeding risk categories: (1) no clinically important bleed risk, (2) low risk, (3) uncertain risk, or (4) intermediate/high risk [36]. Table 9.6 categorizes common surgical procedures by bleeding risk.

Table 9.6 Procedural bleeding risks

High bleeding risk	Intermediate bleeding risk	Low bleeding risk	Uncertain bleeding risk
Prostate biopsy	Visceral surgery	Endoscopy	Pericardiocentesis
Bladder biopsy	Orthopedic surgery	Dental extraction	Exploratory thoracotomy
Intracranial neurosurgery	Abdominal hysterectomy	Peripheral surgery/biopsy	Esophageal biopsy
Spinal canal surgery	PEG placement	Cataract surgery	Endovascular stent graft of the descending aorta
Kidney biopsy	Some AF/VT ablations	Most AF/VT ablations	
Liver biopsy	Lobectomy	SVT ablation	
Vascular surgery	Bronchoscopy with biopsy	Bronchoscopy with BAL	
Valve replacement	VATS	Dilatation and curettage	
		Cholecystectomy	
		Skin biopsy/surgery	

Key: AF atrial fibrillation, *VT* ventricular tachycardia, *VATS* video-assisted thoracoscopic surgery, *SVT* supraventricular tachycardia, *BAL* bronchoalveolar lavage

Further, there is some disagreement in recommendations for perioperative anticoagulation management for specific commonly performed procedures such as hysterectomy and hip/knee replacement between the various professional societies and the ACC expert consensus [36]. When evaluating patients, clinicians should be mindful that surgical procedures involving highly vascularized organs (e.g., kidney, liver, and most vascular and cardiothoracic procedures) or closed spaces (e.g., neurosurgical procedures involving the brain or spine) are considered high risk, and excessive bleeding risk often necessitates interruption of both anticoagulant and antiplatelet therapies. Indeed, the potential to bleed even a small amount under certain circumstances, such as instances involving neuraxial anesthesia, or after intraocular, intracranial, or spinal surgeries, may lead to substantial morbidity and mortality.

In general, when therapeutic indications remain present, anticoagulant and antiplatelet therapies should be continued peri- and postoperatively for low bleeding risk procedures. Oral anticoagulant therapies are often interrupted prior to most moderate and high bleeding risk procedures, after initiating short-term parenteral therapy in patients with elevated thromboembolic risk. Depending on proceduralists' preferences and the specific type of procedure, and after careful review of risks and benefits with patients, moderate bleeding risk surgeries can be performed without interruption of antiplatelet therapy. Antiplatelet therapies are typically held prior to surgeries with high bleeding risk.

Assessing Patient-Related Bleed Risk

The clinician should then obtain a comprehensive medical and bleeding history, as this is also an essential component in the assessment of peri-procedural bleeding risk (Table 9.7). A thorough history should include a comprehensive review of risk factors and comorbid conditions (i.e., advanced age greater than 55 years old, renal and hepatic dysfunction, cancer), family history of bleeding, prior minor and major bleeding events while on anticoagulation, and prior postsurgical bleeding events. If the patient's medical and bleeding history is unrevealing, routine coagulation tests (i.e., prothrombin time, partial thromboplastin time, and international normalized ratio [INR]) should not be performed for patients that are not on anticoagulation [37]. On the other hand, for patients that are on anticoagulation such as warfarin, coagulation testing may provide further insight into a patient's bleeding risk and help estimate when warfarin will need to be discontinued in the event of supratherapeutic INR values.

Table 9.7 Patient-related medical risk factors [4, 36, 53, 66]

Medical risk factors
Age >55 years
Prior CVA or vascular disease
Creatinine clearance <90 mL/min
Hepatic dysfunction
Congestive heart failure
Anemia (Hct < 30%) [66]
Cancer
Systolic blood pressure <100 mm of Hg
Systolic blood pressure >200 mm of Hg
Female gender
Diabetes mellitus
Prior history of bleeding

For patients with atrial fibrillation who are on anticoagulation, several risk scores have been devised in attempts to identify bleeding risk [38–40]. The most widely used risk score is the HAS-BLED (*H*ypertension, *A*bnormal Renal/Liver Function, *S*troke, *B*leeding History or Predisposition, *L*abile INR, *E*lderly, *D*rugs/Alcohol Concomitantly) scoring system that helps predict 1-year risk of major bleeding [40]. Data for the HAS-BLED scoring system was derived from analysis of 3978 patients who were evaluated in the Euro Heart Survey. Major bleeding is defined as a significant hemoglobin decrease of greater than 2 g/dL, the need for blood transfusion, intracranial bleeding, and hospitalization. Table 9.8 summarizes this clinical prediction tool. A calculated HAS-BLED score can range from 0 to 9 and is based on eight different parameters, with varying weighted scores of 0 to 2 for each.

Of note, although HAS-BLED can provide information regarding a patient's bleeding risk based on comorbid conditions (Table 9.8), the scoring system is limited by its modest

Table 9.8 HAS-BLED score [40]

HAS-BLED	Points
Hypertension	1
Abnormal renal function/abnormal liver function	1–2
Hemorrhagic stroke	1
Bleeding history	1
Labile INRs	1
Elderly (≥65)	1
Drugs (NSAIDS and antiplatelet)/alcohol use	1–2
Total possible score	9

Table 9.9 HAS-BLED bleeding risk [40]

HAS-BLED score	Yearly major bleed risk (%)
0	1.13
1	1.02
2	1.88
3	3.74
4	8.7
5	12.5

predictive value in the periprocedural setting and has not been endorsed by current guidelines for this purpose in patients with AF [40, 41] (Table 9.9).

Perioperative Management of Patients on Warfarin

Evidence supporting the use of warfarin in the treatment and prevention of VTE and ATE is well-established. In 1948, Karl Paul Link developed warfarin, a more potent derivative of dicoumarol, with the intent to use it as a rodenticide [42]. In 1954, warfarin was approved for use in humans as an anticoagulant for the treatment of myocardial infarction and stroke [42–44]. Warfarin acts by preventing synthesis of the active forms of the vitamin K-dependent factors, which include II, VII, IX, and X, as well as anticoagulant proteins C and S. Its therapeutic level is measured using the prothrombin time (PT) and international normalized ratio (INR). In most clinical scenarios involving venous and arterial thromboembolism, the therapeutic INR target range is between 2 and 3. The half-life of warfarin is 36–42 h, and it takes about 5 days to lose its anticoagulant effect when discontinued at a therapeutic INR [6, 45].

If the patient undergoing surgical procedure is deemed to have high thromboembolic risk, the next step is to determine the bleeding risk of the procedure. For low bleeding risk surgeries such as minor dental procedures, skin biopsies, and cataract removal, the risk of thromboembolism outweighs the potential risk of bleeding. In these cases, interruption of warfarin therapy is not recommended [45]. Studies of patients on warfarin undergoing low bleeding risk procedures have demonstrated a threefold increased risk of bleeding, although the bleeding events were predominantly minor and self-limited events [46, 47].

Managing patients undergoing moderate or high bleeding risk surgical procedures is more complex. Continuing warfarin therapy during these procedures increases the risk of major bleeding events, while interrupting anticoagulation during the perioperative period increases the risk of thromboembolism. In these instances, initiating short-term parenteral or bridge therapy with unfractionated heparin (UFH) or low-molecular-weight heparin (LMWH) should be considered [20, 25].

High Bleeding Risk

In patients undergoing high bleeding risk procedures, bridging therapy should not be attempted [6]. The bleeding risk of bridging therapy outweighs the risk of developing a thromboembolic event. Warfarin therapy should be discontinued 5 days prior to the procedure to allow the INR to come down to an acceptable level for the procedure. Warfarin should then be restarted at the patient's home dose as soon as possible postoperatively [4].

Short-Term Parenteral or "Bridge" Therapy

When short-term parenteral therapy is initiated to reduce both periprocedural bleeding and thromboembolic risks, the first step is to obtain a baseline INR measurement as early as 10–14 days prior to the elective procedure (obtaining an INR level closer to the date of surgery may lead to delays in perioperative planning). If the INR is subtherapeutic (1.5–1.9), the patient should stop taking warfarin 3–4 days prior to the procedure. If the INR is within the therapeutic range (between 2 and 3), the patient should stop taking warfarin 5 days prior to the procedure. If the INR is elevated, between 3 and 4.5, then warfarin should be stopped 6 days prior to the procedure [15, 25]. INR that is above 4.5 may require postponement of the surgical procedure to allow for INR normalization. Generally, the INR should be rechecked within 24 h before the procedure, especially if a normal INR is preferred. Most proceduralists prefer an INR that is less than 1.5 at the time of surgery. Approximately 36 h after the last dose of warfarin is given (approximately when the INR will fall below the target range); a therapeutic dose of either UFH or LMWH should be started [25, 45]. In the inpatient setting, therapeutic dosing of UFH or LMWH can be started once the INR is measured to be subtherapeutic (i.e., when INR is below 2.0). Barring contraindications such as renal failure and obesity, LMWH is generally preferred due to its low cost, ease of administration, and clinical efficacy, including for patients with mechanical valve replacement [46]. For patients being bridged with LMWH, the last dose should be given 24 h prior to surgery. For patients being bridged with UFH, the infusion should be stopped 6 h prior to the procedure.

The most appropriate time to restart warfarin during postoperative period should be performed after thoughtful discussion with the surgeon or proceduralist. In most cases, warfarin can be safely restarted the evening after an uncomplicated procedure with low bleeding risk. Warfarin should typically be restarted at the pre-procedural maintenance dose. Depending on the post-procedural level of hemostasis, resumption of LMWH or UFH can be considered 24–72 h after the procedure and continued until the INR is therapeutic [19, 25, 45].

Instituting periprocedural parenteral therapy comes at the cost of an increased risk of bleeding (Fig. 9.2). Siegel and colleagues reported in their meta-analysis that the overall incidence of bleeding in patients bridged with LMWH was 13.1%, while the incidence of overall bleeding in patients that were not bridged was 3.4% [20]. On the other hand, bridge therapy has been shown to reduce the risk of thromboembolism postoperatively from 1.5% to less than 0.5% [25]. Although the overall incidence may seem low, one should be mindful that a recurrent VTE can be fatal in 5–10% of cases [48] and ATE can lead to a fatality rate as high as 20% [49].

Fig. 9.2 Overall bleeding risk in bridged and not bridged patients [20]

Perioperative Management of Patients on Direct Oral Anticoagulants

DOACs, also known as novel anticoagulants (NOACs), oral direct inhibitors, target-specific oral anticoagulants (TSOACs), or non-vitamin K oral anticoagulants, are increasingly becoming the agents of choice for anticoagulation. These agents include direct thrombin inhibitors such as dabigatran and factor Xa inhibitors such as rivaroxaban, apixaban, and edoxaban [50–52]. Anticoagulation therapy using DOACs is indicated for patients with VTE and non-valvular atrial fibrillation [53, 54]. DOACS have a rapid onset of action, and most are rapidly cleared primarily by the kidneys [51]. The pharmacokinetics of these drugs is very predictable, which eliminates the need for routine testing to evaluate therapeutic levels [51]. Perioperative management of DOAC therapy relies on the patient's renal function and the pharmacokinetics of the specific oral anticoagulant. Renal function should be assessed with creatinine clearance calculated via Cockcroft-Gault equation. In addition, compared to warfarin, these agents have a more predictable anticoagulation response. *Due to the rapid onset and clearance, no preoperative bridging therapy with parenteral agents is recommended.* The only roles for UFH in DOAC-treated patients are (1) for cases where rapid reversibility of anticoagulation may be necessary and (2) in postoperative situations when the patient is unable to tolerate oral intake which would require the use of parenteral anticoagulation. In this scenario, postoperative patients who possess high post-procedural bleed risk should be started on parenteral agents 48–72 h following surgery, and those with low post-procedural bleed risk should be started on parenteral agents 24 h afterward. When the patient is able to tolerate oral intake, the switch from parenteral agent to DOAC can be made. The management of DOACs in the perioperative period is still based mostly on expert opinion.

Dabigatran

Of the DOACs, dabigatran is the only Food Drug Administration (FDA)-approved oral direct thrombin inhibitor. It is a prodrug, and its plasma concentration reaches a therapeutic level 1.52 h after ingestion [50]. The half-life of dabigatran is 12–17 h, and it is primarily excreted through the kidneys (80%) [4, 52, 53].

As stated, deciding the best time to stop therapy depends upon the patient's renal function, as determined by Cockcroft-Gault creatinine clearance (CrCl). For patients undergoing low bleeding risk surgery with a CrCl greater than 30 mL/min, dabigatran should be stopped 24–48 h prior to the procedure. For patients with CrCl less than 30 mL/min undergoing a low bleeding risk procedure, ≥72 h should be allowed to let the drug clear. In patients undergoing low bleeding risk procedures, dabigatran can be restarted 24 h after the surgery (Table 9.10) [4, 15].

Table 9.10 Summary of perioperative recommendation for DOACs [15, 53]

	Low bleeding risk procedure	Uncertain/ intermediate/high bleeding risk procedure
Dabigatran	CrCl > 30: Hold for ≥24–48 h	CrCl > 30: Hold for ≥48–96 h
	CrCl < 30: Hold ≥72 h	CrCl < 30: Hold for ≥120 h
Rivaroxaban	CrCl > 30: Hold for ≥24 h	CrCl > 30: Hold for ≥48 h
	CrCl < 30: Hold for ≥36–48 h	CrCl < 30: No data. Consider measuring anti-Xa level and/or holding for ≥72 h
Apixaban	CrCl > 30: Hold for ≥24 h	CrCl > 30: Hold for ≥48 h
	CrCl < 30: Hold for ≥36–48 h	CrCl < 30: No data. Consider measuring anti-Xa level and/or holding for ≥72 h
Edoxaban	CrCl > 30: Hold for ≥24 h	CrCl > 30: Hold for ≥48 h
	CrCl < 30: Hold for ≥36–48 h	CrCl < 30: Consider measuring anti-Xa level and/or holding for ≥72 h

For uncertain, intermediate, or high bleeding risk procedures, additional time should be allowed for the drug to clear, thereby reducing the risk of major bleed events during the perioperative period. For patients with a CrCl greater than 30 mL/min undergoing high bleeding risk surgery, dabigatran should be held 48–96 h prior to the procedure. For CrCl less than 30 mL/min, the oral anticoagulant should be held for ≥120 h prior to the procedure. To determine when to reinitiate anticoagulation postoperatively, it is most important to assess hemostasis at the procedural site. Usually, dabigatran can be restarted the night of the procedure in most low bleeding risk surgeries. For higher bleeding risk surgeries, it is recommended to wait 48–72 h [4, 15].

Rivaroxaban

Rivaroxaban is a direct oral factor Xa inhibitor that is rapidly absorbed and has high oral bioavailability (10 mg, 80–100%; 20 mg, 66%). Although primarily cleared via the kidneys (66%), the drug is also partially cleared via the gastrointestinal tract (33%) [50]. Its half-life is approximately 5–9 h [4, 52].

For patients undergoing low bleeding risk surgery with a CrCl greater than 30 mL/min, rivaroxaban should be stopped at least 36–48 h prior to the procedure. For patients with a CrCl of 25–30 mL/min undergoing the same procedure, rivaroxaban should be discontinued at least 36 h before the procedure. In patients undergoing low bleeding risk procedures, rivaroxaban can be restarted 24 h after the surgery [4, 53].

For uncertain, intermediate, or high bleeding risk procedures, additional time should be allowed for the drug to clear. For patients with a CrCl of greater than 30 mL/min undergoing high bleeding risk surgery, rivaroxaban should be held at least 48 h prior to the procedure. For CrCl 15–30 mL/min, the drug should be held at least 72 h prior to the procedure. However, there is limited data in patients with a CrCl less than 30 on any factor Xa inhibitor. Therefore, in these patients, checking an agent-specific anti-Xa level may be beneficial prior to surgery. Reinitiation of anticoagulant therapy can be considered 24–48 h postoperatively [4, 53], with this approach associated with a 1.2% rate of major bleeding within 30 days following the procedure [15]. It should be noted that there is very limited data with the best strategies on anticoagulation management in high-risk procedures such as neurosurgery.

Apixaban

Like rivaroxaban, apixaban is a direct factor Xa inhibitor. It also has a high oral bioavailability (~50%), and absorption is not affected by food. Unlike the other DOACs, apixaban is mostly excreted by the gastrointestinal tract, as renal clearance only accounts for only about 25% of its excretion. Nevertheless, perioperative management of apixaban still depends upon the patient's renal function. The half-life of apixaban is highly variable but is estimated to be 8–15 h [52].

For patients undergoing low bleeding risk surgery with a CrCl greater than 30 mL/min, apixaban can be stopped 24 h prior to the surgery. For patients with CrCl less than 30 mL/min undergoing the same procedure, 36–48 h should be allowed to let the drug clear. In patients undergoing low bleeding risk procedures, reinitiation of apixaban can be considered 24 h after the surgery [4, 53].

For patients with a CrCl of greater than 30 mL/min undergoing uncertain, intermediate, or high bleeding risk surgery, apixaban should be held for ≥48 h prior to the procedure. For CrCl less than 30 mL/min, it should be held at least 72 h prior to the procedure. Although the data is sparse in patients with a low CrCl, checking an agent-specific anti-Xa level may be beneficial. Reinitiation of anticoagulation in these patients can be considered 48–72 h following surgery [4].

Edoxaban

Edoxaban is a reversible direct factor Xa inhibitor. It also has a good oral bioavailability (~60%), and renal clearance accounts for about 50% of its excretion. The half-life of edoxaban is highly variable but is estimated to be 8–10 h.

For patients undergoing low bleeding risk surgery with a CrCl greater than 30 mL/min, edoxaban can be stopped ≥24 h prior to the surgery. For patients with CrCl less than 30 mL/min undergoing the same procedure, ≥36 h should be allowed to let the drug clear.

For patients with a CrCl of greater than 30 mL/min undergoing uncertain, intermediate, or high bleeding risk surgery, edoxaban should be held for ≥48 h prior to the procedure. For CrCl less than 30 mL/min, the data is sparse, but consider withholding edoxaban for at least 72 h or checking an agent-specific anti-Xa level, prior to procedure.

Periprocedural Assessment of Patients on Antiplatelet Agents

Perioperative management in patients with a history of coronary artery disease (CAD), especially those with previous history of myocardial infarction (MI), can be complex. In fact, the perioperative mortality for patients with CAD undergoing non-cardiac surgery can range from 1% to 5%, and of those cases, 20–35% are attributable to cardiovascular complications [36]. The use of antiplatelet agents for both primary and secondary prevention has grown over the past two decades due to the increasing age of the population and the increasing number of percutaneous coronary interventions [55]. In this section, the perioperative management of antiplatelet agents including aspirin, clopidogrel, and ticagrelor will be reviewed.

Aspirin

Aspirin irreversibly inhibits cyclooxygenase 1 (COX-1) and cyclooxygenase 2 (COX-2) [36]. These enzymes are responsible for the synthesis of thromboxanes that promote platelet activation and vasoconstriction. Since aspirin is an irreversible inhibitor of cyclooxygenase, platelets are inactivated for the duration of their life span, which is 7–10 days. Since 10% of the circulating platelet mass is produced by the bone marrow each day, platelet function can recover at a rate of about 10% per day that aspirin is held [36]. Understanding this timing is important in determining the perioperative management strategy for aspirin.

Aspirin for Primary Prevention

One of the most common uses for aspirin is in the primary prevention of CAD and MI. The United States Preventive Services Task Force (USPSTF) has recommended that men ages 45–79 and women ages 55–79 be started on aspirin when there is not a high risk of gastrointestinal hemorrhage [56]. Patients on aspirin for primary prevention CAD and MI are at relatively lower risk of having an ischemic cardiac event compared to those on aspirin for secondary prevention. Therefore, in a patient on aspirin for primary prevention, aspirin can simply be stopped 7–10 days prior to the surgery [57]. This will minimize any bleeding risk associated with surgery. Aspirin can be reinitiated when the bleeding risk from the surgery is no longer present.

Aspirin for Secondary Prevention

Aspirin is also used as a monotherapy for secondary prevention of MI, stroke, and thromboembolism in patients with atrial fibrillation. This section will focus on perioperative management of aspirin in patients taking it for secondary prevention of stroke and MI. Discontinuation of aspirin in these patients is associated with an increased risk of stroke and MI within 7–14 days postoperatively [36]. Therefore, the discontinuation of aspirin must be weighed against the bleeding risk of the procedure. The practictioner must first determine if the procedure places the pateint at a low, moderate, or high bleeding risk.

Low Bleeding Risk Procedure

Low bleeding risk procedures, including endoscopy, dental extraction, peripheral plastic surgery, and biopsies, put the patient at little risk for bleeding. Although this bleeding risk is higher in patients taking aspirin than that of the general population, the increase is minimal [36]. Therefore, patients on aspirin for secondary prevention undergoing low bleeding risk procedures should be advised to continue aspirin.

Moderate Bleeding Risk Procedure

Moderate bleeding risk procedures include visceral surgery, major orthopedic surgery, and cardiovascular surgery. Studies have shown that patients that continue to take aspirin before a moderate bleeding risk procedure are more likely to have increased blood loss and require a blood transfusion [55]. In patients undergoing urological surgery, there was almost a threefold increase in blood transfusion need in those who continued aspirin perioperatively [58]. However, almost all studies have shown that there is no increase in mortality related to bleeding in patients who continue aspirin versus those who did not [36]. Furthermore, there is a decrease in the risk for major adverse cardiovascular events (MACE) in patients who continued aspirin [55]. Therefore, patients on aspirin for secondary prevention of MI or stroke should be advised to continue aspirin perioperatively as the benefit outweighs the risk. Patients should, however, be advised of the increased possibility for a blood transfusion.

High Bleeding Risk Procedure

High bleeding risk surgeries can cause significant amount of bleeding even in patients who are not on any antithrombotic therapy. Examples of these procedures include intracranial surgery, spinal canal surgery, prostate resections, and catheter-based neurological interventions. Patients continued on aspirin during these procedures had an increased rate of reoperation, internal hemorrhage, and increased mortality [59]. Therefore, patients undergoing high bleeding risk procedures should be advised to stop aspirin 7 days prior to the procedure and to resume use postoperatively when bleeding risk has been minimized.

Dual Antiplatelet Therapy

Dual antiplatelet therapy (DAPT) usually involves the use of aspirin with the addition of an adenosine diphosphate (ADP) receptor inhibitor. These medications block ADP from binding to its receptor on the platelet. ADP binding to its receptor is a key step in the activation of platelets, and interrupting it renders platelets ineffective [36, 59]. The most common ADP receptor inhibitors used in practice are clopidogrel and prasugrel, which irreversibly inhibit the ADP receptor, and ticagrelor, which reversibly inhibits platelets. Although ticagrelor and prasugrel have quicker antiplatelet onset than clopidogrel, they have similar elimination half-lives [59].

Patients on DAPT are usually at higher cardiovascular risk because they have known CAD, previous MIs, and, in many cases, coronary artery stents. They are also at a much higher risk of bleeding, due to nearly complete loss of platelet function. In fact, one study showed that patients on DAPT are up to eight times more likely to suffer a bleeding complication after intermediate bleeding risk procedures when compared to patients on aspirin monotherapy undergoing the same procedure [60]. Therefore, it is important to carefully manage patients on DAPT undergoing surgery.

High-Risk Patients on DAPT

The criteria defining a high-risk patient on DAPT are defined in Table 9.11. These patients are at extremely high risk of developing postoperative

Table 9.11 High-risk patients on DAPT [36, 55, 67]

High-risk patients on DAPT
• Percutaneous transluminal coronary angioplasty <2 weeks ago
• Myocardial infarction <6 weeks ago
• Bare metal stent <6 weeks ago
• Drug-eluting stent <6 months ago
• High-risk (i.e., after STEMI) drug-eluting stent <12 months ago

cardiovascular complications such as MI, in-stent thrombosis, and sudden cardiac death. Therefore, the practitioner must first question the need for the surgery. If possible, elective surgery should be delayed until the patient is no longer considered at high risk for stopping DAPT [61]. On the other hand, emergent surgery should be carried out regardless of DAPT. In some cases, platelet transfusion has been used to counteract the effects of antiplatelet therapy. However, platelet transfusion has only been demonstrated to reverse the effect of aspirin and not that of clopidogrel or other agents [62].

Low Bleeding Risk Surgery

In patients taking DAPT undergoing non-emergent surgery that cannot wait until the patient is no longer considered at high risk, the first step is to assess the patients' bleeding risk. In patients undergoing low bleeding risk surgery, the risk of MACE (including in-stent thrombosis) is higher than the risk of having a major bleed. Therefore, the patient should be advised to continue taking DAPT until the day prior to the surgery. DAPT should be resumed immediately after the procedure is completed as long as no major bleed has occurred [36, 55].

High Bleeding Risk Surgery

High-risk patients on DAPT that are undergoing high bleeding risk procedures should be bridged with short-acting intravenous antiplatelet therapy. This method is similar to bridging patients on vitamin K antagonists with heparin, but rather than using heparin, a glycoprotein (GP) IIb/IIIa inhibitor such as tirofiban or eptifibatide is used. Bridging is performed as follows: aspirin is stopped 7 days prior to the procedure, while the ADP receptor antagonist is stopped 5 days prior to the procedure. Once the ADP receptor antagonist is stopped, a GP IIb/IIIa inhibitor infusion is initiated. The GP IIb/IIIa inhibitor infusion is then stopped a few hours before the start of the surgical procedure [36, 61]. (Tirofiban is stopped 3–6 h before the procedure, and eptifibatide is stopped 4–12 h before the procedure [59].) DAPT should be restarted immediately after the surgical procedure. Chou and colleagues showed no change in thrombotic risk when bridging was used [63], while Savonitto and colleagues and Lizza and colleagues showed complete protection against in-stent thrombosis with no change in perioperative bleeding risk [64, 65]. Large prospective randomized trials are needed to confirm which strategy is best.

Moderate Bleeding Risk Surgery

Patients at high risk with DAPT discontinuation and moderate bleeding risk procedures including urological surgeries and abdominal surgeries should be further risk stratified based on cardiovascular risk [36]. The exact parameters of this risk stratification are not well defined. Therefore, the clinician's knowledge of the individual patient's history becomes an invaluable tool in determining which patients should be considered at very high cardiovascular risk. Moreover, if the patient is determined to be a very high-risk patient and is undergoing a moderate bleeding risk surgery, they should be treated as if they are undergoing high bleeding risk surgery [36]. That is, they should be bridged with a short-acting antiplatelet infusion as described above.

On the other hand, if a patient is not at very high cardiovascular risk, the ADP receptor antagonist should be stopped 5 days prior to the procedure. After the procedure is completed, the ADP receptor antagonist should be reinitiated right away starting with a full loading dose. Aspirin should be continued throughout the entire perioperative period [36, 55].

Low- to Moderate-Risk Patients on DAPT

Patients on DAPT considered to be at low to moderate cardiovascular risk are still at relatively high risk of perioperative MACE compared to the general population. In these patients, the risk of bleeding tends to be higher than the risk of MACE. Therefore, any patient in this group undergoing surgery should stop their ADP receptor antagonist 5 days prior to the procedure and continue aspirin throughout the perioperative period. After the procedure, the ADP receptor antagonist should be restarted with or without a loading dose [55].

Clinical Vignette 1 Discussion

This patient's history is significant for chronic atrial fibrillation with a CHA_2DS_2-VASc score of 1 and coronary artery disease with recent placement of a drug-eluting stent. The patient is on both anticoagulation and dual antiplatelet therapy. Given the urgent need for ERCP and the low bleeding risk associated with the procedure, the patient should proceed without modification of anticoagulation or antiplatelet therapy. However, since the cholecystectomy is elective and is associated with moderate bleeding risk, it should be postponed for 3 more months (or a total of 6 months following stent placement) to minimize the risk of stent thrombosis. At that point, clopidogrel and warfarin can be discontinued 5 days prior to the procedure and resumed postoperatively as soon as permissible, without the need for a loading dose.

Clinical Vignette 2 Discussion

In this clinical scenario, the patient with a recent history of unprovoked bilateral pulmonary embolism and lower extremity DVT (diagnosed 2 months prior) will undergo intra-abdominal surgery (appendectomy). The patient is currently taking apixaban. Because the thrombotic event occurred within the past 3 months, he is considered to have high perioperative thrombotic risk for recurrent VTE. If the surgery is emergent (e.g., perforated viscous), the patient should proceed to surgery immediately. However, assuming that the patient's renal function is normal (i.e., creatinine clearance is greater than 50), the surgery can be postponed by 48 h after the last dose of apixaban was taken to minimize the bleeding risk. Use of a parenteral agent for preoperative bridging is not indicated for patients who are on DOACs. To minimize perioperative thrombotic risk, the patient can be placed on heparin "bridge" therapy immediately following the appendectomy. Oral anticoagulation with apixaban can be resumed postoperatively when hemostasis is confirmed.

Conclusion

The management of perioperative anticoagulation is a daunting task. With the advent of newer anticoagulants come new risks and benefits especially in the operative setting. Despite the proper precautions, the line between thrombotic risk and bleeding is small. As with any medical condition, the risks and benefits should be thoroughly discussed with the patient so that an informed joint decision can be made. Moreover, it is increasingly important for the clinician to be well versed in risk stratification of patients and anticoagulants so that the best decision is made for every patient.

Key Points

- The first step in managing perioperative anticoagulation is to consider the need and timing of the surgical or invasive procedure.
- The clinician should determine the periprocedural thromboembolic risk for the patient using available risk stratification tools (Fig. 9.1 and Table 9.1).
- Thromboembolic risk stratification for patients with atrial fibrillation can be determined using the CHA_2DS_2-VASc score (Tables 9.2 and 9.3).
- Next, the clinician should determine the periprocedural risk of bleeding (Tables 9.7, 9.8, 9.9, and 9.10).
- Patients on anticoagulant therapy with the highest thromboembolic risk should be started on short-term parenteral or "bridge" therapy upon cessation of oral anticoagulant therapies during the perioperative period.
- Patients on anticoagulant therapies with low and intermediate thrombotic risk are unlikely to benefit from perioperative bridge therapy.

Self-Assessment Questions

1. A 58-year-old man presents to the emergency room with 3 days of black tar-like stools. He

has also been feeling weak during the past few days. His past medical history is significant for atrial fibrillation, hypertension, and a transient ischemic attack 1 year prior. His current medications include metoprolol 25 mg twice daily, lisinopril 10 mg daily, amlodipine 10 mg daily, and warfarin 5 mg daily.

His initial vitals are as follows: T, 98.7F; BP, 102/61 mmHg; HR, 121 bpm; RR, 16; and O_2 sat, 98% on room air. He has conjunctival pallor and an irregularly irregular heart rate. On rectal exam, he is found to have black stool that is positive for occult blood.

Initial labs are remarkable for a hemoglobin of 6.2 g/dL (down from a baseline of 12.3 g/dL) and an INR of 3.2. The patient is given intravenous vitamin K and two units of packed red blood cells. He goes for an upper endoscopy and a visible vessel is clipped. Three days post-procedure, the patient is cleared to restart anticoagulation. The INR at this time is 1.2.

What is the best strategy for post-procedural therapeutic anticoagulation?

(a) Start heparin drip for 3 days prior to starting warfarin, and overlap the two till patient has an INR >2.
(b) Start warfarin alone at the patient's home dose.
(c) Start warfarin alone at half the patient's home dose.
(d) Start heparin drip and warfarin at the same time and overlap the two till the INR is >2.
(e) Start heparin drip and warfarin at the same time and overlap the two for 5 days after the INR is >2.

2. A 78-year-old woman with a history of hypertension presents to your cardiology office for a preoperative evaluation. She is supposed to undergo a total abdominal hysterectomy with bilateral salpingo-oophorectomy for uterine cancer. Her past medical history is significant for aortic stenosis for which she has a mechanical tilting disc valve replacement. Her only medication is warfarin 5 mg daily. She has been on this dose for years with a stable INR.

Her vitals and physical exam are normal. Her labs are unremarkable except for an INR of 3.1.

After speaking to the surgeon, you become aware that he will be stopping the patient's warfarin 5 days prior to the surgery during which time the patient will be on heparin. The surgeon requests your opinion on how to restart the patient's anticoagulation therapy.

Which of the following is the best approach?

(a) Restart warfarin at the patient's home dose without a heparin bridge, because tilting disc aortic valves are at low risk for thromboembolic complications.
(b) Start heparin drip for 3 days prior to starting warfarin, and overlap the two till the INR is therapeutic.
(c) Start therapeutic low-molecular-weight heparin and warfarin at the same time and overlap them till the patient's INR is therapeutic.
(d) Restart the patient's home dose of warfarin, because the bleeding risk of bridging outweighs the thromboembolic risks.

3. A 66-year-old man presents to your office with stable substernal chest pain that radiates down his left arm. The pain began while he was out for a morning walk and subsided after he rested for about 5 min. He has had this pain before, but it seems to be worsening. He has a history of hypertension, hyperlipidemia, and prostate cancer. He is scheduled to have a prostatectomy for his prostate cancer in 6 weeks.

He is a former smoker and quit 23 years ago. His father died of a massive heart attack at age 58. His physical exam and laboratory work are unremarkable including cardiac enzymes.

Given his symptoms, he is referred for cardiac angiogram which shows an 85% blockage in the mid right coronary artery (RCA). The rest of the angiogram is unremarkable.

Knowing that the patient will have a necessary surgical procedure in 6 weeks, which of the following is the best intervention for him?

(a) No intervention till after his prostate surgery

(b) Drug-eluting stent of his RCA
(c) Bare metal stent of his RCA
(d) Balloon angioplasty of his RCA

4. A 32-year-old man is brought in by EMS after three episodes of hematemesis at home. He has a history of atrial fibrillation and is on daily warfarin. He also has hypertension, peripheral vascular disease, and is a daily drinker.

   His vitals are notable for a heart rate of 134 beats/min and a blood pressure of 82/52 mmHg. He is lethargic but arousable and has scleral icterus. His abdomen is soft, non-tender, and moderately distended. There is a positive fluid wave and shifting dullness. The remainder of his physical exam is unremarkable.

   Initial labs show a hemoglobin of 6.3 g/dL and an INR of 8.5. The patient is ordered for IV fluids, two units of packed red blood cells, and IV vitamin K. He is also started on antibiotics for a suspected esophageal bleed.

   Which of the following would be the most appropriate next step in this patient?
   (a) Two units of FFP followed by emergent endoscopy.
   (b) An additional dose of IV vitamin K followed by emergent endoscopy.
   (c) First four-factor prothrombin complex concentrate followed by emergent endoscopy.
   (d) Hold the patients warfarin and allow the patients INR to come down and perform endoscopy in 48 h.
   (e) First four-factor prothrombin complex concentrate followed by heparin drip to maintain full anticoagulation in preparation for endoscopy.

5. A 78-year-old man presents for a routine preoperative evaluation for hernia repair. The procedure is scheduled to happen in 3 days. He has a history of atrial fibrillation and type 2 diabetes. His current medications are rivaroxaban, insulin, and lisinopril. His vitals and physical exam are normal, except for a reducible inguinal hernia. His labs show slightly decreased renal function or kidney function with a creatinine clearance of 35 mL/min.

   Which of the following is the most appropriate perioperative management of his anticoagulation therapy?
   (a) Stop rivaroxaban 5 days prior to surgery with no heparin bridge postoperatively.
   (b) Stop rivaroxaban 5 days prior to surgery and bridge the patient with heparin 5 days postoperatively.
   (c) Do not take rivaroxaban on the day of the surgery, and restart 1 day postoperatively.
   (d) Stop the rivaroxaban 48 h prior to surgery and restart anticoagulation 24 h postoperatively.

Self-Assessment Answers

1. (b) Start warfarin alone at the patient's home dose.

   Patients with atrial fibrillation do not need routine bridging anticoagulation. Given his recent gastrointestinal bleed, allowing his INR to reach the target range over 5–10 days without any heparin bridging is reasonable to avoid recurrent bleeding.

2. (c) Start therapeutic low-molecular-weight heparin and warfarin at the same time and overlap them till the patient's INR is therapeutic.

   Patients with mechanical aortic or mitral valve replacement who have risk factors for thromboembolism (including hypertension) are at moderate risk for thrombotic complications and likely should receive bridging anticoagulation while warfarin is reinitiated. Use of low-molecular-weight heparin is appropriate to avoid prolonged hospitalization.

3. (d) Balloon angioplasty of his RCA.

   For patients in whom surgery cannot be delayed, use of balloon angioplasty allows a temporary hold of dual antiplatelet therapy as soon as 2 weeks following the procedure.

4. (c) First four-factor prothrombin complex concentrate followed by emergent endoscopy.

   Four-factor prothrombin concentrate complex allow for a more rapid reversal of warfarin than fresh frozen plasma prior to emergent procedures. Anticoagulation should be held until a bleeding source is identified and resolved.

5. (d) Stop the rivaroxaban 48 h prior to surgery and restart anticoagulation 24 h postoperatively.

   In patients with normal renal function, rivaroxaban can be stopped 48 h prior to surgery and restarted as soon as the surgical site is no longer at risk for bleeding. This often occurs at 24 h postoperatively for surgeries with a low risk of bleeding.

References

1. Gallego P, Apostolakis S, Lip GY. Bridging evidence-based practice and practice-based evidence in periprocedural anticoagulation. Circulation. 2012;126(13):1573–6.
2. Guyatt GH, Akl EA, Crowther M, Schunemann HJ, Gutterman DD, Zelman Lewis S, et al. Introduction to the ninth edition: antithrombotic therapy and prevention of thrombosis, 9th ed: American College of Chest Physicians Evidence-Based Clinical Practice Guidelines. Chest. 2012;141(2 Suppl):48S–52S.
3. Douketis JD, Berger PB, Dunn AS, Jaffer AK, Spyropoulos AC, Becker RC, et al. The perioperative management of antithrombotic therapy: American College of Chest Physicians Evidence-Based Clinical Practice Guidelines (8th Edition). Chest. 2008;133(6 Suppl):299S–339S.
4. Spyropoulos AC, Douketis JD. How I treat anticoagulated patients undergoing an elective procedure or surgery. Blood. 2012;120(15):2954–62.
5. Dincq AS, Lessire S, Douxfils J, Dogne JM, Gourdin M, Mullier F. Management of non-vitamin K antagonist oral anticoagulants in the perioperative setting. Biomed Res Int. 2014;2014:385014.
6. Douketis JD, Spyropoulos AC, Spencer FA, Mayr M, Jaffer AK, Eckman MH, et al. Perioperative management of antithrombotic therapy: antithrombotic therapy and prevention of thrombosis, 9th ed: American College of Chest Physicians Evidence-Based Clinical Practice Guidelines. Chest. 2012;141(2 Suppl):e326S–50S.
7. Kearon C, Hirsh J. Management of anticoagulation before and after elective surgery. N Engl J Med. 1997;336(21):1506–11.
8. January CT, Wann LS, Alpert JS, Calkins H, Cigarroa JE, Cleveland JC Jr, et al. 2014 AHA/ACC/HRS guideline for the management of patients with atrial fibrillation: a report of the American College of Cardiology/American Heart Association Task Force on Practice Guidelines and the Heart Rhythm Society. J Am Coll Cardiol. 2014;64(21):e1–76.
9. Wolf PA, Abbott RD, Kannel WB. Atrial fibrillation as an independent risk factor for stroke: the Framingham Study. Stroke. 1991;22(8):983.
10. Lin HJ, Wolf PA, Kelly-Hayes M, et al. Stroke severity in atrial fibrillation: the Framingham study. Stroke. 1996;27:1760–4.
11. Gage BF, van Walraven C, Pearce L, Hart RG, Koudstaal PJ, Boode BS, et al. Selecting patients with atrial fibrillation for anticoagulation: stroke risk stratification in patients taking aspirin. Circulation. 2004;110(16):2287–92.
12. Gage BF, Waterman AD, Shannon W, Boechler M, Rich MW, Radford MJ. Validation of clinical classification schemes for predicting stroke: results from the national registry of atrial fibrillation. JAMA. 2001;285(22):2864–70.
13. Mason PK, Lake DE, DiMarco JP, Ferguson JD, Mangrum JM, Bilchick K, et al. Impact of the CHA2DS2-VASc score on anticoagulation rec ommendations for atrial fibrillation. Am J Med. 2012;125(6):603.e1–6.
14. Kirchhof P, Benussi S, Kotecha D, Ahlsson A, Atar D, Casadei B, et al. 2016 ESC guidelines for the management of atrial fibrillation developed in collaboration with EACTS. Europace. 2016;18(11):1609–78.
15. Doherty JU, Gluckman TJ, Hucker WJ, Januzzi JL Jr, Ortel TL, Saxonhouse SJ, Spinler SA. 2017 ACC expert consensus decision pathway for periprocedural management of anticoagulation in patients with nonvalvular atrial fibrillation: a report of the American College of Cardiology Clinical Expert Consensus Document Task Force. J Am Coll Cardiol. 2017;69(7):871–98.
16. Olesen JB, Lip GY, Hansen ML, Hansen PR, Tolstrup JS, Lindhardsen J. Validation of risk stratification schemes for predicting stroke and thromboembolism in patients with atrial fibrillation: nationwide cohort study. BMJ. 2011;342:d124.
17. Friberg L, Rosenqvist M, Lip GY. Evaluation of risk stratification schemes for ischaemic stroke and bleeding in 182,678 patients with atrial fibrillation: the Swedish Atrial Fibrillation cohort study. Eur Heart J. 2012;33(12):1500–10.
18. Friberg L, Skeppholm M, Terent A. Benefit of anticoagulation unlikely in patients with atrial fibrillation and a CHA2DS2-VASc score of 1. J Am Coll Cardiol. 2015;65(3):25–32.
19. Douketis JD, Spyropoulos AC, Kaatz S, Becker RC, Caprini JA, Dunn AS, et al. Perioperative bridging anticoagulation in patients with atrial fibrillation. N Engl J Med. 2015;373(9):823–33.
20. Siegal D, Yudin J, Kaatz S, Douketis JD, Lim W, Spyropoulos AC. Periprocedural heparin bridging in patients receiving vitamin K antagonists: systematic review and meta-analysis of bleeding and thromboembolic rates. Circulation. 2012;126(13):1630–9.
21. Kovacs MJ, Kearon C, Rodger M, Anderson DR, Turpie AG, Bates SM, et al. Single-arm study of bridging therapy with low-molecular-weight heparin for patients at risk of arterial embolism who require temporary interruption of warfarin. Circulation. 2004;110(12):1658–63.

22. Cannegieter SC, Rosendaal FR, Briët E. Thromboembolic and bleeding complications in patients with mechanical heart valve prosthesis. Circulation. 1994;89:635–41.
23. Andersen PV, Alstrup P. Long-term survival and complications in patients with mechanical aortic valves without anticoagulation. A follow-up study from 1 to 15 years. Eur J Cardiothorac Surg. 1992;6(2):62–5.
24. McKenzie DB, Wong K, Edwards T. The management of patients with mechanical heart valves and intracerebral haemorrhage. Br J Cardiol. 2008;15:145–8.
25. Jaffer AK. Perioperative management of warfarin and antiplatelet therapy. Cleve Clin J Med. 2009;76(Suppl 4):S37–44.
26. Perry DJ, Noakes TJ, Helliwell PS. Guidelines for the management of patients on oral anticoagulants requiring dental surgery. Br Dent J. 2007;203(7):389–93.
27. Malloy PC, Grassi CJ, Kundu S, Gervais DA, Miller DL, Osnis RB, et al. Standards of Practice Committee with Cardiovascular and Interventional Radiological Society of Europe (CIRSE) Endorsement. Consensus guidelines for periprocedural management of coagulation status and hemostasis risk in percutaneous image-guided interventions. J Vasc Interv Radiol. 2009;20(7 Suppl):S240–9.
28. Gogarten W, Vandermeulen E, Van Aken H, Kozek S, Llau JV, Samama CM, European Society of Anaesthesiology. Regional anaesthesia and antithrombotic agents: recommendations of the European Society of Anaesthesiology. Eur J Anaesthesiol. 2010;27(12):999–1015.
29. Horlocker TT. Regional anaesthesia in the patient receiving antithrombotic and antiplatelet therapy. Br J Anaesth. 2011;107(Suppl 1):i96–106.
30. Zaca V, Marcucci R, Parodi G, Limbruno U, Notarstefano P, Pieragnoli P, et al. Management of antithrombotic therapy in patients undergoing electrophysiological device surgery. Europace. 2015;17(6):840–54.
31. Narouze S, Benzon HT, Provenzano DA, Buvanendran A, De Andres J, Deer TR, et al. Interventional spine and pain procedures in patients on antiplatelet and anticoagulant medications: guidelines from the American Society of Regional Anesthesia and Pain Medicine, the European Society of Regional Anaesthesia and Pain Therapy, the American Academy of Pain Medicine, the International Neuromodulation Society, the North American Neuromodulation Society, and the World Institute of Pain. Reg Anesth Pain Med. 2015;40(3):182–212.
32. Burnett AE, Mahan CE, Vazquez SR, Oertel LB, Garcia DA, Ansell J. Guidance for the practical management of the direct oral anticoagulants (DOACs) in VTE treatment. J Thromb Thrombolysis. 2016;41(1):206–32.
33. Witt DM, Clark NP, Kaatz S, Schnurr T, Ansell JE. Guidance for the practical management of warfarin therapy in the treatment of venous thromboembolism. J Thromb Thrombolysis. 2016;41(1):187–205.
34. ASGE Standards of Practice Committee, Acosta RD, Abraham NS, Chandrasekhara V, Chathadi KV, Early DS, Eloubeidi MA, et al. The management of antithrombotic agents for patients undergoing GI endoscopy. Gastrointest Endosc. 2016;83(1):3–16.
35. Veitch AM, Vanbiervliet G, Gershlick AH, Boustiere C, Baglin TP, Smith L-A, et al. Endoscopy in patients on antiplatelet or anticoagulant therapy, including direct oral anticoagulants: British Society of Gastroenterology (BSG) and European Society of Gastrointestinal Endoscopy (ESGE) guidelines. Endoscopy. 2016;48(4):c1.
36. Oprea AD, Popescu WM. Perioperative management of antiplatelet therapy. Br J Anaesth. 2013;111(Suppl 1):i3–17.
37. Chee YL, Crawford JC, Watson HG, Greaves M. Guidelines on the assessment of bleeding risk prior to surgery or invasive procedures. British Committee for Standards in Haematology. Br J Haematol. 2008;140(5):496–504.
38. Fang MC, Go AS, Chang Y, Borowsky LH, Pomernacki NK, Udaltsova N, Singer DEA. new risk scheme to predict warfarin-associated hemorrhage: the ATRIA (Anticoagulation and Risk Factors in Atrial Fibrillation) Study. J Am Coll Cardiol. 2011;58(4):395–401.
39. Gage BF, Yan Y, Milligan PE, Waterman AD, Culverhouse R, Rich MW, Radford MJ. Clinical classification schemes for predicting hemorrhage: results from the National Registry of Atrial Fibrillation (NRAF). Am Heart J. 2006;151(3):713–9.
40. Pisters RLD, Nieuwlaat R, de Vos CB, Crijns HJ, Lip GY. A novel user-friendly score (HAS-BLED) to assess 1-year risk of major bleeding in patients with atrial fibrillation: the Euro Heart Survey. Chest. 2010;138(5):1093–100.
41. Omran H, Bauersachs R, Rübenacker S, Goss F, Hammerstingl C. The HAS-BLED score predicts bleedings during bridging of chronic oral anticoagulation. Results from the national multicentre BNK Online bRiDging REgistRy (BORDER). Thromb Haemost. 2012;108(1):65–73.
42. Link KP. The discovery of dicumarol and its sequels. Circulation. 1959;19(1):97–107.
43. Pirmohamed M. Warfarin: almost 60 years old and still causing problems. Br J Clin Pharmacol. 2006;62(5):509–11.
44. Campbell HA, et al. Studies on the hemorrhagic sweet clover disease. J Biol Chem. 1940;136:47–55.
45. Douketis JD. Perioperative management of patients who are receiving warfarin therapy: an evidence-based and practical approach. Blood. 2011;117(19):5044–9.
46. Syed S, Adams BB, Liao W, Pipitone M, Gloster H. A prospective assessment of bleeding and international normalized ratio in warfarin-anticoagulated patients having cutaneous surgery. J Am Acad Dermatol. 2004;51(6):955–7.
47. Jamula E, Anderson J, Douketis JD. Safety of continuing warfarin therapy during cataract surgery: a systematic review and meta-analysis. Thromb Res. 2009;124(3):292–9.
48. Linkins L, Choi PT, Douketis JD. Clinical impact of bleeding in patients taking oral anticoagulant therapy

for venous thromboembolism: a meta-analysis. Ann Intern Med. 2003;139:893–900.
49. Schulman S, Rhedin AS, Lindmarker P, Carlsson A, Larfars G, Nicol P, et al. A comparison of six weeks with six months of oral anticoagulant therapy after a first episode of venous thromboembolism. Duration of Anticoagulation Trial Study Group. N Engl J Med. 1995;332(25):1661–5.
50. Mekaj YH, Mekaj AY, Duci SB, Miftari EI. New oral anticoagulants: their advantages and disadvantages compared with vitamin K antagonists in the prevention and treatment of patients with thromboembolic events. Ther Clin Risk Manag. 2015;11:967–77.
51. Raval AN, Cigarroa JE, Chung MK, Diaz-Sandoval LJ, Diercks D, Piccini JP, et al. Management of patients on non-vitamin K antagonist oral anticoagulants in the acute care and periprocedural setting: a scientific statement from the American Heart Association. Circulation. 2017;135(10):e604–e33.
52. Makaryus JN, Halperin JL, Lau JF. Oral anticoagulants in the management of venous thromboembolism. Nat Rev Cardiol. 2013;10(7):397–409.
53. Imberti D, Ambrosoli A, Cimminiello C, Compagnone C, Fanelli A, Tripodi A, et al. Periprocedural management of rivaroxaban-treated patients. Expert Opin Pharmacother. 2015;16(5):685–91.
54. Baker WL, Phung OJ. Systematic review and adjusted indirect comparison meta-analysis of oral anticoagulants in atrial fibrillation. Circ Cardiovasc Qual Outcomes. 2012;5(5):711–9.
55. Di Minno MN, Milone M, Mastronardi P, Ambrosino P, Di Minno A, Parolari A, et al. Perioperative handling of antiplatelet drugs. A critical appraisal. Curr Drug Targets. 2013;14(8):880–8.
56. Wolff T, Miller T, Ko S. Aspirin for the primary prevention of cardiovascular events: an update of the evidence for the US Preventive Services Task Force. U.S. Preventive Services Task Force Evidence Syntheses, formerly Systematic Evidence Reviews. Rockville: Agency for Healthcare Research and Quality (US); 2009.
57. Biondi-Zoccai GG, Lotrionte M, Agostoni P, Abbate A, Fusaro M, Burzotta F, et al. A systematic review and meta-analysis on the hazards of discontinuing or not adhering to aspirin among 50,279 patients at risk for coronary artery disease. Eur Heart J. 2006;27(22):2667–74.
58. Thurston AV, Briant SL. Aspirin and post-prostatectomy hemorrhage. Br J Urol. 1993;71(5):574–6.
59. Oprea AD, Popescu WM. ADP-receptor inhibitors in the perioperative period: the good, the bad, and the ugly. J Cardiothorac Vasc Anesth. 2013;27(4):779–95.
60. Cook-Norris RH, Michaels JD, Weaver AL, Phillips PK, Brewer JD, Roenigk RK, et al. Complications of cutaneous surgery in patients taking clopidogrel-containing anticoagulation. J Am Acad Dermatol. 2011;65(3):584–91.
61. Brilakis ES, Banerjee S, Berger PB. Perioperative management of patients with coronary stents. J Am Coll Cardiol. 2007;49(22):2145–50.
62. Taylor GMO, Diane MD, Thevenin AMD, Devys J-MMD. Is platelet transfusion efficient to restore platelet reactivity in patients who are responders to aspirin and/or clopidogrel before emergency surgery? J Trauma Acute Care Surg. 2013;74(5):1367–9.
63. Chou S, Eshaghian S, Lamer A, Tran H, Dohad S, Kaul S. Bridging therapy in the perioperative management of patients with drug-eluting stents. Rev Cardiovasc Med. 2009;10(4):209–18.
64. Savonitto S, D'Urbano M, Caracciolo M, Barlocco F, Mariani G, Nichelatti M, et al. Urgent surgery in patients with a recently implanted coronary drug-eluting stent: a phase II study of 'bridging' antiplatelet therapy with tirofiban during temporary withdrawal of clopidogrel. Br J Anaesth. 2010;104(3):285–91.
65. Lizza BD, Kauflin MJ. Extended-infusion eptifibatide to prevent stent thrombosis in a patient undergoing orthopedic surgery. Ann Pharmacother. 2011;45(5):e28.
66. Shireman TI, Howard PA, Kresowik TF, Ellerbeck EF. Combined anticoagulant-antiplatelet use and major bleeding events in elderly atrial fibrillation patients. Stroke. 2004;35(10):2362–7.
67. Llau JV, Ferrandis R, Sierra P, Gomez-Luque A. Prevention of the renarrowing of coronary arteries using drug-eluting stents in the perioperative period: an update. Vasc Health Risk Manag. 2010;6:855–67.

Acute Coronary Syndromes

10

Nilay K. Patel and Sammy Elmariah

Clinical Vignette

A 48-year-old man presents to the emergency department with 36 h of intermittent chest discomfort. He reports his symptoms as substernal chest pressure with radiation into his left arm that occurs primarily while he has been walking and is relieved with rest. On the evening of presentation, his symptoms began while at rest watching television. His past medical history includes hypertension, hyperlipidemia, and 20-pack-year smoking, although he quit 10 years ago. An electrocardiogram is obtained and reveals normal sinus rhythm with T-wave inversions in leads V3–V6. His initial troponin T is 0.36 mg/dL (reference range <0.01 mg/dL). He is admitted to the cardiac care unit for further care.

Introduction

Definitions of Acute Coronary Syndromes

Acute coronary syndromes (ACS) refer to a group of clinical syndromes leading to acute myocardial ischemia related to reduced coronary artery blood flow. These syndromes include ST-segment elevation myocardial infarction (STEMI) and non-ST-segment acute coronary syndromes (NSTE-ACS). STEMI is characterized by the presence of ST-segment elevation or new left bundle branch block (LBBB) on initial electrocardiogram (ECG). NSTE-ACS can be further stratified by the presence of elevated cardiac biomarkers of myocardial necrosis. If cardiac biomarkers are positive, ischemia was severe enough to cause myocyte death and is labeled as a non-ST-segment elevation myocardial infarction (NSTEMI). If cardiac biomarkers are negative, but the patient has either angina at rest, new-onset angina, or worsening of prior angina, the patient is deemed to have unstable angina (UA). ECGs in NSTE-ASCS may reveal ST depressions, T-wave inversions, or no abnormalities. Acute coronary syndromes are common manifestations of coronary artery disease and are an important cause of morbidity and mortality in

N. K. Patel · S. Elmariah (✉)
Division of Cardiology, Department of Medicine, Massachusetts General Hospital, Boston, MA, USA
e-mail: npatel28@partners.org; selmariah@mgh.harvard.edu

J. F. Lau et al. (eds.), *Anticoagulation Therapy*, https://doi.org/10.1007/978-3-319-73709-6_10

the United States and worldwide [1, 2]. In this chapter we will:

1. Describe the role of anticoagulant therapy in acute coronary syndromes (ACS).
2. Discuss mechanism of action of various anticoagulants available for treating ACS.
3. Review available data of comparative outcomes of use of various anticoagulants.
4. Delineate roles of anticoagulant therapy in secondary prevention of ACS.

Pathogenesis of the Acute Coronary Syndrome

The "Third Universal Definition of Myocardial Infarction" defines myocardial infarction (MI) as being caused by a reduction in myocardial oxygen consumption [2]. This can be related to a primary abrupt reduction in coronary artery blood flow, as in the case of spontaneous plaque rupture MI (type 1), the focus of this chapter. Alternatively, disease states that reduce myocardial oxygen supply relative to demand may also lead to myocardial infarction, as in the case of severe anemia or malignant hypertension.

Atherosclerosis describes the typically indolent development of intimal plaque in arteries throughout the body. Many risk factors are known to influence this process, including hyperlipidemia, hypertension, smoking, and diabetes. Eventually, endothelial dysfunction leads to migration of inflammatory cells into the subendothelium. These cells mediate the process of plaque development by consuming oxidized low-density lipoprotein (LDL) and recruiting vascular smooth muscle cells. This process is often unpredictable leaving some plaque more vulnerable with a higher propensity for rupture [3]. Coronary artery plaques, especially those at high risk, e.g., those with a large lipid core or thin fibrous caps, can rupture triggering local platelet activation and aggregation. As this process continues, thrombi form that can partially or totally occlude the coronary artery resulting in ACS (Fig. 10.1).

Initial Management of Patients with ACS

Clinical outcomes in ACS can be improved by a combination of medical therapy with appropriately timed revascularization to restore blood flow to viable myocardium. Revascularization can be achieved pharmacologically, with fibrinolytic therapy or with percutaneous coronary intervention (PCI). Acute medical therapy typically includes anti-ischemic, antiplatelet, anticoagulant, and lipid-lowering therapy. A wide array of large-scale randomized controlled trials has been performed evaluating the efficacy and safety of these therapies in the acute and long-term care of patients who suffer from ACS events.

Patients with STEMI often have total or near-total occlusion of a coronary artery leading to transmural ischemia of myocardium subtended by the blood vessel. The goal of therapy is immediate pharmacological or catheter-based reperfusion to restore normal coronary blood flow. The initial goal of therapy in NSTE-ACS is often to prevent further thrombosis and augment endogenous fibrinolysis. Eventual revascularization may often still be pursued to reduce the degree of coronary stenosis and to prevent reocclusion and ongoing ischemia [5, 6]. Antiplatelet and anticoagulant therapy is essential to achieving both goals. Antiplatelet therapy ensures reduction in platelet activation and aggregation, which are fundamental initial steps in the formation of thrombus. Anticoagulant therapy targets the clotting cascade to prevent fibrin strand deposits.

The American College of Cardiology (ACC) and American Heart Association (AHA) jointly published two separate evidence-based clinical practice guidelines about the management of patients presenting with STEMI and NSTE-ACS [5, 6]. In both cases, prompt initiation of anticoagulation is recommended irrespective of the initial treatment strategy. Thrombin activity at the site of coronary artery plaque rupture mediates formation of thrombus by further activating platelets, converting fibrinogen to fibrin, and augmenting fibrin cross-linking. All anticoagulant

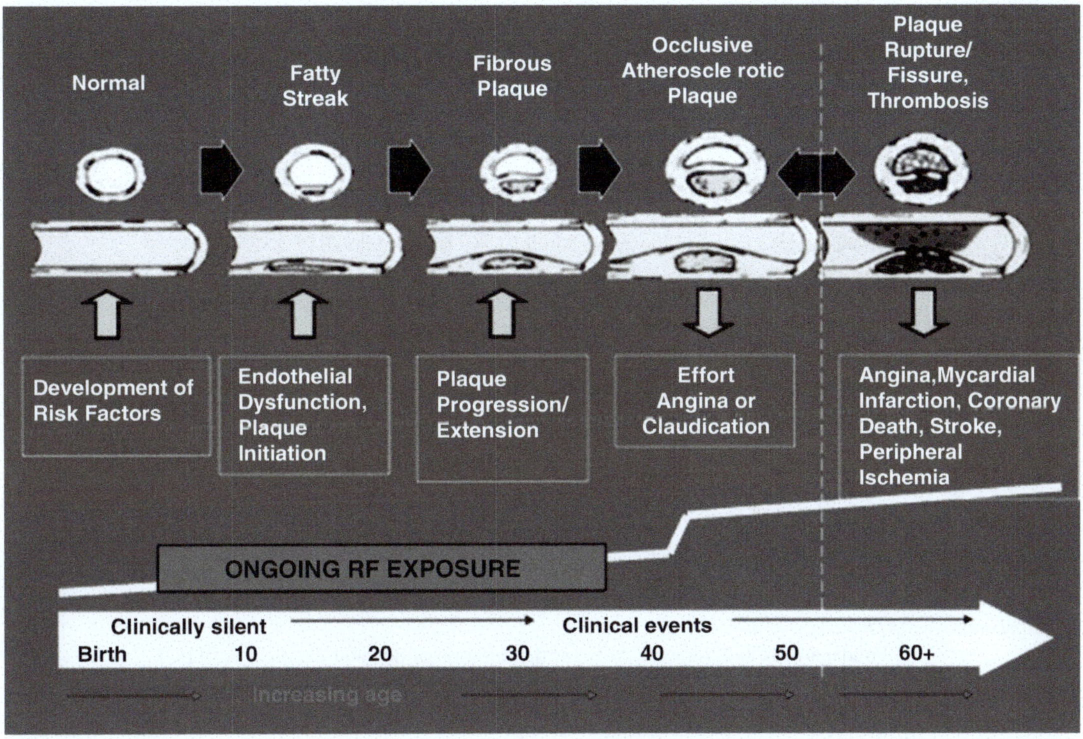

Fig. 10.1 Progression of atherosclerosis—pathologic progression of atherosclerosis starts with subclinical plaque formation between the first and second decade of life. The process can be hastened by exposure to risk factors. Over time, this disease can become clinically apparent with development of angina, myocardial infarction, or sudden cardiac death [4]. Source: National Heart, Lung, and Blood Institute, National Institutes of Health

Table 10.1 Anticoagulant medications utilized in treatment of patients with acute coronary syndromes

Drug	Mechanism of action	Half-life (h)	Route of administration
Unfractionated heparin	Binds to antithrombin III (ATIII), which functions to inactivate thrombin. Heparin-AT binding accelerates thrombin, factor Xa, XIIa, XIa, and IXa inactivation	0.5–2.5 (dose-dependent)	SC, IV
Enoxaparin (LMWH)	Binds to AT, facilitating inactivation of thrombin, factors Xa, XIIa, XIa, and IXa	4.5	SC, IV
Fondaparinux	A synthetic pentasaccharide that is biochemically identical to the high-affinity binding site for antithrombin III (ATIII), leading to inhibition of factor Xa but not thrombin	17	SC, IV
Bivalirudin	Thrombin inhibitors directly without need for antithrombin	0.5	IV

PO per os (by mouth), *IV* intravenous, *SC* subcutaneous

therapy is aimed at reducing thrombin activity or factors upstream from thrombin. Available anticoagulants with data in treatment of patients with ACS are summarized in Table 10.1. Recommendations about the clinical utility of parenteral anticoagulants targeted in the acute care of patients with ACS are summarized in Table 10.2.

Unfractionated Heparin

Mechanism of Action, Dose, and Monitoring

Unfractionated heparin (UFH) binds to the enzyme inhibitor antithrombin III (AT) which activates it and allows it to work more rapidly.

Table 10.2 Summary of recommendations for parenteral anticoagulation therapy for acute coronary syndromes [5, 6]

	Recommendation	COR	LOE
Unfractionated heparin (UFH)	*NSTE-ACS* • Intravenous UFH for 48 h or until PCI is performed with initial loading dose of 60 IU/kg (maximum dose 4000 IU) followed by initial infusion of 12 IU/kg/h (maximum dose 1000 IU/h)	I	B
	• Intravenous UFH is useful in patients with NSTE-ACS undergoing PCI	I	C
	STEMI • Standard dose IV UFH should be administered to maintain aPTT at 1.5–2.0 times control for 48 h or until PCI	I	C
	• Continue UFH through PCI, administering additional IV boluses needed to maintain therapeutic ACT according to institutional protocol	I	C
Enoxaparin (LMWH)	*NSTE-ACS* • Enoxaparin at 1 mg/kg SC every 12 h for duration of hospitalization or until PCI is performed	I	A
	STEMI • If age <75 years, administer 30 mg IV bolus followed by 1 mg/kg SC every 12 h after 15 min (adjust to daily dosing if CrCl < 30 mL/min). If age >75 years, administer 0.75 mg/kg subcutaneously every 12 h. Therapy should continue for up to 8 days or until revascularization	I	A
	• LMWH can be continued through PCI. No additional drug is needed if last dose was within 8 h, and 0.3 mg/kg IV bolus is needed if last dose was 8–12 h earlier	I	B
Fondaparinux	*NSTE-ACS* • Fondaparinux at 2.5 mg SC daily for the duration of hospitalization or until PCI is performed	I	B
	• Administer additional anticoagulant with anti-IIa activity if PCI is performed while patient is on fondaparinux	I	B
	STEMI • Fondaparinux 2.5 mg IV once followed by SC daily for the duration of hospitalization or until PCI is performed	I	B
	• Administer additional anticoagulant with anti-IIa activity if PCI is performed while patient is on fondaparinux	I	B
Bivalirudin	*NSTE-ACS* • Bivalirudin until diagnostic angiography or PCI is performed in patients undergoing and early invasive strategy with loading dose of 0.10 mg/kg followed by 0.25 mg/kg/h	I	B
	• Bivalirudin is useful as an anticoagulant with or without prior treatment with UFH in patients with NSTE-ACS undergoing PCI	I	B
	• In patients with NSTE-ACS with high risk of bleeding, it is reasonable to use bivalirudin monotherapy in preference to UFH and GP IIb/IIIa receptor antagonists	IIa	B
	STEMI: • When using bivalirudin as adjunctive anticoagulant therapy to support primary PCI, administer 0.75 mg/kg IV bolus followed by 1.75 mg/kg/h infusion	I	B

COR class of recommendation, *LOE* level of evidence, *SC* subcutaneous, *PCI* percutaneous coronary intervention, *aPTT* activated partial thromboplastin time

Activated AT is then able to inactivate thrombin, factor Xa, as well as factors XIIa, Xia, and IXa. It is worthwhile to note that the heparin-bound antithrombin complex is not able to inactivate thrombin that is deposited in clot [7].

In the setting of ACS, patients are recommended to receive an initial loading dose of 60 IU/kg with a maximum of 4000 IU and an initial infusion of 12 IU/kg/h with a maximum of 1000 IU/h. Adjustments should be made to the infusion rate based on activated partial thromboplastin time (PTT) to maintain therapeutic anticoagulation according to institutional protocol. Therapy is typically continued for 48 h or until PCI is performed in NSTE-ACS. Patients with STEMI or NSTE-ACS referred for revascularization with PCI can be further treated with unfractionated heparin titrated to achieve an appropriate activated clotting time (ACT) to support the procedure [5, 6].

Patients should have complete blood cell counts monitored daily while receiving therapy to monitor for bleeding and acquired heparin-induced thrombocytopenia (HIT) [8]. Patients with STEMI undergoing reperfusion with fibrinolytic therapy should also receive therapeutic anticoagulation. Therapy should be administered for a minimum of 48 h, preferably for the duration of the hospitalization (up to 8 days) [5].

UFH in ACS

The use of unfractionated heparin became one of the cornerstones of therapy for patients with ACS following early, small, randomized trials. A meta-analysis of 6 randomized trials between 1988 and 1995 comparing aspirin and heparin versus aspirin alone in 1353 patients with unstable angina was performed. As seen in Table 10.3, the analysis revealed that there was a 33% reduction in the risk of myocardial infarction (MI) or death at 3 months in patients with unstable angina receiving combination therapy compared to aspirin alone (7.9% and 10.4%, respectively); however, this finding did not meet statistical significance (confidence interval 0.44–1.02; $p = 0.06$). A nonsignificant decrease in recurrent ischemia of 32% was also seen. The risk of major bleeding doubled for those on combination therapy [9] (Table 10.3).

Complications of Heparin Therapy

While evidence suggests improved cardiovascular endpoints with heparin therapy in acute coronary syndromes with or without revascularization, major bleeding and heparin-induced thrombocytopenia remain important complications.

The risk of major bleeding on heparin therapy does not clearly correlate with the dose administered [16]. Bleeding that complicated acute coronary syndromes is independently associated with recurrent MI, CVA, death, and increased length and cost of hospitalizations [17]. In selected situations for patients on heparin, reversal of the anticoagulant effect may be desired. Given the short half-life of UFH, it may be reasonable to stop the infusion and wait for the anticoagulant effect to wean. In cases of life-threatening bleeding, protamine can be administered to bind to heparin molecules and form an inactive salt. Protamine's onset of action is within 5 min and is irreversible once administered. Approximately 100 units of heparin are neutralized by 1 mg of protamine.

Heparin-induced thrombocytopenia (HIT) is a potentially devastating complication of heparin therapy and is caused by an immune-mediated reaction to drug exposure. While laboratory testing often reveals thrombocytopenia, HIT is strongly associated with thrombotic complications in both the arterial and venous system. Typically, the onset of HIT occurs 5–10 days after heparin initiation, and complications can include venous and arterial thrombosis, skin necrosis, limb gangrene, and visceral organ ischemia and infarction. The diagnosis of HIT typical requires the presence of clinical and laboratory features consistent with the diagnosis [18].

Clinical criteria include the 4T's score which is further delineated in Fig. 10.2.

Table 10.3 Characteristics of six randomized trials of aspirin versus aspirin and heparin and results of relative risk of myocardial infarction or death during hospitalization [9–15]

Source	Total no. of patients	Aspirin dose	Heparin goal	RR (95% CI)
Theroux et al. [10]	243	325 mg twice daily	PTT 1.5–2× normal	0.50 (0.18–2.66)
RISC group [11]	399	75 mg daily	Not stated	0.39 (0.18–1.47)
Cohen et al. [12]	69	80–325 mg daily	PTT 2× normal	0.29 (0.06–6.87)
Cohen et al. [13]	214	162.5 mg daily	PTT 2× normal	0.46 (0.24–1.45)
Holdright et al. [14]	285	150 mg daily	PTT 1.5–2× normal	0.89 (0.66–1.29)
Gurfinkel et al. [15]	143	200 mg daily	PTT 2× normal	0.60 (0.29–1.95)
Summary	1353			0.67 (0.44–1.02)

	Score = 2	Score = 1	Score = 0
Thrombocytopenia Compare the highest platelet count within the sequence of declining platelet counts with the lowest count to determine the % of platelet fall. (Select only 1 option)	o > 50% platelet fall AND nadir of ≥ 20 AND no surgery within preceding 3 days	o > 50% platelet fall BUT surgery within preceding 3 days OR o any combination of platelet fall and nadir that does not fit criteria for Score 2 or Score 0 (eg, 30-50% platelet fall or nadir 10-19)	o < 30% platelet fall o any platelet fall with nadir < 10
Timing (of platelet count fall or thrombosis*) Day 0 = first day of most recent heparin exposure (Select only 1 option)	o platelet fall day 5-10 after start of heparin o platelet fall within 1 day of start of heparin AND exposure to heparin within past 5-30 days	o consistent with platelet fall days 5-10 but not clear (eg, missing counts) o platelet fall within 1 day of start of heparin AND exposure to heparin in past 31-100 days o platelet fall after day 10	o platelet fall ≤ day 4 without exposure to heparin in past 100 days
Thrombosis (or other clinical sequelae) (Select only 1 option)	o confirmed new thrombosis (venous or arterial) o skin necrosis at injection site o anaphylactoid reaction to IV heparin bolus o adrenal hemorrhage	o recurrent venous thrombosis in a patient receiving therapeutic anticoagulants o suspected thrombosis (awaiting confirmation with imaging) o erythematous skin lesions at heparin injection sites	o thrombosis suspected
oTher cause for Thrombocytopenia** (Select only 1 option) **Drugs implicated in drug-induced immune thrombocytopenia (D-ITP)** **Relatively Common:** glycoprotein IIb/IIIa antagonists (abciximab, eptifibatide, tirofiban); quinine, quinidine, sulfa antibiotics, carbamazepine, vancomycin **Less Common:** actinomycin, amitriptyline, amoxicillin/piperacillin/nafcillin, cephalosporins (cefazolin, ceftazidime, ceftriaxone), celecoxib, ciprofloxacin, esomeprazole, fexofenadine, fentanyl, fucidic acid, furosemide, gold salts, levofloxacin, metronidazole, naproxen, oxaliplatin, phenytoin, propranolol, propoxyphene, ranitidine, rifampin, suramin, trimethoprim. Note: This is a partial list.	o no alternative explanation for platelet fall is evident	**Possible other cause is evident:** o sepsis without proven microbial source o thrombocytopenia associated with initiation of ventilator o other	**Probable other cause present:** o within 72 h of surgery o confirmed bacteremia/ fungemia o chemotherapy or radiation within past 20 days o DIC due to non-HIT cause o posttransfusion purpura (PTP) o platelet count < 20 AND given a drug implicated in causing D-ITP (see list) o non-necrotizing skin lesions at LMWH injection site (presumes DTH) o other

Fig. 10.2 The "4T score" for diagnosis of heparin-induced thrombocytopenia. Reprinted from CHEST, Vol. 141/Issue 2 Supp), Linkins LA, Dans AL, Moores LK, Bona R, Davidson BL, Schulman S, Crowther M, Treatment and prevention of heparin-induced thrombocytopenia: antithrombotic therapy and prevention of thrombosis 9th ed.: American College of Chest Physicians Evidence-based Clinical Practice Guidelines, pages e495s-e530s, © 2012, with permission from Elsevier [19]

Laboratory testing includes HIT antibody testing. The risk of HIT is lower with LMWH than with UFH. Once this diagnosis is presumed, heparin therapy should be withheld until the diagnosis is confirmed. If a presumptive diagnosis is made, immediate anticoagulation with a non-heparin anticoagulant is typically recommended unless there is a strong contraindication given the high risk of thrombosis associated with HIT. For patients who present with STEMI or NSTE-ACS but have a history of HIT, patients can still undergo cardiac catheterization or fibrinolytic therapy with use of an alternative non-heparin anticoagulant. For patients referred for PCI, bivalirudin and argatroban can be used [5, 6].

Low-Molecular-Weight Heparins

Mechanism of Action, Dose, and Monitoring

Rates of recurrent ischemia were high even with prompt initiation of UFH, prompting advancements in anticoagulant therapy and the development of low-molecular-weight heparins (LMWHs). Akin to UFH, LMWH binds to the enzyme inhibitor antithrombin III, activating it and accelerating its action. AT functions to inactivate thrombin, factors Xa, XIIa, XIa, and IXa. The molecular weight of LMWH is approximately one third of heparin and is readily absorbed in subcutaneous tissue. Unlike heparin, LMWH does not require routine monitoring [20].

Although a number of different LWMHs have been created, enoxaparin has been most extensively studied in comparison to UFH. The dose of enoxaparin recommended in NSTE-ACS is 1 mg/kg subcutaneously every 12 h [6]. In select patients, an initial IV loading dose of 30 mg can be used. For patients with impaired renal function (CrCl <30 mL/min), dose reduction to 1 mg/kg once daily is recommended. In this setting, consideration of transitioning to UFH is also recommended. Unlike heparin, protamine only partially reverses the anticoagulant effect of LMWH.

LMWH in NSTE-ACS

Enoxaparin has been compared to UFH in four large randomized trials. The ESSENCE trial compared enoxaparin to continuous infusion UFH in 3171 patients treated for NSTE-ACS for a total duration of at least 2 days and up to 8 days [21]. At 30 days of follow-up, a significantly lower rate of a composite endpoint of death, MI, and recurrent angina was seen in the group receiving LMWH compared to UFH (19.8% and 23.3%, respectively) with no significant difference in the rate of major bleeding. Of note, the ESSENCE trial did not require coronary angiography, and there was a significant reduction in eventual revascularization procedures with PCI or coronary artery bypass graft (CABG) surgery in patients receiving LMWH compared to UFH (27.0 and 32.2, respectively) [21]. These benefits were sustained at 1-year follow-up [22].

Further confirmation of these results was presented in the TIMI 11B trial, a second large randomized trial of LMWH compared to UFH therapy in patients with NSTE-ACS [23]. Diagnostic or therapeutic coronary intervention was not planned in this trial. A composite primary endpoint of death, MI, or urgent revascularization was significantly lower in patients receiving enoxaparin compared to those receiving UFH at 8 days of follow-up; however, this result appeared to be most evident in patients with positive biomarkers of myocardial necrosis.

Both of these trials were conducted before more widespread use of routine diagnostic coronary angiography, PCI, and dual antiplatelet therapy (DAPT) in NSTE-ACS. The first trial with closest similarity to contemporary invasive evaluation and dual antithrombotic regimens was the SYNERGY trial [24]. Approximately 10,000 patients with NSTE-ACS were randomized to receive enoxaparin or UFH. Patients were intended to undergo coronary angiography with 47% ultimately receiving PCI and 19% undergoing CABG. A total of 95% of patients received aspirin, 66% received $P2Y_{12}$ inhibitors, and 57% received glycoprotein IIb/IIIa inhibitors. All anticoagulant therapy was discontinued following PCI. The trial results are notable for no significant different in the primary composite endpoint of death or nonfatal MI at 6 months occurring in 17.6% of patients receiving enoxaparin and 17.8% of patients receiving UFH. There was a significant increase in the risk of in-hospital major bleeding for those treated with enoxaparin.

Following the publication of these trials and subsequent meta-analyses, enoxaparin and UFH are frequently cited as having similar clinical efficacy as reflected in ACC/AHA 2014 NSTE-ACS clinical practice guidelines [6, 25]. No other LMWH have proven clinical efficacy in ACS.

LMWH in STEMI

Whereas multiple trials exist comparing UFH and LMWH in NSTE-ACS, less data is available supporting the use of LMWH in STEMI for patients who are treated with primary PCI. In the ATOLL trial, intravenous enoxaparin was compared to UFH but failed to meet its primary composite endpoint. Notably, this trial included only 910 STEMI patients, and approximately 80% received glycoprotein IIb/IIIa inhibitors [26].

In patients with STEMI undergoing reperfusion with fibrinolytic therapy, enoxaparin can be administered as an intravenous bolus followed by subcutaneous injections and is preferred over UFH when therapy extends beyond 48 h. A number of large clinical trials have been performed evaluating the efficacy of enoxaparin in this setting. A meta-analysis of these trials published in 2007 included approximately 27,000 patients with STEMI undergoing fibrinolytic therapy combined with either UFH or enoxaparin [27]. The composite primary endpoint of death, myocardial infarction, and major bleeding at 30 days was significantly less frequent in patients receiving enoxaparin compared to UFH (11.1% and 12.9%, respectively). This difference was driven by a reduction in myocardial infarction; however, the benefit was offset modestly by a significant increase in the rate of major bleeding in patients receiving enoxaparin.

Fondaparinux

Mechanism of Action, Dose, and Monitoring

Fondaparinux is a synthetic pentasaccharide which is biochemically identical to the high-affinity binding site for antithrombin III. In contrast to heparin binding to AT, fondaparinux inhibits factor Xa and does not have an effect on thrombin. No routine monitoring is required for patients on fondaparinux therapy. Fondaparinux is unique for a number of reasons including its long half-life which facilitates once-daily dosing as well as the consistency of its effect. Fondaparinux is excreted renally and is contraindicated in patients with a CrCl <30 mL/min.

Fondaparinux in NSTE-ACS

The OASIS-5 trial primarily provided the evidence supporting the use of fondaparinux in NSTE-ACS. This trial included 20,078 patients with high-risk unstable angina or NSTEMI and compared subcutaneous fondaparinux 2.5 mg daily to standard-dose enoxaparin. Patients were treated for a mean of 6 days and evaluated for development of a primary composite outcome that included death, myocardial infarction, or refractory ischemia at 9 days of follow-up. Primary outcome events occurred in 5.8% of patients on fondaparinux and 5.7% of patients on enoxaparin, suggesting non-inferiority of the fondaparinux compared to enoxaparin. The rate of major bleeding after 9 days was significantly reduced at 9 days in patients receiving fondaparinux compared to enoxaparin (2.2% versus 4.1%). Further, a statistically significant reduction in death was also noted in patients treated with fondaparinux at 1 and 6 months of follow-up. If PCI was pursued, anticoagulation was typically stopped following the procedure. A near-threefold increase in catheter-related thrombi was reported in patients receiving fondaparinux; however, this risk was mitigated by additional intravenous heparin boluses during procedures [28]. In cases of NSTE-ACS where PCI is planned, additional anticoagulant therapy with anti-IIa therapy, such as UFH or bivalirudin, is indicated. Approximately 30% of patients in the OASIS-5 trial underwent PCI with significant reduction in major bleeding noted in patients receiving fondaparinux compared to enoxaparin (2.4% versus 5.1%) and similar rates of the primary composite outcome.

Fondaparinux in STEMI

The OASIS-6 trial serves as the basis for clinical use of fondaparinux in STEMI. The OASIS-6 trial included 12,092 patients with STEMI who were assigned to subcutaneous fondaparinux 2.5 mg daily compared to UFH (stratum 1) or placebo (stratum 2) if patients had no indication for heparin [29]. Anticoagulation was administered for up to 8 days. Stratum 1 consisted of 5658 patients without planned PCI who had no indication for heparin and were assigned to fondaparinux or placebo. Most of these patients (78%) were treated with streptokinase. Stratum 2 consisted of 6434 patients with an indication for heparin and included patients receiving fibrin-specific fibrinolytic therapy, primary PCI, or no reperfusion. At 30 days, there was a significant reduction in the primary composite endpoint of death or reinfarction for the entire clinical trial population including both strata. When evaluated separately, stratum 1 revealed a significant reduction in death or reinfarction, but this difference was not seen in stratum 2 (those that received heparin). The benefit of fondaparinux was most evident in patients receiving fibrinolytic therapy or for patients not undergoing reperfusion therapy. Among patients undergoing PCI, fondaparinux was associated with an increase in guide-catheter thrombosis and coronary complications. The 2013 ACC/AHA STEMI clinical practice guidelines recommend against the use of fondaparinux as the sole anticoagulant to support primary PCI in STEMI. For patients undergoing reperfusion with fibrinolytic therapy however, fondaparinux is an appropriate alternative when administered with an initial intravenous dose followed by daily subcutaneous injections for up to 8 days [5].

Direct Thrombin Inhibitors (DTI)

Mechanism of Action, Dose, and Monitoring

Direct thrombin inhibitors do not require a cofactor, namely, antithrombin III, to inhibit thrombin (see Fig. 10.3). They are capable of binding to clot-bound thrombin, a pitfall of heparin and LMWH therapy. An immune-mediated thrombocytopenia has not been reported secondary to direct thrombin inhibitor therapy. These differences account for some of the potential advantages of DTIs compared to UFH or LMWH [30].

There are two forms of DTIs: bivalent and univalent. Bivalent DTIs, such as hirudin and bivalirudin, bind to both the active site of thrombin in addition to exosite-1. Univalent DTIs, such as argatroban, bind to only the active site. There is no therapeutic drug monitoring routine available for DTIs. Given poor oral bioavailability, bivalirudin is available as an IV medication with a short half-life of approximately 25 min.

Bivalirudin in NSTE-ACS

While a multitude of DTIs are clinically available, bivalirudin has been the most widely studied and will be the focus of this section. While earlier trials were performed evaluating the use of bivalirudin, these were largely completed prior to the widespread use of PCI or $P2Y_{12}$ receptor blockers. More recent large randomized trials have confirmed the clinical utility of bivalirudin in the setting of contemporary antithrombotic treatment paradigms.

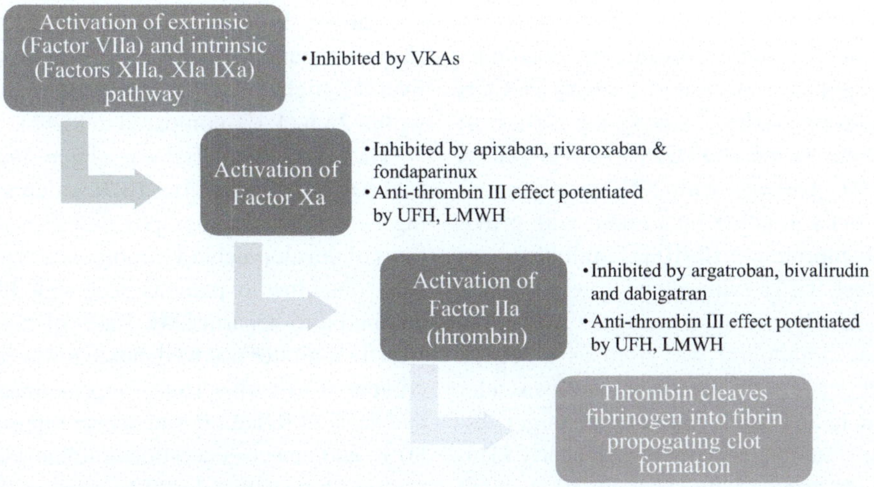

Fig. 10.3 Activation of the coagulation cascade via the extrinsic or intrinsic pathway leads to activation of Factors Xa and finally IIa (thrombin). Pharmacologic targets have been found at multiple levels in this pathway

In the ACUITY trial, a total of 13,819 patients with moderate- or high-risk NSTE-ACS were treated with UFH or enoxaparin with a glycoprotein IIb/IIIa inhibitor, bivalirudin with a glycoprotein IIb/IIIa inhibitor, or bivalirudin alone. Patients were followed for development of a primary composite endpoint of death, MI, or unplanned revascularization at 30 days of follow-up. Patients receiving UFH or enoxaparin with a glycoprotein IIb/IIIa inhibitor compared to bivalirudin with a glycoprotein IIb/IIIa inhibitor had a similar rate of primary outcome events (7.3% and 7.7%, respectively) with a similar rate of bleeding [31]. Bivalirudin alone was associated with similar rates of the primarily endpoint as either strategy including glycoprotein IIb/IIIa inhibition, however, with significantly lower rates of bleeding. Notably, most patients in the ACUITY trial were also treated with clopidogrel. Further discussion about the use of bivalirudin to support primary PCI can be found in the next section.

Bivalirudin in STEMI

The use of bivalirudin as adjunctive anticoagulation to support reperfusion therapy with fibrinolytic medications has not been clinically validated. The ACC/AHA clinical practice guidelines for management of STEMI favor the use of heparin over any direct thrombin inhibitor in this setting.

In contrast, the role of bivalirudin as adjunctive anticoagulation to support primary PCI has been extensively studied. Among the earliest of the large trials is the HORIZONS-AMI trial. A total of 3602 patients with STEMI were randomly assigned to either bivalirudin with provisional glycoprotein IIb/IIIa inhibition or standard-dose UFH with glycoprotein IIb/IIIa inhibition in advance of primary PCI [32]. In most cases, clopidogrel was used as a second antiplatelet agent. A composite cardiovascular endpoint including death, reinfarction, target vessel revascularization, and stroke was nearly identical in both arms of the trial at 30 days of follow-up; however, there was a significantly higher rate of stent thrombosis at 24 h in patients receiving bivalirudin (1.3% compared to 0.3%). In contrast to contemporary management strategies, most cases were performed through femoral arterial access and used primarily clopidogrel instead of newer-generation antiplatelets, and UFH was used with mandated glycoprotein IIb/IIIa inhibitors.

To further establish the role of bivalirudin, the European Ambulance Acute Coronary Syndrome (EUROMAX) was conducted involving 2218 patients with STEMI transported for primary PCI and received either bivalirudin compared to UFH or LMWH [33]. The EUROMAX trial was conducted with notable differences compared to HORIZONS-AMI, including:

1. More frequent radial arterial access (approximately 47% of procedures)
2. Optional glycoprotein IIb/IIIa inhibition (utilized in approximately 60% of patients receiving heparins)
3. Frequent use of newer-generation $P2Y_{12}$ inhibitors (ticagrelor or prasugrel used in approximately 50% of patients)
4. Continued use of bivalirudin for 4 h after PCI to reduce the risk of stent thrombosis

Bivalirudin compared to UFH or LWMH reduced the risk of the primary composite endpoint of death or major bleeding at 30 days (5.1% and 8.5%, respectively), though this difference was driven by a reduction in major bleeding. However, patients treated with bivalirudin had a fivefold higher risk of acute stent thrombosis within 24 h (1.1% compared to 0.2%).

The HEAT-PPCI trial was a large single-center trial performed involving 1829 patients undergoing emergency angiography and showed similar rates of development of a composite primary efficacy outcome in patients receiving bivalirudin compared to heparin [34]. Rates of glycoprotein IIb/IIIa inhibitor use were much lower in this trial compared to earlier trials (approximately 15%), and rates of radial arterial access (approximately 80%) and newer-generation antiplatelet administration (approximately 90%) were much higher. Safety outcomes were similar; however, definite or probable stent thrombosis occurred more often in patients receiving bivalirudin (3.4% compared to 0.9%).

A 2014 meta-analysis was conducted including 16 trials and 33,958 patients treated with bivalirudin compared to heparin in patients planned for PCI. Overall, there was a 9% increase in risk of major adverse cardiac events at 30 days for patients receiving bivalirudin-based regimens compared with heparin-based regimens. There was a significant 38% increase in risk of stent thrombosis for patients treated with bivalirudin. From a safety perspective, bivalirudin did reduce the risk of major bleeding; however, the degree of reduction varied related to concomitant use of glycoprotein IIb/IIIa inhibitors [35].

ACC/AHA clinical practice guidelines support the use of bivalirudin as adjunctive anticoagulant therapy to support primary PCI with or without prior administration of UFH. Caution however should be exercised in patients with CrCl <30 mL/min. Bivalirudin can also be used in patients with STEMI with a prior history of HIT as well as those who receive fibrinolytic therapy who ultimately develop HIT.

Oral Anticoagulant Therapy

Introduction

For a subgroup of patients with acute coronary syndromes, patients may warrant chronic or long-term anticoagulant therapy in addition to traditional dual antithrombotic regimens. Indications for combined dual antithrombotic and anticoagulant therapy, or so-called triple oral anticoagulant therapy (TOAT), exist in patients who experience ACS with or without revascularization and also carry a diagnosis of atrial fibrillation, left ventricular thrombus complicating ACS, history of pulmonary embolism, or a prosthetic heart valve.

The possibility of benefit to oral anticoagulant (OAC) therapy after ACS has also been raised to reduce the risk of recurrent cardiovascular events independent of an alternate indication. The plausibility of this concept is based on the finding that patients who experience ACS have increased activation of the coagulation cascade likely as a result of plaque disruption which exposes tissue factor to the blood vessel lumen. Some data suggests a prolonged period of increased activation of the coagulation cascade beyond the acute insult, suggesting a role for long-term anticoagulation to reduce the risk of recurrent ischemic events [36]. These questions and related evidence supporting clinical practice guidelines will be addressed in the remainder of this chapter.

Mechanism of Action, Dose, and Monitoring of Vitamin K Antagonists

Vitamin K antagonists (VKAs) are a common class of medications used for oral anticoagulant therapy. The prototypical VKA is warfarin and is commonly used in the United States and worldwide. Warfarin functions by inhibiting vitamin K-dependent synthesis of the active forms of clotting factors II, VII, IX, and X and additional regulatory proteins. These clotting factors require gamma carboxylation in order to function through the vitamin-K-dependent enzyme gamma-glutamyl carboxylase. The availability of vitamin K is dependent on the function of a different enzyme, vitamin K epoxide reductase, which is inhibited by warfarin.

VKAs have multiple shortcomings including a narrow therapeutic range, frequent drug-drug interactions, and dosing that is influenced by a multitude of factors including diet and genetics. Anticoagulation with VKAs therefore requires close monitoring. Warfarin is monitored using the prothrombin time with international normalized ratio (INR), which ensures an adequate degree of anticoagulation by reduction in circulating vitamin K-dependent clotting factors. Therapeutic targets for INR are determined by the indication and typical fall between a therapeutic range of values [37]. Time spent below the therapeutic range has been shown to correlate to increased risk of cardiovascular events, and time spent above the therapeutic range has been shown to correlate with increased risk of major bleeding.

VKAs after ACS

The role chronic VKA therapy in the secondary prevention of ACS remains unclear. Two meta-analyses reviewed the use of aspirin plus warfarin versus aspirin alone. The first analysis reviewed 14 trials including over 25,000 patients with follow-up ranging from 3 months to 5 years. Major adverse cardiovascular events including death, nonfatal MI, and nonfatal stroke were reduced in patients who maintained an INR of 2–3 by approximately 27%; however, warfarin also doubled the risk of major bleeding [38]. The second smaller meta-analysis compared the same therapies in approximately 6000 patients across 10 trials; however, most data came from only two trials and patients who underwent PCI were excluded from the analysis. The authors concluded benefit for reduction in cardiovascular events for those at low-intermediate risk of bleeding [39]. National clinical practice guidelines do not provide clear recommendations for the use of aspirin and warfarin for secondary prevention of cardiovascular events given widespread recommendation for using dual antiplatelet therapies with aspirin and $P2Y_{12}$ inhibitors.

Triple Oral Anticoagulant Therapy (TOAT) After ACS

Patients with an indication for long-term anticoagulation, such as atrial fibrillation, history of pulmonary embolism, or a prosthetic heart valve, that have ACS may warrant triple oral anticoagulant therapy. Across the United States, these types of independent indications coexist in 5–10% of patients who undergo coronary artery stenting. The best combination and duration of combined antithrombotic and anticoagulant therapy remains unclear.

The WOEST trial was published in 2013 and included 573 patients who were receiving long-term OAC who were undergoing PCI. Notably, only 25% of patients had a history of ACS events in the study population, and the indication for OAC in 69% of patients was for stroke prophylaxis in atrial fibrillation [40]. Trial patients were randomized to receive aspirin, clopidogrel, and OAC compared to clopidogrel and OAC. Duration of antiplatelet therapy was determined by the type of stent placed per the study protocol. After a median follow-up of almost 1 year, bleeding episodes more than doubled in patients receiving clopidogrel plus OAC compared to patients receiving TOAT (19.4 versus 44.4%). While the study was not powered to assess adequacy in prevention of major adverse cardiovascular events, there was a significant reduction in a combined endpoint of death, MI, stroke, target vessel revascularization, and stent thrombosis. There was also a significant reduction in all-cause death in patients receiving clopidogrel and OAC (2.5 versus 6.3%, CI 0.16–0.93), though this finding has been questioned given the study was not powered to detect this difference.

Other clinical trials have evaluated use of short-term TOAT following stent implantation given the higher risk of stent thrombosis in the first month after placement. In the ISAR-TRIPLE trial, 614 patients undergoing drug-eluting stent placement were randomized to a strategy of aspirin, clopidogrel, and OAC for 6 weeks versus 6 months [41]. After completion of TOAT, patients were planned to receive aspirin and OAC indefinitely. Approximately 70% of patients underwent stent implantation for stable angina, and 84% maintained an indication for oral anticoagulation because of atrial fibrillation. The primary endpoint was a composite of death, MI, stent thrombosis, stroke, or TIMI major bleeding at 9 months with no significant difference found between those receiving TOAT in the 6-week versus 6-month arm (9.8 versus 8.8%).

Based on these trials, some have suggested that prolonged use of triple therapy after stent implantation for patients with an independent indication for oral anticoagulation may not be necessary. But the choice of antiplatelets and anticoagulants and duration of TOAT remain contested, especially in patients with ACS who represented small proportions of patients in these larger trials. ACC/AHA clinical practice guidelines suggest that the duration of triple antithrombotic therapy with a VKA, aspirin, and $P2Y_{12}$ inhibitor should be minimized to the extent possible to limit the risk of bleeding. Patients receiving VKAs should have INR values targeted to lower INR goals, e.g., 2.0–2.5, if possible. Clinicians typically make decisions based on bleeding risk, thromboembolic risk, and type of stent.

Bleeding Risk

While potent and multipronged antithrombotic and anticoagulant therapy has helped to reduce the risk of recurrent ischemic events, implementation of these therapies has strongly predicted risk of bleeding. Multiple predictive models for bleeding risk have been created. The CRUSADE bleeding risk score was developed using eight independent predictors of in-hospital major bleeding for patients admitted with NSTEMI [42] and subsequently has been validated in patients with STEMI. The score combines baseline patient characteristics (sex, history of diabetes, history of peripheral vascular disease) with admission variables (heart rate, blood pressure, signs of CHF, hematocrit, and creatinine clearance) to determine the risk of bleeding. As seen in Fig. 10.4, patients starting with very low CRUSADE scores (≤20) had a risk of major in-hospital bleeding of 3.5% in the validation cohort, while those with very high CRUSADE scores (41–50) had a risk of major in-hospital bleeding of 19.3% (Fig. 10.4).

The European Society of Cardiology (ESC) also advocates use of the Hypertension, Abnormal Renal or Liver Function, Stroke, Bleeding History of Predisposition, Labile International Normalized Ratio, Elderly, Drugs/Alcohol Concomitantly (HAS-BLED) score for patients with atrial fibrillation who require dual antiplatelet therapy and OAC for risk stratification. The HAS-BLED score established a risk score in over 5000 ambulatory patients utilizing clinical features including history of hypertension, stroke, labile INRs, alcohol use prior bleeding, renal disease, liver disease, or age >65 years to determine bleeding risk at 1 year. A number of antithrombotic and anticoagulant recommendations have been created, stratified by low-moderate HAS-BLED scores (0–2 clinical variables are present) and high HAS-BLED scores (≥3 clinical variables are present), as illustrated in Fig. 10.5. For example, a patient who presents with ACS and has an indication for anticoagulation due to atrial fibrillation that has a high HAS-BLED score would receive 4 weeks of triple therapy with aspirin, clopidogrel, and OAC, followed by up to 12 months of clopidogrel and OAC, followed by reversion to OAC indefinitely [43] (Fig. 10.5).

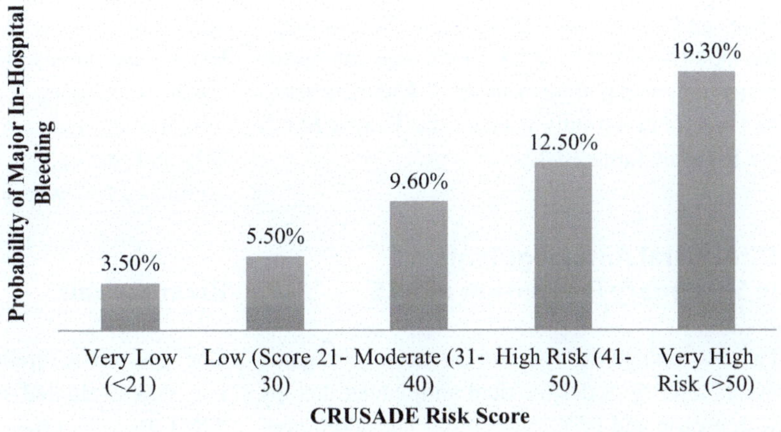

Fig. 10.4 The CRUSADE score predicts the risk of in-hospital major bleeding in patients who present to the hospital for non-ST-segment elevation MI [42]

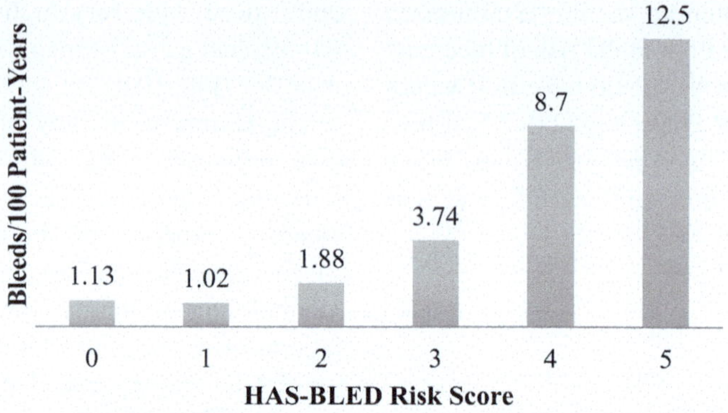

Fig. 10.5 The HAS-BLED risk score predicts risk of bleeding in anticoagulated patients with atrial fibrillation. The score incorporates clinical variables including hypertension, stroke, labile INRs, alcohol use prior bleeding, renal disease, liver disease, or age >65 years to determine bleeding risk at 1 year [43]

Direct Oral Anticoagulants

Mechanism of Action, Dose, and Monitoring

Recent development of newer-generation, direct oral anticoagulants have been clinically validated to help overcome shortcomings of VKA therapy. These medications largely have a more stable pharmacokinetic profile allowing once- or twice-daily administration without routine monitoring. Drug-drug interactions are reduced, and these drugs can be utilized in select patients with chronic kidney disease. Mechanisms of action of DOACs directly inhibit different portions of the coagulation cascade. Dabigatran functions by direct inhibition of thrombin. Rivaroxaban, apixaban, and edoxaban inhibit factor Xa, although the latter does not have an established role in the management of patients with ACS. Characteristics of DOACs commonly used in the United States are listed in Table 10.4.

Direct Oral Anticoagulants in Secondary Prevention of ACS

Patients remain at risk for recurrent ischemic events after ACS despite dual antiplatelet therapy with aspirin and $P2Y_{12}$ inhibition. The addition of vitamin K antagonists has been shown to portend a significant risk of bleeding, with at least two trials suggesting 30–40% of patients on TOAT will have bleeding events within 9–12 months. Since their development, direct oral anticoagulants have also been utilized in the treatment of patients with ACS to reduce recurrent ischemic events.

Dabigatran

In the RE-DEEM trial, 1861 patients with STEMI or NSTEMI on dual antiplatelet therapy were randomized to receive dabigatran at one of four doses (50, 75, 110, and 150 mg) or placebo. Patients were followed for development of major or clinically relevant minor bleeding. At 6 months of follow-up, there was a clear dose-dependent increase in the primary bleeding outcome with odds ratio ranging from 1.82 to 3.88 across escalating dose ranges [45]. There was a trend toward fewer secondary composite outcome events, which included cardiovascular death, nonfatal MI, and stroke, on higher doses of dabigatran compared to lower doses.

Rivaroxaban

The role of the direct oral Xa inhibitor rivaroxaban was evaluated in two ACS trials: ATLAS-TIMI-46, a phase II trial, and ATLAS-ACS2-TIMI-51, a phase III trial. The latter

Table 10.4 Characteristics of direct oral anticoagulants [44]

	Dabigatran	Rivaroxaban	Apixaban
Target	Factor IIa (thrombin)	Factor Xa	Factor Xa
Bioavailability	7%	80%	66%
Renal elimination	80%	66%	27%
Prodrug	Yes	No	No
Half-life	12–14 h	9–13 h	8–15 h
Time to peak action	1–2 h	2–4 h	1–3 h
Dosing in PE and AF	Twice daily	Daily	Twice daily
Available reversal agent?	Yes (idarucizumab)	No	No

PE pulmonary embolism, *AF* atrial fibrillation

included 15,526 patients with recent ACS receiving aspirin and $P2Y_{12}$ inhibitors who were randomized to a low dose of rivaroxaban at either 2.5 mg twice daily, 5 mg twice daily, or placebo. For reference, patients with normal renal function on maintenance doses for stroke prevention in atrial fibrillation or prevention of recurrent pulmonary embolism receive 20 mg daily. This low-dose strategy was determined by ATLAS-ACS-TIMI-46, a phase 2 dose-finding trial involving 3491 patients. The phase III trial followed patients for a mean of 13 months for development of a primary composite endpoint of cardiovascular death, MI, or stroke. Rivaroxaban resulted in a significant reduction in the frequency of the primary outcome to 8.9 versus 10.7% at both doses compared to placebo. Death from any cause was also significantly reduced for those treated with rivaroxaban 2.5 mg twice daily (2.9 versus 4.5%), though this was not seen for the higher dose. Major bleeding and intracranial bleeding was significantly higher in patients receiving rivaroxaban; however, there was no increase in fatal bleeding [46, 47]. Low-dose rivaroxaban was approved by the European Medicines Agency in March of 2013 though not yet by the US Food and Drug Administration.

With regard to stable atherosclerotic disease, the double-blind randomized controlled COMPASS trial evaluated the use of rivaroxaban in patients with stable atherosclerotic vascular disease. The primary outcome consisted of a composite of cardiovascular death, stroke, or myocardial infarction. A total of 27,395 patients were randomized to one of three arms receiving either rivaroxaban 2.5 mg twice daily plus aspirin 100 mg/day ($n = 9152$), rivaroxaban 5 mg daily ($n = 9117$), or aspirin 100 mg/day ($n = 9126$) [48]. To be included in the study, patients had to demonstrate stable atherosclerotic vascular disease, or specifically, atherosclerosis identified in two or more vascular beds, or have two additional risk factors that included tobacco use, diabetes mellitus, congestive heart failure, renal insufficiency, and nonlacunar ischemic stroke ≥1 month. The mean follow-up period was only 23 months, but because the primary endpoint for major adverse cardiovascular events met its pre-specified criteria for superiority in the rivaroxaban-plus-aspirin group, the trial was stopped earlier than planned. Within the rivaroxaban-plus-aspirin group, the primary outcome was met in 4.1%. In comparison, the primary outcome occurred in 4.9% within the rivaroxaban-alone group and in 5.4% within the aspirin-alone group ($p < 0.001$ for rivaroxaban-plus-aspirin versus aspirin alone; $p = 0.12$ for rivaroxaban alone versus aspirin alone) [48].

However, the significant comparative decrease in primary outcome within the rivaroxaban-plus-aspirin group was counterbalanced by a notable increase in major bleeding events, with 3.1% within the rivaroxaban-plus-aspirin group. The rate was 2.8% within the rivaroxaban-alone cohort and 1.9% within the aspirin-alone group ($p < 0.001$ for both rivaroxaban-plus-aspirin versus aspirin alone and rivaroxaban alone versus aspirin alone). Although major bleeding events were significantly higher for the rivaroxaban-plus-aspirin group, events such as fatal or critical organ bleeding were not higher. Further analyses are still needed to determine the role of anticoagulants such as rivaroxaban and other DOACs in the treatment of atherosclerotic vascular disease. The identification of appropriate patients who will benefit from addition of low-dose oral anticoagulants to antiplatelet therapy will be likely be an important factor should guidelines change to reflect findings from COMPASS [48].

Apixaban

Apixaban, another oral factor Xa inhibitor, has been studied in patients with acute coronary syndromes as well. The APPRAISE-2 trial included 7392 patients with a recent acute coronary syndrome at high risk for a recurrent event already taking standard antiplatelet therapy. Patients were randomized to receive placebo or apixaban 5 mg twice daily, which is equivalent to standard-dose therapeutic anticoagulation for stroke prophylaxis for patients with atrial fibrillation with normal renal function [49]. Patients were followed for development of a primary composite cardiovascular efficacy outcome that included cardiovascular death, MI, and ischemic stroke; however, the trial was stopped early due to an increase in major bleeding events for patients receiving apixaban, including intracranial and fatal bleeding.

Current national clinical practice guidelines do not provide recommendations about use of any DOAC for prevention of recurrent cardiovascular events in patients who do not have an independent indication for OAC.

The use of DOACs in patients for stroke prophylaxis in non-valvular atrial fibrillation and prevention of recurrent venous thromboembolism (VTE) is well-established. When patients taking these medications develop an ACS, clinical practice varies significantly about the appropriate choice and duration of a combined antithrombotic and anticoagulant strategy. The first DOAC studied in a large, randomized trial involving patients with ACS with independent indications for OAC was rivaroxaban in the PIONEER-AF-PCI trial [50]. A total of 2124 patients with non-valvular atrial fibrillation undergoing PCI were randomized 1:1:1 to receive a $P2Y_{12}$ inhibitor plus rivaroxaban 15 mg daily (group 1), aspirin plus $P2Y_{12}$ inhibitor plus rivaroxaban 2.5 mg twice daily (group 2, similar to the ATLAS-TIMI-51 strategy), or standard therapy with dose-adjusted VKA therapy (group 3). Patients were followed for development of clinically significant bleeding, which occurred significantly less often in patients receiving any strategy with rivaroxaban compared to those receiving standard therapy (16.8% in group 1, 18.0% in group 2 and 26.7% in group 3). The rate of development of cardiovascular events was similar in all groups. Notably, NSTE-ACS occurred in approximately 50% of trial patients.

Forthcoming clinical trials will provide clarity and add to the growing evidence base about anticoagulant strategies incorporating DOACs in patients undergoing PCI who have other indications for OAC. The REDUAL-PCI trial will randomize patients undergoing PCI to receive dabigatran plus a $P2Y_{12}$ inhibitor (clopidogrel or ticagrelor) compared to aspirin, warfarin plus $P2Y_{12}$ inhibitor. Patients undergoing PCI electively or for ACS will be included in this trial and will be followed for the development of major or clinical relevant non-major bleeding events [51]. The AUGUSTUS trial of apixaban (NCT02415400) and the ENTRUST-PCI trial of edoxaban (NCT02866175) have also been designed to test their safety and efficacy in combined antithrombotic and anticoagulant regimens following PCI. Similar trials including apixaban and edoxaban have also been announced.

Key Points

- Acute coronary syndromes (ACS) refer to a group of clinical syndromes leading to acute myocardial ischemia related to reduced coronary artery blood flow and include STEMI and NSTE-ACS.
- All patients with STEMI and NSTE-ACS should be treated with prompt initiation of anticoagulation therapy. Choice of anticoagulation with unfractionated heparin, enoxaparin,

fondaparinux, or bivalirudin should be based on therapeutic strategy, e.g., emergent revascularization, fibrinolytic therapy, delayed invasive therapy, or lack of reperfusion.

- Patients with an indication for long-term anticoagulation, such as atrial fibrillation, history of venous thromboembolism, or a prosthetic heart valve that have ACS, may warrant TOAT. The need for and duration of TOAT have been the topic of much research and discussion. In general, limited courses of TOAT are desired to reduce bleeding risk.
- DOACs have recently been evaluated in secondary prevention of ACS. While no trials have demonstrated a safe and effective dose, further studies are ongoing. Clinical practice continues to vary significantly about the appropriate choice and duration of a combined antithrombotic and anticoagulant strategy when utilizing DOACs.

Self-Assessment Questions

1. A 50-year-old man with a history of hyperlipidemia presents to the emergency department with substernal chest discomfort. ECG reveals lateral T-wave inversions. Laboratory testing is notable for a normal CBC and troponin T of 0.16 mg/dL (ref range, <0.01 mg/dL). He is administered aspirin 325 mg, clopidogrel 300 mg, atorvastatin 80 mg, and intravenous heparin 4000 IU followed by a drip at 1000 IU/h. You recommend admission to the cardiology floor. Over the following 5 days, he remains free of angina and has no symptoms of heart failure. His physical exam is notable for new asymmetric left lower extremity swelling. Complete blood count reveals a platelet count of 90,000 × 10^9/L (ref range, 150–450 × 10^9/L). What is the next step in management?
   (a) Continue intravenous unfractionated heparin.
   (b) Discontinue intravenous unfractionated heparin.
   (c) Discontinue intravenous unfractionated heparin and start intravenous argatroban.
   (d) Add aspirin 325 mg daily to his regimen.
2. A 59-year-old man with a history of gastroesophageal reflux disease and osteoarthritis presents to the emergency department with crushing substernal chest pain for the past 12 h. ECG reveals anterior ST elevations in leads V2–V5. Laboratory testing is notable for troponin T of 1.21 mg/dL (ref range, <0.01 mg/dL). He is administered aspirin 325 mg, clopidogrel 300 mg, and atorvastatin 80 mg. Cardiology consultation is requested, and the patient is referred for emergent coronary angiography and primary PCI. While examining his medical history, you notice he has a remote history of heparin-induced thrombocytopenia. Which of the following is an acceptable alternative as adjunctive anticoagulation for this patient?
   (a) Enoxaparin
   (b) Bivalirudin
   (c) Fondaparinux
   (d) Unfractionated heparin with glycoprotein IIb/IIIa inhibition
   (e) Primary PCI is contraindicated in this patient
3. A 46-year-old woman with a family history of coronary artery disease presents to the emergency department with indigestion for the past 6 h. ECG reveals inferolateral ST elevations. Laboratory testing is notable for troponin T of 0.86 mg/dL (ref range, <0.01 mg/dL). She receives aspirin 325 mg, clopidogrel 300 mg, atorvastatin 80 mg, and fondaparinux 2.5 mg IV. Cardiology consultation is requested, and the patient is referred for emergent coronary angiography and primary PCI. Which of the following is an acceptable adjunctive anticoagulation strategy to support primary PCI for this patient?
   (a) Administer fondaparinux 2.5 mg IV
   (b) Administer fondaparinux 2.5 mg SC

(c) Administer weight-based Lovenox SC
(d) Administer IV bolus of unfractionated heparin
(e) Primary PCI is contraindicated in this patient

4. A healthy 39-year-old man with no significant past medical history presents to the emergency department with substernal chest discomfort for the past 3 h. ECG reveals anterolateral ST depressions. Laboratory testing is notable for troponin T of 0.16 mg/dL (ref range, <0.01 mg/dL). He receives aspirin 325 mg, clopidogrel 300 mg, atorvastatin 80 mg, and UFH 4000 U IV followed by a drip at 1000 U/h. Coronary angiography is pursued, and the patient receives a drug-eluting stent to the left anterior descending coronary artery and he is started on maintenance aspirin and clopidogrel. He has no history of bleeding. Transthoracic echocardiography reveals an anterior and apical wall motion abnormality with evidence of left ventricular thrombus. Which of the following anticoagulation strategies is supported by clinical practice guidelines?
(a) Discontinue clopidogrel and start warfarin for 6 months
(b) Apixaban 5 mg twice daily for 1 year
(c) Rivaroxaban 20 mg daily for 1 year
(d) Initial triple antithrombotic therapy with aspirin, clopidogrel, and warfarin for the minimal duration possible to limit bleeding risk
(e) Oral anticoagulation is contraindicated given the patient is receiving dual antiplatelet therapy

Self-Assessment Answers

1. (c) Discontinue intravenous unfractionated heparin and start intravenous argatroban

   Patients with heparin-induced thrombocytopenia frequently present with falling platelet levels after 5–10 days of heparin therapy. They may also present with an acute thrombus, such as a deep vein thrombosis.

2. (b) Bivalirudin

   In patients with a history of heparin-induced thrombocytopenia who present with an acute coronary syndrome, use of bivalirudin is the preferred anticoagulant. Fondaparinux has been associated with increased risk of catheter-associated thrombosis during cardiac catheterization.

3. (d) Administer IV bolus of unfractionated heparin

   Unfractionated heparin is the first-line anticoagulant for patients presenting with STEMI who are planning to undergo primary PCI.

4. (d) Initial triple antithrombotic therapy with aspirin, clopidogrel, and warfarin for the minimal duration possible to limit bleeding risk

   Patient with indications for both anticoagulant therapy and DAPT should be treated with TOAT for as short a period of time as necessary following PCI.

References

1. Newby LK, Jesse RL, Babb JD, et al. ACCF 2012 expert consensus document on practical clinical considerations in the interpretation of troponin elevations: a report of the American College of Cardiology Foundation Task Force on Clinical Expert Consensus Documents. J Am Coll Cardiol. 2012;60:2427–63.
2. Thygesen K, Alpert JS, Jaffe AS, et al. Third universal definition of myocardial infarction. J Am Coll Cardiol. 2012;60:1581–98.
3. Davies M. The pathophysiology of acute coronary syndromes. Heart. 2000;83:361–6.
4. National Heart, Lung, and Blood Institute; National Institutes of Health; U.S. Department of Health and Human Services.
5. O'Gara PT, Kushner FG, Ascheim DD, Casey DE Jr, Chung MK, de Lemos JA, et al. 2013 ACCF/AHA guideline for the management of ST-elevation myocardial infarction: a report of the American College of Cardiology Foundation/American Heart Association Task Force on Practice Guidelines. Circulation. 2013;127(4):e362.
6. Amsterdam EA, Wenger NK, Brindis RG, Casey DE Jr, Ganiats TG, Holmes DR Jr, et al. 2014 AHA/ACC guideline for the management of patients with non-ST-elevation acute coronary syndromes: executive summary: a report of the American College of Cardiology/American Heart Association Task Force on Practice Guidelines. Circulation. 2014;130(25):2354.
7. Wietz J, Hudoba M, Massel D, Maragnore J, Hirsh J. Clot-bound thrombin is protected from inhibition by heparin-antithrombin III but is susceptible to inactivation by antithrombin III-independent inhibitors. J Clin Invest. 1990;86(2):385.

8. Warkentin TE, Greinacher A, Koster A, Lincoff AM, American College of Chest Physicians. Treatment and prevention of heparin-induced thrombocytopenia: American College of Chest Physicians Evidence-Based Clinical Practice Guidelines (8th edition). Chest. 2008;133(6 Suppl):340S.
9. Oler A, Whooley MA, Oler J, Grady D. Adding heparin to aspirin reduces the incidence of myocardial infarction and death in patients with unstable angina. A meta-analysis. JAMA. 1996;276(10):811–5.
10. Theroux P, Ouimet H, McCans J, et al. Aspirin, heparin, or both to treat acute unstable angina. N Engl J Med. 1988;319:1105–11.
11. The RISC Group. Risk of myocardial infarction and death during treatment with low dose aspirin and intravenous heparin in men with unstable coronary artery disease: the RISC Group. Lancet. 1990;336:827–30.
12. Cohen M, Adams PC, Hawkins L, Bach M, Fuster V. Usefulness of antithrombotic therapy in resting angina pectoris or non-Q-wave myocardial infarction in preventing death and myocardial infarction (a pilot study from the Antithrombotic Therapy in Acute Coronary Syndromes Study Group). Am J Cardiol. 1990;66:1287–92.
13. Cohen M, Adams PC, Parry G, et al. Combination antithrombotic therapy in unstable rest angina and non-Q-wave infarction in nonprior aspirin users: primary end points analysis from the ATACS trial: Antithrombotic Therapy in Acute Coronary Syndromes Research Group. Circulation. 1994;89:81–8.
14. Holdright D, Patel D, Cunningham D, et al. Comparison of the effect of heparin and aspirin versus aspirin alone on transient myocardial ischemia and in-hospital prognosis in patients with unstable angina. J Am Coll Cardiol. 1994;24:39–45.
15. Gurfinkel EP, Manos EJ, Mejail RI, et al. Low molecular weight heparin versus regular heparin or aspirin in the treatment of unstable angina and silent ischemia. J Am Coll Cardiol. 1995;26:313–8.
16. Juergens CP, Semsarian C, Keech AC, Beller EM, Harris PJ, et al. Hemorrhagic complications of intravenous heparin use. Am J Cardiol. 1997;80(2):150.
17. Fitchett D. The impact of bleeding in patients with acute coronary syndromes: how to optimize the benefits of treatment and minimize the risk. Can J Cardiol. 2007;23(8):663–71.
18. Greinacher A. Heparin-induced thrombocytopenia. N Engl J Med. 2015;373:252–61.
19. Linkins LA, Dans AL, Moores LK, Bona R, Davidson BL, Schulman S, et al. Treatment and prevention of heparin-induced thrombocytopenia: antithrombotic therapy and prevention of thrombosis 9th ed: American College of Chest Physicians Evidence-Based Clinical Practice Guidelines. Chest. 2012;141(2 Suppl):e495S–530S.
20. Hirsh J, Levine MN. Low molecular weight heparin. Blood. 1992;79(1):1.
21. Cohen M, Demers C, Gurfinkel EP, Turpie AG, Fromell GJ, Goodman S, et al. A comparison of low-molecular-weight heparin with unfractionated heparin for unstable coronary artery disease. Efficacy and Safety of Subcutaneous Enoxaparin in Non-Q-Wave Coronary Events Study Group. N Engl J Med. 1997;337(7):447.
22. Goodman SG, Cohen M, Bigonzi F, Gurfinkel EP, Radley DR, Le Iouer V, et al. Randomized trial of low molecular weight heparin (enoxaparin) versus unfractionated heparin for unstable coronary artery disease: one-year results of the ESSENCE Study. Efficacy and Safety of Subcutaneous Enoxaparin in Non-Q Wave Coronary Events. J Am Coll Cardiol. 2000;36(3):693.
23. Antman EM, McCabe CH, Gurfinkel EP, Turpie AG, Bernink PJ, Salein D, et al. Enoxaparin prevents death and cardiac ischemic events in unstable angina/non-Q-wave myocardial infarction. Results of the thrombolysis in myocardial infarction (TIMI) 11B trial. Circulation. 1999;100(15):1593.
24. Ferguson JJ, Califf RM, Antman EM, Cohen M, Grines CL, Goodman S, et al. Enoxaparin vs unfractionated heparin in high-risk patients with non-ST-segment elevation acute coronary syndromes managed with an intended early invasive strategy: primary results of the SYNERGY randomized trial. JAMA. 2004;292(1):45.
25. Silvain J, Beygui F, Barthélémy O, Pollack C Jr, Cohen M, Zeymer U, et al. Efficacy and safety of enoxaparin versus unfractionated heparin during percutaneous coronary intervention: systematic review and meta-analysis. BMJ. 2012;344:e553.
26. Montalescot G, Zeymer U, Silvain J, Boulanger B, Cohen M, Goldstein P, et al. Intravenous enoxaparin or unfractionated heparin in primary percutaneous coronary intervention for ST-elevation myocardial infarction: the international randomised open-label ATOLL trial. Lancet. 2011;378(9792):693–703.
27. Murphy SA, Gibson CM, Morrow DA, Van de Werf F, Menown IB, Goodman SG, et al. Efficacy and safety of the low-molecular weight heparin enoxaparin compared with unfractionated heparin across the acute coronary syndrome spectrum: a meta-analysis. Eur Heart J. 2007;28(17):2077.
28. Yusuf S, Mehta SR, Chrolavicius S, Afzal R, Pogue J, Granger CB, et al. Comparison of fondaparinux and enoxaparin in acute coronary syndromes. N Engl J Med. 2006;354(14):1464.
29. Yusuf S, Mehta SR, Chrolavicius S, Afzal R, Pogue J, Granger CB, et al. Effects of fondaparinux on mortality and reinfarction in patients with acute ST-segment elevation myocardial infarction: the OASIS-6 randomized trial. JAMA. 2006;295(13):1519.
30. Van De Car DA, Rao SV, Ohman EM. Bivalirudin: a review of the pharmacology and clinical application. Expert Rev Cardiovasc Ther. 2010;8(12):1673–81.
31. Stone GW, McLaurin BT, Cox DA, Bertrand ME, Lincoff AM, Moses JW, et al. Bivalirudin for patients with acute coronary syndromes. N Engl J Med. 2006;355(21):2203.
32. Stone GW, Witzenbichler B, Guagliumi G, Peruga JZ, Brodie BR, Dudek D, et al. Bivalirudin during primary PCI in acute myocardial infarction. N Engl J Med. 2008;358(21):2218.
33. Steg PG, van't Hof A, Hamm CW, Clemmensen P, Lapostolle F, Coste P, et al. Bivalirudin started during

emergency transport for primary PCI. N Engl J Med. 2013;369(23):2207.
34. Shahzad A, Kemp I, Mars C, Wilson K, Roome C, Cooper R, et al. Unfractionated heparin versus bivalirudin in primary percutaneous coronary intervention (HEAT-PPCI): an open-label, single centre, randomised controlled trial. Lancet. 2014;384(9957):1849–58.
35. Cavender MA, Sabatine MS. Bivalirudin versus heparin in patients planned for percutaneous coronary intervention: a meta-analysis of randomised controlled trials. Lancet. 2014;384(9943):599–606.
36. Williams MJ, Morison IM, Parker JH, Stewart RA. Progression of the culprit lesion in unstable coronary artery disease with warfarin and aspirin versus aspirin alone: preliminary study. J Am Coll Cardiol. 1997;30(2):364.
37. Oake N, Jennings A, Forster AJ, Fergusson D, Doucette S, van Walraven C. Anticoagulation intensity and outcomes among patients prescribed oral anticoagulant therapy: a systematic review and meta-analysis. CMAJ. 2008;179(3):235.
38. Andreotti F, Testa L, Biondi-Zoccai GG, Crea F. Aspirin plus warfarin compared to aspirin alone after acute coronary syndromes: an updated and comprehensive meta-analysis of 25,307 patients. Eur Heart J. 2006;27(5):519.
39. Rothberg MB, Celestin C, Fiore LD, Lawler E, Cook JR. Warfarin plus aspirin after myocardial infarction or the acute coronary syndrome: meta-analysis with estimates of risk and benefit. Ann Intern Med. 2005;143(4):241.
40. Dewilde WJ, Oirbans T, Verheugt FW, Kelder JC, De Smet BJ, Herrman JP. Use of clopidogrel with or without aspirin in patients taking oral anticoagulant therapy and undergoing percutaneous coronary intervention: an open-label, randomised, controlled trial. Lancet. 2013;381(9872):1107.
41. Fiedler KA, Maeng M, Mehili J, et al. Duration of triple therapy in patients requiring oral anticoagulation after drug-eluting stent implantation: The ISAR-TRIPLE Trial. J Am Coll Cardiol. 2015;65:1619–29.
42. Subherwal S, Bach RG, Chen AY, Gage BF, Rao SV, Newby K, et al. Baseline risk of major bleeding in non-ST-segment-elevation myocardial infarction: the CRUSADE bleeding score. Circulation. 2009;119:1873–182.
43. Roffi M, Patrono C, Collet JP, Mueller C, Valgimigli M, Andreotti F, et al. 2015 ESC guidelines for the management of acute coronary syndromes in patients presenting without persistent ST-segment elevation: Task Force for the Management of Acute Coronary Syndromes in Patients Presenting without Persistent ST-Segment Elevation of the European Society of Cardiology (ESC). Eur Heart J. 2016;37(3):267.
44. Kaatz S, Kouides PA, Garcia DA, Spyropoulous AC, Crowther M, Douketis JD. Guidance on the emergent reversal of oral thrombin and factor Xa inhibitors. Am J Hematol. 2012;87(Suppl 1):S141–5.
45. Oldgren J, Budaj A, Granger CB, Khder Y, Roberts J, Siegbahn A, et al. Dabigatran vs. placebo in patients with acute coronary syndromes on dual antiplatelet therapy: a randomized, double-blind, phase II trial. Eur Heart J. 2011;32(22):2781–9.
46. Mega JL, Braunwald E, Mohanavelu S, et al. Rivaroxaban versus placebo in patients with acute coronary syndromes (ATLAS ACS-TIMI 46): a randomised, double-blind, phase II trial. Lancet. 2009;374:29–38.
47. Mega J, Braunwald E, Wiviott S, Bassand J, Bhatt D, Bode C, et al. Rivaroxaban in patients with a recent acute coronary syndrome. N Engl J Med. 2012;366:9–19.
48. Eikelboom JW, Connolly SJ, Bosch J, Dagenais GR, Hart RG, Shestakovska O, COMPASS Investigators, et al. Rivaroxaban with or without aspirin in stable cardiovascular disease. N Engl J Med. 2017;377(14):1319–30.
49. Alexander JH, Lopes RD, James S, Kilaru R, He Y, Mohan P, Bhatt DL, et al. Apixaban with antiplatelet therapy after acute coronary syndrome. N Engl J Med. 2011;365(8):699.
50. Gibson CM, Mehran R, Bode C, Halperin J, Verheugt FW, Wildgoose P, et al. Prevention of bleeding in patients with atrial fibrillation undergoing PCI. N Engl J Med. 2016;375:2423–34.
51. Cannon CP, Gropper S, Bhatt DL, Ellis SG, Kimura T, Lip GY, et al. Design and rationale of the RE-DUAL PCI trial: a prospective, randomized, phase 3b study comparing the safety and efficacy of dual antithrombotic therapy with dabigatran etexilate versus warfarin triple therapy in patients with nonvalvular atrial fibrillation who have undergone percutaneous coronary intervention with stenting. Clin Cardiol. 2016;39(10):555–64.

11 Antithrombotic Therapy for Patients with Atrial Fibrillation

Kyla M. Lara and Jonathan L. Halperin

Clinical Vignettes

Case 1: *A 78-year-old woman with no known medical problems is found on a routine office visit to have asymptomatic atrial fibrillation. The ventricular rate is ~88 bpm and blood pressure is normal. There are no abnormalities on cardiovascular examination aside from the rhythm. In anticipation of cardioversion, she undergoes transesophageal echocardiography, which reveals left atrial enlargement and dense spontaneous echo-contrast in the left atrium. Ventricular and valvular function is normal. Before electrical cardioversion is performed, sinus rhythm transiently resumes, but atrial fibrillation then recurs, all without her symptomatic awareness of the changes in rhythm.*

Case 2: *A 58-year-old overweight man with a history of hypertension, obstructive sleep apnea, and recent deployment of a drug-eluting coronary stent complains of palpitations. He is currently taking aspirin, clopidogrel, metoprolol, and atorvastatin. The electrocardiogram shows atrial fibrillation with controlled ventricular response and no evidence of ischemia. Transthoracic echocardiography shows mild left ventricular hypertrophy with preserved systolic function and considerable left atrial enlargement.*

Introduction

As early as 1658, Johann Jakob Wepfer described a link between an irregular pulse and stroke. Today, atrial fibrillation (AF) is recognized as the most common clinically significant cardiac arrhythmia, affecting some 3 million Americans—about 1% of the population—and countless millions more worldwide [1]. Both the prevalence and risk associated with AF increase with age, with 70% of affected patients between 65 and 85 years old. A substantial portion of AF goes unrecognized due to under-sampling, asymptomatic, and paroxysmal forms, and ischemic stroke is often its first clinical manifestation [2]. The risk of stroke among patients with AF varies with genetic factors and ethnicity and with comorbidities that include hypertension, diabetes, structural heart disease,

K. M. Lara
Department of Medicine, The Icahn School of Medicine at Mount Sinai, New York, NY, USA
e-mail: kyla.lara@mountsinai.org

J. L. Halperin (✉)
The Cardiovascular Institute, Mount Sinai Medical Center, New York, NY, USA
e-mail: jonathan.halperin@mssm.edu

J. F. Lau et al. (eds.), *Anticoagulation Therapy*, https://doi.org/10.1007/978-3-319-73709-6_11

and heart failure, while the risk in patients with AF without other risk factors is barely distinguishable from that of patients with normal sinus rhythm. The average risk of stroke may be lower than the 5% annual rate observed in the placebo arms of randomized trials conducted a generation ago but is at least twice as high among those with prior stroke. Beyond its significance as a risk factor for ischemic stroke, AF is also associated with an incremental risk of mortality that persists even when effective stroke prevention therapy is employed.

The fundamental circulatory defect associated with AF is ineffective atrial contraction resulting in stasis of blood that can lead to thrombus formation, most often in the left atrial appendage (LAA). Mechanisms other than stasis, however, must contribute to the occurrence of thromboembolic events, which require propulsion of thrombus into the systemic circulation. The pathogenesis involves a complex interplay of endothelial dysfunction, procoagulant factors, inflammation, neurohumoral activation, structural pathology of the atrial myocardium, and abnormal flow patterns in the LAA [3]. The fundamental atrial pathology associated with AF is fibrosis that arises as a nonspecific response to remodeling, apoptosis, and/or necrosis of atrial myocytes and involves the complex interplay of several fibroproliferative signaling pathways [4]. Whether and how the development of the fibrotic atrial cardiomyopathy that characterizes AF histologically mediates the relationship between the arrhythmia and clinical events remains speculative, as do the mechanisms underlying the relationship between aging and the sequelae of AF (Fig. 11.1).

Strategies for clinical management of patients with AF involve control of the ventricular rate, anticoagulation, and, in patients who remain symptomatic, measures to restore and maintain sinus rhythm. Rate control reduces the risk of ischemia, ventricular dysfunction, and heart failure, which promote stasis and adversely impact prognosis. Early cardioversion is essential in patients who develop hemodynamic instability (myocardial ischemia, pulmonary edema, or cardiogenic shock) in response to the onset of AF, whereas in those with more stable presentations or AF of longer duration, the decision to pursue a rate control vs. rhythm control strategy should acknowledge that neither survival nor the risk of thromboembolism is necessarily enhanced by targeting the rhythm alone [5–8]. The failure of a rhythm control strategy to improve outcomes other than arrhythmia symptoms in clinical trials may be related to recurrent AF, atrial electrical-mechanical discordance, pro-arrhythmic toxicity of anti-arrhythmic drugs, and the risks associated with catheter-based or surgical ablation procedures. Conversely, a rate control strategy fails to ameliorate progressive anatomical and electrical remodeling of the atria that diminishes the likelihood of restoring and maintaining sinus rhythm over time and typically commits the patient to long-term anticoagulation with its attendant risks.

Preventing Thromboembolism: Anticoagulant Versus Antiplatelet Therapy

Trials pioneering antithrombotic therapy with anticoagulant and antiplatelet drugs to reduce the risk of stroke in patients with non-valvular AF have had a lasting impact on clinical care. Meta-analysis of 29 randomized trials testing long-term (>12 weeks) therapy with antithrombotic agents in a total of 28,044 patients found a composite relative risk reduction of 64% in groups managed with adjusted-dose warfarin, absolute risk reduction of 2.7% per year for primary prevention and 8.4% for secondary prevention, compared to control groups receiving placebo or no antithrombotic therapy [9]. Compared to placebo, antiplatelet therapy with aspirin produced absolute risk reductions of 0.8% per year for primary prevention and 2.5% per year for secondary prevention. Warfarin was associated with a 37% greater reduction in stroke than aspirin and was

PROMOTERS	TRIGGERS	SUBSTRATE REMODELING	SEQUELAE
Genetic Factors • PITX2 • ZFHX3 • KCNN3 • Ion channels • Gap junction proteins • Signaling molecules	**Exogenous Factors** • Alcohol • Caffeine • Sympathomimetics • Metabolic imbalance • Hypoxia • Sleep apnea	**Inflammatory Markers** • Interleukins • TNF-α • CRP • Cytokines • Profibrotic signaling	**Heart Failure** • Systolic • Diastolic • Atrial dysfunction • Neurohumoral adaptation
Hemodynamic Forces • Cardiac • Pulmonary • Systemic	**Inflammation** • Systemic • Pericardial • Endocardial	**Electrical** • Ion channels • Re-entry • Refractoriness	**Thromboembolism** • Ischemic stroke
Autonomic Activity • Adrenergic • Vagal • Automaticity • Refractoriness	**Anatomical Distension** • Perivascular • Pulmonary veins • Vena Cava • Ligament of Marshall	**Structural** • Obesity • Angiotensin-II • TGF-β • Tachycardia-related • Fibrosis	**Cognitive Decline** • Vascular dementia **Impaired Quality of Life** • Comorbidities
NSR →	**Paroxysmal AF** →	**Persistent AF** →	**Influence of Aging**

Fig. 11.1 Atrial fibrillation in context: promoters, triggers, substrate remodeling and sequelae of atrial fibrillation and the influence of aging. *PITX2* paired-like homeodomain 2, *ZFHX3* zinc finger homeobox protein 3, *KCNN3* potassium calcium-activated channel subfamily N member 3, *TNF-α* tumor necrosis factor alpha, *CRP* C-reactive protein, *TGF-β* transforming growth factor beta, *AF* atrial fibrillation. Republished with permission of John Wiley and Sons, Inc., Journal of Biomedical Materials Research Part A, Atrial Fibrillation, Thomas M. Munger, Li-Qun Wu, and Win K, Vol. 28/No. 1, pages 1-17, © 2014; permission conveyed through Copyright Clearance Center, Inc [3]

more effective than the combination of low-dose warfarin plus aspirin. While a combination of aspirin plus clopidogrel (dual antiplatelet therapy, DAPT) was more effective than aspirin monotherapy in preventing ischemic stroke and systemic embolism, DAPT proved inferior to and no safer than anticoagulation with a VKA in patients with AF.

Balancing the Benefit and Risk of Anticoagulation

Trials demonstrating the efficacy of oral anticoagulation generally excluded patients in whom AF was complicated by rheumatic mitral stenosis of varying severity or those with mechanical or biological prosthetic heart valves. Patients who had undergone valve repair surgery were represented infrequently, if at all, in the trials conducted between 1987 and 1994. More recent studies of alternative anticoagulant drugs generally employed active-controlled, non-inferiority statistical designs, requiring preservation of the entry criteria used in the index trials of warfarin versus placebo. Only recently have sufficient data become available to prompt reconsideration of the term "non-valvular" AF, which today excludes mainly patients with more than moderate rheumatic mitral stenosis, those with mechanical prosthetic heart valves, and those within the first 3 months following heart valve surgery (Table 11.1) [10, 11]. Antithrombotic therapy for patients with other forms of left- or right-sided native valve disease who have AF or atrial flutter is managed in the same general way as for those with AF without valvular heart disease.

Table 11.1 Valvular heart disease

	Eligible for DOAC	DOAC contraindicated
Mechanical prosthetic valve		✓
Moderate to severe mitral stenosis		✓
Other native valve disease	✓	
Severe aortic stenosis	✓	
Bioprosthetic valve[a]	✓[a]	
Mitral valve repair[a]	✓[a]	
PTAV and TAVR[a]	✓[a]	
Hypertrophic cardiomyopathy	✓	
Intraoperative MAZE procedures[a]	✓[a]	
Surgical left atrial appendage ligation, plication, or amputation[a]	✓[a]	
Other cardiac surgery[a]	✓[a]	

PTAV percutaneous transluminal aortic valvuloplasty, *TAVR* transcatheter aortic valve replacement
[a]DOACs are not recommended during the first 3 months following procedure

Table 11.2 $CHADS_2$ risk assessment

Risk criteria	Score (points)
Congestive heart failure	1
Hypertension	1
Age ≥75	1
Diabetes	1
Stroke or TIA in the past	2

Notes: Congestive heart failure defined as an ejection fraction of less than 35–40%, hypertension defined as systolic blood pressure >150–160 or requiring sustained antihypertensive medication, stroke including TIA or systemic embolism
TIA transient cerebral ischemic attack

Table 11.3 $CHADS_2$ index with estimated stroke risk per year [17]

Score (total points)	Risk of stroke (%/year)
0	1.9
1	2.8
2	4.0
3	5.9
4	8.5
5	12.5
6	18.2

Notes: Approximate risk threshold for anticoagulation of 3% annual stroke risk occurs between a score of 1 and 2

The decision to initiate long-term anticoagulant therapy in a patient with AF requires estimating the risks of thromboembolism and bleeding. This is particularly pertinent to the use of VKAs because of their unpredictable pharmacokinetics, genetic variations affecting drug metabolism, interactions with food and other drugs, and the narrow therapeutic margin between antithrombotic efficacy and hemorrhagic toxicity [12]. Intracerebral hemorrhage (ICH) occurs at a rate of approximately 0.5% per year, even in carefully managed patients with AF taking warfarin at recommended therapeutic intensity [13, 14]. The first widely accepted risk stratification scheme, the $CHADS_2$ score, allocated one point each for a history of clinical heart failure, impaired left ventricular systolic function (generally taken as an ejection fraction below 35–40%), hypertension (not clearly defined in terms of severity but generally interpreted as systolic blood pressure >150–160 mmHg or requiring sustained antihypertensive medication), age ≥75 years, or diabetes mellitus and two points for a history of ischemic stroke, transient cerebral ischemic attack (TIA), or systemic embolism (Table 11.2) [15]. A score ≥2 is associated with an annual risk of stroke >3% when patients are not anticoagulated, a level of risk deemed high enough by most guideline writing groups to warrant warfarin despite the associated risk of bleeding and the inconvenience of anticoagulation monitoring and dose adjustments (Table 11.3) [16, 17].

The $CHADS_2$ scheme categorizes a relatively large proportion (up to 40%) of patients at intermediate risk, and because the advent of newer anticoagulants provides alternatives that offer greater ease of use and significantly lower risk of intracerebral hemorrhage than VKAs, the CHA_2DS_2-VASc score has become preferred. This enhanced tool addresses age as a continuous variable, allocating 1 point to patients 65–74 years old and 2 to those older; the incremental risk in women compared to men, allocating 1 point for female sex; and the prognostic

Table 11.4 CHA_2DS_2VASc risk assessment

Risk criteria	Score
Congestive heart failure or LVEF ≤35%	1
Hypertension	1
Age >75 years	2
Diabetes	1
Stroke/TIA/systemic embolism	2
Vascular disease (MI/PAD/aortic plaque)	1
Age 65–74 years	1
Sex category (female)	1

LVEF left ventricular ejection fraction, *TIA* transient ischemic attack, *MI* myocardial infarction, *PAD* peripheral arterial disease

Table 11.5 CHA_2DS_2VASc index with stroke risk score [17, 18]

	Score (total points)	Risk of stroke (%/year)
Low risk	0	0.2
Intermediate risk	1	0.6
High risk	2–9	2.2–12.2

Notes: CHA_2DS_2VASc score more accurately identifies the truly low risk patients with atrial fibrillation than $CHADS_2$. These stroke rates are estimates derived from cohorts in 2012 and may vary from more recent cohorts

importance of atherosclerosis, assigning another point for patients with vascular disease defined as prior myocardial infarction (MI), clinical peripheral artery disease (claudication, revascularization, or amputation), or complex (mobile, ulcerated, or >4 mm thick) atheromatous plaque in the thoracic aorta detected by vascular imaging (Table 11.4). Patients with a CHA_2DS_2-VASc score of 0 face an approximately 0.2% annual risk of stroke without anticoagulation, while those with scores ≥2 have at least tenfold greater risk (Table 11.5) [18].

Other predictors of stroke in patients with non-valvular AF include elevated blood levels of N-terminal pro-B-type natriuretic peptide (NT-proBNP) or troponin and evidence of atrial fibrosis detected by cardiac magnetic resonance imaging (CMR) [4, 19, 20]. The ABC score, denoting age, biomarkers, and clinical history, consistently predicted stroke risk with greater accuracy than the CHA_2DS_2-VASc score but is less convenient to use, requiring a calculator to predict 1- and 3-year risks of stroke or systemic embolism [21]. Direct assessment of the severity of atrial fibrosis could potentially have high predictive value for a number of the clinical correlates and consequences of AF, but current technology requires gadolinium-enhanced gated cardiac magnetic resonance imaging [20, 22]. Standardized methodology for this assessment has not been established, and the cost of the technology prohibits its use on a population basis outside of investigational settings.

The anticoagulation decision must also consider the patient's risk of bleeding, but available stratification tools are not specific for ICH, which generally has the most overwhelming clinical consequences compared to ischemic stroke. The HAS-BLED score, recommended in European and Canadian guidelines, comprises seven variables including hypertension (SBP >160 mmHg), abnormal renal and/or hepatic function, stroke, bleeding tendency or anemia, labile INR on warfarin, age >65 years, and drugs (aspirin or nonsteroidal anti-inflammatory drugs [NSAIDS]) and/or alcohol [23]. Additional bleeding risk scores, including ATRIA, ORBIT, and HEMORR2HAGES, have been less well validated and not widely adopted [24–28]. Overall, trial and registry data have shown that major bleeding events are five to eight times less frequent than ischemic strokes among patients with AF, so except at the upper extreme, bleeding risk is considered a modifier rather than primary determinant of the decision to anticoagulate a patient.

Direct Oral Anticoagulants

Warfarin is highly effective in reducing the risk of stroke in patients with AF, but the disutility and bleeding issues described above sparked the development of direct oral anticoagulants (DOACs), also known as novel oral anticoagulants (NOACs), target-specific oral anticoagulants (TSOACs), oral direct inhibitors, and non-vitamin K antagonist oral anticoagulants

Table 11.6 Direct oral anticoagulants: phase 3 trials for stroke prevention in patients with atrial fibrillation [29–32]

Drug	Trial acronym	Dose (mg)	Design	*N*	Risk factors (#)	Dose adjustment
Dabigatran	RE-LY [29]	150 BID 110 BID	Probe	18,113	1	None
Rivaroxaban	ROCKET AF [30]	20 QD 15 QD[a]	Blinded	14,264	≥2	21% at baseline
Apixaban	ARISTOTLE [31]	5 BID 2.5 BID[a]	Blinded	18,206	≥1	5% at baseline
Edoxaban	ENGAGE-AF TIMI 48 [32]	60 QD 30 or 15 QD[a]	Blinded	21,105	≥2	25% at baseline >9% after

[a]Adjusted based on renal function or other factors associated with reduced drug clearance

(NOACs). These drugs, which include direct thrombin inhibitors and direct factor Xa inhibitors, offer the convenience of once or twice daily dosing without the need for laboratory monitoring of coagulation activity or routine dose adjustment. All are relatively small molecules (molecular weights 436–628 g/mol) that can cross the placental barrier, essentially precluding safe use during pregnancy. Their bioavailability is variable, but pharmacodynamics and kinetics are broadly overlapping, such that the onset of peak anticoagulant effect occurs 1–3 h after oral administration and half-lives range from 8 to 17 h. All have potential interactions with drugs that are p-glycoprotein inducers or inhibitors, and several are subject to cytochrome 3A4 metabolic interactions, but the frequency of clinically significant interactions with foods and other drugs is substantially less than exhibited by VKA anticoagulants, yielding considerably more predictable responses. Renal excretion varies among the DOACs, greatest for dabigatran and least for betrixaban, which has not been approved for clinical use in patients with AF. Pivotal trials proved their non-inferiority to warfarin in reducing the risk of stroke or systemic embolism, and each was associated with substantially lower rates of ICH than well-adjusted warfarin (Table 11.6).

Oral Direct Thrombin Inhibitors

Ximelagatran

The first oral direct thrombin inhibitor, ximelagatran (Exanta®, AstraZeneca), studied in a fixed dose in the international SPORTIF trials, proved non-inferior to warfarin for prevention of all stroke (ischemic or hemorrhagic) or systemic embolism and at least as safe in terms of major bleeding [33, 34]. The compound was withdrawn from clinical development because of hepatotoxicity in about 6% of patients and will not be discussed further in this chapter.

Dabigatran Etexilate

Dabigatran (Pradaxa®, Boehringer Ingelheim), an oral direct thrombin inhibitor, was non-inferior to adjusted-dose warfarin in preventing all stroke and systemic embolism in patients with non-valvular AF in the RE-LY trial [29]. The investigators randomized 18,113 patients to one of two fixed, blinded doses of dabigatran, 110 mg BID or 150 mg BID, or adjusted-dose warfarin (target INR 2–3) in an unblinded fashion with stroke or systemic embolism as the primary efficacy outcome. The trial was a multicenter, parallel-group, randomized control study in 951 centers in 44 countries with a median follow-up of 2 years with an intention-to-treat, non-inferiority analysis. The low-dose dabigatran group included 64% males with a mean age of 74 years, persistent, paroxysmal, or permanent atrial fibrillation, and low, intermediate, and high $CHADS_2$ scores (mean 2.2), with about 50% of patients previously taking VKA therapy. Low-dose dabigatran was non-inferior and high-dose dabigatran was superior to warfarin; both doses were associated with significantly lower rates of hemorrhagic stroke than warfarin. The rates of major hemorrhage were similar in the high-dose dabigatran and warfarin groups and lower in the low-dose dabigatran group; gastrointestinal bleeding was more frequent with dabigatran. Patients in the warfarin arm reached therapeutic INR 64% of the time, comparable to performance at higher-quality anticoagulation clinics in the USA. The incidence of MI was initially reported as higher in patients randomized to high-dose dabigatran, but in a reanalysis that included clinically silent MI events detected upon review of electrocardiograms collected during the trial, the difference was no longer statistically significant [35]. The side effect of dyspepsia was more frequent among patients in the dabigatran groups. Since 80% of absorbed dabigatran is excreted by the kidneys, dosing of dabigatran should be adjusted for creatinine clearance (CrCl, estimated by the Cockcroft-Gault equation). Worldwide, dabigatran 110 mg BID is the most commonly prescribed dose for patients with AF. The US Food and Drug Administration approved dabigatran in a dose of 150 mg BID for patients with AF and CrCl ≥30 mL/min, but the dose of 110 mg BID is approved only for prophylaxis of venous thromboembolism in patients undergoing major orthopedic surgery of the hip or knee. In addition, a dose of 75 mg BID is labeled in the USA for use in patients with AF who have CrCl 15–29 mL/min, based on pharmacokinetic modeling that predicted blood levels of dabigatran comparable to those achieved with 150 mg BID in patients with normal renal function. Post-marketing studies have validated the models in terms of blood levels, but clinically meaningful outcome data are not available for the 75 mg BID dose [36].

Oral Factor Xa Inhibitors

Rivaroxaban

Rivaroxaban (Xarelto®, Bayer, Johnson & Johnson), the first oral factor Xa inhibitor approved for stroke prevention in patients with AF, was non-inferior to warfarin in the ROCKET AF trial [30]. This multicenter, double-blind trial included 14,264 patients randomized to rivaroxaban, 20 mg daily (15 mg daily for those with baseline CrCl 30–49 mL/min), or adjusted-dose warfarin (target INR 2–3) at 1178 centers in 45 countries. The study population was 39% women with a mean age of 73 years and a predominance of persistent or permanent (rather than paroxysmal) AF. About two-thirds of the patients had been previously treated with a VKA, while a third were deemed warfarin-naïve, a term defined variably across the various DOAC trials. The mean $CHADS_2$ score was 3.5—considerably higher than in the other studies—and mean CrCl was 67 mL/min. The warfarin group achieved therapeutic INR 55% of the time, a time in therapeutic range (TTR) lower than in the other pivotal trials, to some extent reflecting the clinical complexity and comorbidities of enrolled patients. Over a mean follow-up of 2 years, non-inferior efficacy was demonstrated by both on-treatment and intention-to-treat analyses, but superiority was evident only during the on-treatment period. Unlike the RE-LY trial of dabigatran, treatment with rivaroxaban vs. warfarin was blinded throughout the trial, facilitated by use of a uniform point-of-care coagulation monitoring instrument for most INR measurements at the clinical sites. The device (HemoSense/Alere INRatio PT/INR monitoring system) was later found faulty, yielding artificially lower INR values in patients with hyperfibrinogenemia resulting from inflammatory illness, but an extensive investigation by the investigators and regulatory agencies in Europe and the USA determined that this potential source of error was unlikely to have materially affected the trial [37, 38]. In a prespecified secondary analysis, patients with moderate renal impairment randomized to the reduced rivaroxaban dose of 15 mg daily demonstrated efficacy and safety outcomes against warfarin comparable to those with normal renal function taking the higher dose [39].

Apixaban

Apixaban (Eliquis®, Bristol-Myers Squibb, Pfizer), a factor Xa inhibitor, was associated with significantly lower rates of stroke and bleeding than warfarin in patients with AF in the ARISTOTLE trial [31]. In this multicenter, double-blind, non-inferiority trial, 18,301 patients at 1034 centers in 39 countries were randomized to either adjusted-dose warfarin (target INR 2–3) or apixaban, 5 mg BID. Patients with two or more of the following criteria, age ≥80 years, weight ≤60 kg, or serum creatinine ≥1.5 mg/dL, received a lower dose of apixaban, 2.5 mg BID. The trial population had a mean age of 70 years and was 35.5% females with predominantly persistent or permanent AF; 57.1% reported prior VKA use. The mean $CHADS_2$ score was 2.1 with CrCl >50 mL/min in >80%. The warfarin group achieved therapeutic INR 62% of the time on treatment. Over a median follow-up of 1.8 years, apixaban satisfied criteria for superiority for both the primary efficacy outcome of all stroke or systemic embolism and the primary safety outcome of major bleeding using the International Society of Thrombosis and Hemostasis (ISTH) definition. There was no significant difference in rates of ischemic stroke in patients randomized to apixaban or warfarin. In contrast to the substantially larger proportions of patients receiving reduced doses of dabigatran (110 mg BID) in the RE-LY trial or rivaroxaban (15 mg once daily) in the ROCKET AF trial, only 5% of those randomized to apixaban in the ARISTOTLE trial received the 2.5 mg BID dose (fewer than 500 patients), an inadequate experience upon which to assess the efficacy or safety of the dose reduction scheme, yet most post-marketing surveys have shown substantially larger proportions of patients receiving the low dose in clinical practice [40].

Apixaban was compared to aspirin in patients with AF deemed unsuitable for warfarin therapy in the AVERROES trial [41]. This multicenter, double-blind trial randomized 5599 patients at 522 centers in 36 countries to apixaban, 5 mg BID plus placebo, or aspirin 81–324 mg daily plus placebo, the aspirin dose selected by the investigator. The reasons for VKA unsuitability included inability to maintain the INR in therapeutic range or to measure INR at regular intervals, previous major bleeding, non-bleeding adverse events, difficulty contacting patients for dose adjustments, uncertain adherence, concurrent medications known to interact with warfarin, liver disease, $CHADS_2$ risk score of 1, patient unwillingness to take warfarin, and certain specified medical conditions. Clinical characteristics of the enrolled cohort included a median age of 70 years, 59% males, a mean $CHADS_2$ score of 2, and 14% prior VKA use and 75% prior ASA use within 30 days. The trial was stopped after 1.1 years, when there was clear superiority of apixaban with lower rates of stroke or systemic embolism and no increase in rates of major bleeding. Of patients randomized to aspirin, 91% were prescribed doses ≤162 mg, leaving uncertain whether the higher dose of 325 mg daily that seemed efficacious in the SPAF-1 trial might have yielded different results. Early termination of the study may have inflated the benefit of apixaban or underestimated differences in bleeding complications between apixaban and aspirin.

Edoxaban

Edoxaban (Savaysa®, Daiichi Sankyo), a factor Xa inhibitor, was non-inferior to adjusted-dose warfarin for the primary efficacy outcome of stroke, systemic embolism, or death from cardiovascular causes and associated with lower rates of bleeding in the ENGAGE AF-TIMI 48 trial [32]. This multicenter, double-blind trial included 21,105 patients at 1293 centers in 46 countries randomized to edoxaban in either a high-dose or low-dose regimen or to adjusted-dose warfarin (target INR 2–3). Patients randomized to either edoxaban dose stratum received half the assigned dose when CrCl fell to 30–50 mL/min, body weight was ≤60 kg, or during concurrent treatment with verapamil or quinidine, which increase exposure to the factor Xa inhibitor. The study population consisted of 38% women with a median age of 72; 77% had $CHADS_2$ scores <3 (mean 2.8), and about 59% had previously been treated with a VKA. Patients in the warfarin group had INR values in the therapeutic range 68.4% of the time, better control than in the other DOAC pivotal trials though the methods used to calculate TTR differed across studies. Over a mean follow-up of 2.8 years, both doses of edoxaban were non-inferior to warfarin, but while in the intention-to-treat analysis there was a trend toward superiority of high-dose edoxaban over warfarin, there was a corresponding unfavorable trend with low-dose edoxaban for the primary efficacy outcome. Both doses were associated with significantly lower rates of cardiovascular death than warfarin. Only the higher-dose edoxaban regimen of 60 mg once daily reduced to 30 mg for those meeting criteria for enhanced exposure was brought to market for this indication, and because the relative efficacy of edoxaban diminished with improving renal function, the US label bears a caution to avoid use in patients with CrCl ≥90 mL/min.

Taken together, when compared to warfarin, the DOACs are non-inferior for prevention of all stroke and systemic embolism in patients with AF, reduce the risk of ICH, are associated with better outcomes in those who develop major bleeding, and yield comparable reductions in mortality (~10% per year), mostly related to lower rates of cardiovascular death and fatal bleeding [42, 43]. The apparent differences between the various DOACs are due more to variations in trial designs, dosing, intrinsic risk of enrolled patients, concurrent treatments, and other factors than to the drugs themselves. Notably, in approved doses, which vary by country, factor Xa inhibitors may have less efficacy against ischemic stroke than high-dose dabigatran but also result in less bleeding and are less dependent on renal clearance than dabigatran. When selecting a DOAC or warfarin for individual patients, clinicians should consider the patient's individual characteristics, risks of thromboembolism, bleeding, personal values and preferences, convenience, anticipated adherence, economics, and similarities to profiles of patients enrolled in the clinical trials.

Clinical Practice Guidelines

While there is general concordance across clinical practice guideline recommendations for most aspects of AF patient management, differences exist in certain areas of antithrombotic therapy (Table 11.7).

Table 11.7 Antithrombotic therapy for atrial fibrillation: current guidelines [44, 45]

Risk factors	Recommended therapy	
	ESC [44]	AHA/ACC/HRS [45]
No risk factors CHA_2DS_2-VASc = 0	Prefer neither Or ASA 75–325 mg daily	Neither ASA 75–235 mg daily nor OAC
CHA_2DS_2-VASc = 1	Prefer OAC Or ASA 75–325 mg daily	Neither ASA 75–235 mg daily nor OAC
CHA_2DS_2-VASc ≥2	DOAC > VKA	DOAC or VKA
Mechanical valve (modern)	VKA: INR 2.0–3.0 (AVR) VKA: INR 2.5–3.5 (MVR)	

ESC European Society of Cardiology, *AHA* American Heart Association, *ACC* American College of Cardiology, *HRS* Heart Rhythm Society, *ASA* aspirin, *OAC* oral anticoagulant *DOAC* direct oral anticoagulant, *VKA* vitamin K antagonist, *AVR* aortic valve replacement, *MVR* mitral valve replacement

Among the most controversial is the management of patients with AF and a single intermediate risk factor, men with CHA_2DS_2-VASc scores of 1 or women with scores of 2 (one risk factor other than sex). The 2016 ESC guidelines recommended anticoagulation for males with scores of 1 and females with scores of 2 [44]. The 2014 ACC/AHA/HRS guideline recommended anticoagulation for those with scores ≥2, no antithrombotic therapy for those with scores of 0, and for those with scores of 1, no therapy, aspirin, or an anticoagulant were each deemed acceptable options [45]. The difference could affect the proportion of patients managed with anticoagulation by about 5%—more than a quarter of a million individuals in the USA alone. This controversy is rooted in estimates of the risk of bleeding compared with no antithrombotic therapy among those near the lower pole of the stroke risk spectrum and acknowledges that risk stratification schemes like CHA_2DS_2-VASc entail compromises in terms of accuracy in exchange for convenience. Anticoagulation with VKAs, in particular, compounds the risk of ICH. Approximately 20% of all ICH events have been attributed to warfarin therapy, which also doubles the associated mortality rate. And although major and sometimes fatal extracranial bleeding can occur, much of the effort to attenuate bleeding risk is focused on avoiding ICH. Reduction in intracranial bleeding is the most distinguishing feature of the DOACs compared to warfarin (odds ratio 0.49; 95% CI 0.36–0.65) [46]. The mechanism by which DOACs confer less risk of ICH is uncertain, but the observation is sufficiently robust to make it reasonable to recommend a DOAC over warfarin when anticoagulation is prescribed for patients with CHA_2DS_2-VASc scores of 1, though limited data are available outside of clinical trials to substantiate this recommendation.

Anticoagulation in Specific Patient Subgroups

Patients with Prior Stroke

Patients with AF and prior stroke represent an important subgroup because they face high rates of recurrent ischemic events that are only partly ameliorated by VKAs. In general, the DOACs have proven particularly effective in this situation, though the strength of evidence varies with the prevalence of secondary prevention cohorts in the various trials. Over half the patients enrolled in the ROCKET AF trial of rivaroxaban had previously sustained ischemic stroke or systemic embolism, and the factor Xa inhibitor performed as well against warfarin in this subgroup as in the overall trial population (interaction $p = 0.23$) [47]. This should be considered when choosing among the various DOACs for patients with prior stroke, but the fact that dabigatran, 150 mg BID, was the only one to exhibit superior efficacy for the endpoint of ischemic stroke makes the direct thrombin inhibitor a well-founded alternative. In the RE-LY trial, the efficacy and safety of both doses of dabigatran in patients with previous stroke or TIA also paralleled the outcomes in patients with AF treated for primary stroke prevention [48]. Meta-analysis of 14,527 patients with prior stroke or TIA in the RE-LY, ARISTOTLE, and ROCKET AF trials found that DOACs were associated with a significant reduction in the incidence of stroke and systemic embolism compared with warfarin (odds ratio [OR] 0.85; 95% confidence interval [CI] 0.74–0.99) [49]. The risk of hemorrhagic transformation in those with stroke occurring within 2–3 months earlier is negligible, and DOACs are generally safe. On the other hand, the decision to anticoagulate patients with AF in the setting of acute stroke becomes more complicated, as recommendations are based only on expert opinion considering the interval from and severity of stroke. Patient management in this situation goes beyond the scope of this chapter and requires consultation with a stroke neurologist.

Patients with Impaired Renal Function

The safety and efficacy of the factor Xa inhibitors were assessed in subpopulations with moderately impaired renal function through dose reductions variously and at least partly based on serum creatinine concentration or calculated creatinine clearance [39, 50]. The doses of dabigatran tested in the RE-LY trial, in contrast, were assigned on a randomized basis without regard to renal function [51]. In aggregate, while the dose reductions in the pivotal trials yielded efficacy and safety data consistent with the overall trial findings for patients with CrCl 30–49 mL/min (calculated by the Cockcroft-Gault equation), clinical outcome data are not available on the use of DOACs in patients with CrCl <30 mL/min and in those on hemodialysis, for whom warfarin remains the currently recommended anticoagulant, albeit with considerable limitations [52]. Renal function can be assessed using the creatinine clearance estimated by the Cockcroft-Gault equation, which incorporates body weight, or by estimating the glomerular filtration rate (eGFR) using the Modification of Diet in Renal Disease (MDRD) or Chronic Kidney Disease Epidemiology Collaboration (CKD-EPI) formulas, which do not incorporate body weight. In general, the eGFR may be used to determine the dosing of dabigatran, rivaroxaban and apixaban, when the result is in the normal range (≥ 60 mL/min/1.73 m^2). For patients with lower eGFR levels, the

Cockcroft-Gault equation should be employed. Only the Cockcroft-Gault equation should be used to guide dosing of edoxaban, which is affected at both the upper and lower extremes of renal function.

Elderly Patients

Elderly patients (≥75 years old) with AF face a higher risk of thromboembolism, worse stroke outcomes, and a greater tendency to bleeding during anticoagulation than younger individuals, yet the net clinical benefit of warfarin compared with aspirin or no antithrombotic therapy expands with age [53]. Secondary analyses of trial data found the reduction in intracranial hemorrhage with DOACs independent of patient age, favoring use of the DOACs over warfarin. The effect of dabigatran on extracranial bleeding varied with age, both doses reducing the risk in patients aged <75 years compared to warfarin, but the risk of extracranial bleeding was higher risk in patients aged ≥75 years given the higher (150 mg BID) dose of dabigatran compared to warfarin. In patients <75 years old, dabigatran 150 mg BID is more effective than warfarin, whereas in older patients the lower dose of dabigatran, 110 mg BID, may be preferred, particularly among those at high risk of bleeding. Apixaban, 5 mg twice daily (or 2.5 mg twice daily for patients meeting the protocol criteria for dose reduction), was associated with the lowest risk of bleeding, with relative risk reduction similar to that with the lower dose of dabigatran (110 mg twice daily) compared to warfarin. The ROCKET AF trial of rivaroxaban included a larger proportion of elderly patients than the other trials. In a pre-specified secondary analysis, absolute rates of stroke and systemic embolism and major bleeding were higher among elderly patients than younger patients, and the relative effects of rivaroxaban (20 mg once daily or 15 mg daily for those with moderate renal impairment) compared with adjusted-dose warfarin were consistent among elderly and younger patients for prevention of stroke and systemic embolism and with respect to the risk of major bleeding. The net clinical benefit of rivaroxaban compared to warfarin was greater among older patients [54]. In the ENGAGE AF-TIMI 48 trial of edoxaban (60 mg once daily or 30 mg for those with impaired renal function), age had a greater impact on major bleeding than thromboembolism, and since rates of bleeding and death increased with age, treatment of elderly patients with edoxaban provided a greater safety advantage over warfarin compared to younger patients [55]. Similar advantages, likely related to age, were evident for frail patients prone to falls, a particularly difficult clinical situation that exemplifies the challenges of sustaining long-term anticoagulant therapy in patients with AF and accumulated comorbidities [56].

Patients with Diabetes Mellitus

Both AF and diabetes mellitus are rising in prevalence, these conditions often occur together, and diabetes is an independent risk factor for stroke in patients with AF. Activation of the coagulation system, impaired fibrinolytic activity, alterations in platelet and endothelial function, and higher levels of tissue plasminogen activator antigen and factor VIII activity may contribute to the higher mortality rates of stroke in diabetic than nondiabetic patients with AF [57]. Diabetic patients demonstrate larger left atrial diameters and left atrial appendage sizes and a higher prevalence of left atrial or appendage thrombus than do nondiabetic patients [58]. The presence of diabetes influences stroke risk in patients with AF to an extent similar to the incremental risk of coronary events in diabetic patients with atherosclerosis. The ROCKET AF of rivaroxaban enrolled a greater proportion of patients with diabetes (39.9%) than did other trials of DOACs (23.3% in the RE-LY trial of dabigatran, 25% in the ARISTOTLE and 19.2% in the AVERROES trials of apixaban, and 36% in the ENGAGE AF-TIMI 48 trial of edoxaban). Overall, however, secondary analyses specifically examining patients enrolled in the pivotal trials found the relative efficacy and safety of the DOACs versus warfarin similar in patients with and without diabetes, supporting their use as an alternative to warfarin in diabetic patients with AF.

Heart Failure

Between 12 and 41% of patients with heart failure have AF, the prevalence of the arrhythmia rising with the severity of heart failure [59]. The commonly used thromboembolic risk prediction scores, such as CHA_2DS_2-VASc, incorporate a clinical history of heart failure as an independent risk factor for thromboembolic events in patients with AF. Factors including but not limited to hepatic congestion may account for the observation that patients with heart failure have a lower TTR during anticoagulation with VKA anticoagulants, predisposing to both reduced efficacy and increased risk of bleeding [60]. Among the pivotal DOAC trials, 62.5% of patients randomized in the ROCKET AF trial of rivaroxaban had a history of heart failure or a reduced left ventricular ejection fraction compared to 32.0% of those in the RE-LY trial of dabigatran, 35.4% of the ARISTOTLE trial of apixaban, and 57.4% of the ENGAGE AF-TIMI 48 trial of edoxaban. In general, rates of stroke or systemic embolism and bleeding were similar between patients with and without heart failure, and the treatment effects of the DOACs were similar in patients with and without HF, suggesting that relative efficacy and safety extend to the patients with AF and heart failure, independent of systolic function or functional class.

Pattern of AF and Patients Undergoing Cardioversion

Episodic or intermittent AF that terminates spontaneously within 7 days is classified as paroxysmal, while arrhythmia lasting longer or requiring intervention for termination is designated persistent. Several studies have documented symptomatic, physiological, and anatomical differences between patients with paroxysmal and persistent AF. The relative risk of thromboembolism in patients with paroxysmal versus permanent AF has varied in analyses of various cohorts, but regardless of the pattern of AF, anticoagulation is indicated for patients with additional stroke risk factors, and neither the pattern nor the burden of AF is included in most guideline recommended risk stratification strategies.

In patients undergoing cardioversion (Table 11.8), the X-VeRT trial investigators randomized 1504 patients to rivaroxaban or a VKA in the pericardioversion period and found rivaroxaban associated with a low incidence of thromboembolic events, myocardial infarction, cardiovascular death, or major bleeding [61]. When the conventional strategy (which requires at least 3 consecutive weeks of continuous anticoagulation at therapeutic intensity) was employed, rivaroxaban allowed for earlier cardioversion than VKAs, simply because several additional weeks are typically required to establish a stable dose with the latter. Similar results were found with edoxaban in the ENSURE-AF trial [62]. The protocol of the EMANATE trial of 1500 patients, currently ongoing, encourages an early image-guided approach; the trial is expected to provide the first systematic assessment of the fate of intracardiac thrombus in patients treated with a DOAC prior to cardioversion (Table 11.8) [63] (see Chap. 12).

Patients Undergoing Catheter Ablation

In patients undergoing catheter ablation, uninterrupted anticoagulation is favored to decrease thromboembolic risk, with VKAs used most

Table 11.8 Supplementary studies in atrial fibrillation [61–68]

	Dabigatran	Rivaroxaban	Apixaban	Edoxaban
Cardioversion		X-VERT [61]	EMANATE [63]	ENSURE-AF [62]
Catheter ablation of AF	RE-CIRCUIT [64–66]	VENTURE-AF [65] OCEAN	AXAFA[a]	
PCI/stent	RE-DUAL PCI [67]	PIONEER AF-PCI [66, 68]	AUGUSTUS[a]	ENTRUST-AF[a]

PCI percutaneous coronary intervention, *AF* atrial fibrillation

[a]National Clinical Trial Number (NCT) for ongoing studies: AXAFA, NCT02227550; AUGUSTUS, NCT02415400; ENTRUST-AF, NCT02866175

commonly [69]. Limited observational studies and case series are available to inform use of dabigatran and rivaroxaban in this setting; however, prospective studies using uninterrupted DOAC therapy are underway and may justify these as safe alternatives for patients undergoing catheter ablation of AF.

Patients with Coronary Artery Disease

In general, 35–40% of patients in trials of thc DOACs for AF received concomitant antiplatelet agents, most often because of concurrent coronary disease. Concomitant antiplatelet therapy increased the risk of major bleeding by about 1.6-fold, and the effect was similar with either DOACs or warfarin, such that concomitant antiplatelet therapy did not affect the efficacy and safety of the DOACs relative to warfarin.

Patients with AF who sustain an acute coronary syndrome or undergo percutaneous coronary intervention (PCI) with deployment of drug-eluting stents represent particular clinical challenges because anticoagulation alone is less effective than platelet inhibition for prevention of stent thrombosis, while platelet inhibitors (e.g., aspirin alone or in combination with a thienopyridine—dual antiplatelet therapy, DAPT) have been less effective than warfarin in preventing thromboembolic complications of AF. The combination of DAPT with an anticoagulant ("triple therapy") is associated with relatively high rates of major and clinically relevant non-major bleeding. The WOEST trial compared the safety and efficacy of clopidogrel plus warfarin to clopidogrel plus both aspirin and warfarin (triple therapy) among 573 patients undergoing PCI who required anticoagulation for indications including but not limited to AF [70]. The group receiving clopidogrel plus warfarin had a significantly lower rate of bleeding through 1 year after PCI than did the group receiving triple therapy [70].

Data emerging from the PIONEER AF-PCI trial of rivaroxaban, the RE-DUAL PCI trial of dabigatran, the AUGUSTUS trial of apixaban, and the ENTRUST-AF PCI trial of edoxaban will address each of the DOACs in varying dose combinations with antiplatelet regimens in patients with AF undergoing PCI (Table 11.4). PIONEER AF-PCI, the first completed study to compare DOACs to traditional VKAs plus DAPT in patients with AF receiving antiplatelet therapy after PCI, found that either a regimen of low-dose rivaroxaban plus P_2Y_{12} or very low dose plus DAPT was associated with a lower rate of clinically significant bleeding compared to VKA plus DAPT [66, 68]. Although all three treatment groups had similar rates of death from cardiovascular diseases, myocardial infarction, or stroke, broad confidence intervals limited conclusions regarding efficacy. The investigators randomized 2124 subjects (just over 700 subjects in each treatment strategy) to rivaroxaban 15 mg daily plus clopidogrel or P_2Y_{12} inhibitor; rivaroxaban 2.5 mg BID plus DAPT for 1, 6, or 12 months followed by rivaroxaban 15 mg daily plus low-dose aspirin; or VKA plus DAPT for 1, 6, or 12 months followed by VKA plus low-dose aspirin.

RE-DUAL PCI, a phase 3b randomized, open-label, blinded-endpoint trial randomizes 2500 patients (~833 patients per treatment arm) to dabigatran (110 or 150 mg twice daily) and clopidogrel or ticagrelor to traditional triple therapy after PCI [67]. Patients in both dabigatran arms stop aspirin immediately after PCI, while patients in the warfarin arm stop aspirin 1 month after bare metal stenting and 3 months after deployment of drug-eluting stents. The minimum duration of treatment is 6 months with time to first ISTH major bleeding event or clinically relevant non-major bleeding the primary endpoint. The AUGUSTUS trial, also underway, randomized 4000 patients to either apixaban plus a P_2Y_{12} inhibitor with or without aspirin or warfarin plus a P_2Y_{12} with or without aspirin, beginning within 14 days after ACS and/or PCI. ENTRUST-AF PCI, yet another trial addressing this issue, tests two edoxaban dosing regimens (60 or 30 mg once daily) in addition to DAPT with aspirin plus clopidogrel and edoxaban combined with clopidogrel after stopping aspirin. Taken together, these trials set the stage for direct and indirect comparisons of a wide array of strategies combining various anticoagulant and antiplatelet drug regimens in patients with AF undergoing PCI, but there will likely be only a limited foundation upon which to choose an optimum regimen for an individual patient.

Uncertainties Surrounding the Use of DOACs

Despite the overall net clinical benefit associated with DOAC therapy compared to warfarin in the pivotal trials, uncertainties emerged around how to employ these anticoagulants for specific patients with AF, including those with renal impairment, advanced age, and diabetes mellitus and those undergoing cardioversion, coronary revascularization, or ablation procedures or those with asymptomatic device-detected atrial tachyarrhythmia or prior hemorrhagic stroke. In general, use of DOACs true prospective comparative effective studies for indications including but not limited to AF are unlikely to become available in the foreseeable future, and clinicians will be compelled to base treatment choices on inferences gleaned from matching patients to the most relevant studies (Fig. 11.2). Given the paucity of comparative data, several authors used subgroup analyses of the trials to develop consensus-based advice regarding anticoagulant decisions [11, 71, 72].

Practice-Based and Registry Studies

The outcomes of randomized trials need corroboration in practiced-based settings, and data are emerging from a variety of observational studies and registries. Although the clinical trial data

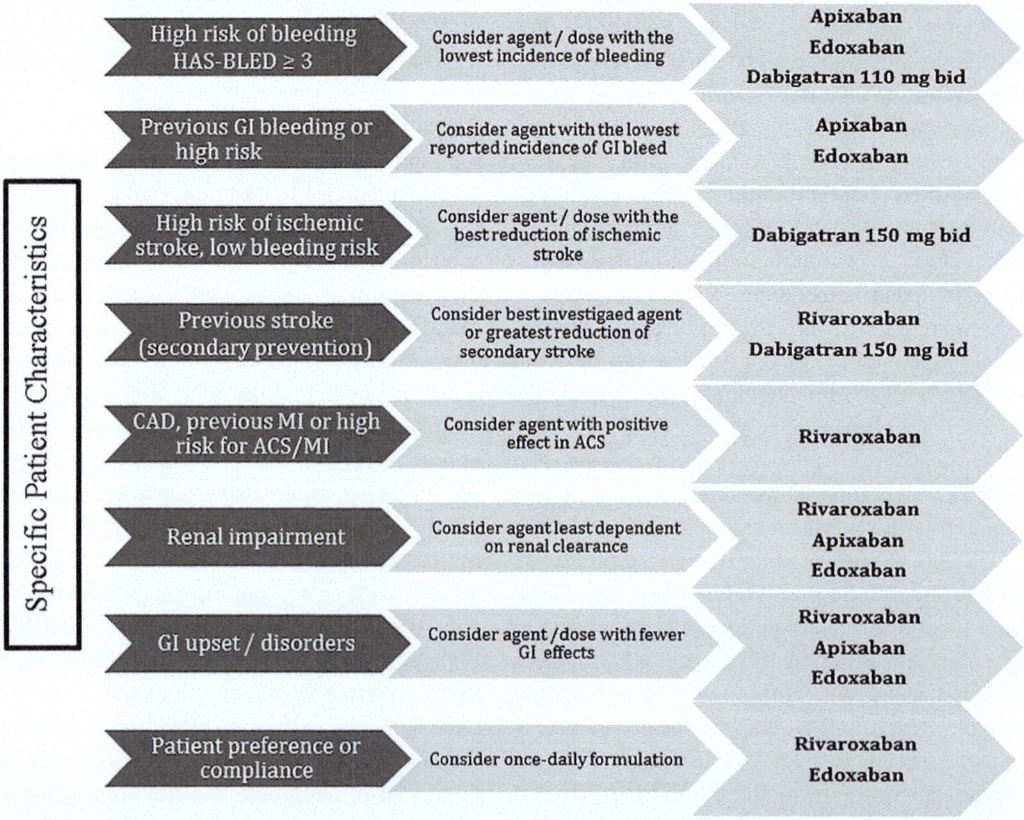

Fig. 11.2 Considerations in DOAC selection for AF: extrapolations from the pivotal trials. *GI* gastrointestinal, *CAD* coronary artery disease, *MI* myocardial infarction, *ACS* acute coronary syndrome

provide integral information for practice guidelines, global registry programs and observational studies (ORBIT, GARFIELD, GLORIA-AF, XANTUS, and PREFER), among others, provide complementary data and insight into the epidemiology and practice patterns involving patients with AF managed in routine clinical practice. Overall, these studies corroborate findings from clinical trials as regards safety and efficacy. A report from the GLORIA-AF (Global Registry on Long-Term Oral Antithrombotic Treatment in Patients with Atrial Fibrillation) registry on ~2900 patients followed at 2 years found a low incidence of life-threatening (0.54%) and major (1.12%) bleeding and effective reduction in stroke (0.63%) with dabigatran compared to VKA therapy. The XANTUS study similarly corroborated the safety profile of rivaroxaban in routine clinical practice. GARFIELD (Global Anticoagulant Registry in the Field) registry capturing the burden of disease recruited >57,000 patients with newly diagnosed non-valvular AF with at least one additional risk factor for stroke followed over 8 years. Because they have less restrictive entry criteria, these studies enhance the generalizability of the knowledge base underpinning the use of DOACs in broad populations of patients with AF and may more comprehensively represent those encountered routinely by practitioners.

Assessment of the Anticoagulant Effect

There are presently no approved coagulation assays to gauge the intensity of anticoagulation with the DOACs, which can be particularly vexing when bleeding occurs or when patients face an urgent need for invasive cardiovascular or surgical procedures that require correction of the anticoagulated state. The aPTT roughly correlates with dabigatran blood levels but varies rapidly with time and cannot be reliably employed to guide dosing. The ecarin clotting time reflects the anticoagulant effect of dabigatran and when normal generally excludes dabigatran effect. A diluted thrombin time assay has shown promise as a method for assessing the effect of dabigatran, but is not commercially available in the USA. During treatment with the oral factor Xa inhibitors, prolongation of the prothrombin time is typical, but does not correlate well with clinical efficacy or risk of bleeding. Measurements of anti-Xa activity can be obtained, but the lag time required to obtain results and relatively rapid kinetics of the factor Xa inhibitors limit the clinical utility of this approach except in steady-state situations.

Anticoagulation Reversal

While all anticoagulants carry a risk of bleeding, hemorrhagic complications in patients managed with the DOACs are associated with generally better outcomes than those that occur on warfarin, mainly because the central nervous system is less frequently involved. Despite this, the unavailability of specific reversal strategies for the DOACs made many physicians hesitate to prescribe these agents and patients reluctant to take them. This situation is changing, as ongoing and planned trials of reversal strategies have shown promising results (Table 11.9).

The first to reach approval for clinical use was idarucizumab, a specific monoclonal antibody fragment that exhibits ~350 times greater affinity for thrombin than does dabigatran [73, 74]. The agent is administered in an initial dose of 5 g, infused intravenously as two successive 50 mL vials of 2.5 g each, and has an immediate onset of action without demonstrated procoagulant or anticoagulant effects. The kinetics are such that dabigatran may be restarted 24 h after administration of idarucizumab in situations when the risk of bleeding has decreased sufficiently and reinstatement of anticoagulation is indicated. Data from the REVERSE-AD trial demonstrated effective reversal of the anticoagulant effect of dabigatran in patients with uncontrolled major bleeding and in those undergoing urgent surgery or invasive procedures, and the agent was approved for clinical use in 2015 [73].

Reversal strategies for the factor Xa inhibitors include andexanet alfa (Portola), under investigation

Table 11.9 Anticoagulant-reversal agents: pharmacologic targets

Anticoagulant	Class	Vitamin K	FFP	Protamine	Idarucizumab	Andexanet alfa	Ciraparantag
Dabigatran	IIa inhibitor				✓		✓
Apixaban	Xa inhibitor					✓	✓
Rivaroxaban	Xa inhibitor					✓	✓
Edoxaban	Xa inhibitor					✓	✓
Unfractionated heparin	Heparin			✓		?	✓
LMWH	Heparin					?	✓
Fondaparinux	AT-III Xa inhibitor					?	✓
Warfarin	VKA	✓	✓				

FFP fresh frozen plasma, *VKA* vitamin K antagonist, *LMWH* low-molecular-weight heparin, *AT-III* antithrombin III inhibitor

in the ANNEXA-R and ANNEXA-A trials, and ciraparantag (PER977, Perisphere), a broad-spectrum reversal agent in an earlier stage of investigation [75, 76]. Both represent novel potential methods to reverse anticoagulation for uncontrolled major bleeding or to reduce the risk of bleeding in anticoagulated patients prior to urgent surgery or invasive procedures [77, 78]. Outcomes of interest include laboratory markers of coagulation activity and clinical bleeding outcomes. Andexanet alfa, a recombinant analogue of factor Xa currently pending FDA approval, acts as a decoy by binding oral direct Xa inhibitors and competes for binding sites of the heparin-antithrombin complex [79, 80]. It is administered as a bolus followed by a 2-h infusion and has a half-life of 30–60 min and based on preliminary data has achieved 79% efficacy in hemostasis. Ciraparantag, currently in phase 2 clinical studies, targets low-molecular-weight heparin, unfractionated heparin, and the direct oral anticoagulants but is not expected to reverse the anticoagulant effect of warfarin [80]. Its mechanism of action has not been fully disclosed.

Conclusions

The robust evidence for anticoagulation in patients with AF to prevent stroke provides an invaluable opportunity for patient care. As the use of DOACs expands, comparative studies will be required for optimal implementation, but these are unlikely to emerge for many years. Additionally, prescriber confidence in effective reversal strategies will be fundamental for the future of anticoagulation in various clinical scenarios. Because the individual DOACs have more similarities than differences, clinicians should focus on identifying patients at risk and assuring appropriate anticoagulation rather than on the selection of one target-specific agent over another. Finally, apart from therapy to prevent stroke, AF is independently associated with increased mortality, which calls for additional studies to improve understanding of the mechanistic links and allow more effective and comprehensive therapeutic approaches.

Key Points

- Warfarin is superior to antiplatelet therapy for primary and secondary stroke prevention in patients with AF.
- The term non-valvular AF refers to patients with AF other than those with moderate to severe rheumatic mitral stenosis, those with mechanical prosthetic heart valves, and those within the first 3 months following heart valve surgery.
- The CHA_2DS_2-VASc score is the most widely accepted stroke risk assessment scheme. Anticoagulation is recommended for patients with non-valvular AF and scores ≥ 2, though alterative risk

predictors including blood biomarkers or atrial fibrosis detected by advanced cardiac imaging have been introduced.

- The HAS-BLED score predicts risk of major bleeding in anticoagulated patients, with scores ≥ 4 associated with high risk. No currently available risk score, however, accurately predicts ICH, the only complication typically associated with clinical outcomes worse than the ischemic strokes anticoagulation is intended to prevent.
- As a group, DOACs are non-inferior to warfarin for prevention of stroke and systemic embolism, are associated with better outcomes of major bleeding, and reduce the risk of ICH compared to warfarin.
- Outcome differences between the DOACs in the pivotal trials may be explained largely on the basis of variations in dosing, study design, intrinsic risk, concurrent treatment, and other factors, rather than the drugs themselves.
- Idarucizumab is indicated for dabigatran reversal and is the only agent currently approved specifically to reverse the anticoagulant effect of a DOAC, though others are under development to reverse the effect of the factor Xa inhibitors.

Self-Assessment Questions

1. A 78-year-old woman with no known medical problems is found to have asymptomatic atrial fibrillation on a routine office visit. The ventricular rate is ~88 bpm and blood pressure is normal. There are no abnormalities on cardiovascular examination aside from the rhythm. In anticipation of cardioversion, she undergoes transesophageal echocardiography, which reveals left atrial enlargement and dense spontaneous echo-contrast in the left atrium. Ventricular and valvular function appears normal. Before electrical cardioversion is performed, sinus rhythm transiently resumes, but atrial fibrillation then recurs, all without her symptomatic awareness of the changes in rhythm. What is the next most appropriate step in management?
   (a) Perform direct current electrical cardio-version.
   (b) Administer ibutilide.
   (c) Begin an oral anticoagulant.
   (d) Begin flecainide.
2. A 58-year-old overweight man with a history of hypertension, obstructive sleep apnea, and recent deployment of a drug-eluting coronary stent complains of palpitation. He is currently taking aspirin, clopidogrel, metoprolol, and atorvastatin. The electrocardiogram shows atrial fibrillation with controlled ventricular response and no ischemia. Transthoracic echocardiography shows mild left ventricular hypertrophy with preserved systolic function and left atrial enlargement. What is the appropriate antithrombotic strategy?
   (a) Add warfarin to dual antiplatelet therapy.
   (b) Add rivaroxaban 20 mg daily to dual antiplatelet therapy.
   (c) Add dabigatran 150 mg daily to dual antiplatelet therapy.
   (d) Add rivaroxaban 15 mg daily to clopidogrel and discontinue aspirin.
3. A 66-year-old woman with type 2 diabetes mellitus presents to the emergency department with palpitation and shortness of breath. The electrocardiogram confirms newly detected atrial fibrillation. She is started on anticoagulation and undergoes cardioversion 1 month later with restoration of sinus rhythm. She presents a month after cardioversion in sinus rhythm. Which antithrombotic strategy is recommended at this time?
   (a) Continue anticoagulation and obtain ambulatory rhythm monitoring.
   (b) Stop anticoagulation and obtain ambulatory rhythm monitoring.
   (c) Stop anticoagulation and start aspirin.
   (d) Stop anticoagulation and start clopidogrel.
4. A 76-year-old man with chronic kidney disease (CrCl 52 mL/min), hypertension, and paroxysmal AF returns to clinic with dyspnea

on exertion and lightheadedness. Given that there have been three documented episodes of AF over the past few months, you prescribe amiodarone on top of his current regimen of lisinopril, 10 mg daily; diltiazem, 180 mg daily; and rivaroxaban, 20 mg daily. Which medication adjustment would you recommend at this time?
   (a) Increase lisinopril to 30 mg daily.
   (b) Decrease rivaroxaban to 15 mg daily.
   (c) Decrease diltiazem to 120 mg daily.
   (d) Increase amiodarone to 400 mg daily.
5. A 92-year-old woman with severe peripheral artery disease and atrial fibrillation, for which she is anticoagulated with warfarin, is admitted to hospital with worsening foot pain. On examination, her weight is 58 kg, the ventricular rate is controlled, and there are no signs of heart failure, but both lower limbs are ischemic, with gangrenous toes. Over the next several days, the INR becomes labile on her usual warfarin regimen, peaking at 3.8, and hemoglobin content falls. Her son reports that she has a history of recurrent GI bleeding requiring temporary interruptions of warfarin and conservative management. The consulting vascular surgeon sees no option for revascularization, and the patient and her family choose hospice care with analgesia. Which anticoagulation regimen would you recommend at discharge?
   (a) Continue warfarin.
   (b) Start apixaban 5 mg BID.
   (c) Start apixaban 2.5 mg BID.
   (d) Start dabigatran 150 mg BID.

Self-Assessment Answers

1. (c) Begin an oral anticoagulant.

   Although she remains asymptomatic, her CHA_2DS_2-VASc score of 3 indicates an increased risk of thromboembolism. Given the spontaneous recurrence of AF, cardioversion would provide no assurance of sustained utility, and the inherent risks of anti-arrhythmic drug therapy outweigh the potential benefits in an asymptomatic patient. It is reasonable to initiate anticoagulation for stroke prevention, and assuming renal function is satisfactory, any of the DOACs or a VKA would be appropriate in this case.
2. (d) Add rivaroxaban 15 mg daily to clopidogrel and discontinue aspirin.

   This symptomatic man with a CHA_2DS_2-VASc score of 2 should be anticoagulated, but his current need for DAPT following recent PCI would increase the risk of bleeding if an anticoagulant were added. Given the results of the PIONEER AF-PCI trial, low-dose rivaroxaban (15 mg daily) + a $P2Y_{12}$ inhibitor or very low-dose rivaroxaban (2.5 mg BID) + DAPT are safer than warfarin + DAPT, with trials studying dabigatran, apixaban, and edoxaban in progress. Since dabigatran should be administered twice daily, the combination of rivaroxaban, 15 mg daily + clopidogrel, 75 mg daily (without aspirin) would be the most reasonable strategy of the listed options, though efficacy compared to other alternatives has not been firmly established.
3. (a) Continue anticoagulation and obtain ambulatory rhythm monitoring.

   Although sinus rhythm seems to have been maintained, the lack of an identified reversible cause of AF and her CHA_2DS_2-VASc score of 3 indicate risks of both recurrence and thromboembolism. Hence, a longer period of anticoagulation is generally recommended, though the optimum duration and role of long-term cardiac rhythm monitoring are uncertain in this situation.
4. (b) Decrease rivaroxaban to 15 mg daily.

   Although the other medication adjustments may be considered, they are all less urgent than reducing the risk of bleeding. Since both amiodarone and diltiazem can increase blood levels of rivaroxaban through interactions involving the P-glycoprotein system and inhibition of hepatic metabolism and renal function is mildly impaired, the dose of rivaroxaban should be decreased to 15 mg daily, and the patient should be monitored for symptoms or signs of bleeding.
5. (c) Start apixaban 2.5 mg BID.

   Given her CHA_2DS_2-VASc score of 4, there is a clear indication for anticoagulation, although the history of recurrent GI blood loss during warfarin treatment places her at risk of further bleeding. Apixaban, 2.5 mg BID, would offer some protection against ischemic stroke and represent a safer alternative than warfarin. This option should be discussed with the patient and her family in the context of establishing the goals of ongoing care.

References

1. Sheikh A, Patel NJ, Nalluri N, Agnihotri K, Spagnola J, Patel A, et al. Trends in hospitalization for atrial fibrillation: epidemiology, cost, and implications for the future. Prog Cardiovasc Dis. 2015;58(2):105–16.
2. Flaker GC, Belew K, Beckman K, Vidaillet H, Kron J, Safford R, et al. Asymptomatic atrial fibrillation: demographic features and prognostic information from the Atrial Fibrillation Follow-up Investigation of Rhythm Management (AFFIRM) study. Am Heart J. 2005;149(4):657–63.
3. Munger TM, LQ W, Shen WK. Atrial fibrillation. J Biomed Res. 2014;28(1):1–17.
4. Hirsh BJ, Copeland-Halperin RS, Halperin JL. Fibrotic atrial cardiomyopathy, atrial fibrillation, and thromboembolism: mechanistic links and clinical inferences. J Am Coll Cardiol. 2015;65(20):2239–51.
5. Wyse DG, Waldo AL, DiMarco JP, Domanski MJ, Rosenberg Y, Schron EB, et al. A comparison of rate control and rhythm control in patients with atrial fibrillation. N Engl J Med. 2002;347(23):1825–33.
6. Corley SD, Epstein AE, DiMarco JP, Domanski MJ, Geller N, Greene HL, et al. Relationships between sinus rhythm, treatment, and survival in the Atrial Fibrillation Follow-Up Investigation of Rhythm Management (AFFIRM) study. Circulation. 2004;109(12):1509–13.
7. Freudenberger RS, Wilson AC, Kostis JB. Comparison of rate versus rhythm control for atrial fibrillation in patients with left ventricular dysfunction (from the AFFIRM study). Am J Cardiol. 2007;100(2):247–52.
8. Van Gelder IC, Hagens VE, Bosker HA, Kingma JH, Kamp O, Kingma T, et al. A comparison of rate control and rhythm control in patients with recurrent persistent atrial fibrillation. N Engl J Med. 2002;347(23):1834–40.
9. Hart RG, Pearce LA, Aguilar MI. Meta-analysis: antithrombotic therapy to prevent stroke in patients who have nonvalvular atrial fibrillation. Ann Intern Med. 2007;146(12):857–67.
10. Eikelboom JW, Connolly SJ, Brueckmann M, Granger CB, Kappetein AP, Mack MJ, et al. Dabigatran versus warfarin in patients with mechanical heart valves. N Engl J Med. 2013;369(13):1206–14.
11. Heidbuchel H, Verhamme P, Alings M, Antz M, Diener HC, Hacke W, et al. Updated European Heart Rhythm Association Practical Guide on the use of non-vitamin K antagonist anticoagulants in patients with non-valvular atrial fibrillation. Europace. 2015;17(10):1467–507.
12. Shen AY, Yao JF, Brar SS, Jorgensen MB, Chen W. Racial/ethnic differences in the risk of intracranial hemorrhage among patients with atrial fibrillation. J Am Coll Cardiol. 2007;50(4):309–15.
13. Hart RG, Boop BS, Anderson DC. Oral anticoagulants and intracranial hemorrhage. Facts and hypotheses. Stroke. 1995;26(8):1471–7.
14. Sjoblom L, Hardemark HG, Lindgren A, Norrving B, Fahlen M, Samuelsson M, et al. Management and prognostic features of intracerebral hemorrhage during anticoagulant therapy: a Swedish multicenter study. Stroke. 2001;32(11):2567–74.
15. van Walraven C, Hart RG, Wells GA, Petersen P, Koudstaal PJ, Gullov AL, et al. A clinical prediction rule to identify patients with atrial fibrillation and a low risk for stroke while taking aspirin. Arch Intern Med. 2003;163(8):936–43.
16. Go AS, Hylek EM, Chang Y, Phillips KA, Henault LE, Capra AM, et al. Anticoagulation therapy for stroke prevention in atrial fibrillation: how well do randomized trials translate into clinical practice? JAMA. 2003;290(20):2685–92.
17. Gage BF, van Walraven C, Pearce L, Hart RG, Koudstaal PJ, Boode BS, et al. Selecting patients with atrial fibrillation for anticoagulation: stroke risk stratification in patients taking aspirin. Circulation. 2004;110(16):2287–92.
18. Lip GY, Halperin JL. Improving stroke risk stratification in atrial fibrillation. Am J Med. 2010;123(6):484–8.
19. Hijazi Z, Wallentin L, Siegbahn A, Andersson U, Christersson C, Ezekowitz J, et al. N-terminal pro-B-type natriuretic peptide for risk assessment in patients with atrial fibrillation: insights from the ARISTOTLE trial (Apixaban for the prevention of stroke in subjects with atrial fibrillation). J Am Coll Cardiol. 2013;61(22):2274–84.
20. Marrouche NF, Wilber D, Hindricks G, Jais P, Akoum N, Marchlinski F, et al. Association of atrial tissue fibrosis identified by delayed enhancement MRI and atrial fibrillation catheter ablation: the DECAAF study. JAMA. 2014;311(5):498–506.
21. Hijazi Z, Lindback J, Alexander JH, Hanna M, Held C, Hylek EM, et al. The ABC (age, biomarkers, clinical history) stroke risk score: a biomarker-based risk score for predicting stroke in atrial fibrillation. Eur Heart J. 2016;37(20):1582–90.
22. Markl M, Schnell S, Wu C, Bollache E, Jarvis K, Barker AJ, et al. Advanced flow MRI: emerging techniques and applications. Clin Radiol. 2016;71(8):779–95.
23. Pisters R, Lane DA, Nieuwlaat R, de Vos CB, Crijns HJ, Lip GYA. novel user-friendly score (HAS-BLED) to assess 1-year risk of major bleeding in patients with atrial fibrillation: the Euro Heart Survey. Chest. 2010;138(5):1093–100.
24. Fang MC, Go AS, Chang Y, Borowsky LH, Pomernacki NK, Udaltsova N, et al. A new risk scheme to predict warfarin-associated hemorrhage: The ATRIA (Anticoagulation and Risk Factors

in Atrial Fibrillation) study. J Am Coll Cardiol. 2011;58(4):395–401.
25. Roldan V, Marin F, Fernandez H, Manzano-Fernandez S, Gallego P, Valdes M, et al. Predictive value of the HAS-BLED and ATRIA bleeding scores for the risk of serious bleeding in a "real-world" population with atrial fibrillation receiving anticoagulant therapy. Chest. 2013;143(1):179–84.
26. Apostolakis S, Lane DA, Guo Y, Buller H, Lip GY. Performance of the HEMORR(2)HAGES, ATRIA, and HAS-BLED bleeding risk-prediction scores in patients with atrial fibrillation undergoing anticoagulation: the AMADEUS (evaluating the use of SR34006 compared to warfarin or acenocoumarol in patients with atrial fibrillation) study. J Am Coll Cardiol. 2012;60(9):861–7.
27. Senoo K, Proietti M, Lane DA, Lip GY. Evaluation of the HAS-BLED, ATRIA, and ORBIT bleeding risk scores in patients with atrial fibrillation taking warfarin. Am J Med. 2016;129(6):600–7.
28. Quinn GR, Singer DE, Chang Y, Go AS, Borowsky LH, Fang MC. How well do stroke risk scores predict hemorrhage in patients with atrial fibrillation? Am J Cardiol. 2016;118(5):697–9.
29. Connolly SJ, Ezekowitz MD, Yusuf S, Eikelboom J, Oldgren J, Parekh A, et al. Dabigatran versus warfarin in patients with atrial fibrillation. N Engl J Med. 2009;361(12):1139–51.
30. Patel MR, Mahaffey KW, Garg J, Pan G, Singer DE, Hacke W, et al. Rivaroxaban versus warfarin in nonvalvular atrial fibrillation. N Engl J Med. 2011;365(10):883–91.
31. Granger CB, Alexander JH, McMurray JJ, Lopes RD, Hylek EM, Hanna M, et al. Apixaban versus warfarin in patients with atrial fibrillation. N Engl J Med. 2011;365(11):981–92.
32. Giugliano RP, Ruff CT, Braunwald E, Murphy SA, Wiviott SD, Halperin JL, et al. Edoxaban versus warfarin in patients with atrial fibrillation. N Engl J Med. 2013;369(22):2093–104.
33. Olsson SB. Stroke prevention with the oral direct thrombin inhibitor ximelagatran compared with warfarin in patients with non-valvular atrial fibrillation (SPORTIF III): randomised controlled trial. Lancet. 2003;362(9397):1691–8.
34. Albers GW, Diener HC, Frison L, Grind M, Nevinson M, Partridge S, et al. Ximelagatran vs warfarin for stroke prevention in patients with nonvalvular atrial fibrillation: a randomized trial. JAMA. 2005;293(6):690–8.
35. Connolly SJ, Ezekowitz MD, Yusuf S, Reilly PA, Wallentin L. Newly identified events in the RE-LY trial. N Engl J Med. 2010;363(19):1875–6.
36. Kooiman J, van der Hulle T, Maas H, Wiebe S, Formella S, Clemens A, et al. Pharmacokinetics and pharmacodynamics of dabigatran 75 mg b.i.d. in patients with severe chronic kidney disease. J Am Coll Cardiol. 2016;67(20):2442–4.
37. Alere INRatio2 PT/INR professional test strips: recall - higher INR when performed by Central Laboratory. http://www.fda.gov/Safety/MedWatch/SafetyInformation/SafetyAlertsforHumanMedicalProducts/ucm396324.htm.
38. Patel MR, Hellkamp AS, Fox KA. Point-of-care warfarin monitoring in the ROCKET AF trial. N Engl J Med. 2016;374(8):785–8.
39. Fox KA, Piccini JP, Wojdyla D, Becker RC, Halperin JL, Nessel CC, et al. Prevention of stroke and systemic embolism with rivaroxaban compared with warfarin in patients with non-valvular atrial fibrillation and moderate renal impairment. Eur Heart J. 2011;32(19):2387–94.
40. Steinberg BA, Shrader P, Thomas L, Ansell J, Fonarow GC, Gersh BJ, et al. Off-label dosing of non-vitamin K antagonist oral anticoagulants and adverse outcomes: The ORBIT-AF II Registry. J Am Coll Cardiol. 2016;68(24):2597–604.
41. Connolly SJ, Eikelboom J, Joyner C, Diener HC, Hart R, Golitsyn S, et al. Apixaban in patients with atrial fibrillation. N Engl J Med. 2011;364(9):806–17.
42. Ruff CT, Giugliano RP, Braunwald E, Hoffman EB, Deenadayalu N, Ezekowitz MD, et al. Comparison of the efficacy and safety of new oral anticoagulants with warfarin in patients with atrial fibrillation: a meta-analysis of randomised trials. Lancet. 2014; 383(9921):955–62.
43. Kittelson JM, Steg PG, Halperin JL, Goldenberg NA, Schulman S, Spyropoulos AC, et al. Bivariate evaluation of thromboembolism and bleeding in clinical trials of anticoagulants in patients with atrial fibrillation. Thromb Haemost. 2016;116(3):544–53.
44. Kirchof P, Benussi S, Kotecha D, Ahlsson A, Atar D, Casadei B, et al. Task Force for the management of atrial fibrillation of the European Society of Cardiology (ESC). 2016 ESC Guidelines for the management of atrial fibrillation developed in collaboration with EACTS. Eur J Cardiothorac Surg. 2016;50(5):e1–e88.
45. January CT, Wann LS, Alpert JS, Calkins H, Cigarroa JE, Cleveland JC Jr, et al. 2014 AHA/ACC/HRS guideline for the management of patients with atrial fibrillation: a report of the American College of Cardiology/American Heart Association Task Force on Practice Guidelines and the Heart Rhythm Society. J Am Coll Cardiol. 2014;64(21):e1–76.
46. Chatterjee S, Sardar P, Biondi-Zoccai G, Kumbhani DJ. New oral anticoagulants and the risk of intracranial hemorrhage: traditional and Bayesian meta-analysis and mixed treatment comparison of randomized trials of new oral anticoagulants in atrial fibrillation. JAMA Neurol. 2013;70(12):1486–90.
47. Hankey GJ, Patel MR, Stevens SR, Becker RC, Breithardt G, Carolei A, et al. Rivaroxaban compared with warfarin in patients with atrial fibrillation and previous stroke or transient ischaemic attack: a subgroup analysis of ROCKET AF. Lancet Neurol. 2012;11(4):315–22.
48. Diener HC, Connolly SJ, Ezekowitz MD, Wallentin L, Reilly PA, Yang S, et al. Dabigatran compared with warfarin in patients with atrial fibrillation and previous transient ischaemic attack or stroke: a sub-

group analysis of the RE-LY trial. Lancet Neurol. 2010;9(12):1157–63.
49. Ntaios G, Papavasileiou V, Diener HC, Makaritsis K, Michel P. Nonvitamin-K-antagonist oral anticoagulants in patients with atrial fibrillation and previous stroke or transient ischemic attack: a systematic review and meta-analysis of randomized controlled trials. Stroke. 2012;43(12):3298–304.
50. Hohnloser SH, Hijazi Z, Thomas L, Alexander JH, Amerena J, Hanna M, et al. Efficacy of apixaban when compared with warfarin in relation to renal function in patients with atrial fibrillation: insights from the ARISTOTLE trial. Eur Heart J. 2012;33(22):2821–30.
51. Hijazi Z, Hohnloser SH, Oldgren J, Andersson U, Connolly SJ, Eikelboom JW, et al. Efficacy and safety of dabigatran compared with warfarin in relation to baseline renal function in patients with atrial fibrillation: a RE-LY (Randomized Evaluation of Long-term Anticoagulation Therapy) trial analysis. Circulation. 2014;129(9):961–70.
52. Shah M, Avgil Tsadok M, Jackevicius CA, Essebag V, Eisenberg MJ, Rahme E, et al. Warfarin use and the risk for stroke and bleeding in patients with atrial fibrillation undergoing dialysis. Circulation. 2014;129(11):1196–203.
53. Singer DE, Chang Y, Fang MC, Borowsky LH, Pomernacki NK, Udaltsova N, et al. The net clinical benefit of warfarin anticoagulation in atrial fibrillation. Ann Intern Med. 2009;151(5):297–305.
54. Halperin JL, Hankey GJ, Wojdyla DM, Piccini JP, Lokhnygina Y, Patel MR, et al. Efficacy and safety of rivaroxaban compared with warfarin among elderly patients with nonvalvular atrial fibrillation in the rivaroxaban once daily, oral, direct factor Xa inhibition compared with vitamin K antagonism for prevention of stroke and embolism trial in atrial fibrillation (ROCKET AF). Circulation. 2014;130(2):138–46.
55. Kato ET, Giugliano RP, Ruff CT, Koretsune Y, Yamashita T, Kiss RG, et al. Efficacy and safety of edoxaban in elderly patients with atrial fibrillation in the ENGAGE AF-TIMI 48 trial. J Am Heart Assoc. 2016;5(5):e003432.
56. Steffel J, Giugliano RP, Braunwald E, Murphy SA, Mercuri M, Choi Y, et al. Edoxaban versus warfarin in atrial fibrillation patients at risk of falling: ENGAGE AF-TIMI 48 analysis. J Am Coll Cardiol. 2016;68(11):1169–78.
57. Wang TD, Chen WJ, SS S, TC S, Chen MF, Liau CS, et al. Increased levels of tissue plasminogen activator antigen and factor VIII activity in nonvalvular atrial fibrillation: relation to predictors of thromboembolism. J Cardiovasc Electrophysiol. 2001;12(8):877–84.
58. Klem I, Wehinger C, Schneider B, Hartl E, Finsterer J, Stollberger C. Diabetic atrial fibrillation patients: mortality and risk for stroke or embolism during a 10-year follow-up. Diabetes Metab Res Rev. 2003;19(4):320–8.
59. Nieminen MS, Brutsaert D, Dickstein K, Drexler H, Follath F, Harjola VP, et al. EuroHeart Failure Survey II (EHFS II): a survey on hospitalized acute heart failure patients: description of population. Eur Heart J. 2006;27(22):2725–36.
60. Witt DM, Delate T, Clark NP, Martell C, Tran T, Crowther MA, et al. Outcomes and predictors of very stable INR control during chronic anticoagulation therapy. Blood. 2009;114(5):952–6.
61. Cappato R, Ezekowitz MD, Klein AL, Camm AJ, Ma CS, Le Heuzey JY, et al. Rivaroxaban vs. vitamin K antagonists for cardioversion in atrial fibrillation. Eur Heart J. 2014;35(47):3346–55.
62. Goette A, Merino JL, Ezekowitz MD, Zamoryakhin D, Melino M, Jin J, et al. Edoxaban versus enoxaparin-warfarin in patients undergoing cardioversion of atrial fibrillation (ENSURE-AF): a randomised, open-label, phase 3b trial. Lancet. 2016;388(10055):1995–2003.
63. Ezekowitz MD, Pollack CV, Sanders P, Halperin JL, Spahr J, Cater N, et al. Apixaban compared with parenteral heparin and/or vitamin K antagonist in patients with nonvalvular atrial fibrillation undergoing cardioversion: rationale and design of the EMANATE trial. Am Heart J. 2016;179:59–68.
64. Calkins H, Gerstenfeld EP, Schilling R, Verma A, Willems S. RE-CIRCUIT study-randomized evaluation of dabigatran etexilate compared to warfarin in pulmonary vein ablation: assessment of an uninterrupted periprocedural anticoagulation strategy. Am J Cardiol. 2015;115(1):154–5.
65. Cappato R, Marchlinski FE, Hohnloser SH, Naccarelli GV, Xiang J, Wilber DJ, et al. Uninterrupted rivaroxaban vs. uninterrupted vitamin K antagonists for catheter ablation in non-valvular atrial fibrillation. Eur Heart J. 2015;36(28):1805–11.
66. Gibson CM, Mehran R, Bode C, Halperin J, Verheugt FW, Wildgoose P, et al. Prevention of bleeding in patients with atrial fibrillation undergoing PCI. N Engl J Med. 2016;375(25):2423–34.
67. Cannon CP, Gropper S, Bhatt DL, Ellis SG, Kimura T, Lip GY, et al. Design and Rationale of the RE-DUAL PCI Trial: a prospective, randomized, phase 3b study comparing the safety and efficacy of dual antithrombotic therapy with dabigatran etexilate versus warfarin triple therapy in patients with nonvalvular atrial fibrillation who have undergone percutaneous coronary intervention with stenting. Clin Cardiol. 2016;39(10):555–64.
68. Gibson CM, Mehran R, Bode C, Halperin J, Verheugt F, Wildgoose P, et al. An open-label, randomized, controlled, multicenter study exploring two treatment strategies of rivaroxaban and a dose-adjusted oral vitamin K antagonist treatment strategy in subjects with atrial fibrillation who undergo percutaneous coronary intervention (PIONEER AF-PCI). Am Heart J. 2015;169(4):472–8.e5.
69. Santangeli P, Di Biase L, Horton R, Burkhardt JD, Sanchez J, Al-Ahmad A, et al. Ablation of atrial fibrillation under therapeutic warfarin reduces periprocedural complications: evidence from a meta-analysis. Circ Arrhythm Electrophysiol. 2012;5(2):302–11.

70. Dewilde WJ, Oirbans T, Verheugt FW, Kelder JC, De Smet BJ, Herrman JP, et al. Use of clopidogrel with or without aspirin in patients taking oral anticoagulant therapy and undergoing percutaneous coronary intervention: an open-label, randomised, controlled trial. Lancet. 2013;381(9872): 1107–15.
71. Diener HC, Aisenberg J, Ansell J, Atar D, Breithardt G, Eikelboom J, et al. Choosing a particular oral anticoagulant and dose for stroke prevention in individual patients with non-valvular atrial fibrillation: part 2. Eur Heart J. 2017;38(12):860–8.
72. Diener HC, Aisenberg J, Ansell J, Atar D, Breithardt G, Eikelboom J, et al. Choosing a particular oral anticoagulant and dose for stroke prevention in individual patients with non-valvular atrial fibrillation: part 1. Eur Heart J. 2017;38(12):852–9.
73. Pollack CV Jr, Reilly PA, Eikelboom J, Glund S, Verhamme P, Bernstein RA, et al. Idarucizumab for dabigatran reversal. N Engl J Med. 2015;373(6): 511–20.
74. Pollack CV Jr, Reilly PA, Bernstein R, Dubiel R, Eikelboom J, Glund S, et al. Design and rationale for RE-VERSE AD: a phase 3 study of idarucizumab, a specific reversal agent for dabigatran. Thromb Haemost. 2015;114(1):198–205.
75. Yeh CH, Fredenburgh JC, Weitz JI. The real decoy: an antidote for factor Xa-directed anticoagulants. Circ Res. 2013;113(8):954–7.
76. Lu G, DeGuzman FR, Hollenbach SJ, Karbarz MJ, Abe K, Lee G, et al. A specific antidote for reversal of anticoagulation by direct and indirect inhibitors of coagulation factor Xa. Nat Med. 2013;19(4):446–51.
77. Costin J, Ansell J, Laulicht B, Bakhru S, Steiner S. Reversal agents in development for the new oral anticoagulants. Postgrad Med. 2014;126(7):19–24.
78. Greinacher A, Thiele T, Selleng K. Reversal of anticoagulants: an overview of current developments. Thromb Haemost. 2015;113(5):931–42.
79. Siegal DM, Curnutte JT, Connolly SJ, Lu G, Conley PB, Wiens BL, et al. Andexanet alfa for the reversal of factor Xa inhibitor activity. N Engl J Med. 2015;373(25):2413–24.
80. Gomez-Outes A, Suarez-Gea ML, Lecumberri R, Terleira-Fernandez AI, Vargas-Castrillon E. Specific antidotes in development for reversal of novel anticoagulants: a review. Recent Pat Cardiovasc Drug Discov. 2014;9(1):2–10.

Anticoagulant Strategies for Electrophysiology Procedures

12

Stuart J. Beldner and David L. Stern

Clinical Vignettes

Case 1: *A 76-year-old woman with a past medical history of hypertension, non-insulin-dependent diabetes, and coronary artery disease status post bypass surgery 9 years ago, maintained on ASA 81 mg daily, a high-dose statin, an ACE inhibitor, and a beta-blocker, has experienced paroxysmal atrial fibrillation over the past 5 years for which she takes warfarin. Her INR is monitored monthly and is usually, but not always, in the therapeutic range, between 2.0 and 3.0. Although she has previously denied symptoms of her paroxysmal atrial fibrillation, upon review of an event monitor, her periods of atrial fibrillation correlated with fatigue and dyspnea on exertion. After discussion of risks, benefits, and alternatives, the decision is made to perform pulmonary vein isolation (PVI) and ablation. You consider how best to manage her anticoagulant and antiplatelet medications before, during, and after the PVI procedure.*

Case 2: *A 33-year-old man in the second year of his cardiovascular disease fellowship develops palpitations while working overnight. He has had palpitations in the past, but they were transient and resolved spontaneously. This episode does not resolve. He has no known risk factors for cardiovascular disease. He checks his own pulse and finds it is approximately 170 beats/min. He reports to the emergency room, at which point he is put on a monitor, and an EKG is performed. He is found to be normotensive at 105/60, and his EKG demonstrates atrial fibrillation with a rapid ventricular rate of 164 beats/min. He tells the emergency room (ER) physician that the last thing he ate was more than 12 h prior, but he has had several cups of coffee and one energy drink (containing caffeine). He denies any other drug use and reports no allergies to medications. In the ER, the fellow/patient receives intravenous atrioventricular (AV) nodal blockers (a calcium channel blocker), with some reduction in heart rate and improvement in symptoms. He is then given an oral equivalent of the calcium channel blocker, and his blood pressure is monitored without evidence of hypotension throughout the night. You consider how best to manage his atrial fibrillation and necessary therapies for stroke prevention.*

S. J. Beldner (✉) · D. L. Stern
Department of Cardiology, Northwell Health, Zucker School of Medicine at Hofstra/Northwell, Manhasset, NY, USA
e-mail: sbelder@northwell.edu; dstern@northwell.edu

J. F. Lau et al. (eds.), *Anticoagulation Therapy*, https://doi.org/10.1007/978-3-319-73709-6_12

Case 3: *A 92-year-old man with a history of heart failure with preserved ejection fraction, EF 70%, non-insulin-dependent diabetes, stage IV chronic kidney disease, and atrial fibrillation for which he is on apixaban 2.5 mg twice daily is admitted to the hospital with syncope. His list of home medications includes a beta-blocker. Admission EKG reveals sinus bradycardia at 48 bpm with first-degree AV delay (PR interval of 230 ms), RBBB with LAFB, and a QRS of 125 ms. The beta-blocker is held. While on telemetry monitoring, he is noted to have paroxysms of atrial fibrillation with ventricular rates in the 130 s while sleeping and conversation pauses of greater than 6 s. He is sleeping during these episodes and reports no symptoms. After discussion with the patient, the decision is made to put in a pacemaker. You consider how best to manage apixaban before, during, and after a pacemaker implantation.*

Risks and Benefits of Anticoagulation in Patients Undergoing Electrophysiology Procedures

The decision to use anticoagulation prior to, during, and/or after an electrophysiology procedure is always based on balancing the risks and benefits for the individual patient and the specific procedure. Atrial fibrillation is the most common arrhythmia requiring the use of anticoagulation, and it is the most common arrhythmia seen in patients presenting for electrophysiology procedures: it affects up to 10% of the population by the time a patient reaches 80 years of age [1]. Based on data from the Framingham Heart Study, a patient's lifetime risk of developing atrial fibrillation is approximately 25% [2]. For patients with atrial fibrillation, therapeutic anticoagulation with warfarin or one of the direct oral anticoagulants remains the gold standard in prevention of thromboembolic events, most notably, stroke. The $CHADS_2$ [3] and CHA_2DS_2-VASc [4] risk calculators provide evidence-based annualized stroke risk estimation for patients with atrial fibrillation while not on anticoagulation therapy (see Table 12.1), and these risk scores help inform our decisions regarding anticoagulation before, during, and after procedures (see Table 12.2 for review of ACC/AHA/HRS guidelines on the management of atrial fibrillation). These scores help reinforce the notion that patients with prior cerebrovascular events are at especially high risk, but they are not comprehensive risk scores; for example, they do not capture the significant risk of thromboembolic events associated with mechanical mitral and aortic valves, which would also require continuous anticoagulation. As such, these risk calculators are helpful guidelines, but are not intended to be absolute rules for anticoagulation. The anticoagulant strategies for electrophysiology procedures are well informed by data but continue to require sound clinical judgment by practitioners.

The risk of thromboembolic events must always be weighed against the risk of bleeding. As the $CHADS_2$ and CHA_2DS_2-VASc schemas predict thromboembolic risk (see Table 12.1), there have been calculators to assess bleeding risk. HAS-BLED is most widely used and assigns risk to *h*ypertension, *a*bnormal renal/liver function, *s*troke, *b*leeding history or predisposition, *l*abile INRs, *e*lderly (>65 years old), and use of *d*rugs that promote bleeding excess or alcohol [4]. An elevated HAS-BLED score (>3) indicates a "high risk" for bleeding and suggests that a patient may receive more harm than benefit from anticoagulation. Similarly, the electrophysiology procedures themselves carry varied risks of thromboembolism and bleeding.

Table 12.1 Evidence-based recommendations for anticoagulation for patients with atrial fibrillation [5]

Class I (Level A) recommendations
1. Warfarin for patients with patients with CHADSVASc ≥ 2
2. Monitoring of INR at least weekly while initiating warfarin
Class I (Level B) recommendations
1. Determination of anticoagulation based on risk of thromboembolism
2. Use of CHADSVASc to assess risk of stroke
3. Warfarin for patients with mechanical heart valves—higher INRs, depending on type of valve
4. Use of direct oral anticoagulants, e.g., dabigatran, rivaroxaban, or apixaban, for patients with CHADSVASc ≥2
5. Assessing renal function prior to initiation of direct oral anticoagulant and repeating assessment annually
Class I (Level C) recommendations
1. Using discussion of risks of stroke and of bleeding and patient's preferences in determining anticoagulation
2. Use of direct oral anticoagulants in patients who cannot maintain therapeutic INR
3. Reevaluating the need for anticoagulation on periodic basis
4. Bridging with heparin or LMWH when a mechanical valve is involved
5. Use of risk/benefit analysis to determine bridging even when no mechanical valve is involved
6. Anticoagulation for atrial flutter
Class IIa (Level A) recommendations: None
Class IIa (Level B) recommendations
1. Not using anticoagulation for patients with CHADSVASc = 0
2. Warfarin for patients with CHADSVASc ≥2 and end-stage kidney disease (CrCl < 15 mL/min)
Class IIb (Level B) recommendation
– Clopidogrel and oral anticoagulation (without ASA) after revascularization in patients with CHADSVASc ≥2
Class IIb (Level C) recommendation
1. Not using anticoagulation, or using ASA, for patients CHADSVASc = 1 who have nonvalvular atrial fibrillation
2. Reducing doses of direct oral anticoagulants for patients with moderate-severe CKD
3. Using bare metal stents for PCI to reduce the duration of DAPT
Class III (Level B)—Harm seen with use of dabigatran in patients with mechanical heart valves
Class III (Level C)—No benefit seen in using dabigatran or rivaroxaban in patients with end-stage CKD or dialysis

As an example, direct current cardioversion to restore normal sinus rhythm should be performed while anticoagulated, because the risks of procedural and post-procedural thromboembolism are high, while the procedural risks of bleeding are nominal; the only bleeding that the authors have seen that can be attributed to cardioversion is the rare event when a patient has bitten his/her tongue, and blood loss has been minimal in those cases. By contrast, the thromboembolic risks of laser lead extraction are dwarfed by the very significant procedural risks of bleeding, and so although there is no published data that specifically addresses the risks and benefits of anticoagulation during laser lead extraction, we would recommend against performing this procedure while on uninterrupted anticoagulation.

The patient-specific risks and benefits may be further complicated by comorbidities and medications that are not included in their $CHADS_2$ and CHA_2DS_2-VASc risk scores, such as coronary artery disease and/or recent percutaneous coronary interventions requiring the use of antiplatelet agents. Published in 2013, the results of WOEST trial suggest that, for patients requiring both anticoagulation and antiplatelet therapy, bleeding events could be reduced by using monotherapy with clopidogrel, rather than dual antiplatelet therapy with clopidogrel and aspirin [6]. In light of the reduced risk of bleeding with single antiplatelet therapy compared with dual antiplatelet therapy, for elective electrophysiology procedures such as generator changes or catheter ablations of atrial fibrillation, atrial flutter, or ventricular tachycardia, our preference is to postpone the procedure until the patient no longer requires dual antiplatelet therapy.

Device implantations, catheter ablations, cardioversions, left atrial appendage occlusion, and all of their variations involve the risk of bleeding. This risk is often amplified by the pre-, peri-, and post-procedural requirements for anticoagulation. The evidence base for current practice of each of anticoagulation strategies for these electrophysiology procedures is discussed here.

Table 12.2 $CHADS_2$ versus CHADSVASc, approximate annualized % risk of CVA without anticoagulation [5]

Score	0	1	2	3	4	5	6	7	8	9
$CHADS_2$	1.9	2.8	4.0	5.9	8.5	12.5	18.2			
CHA_2DS_2-VASc	0	1.3	2.2	3.2	4.0	6.7	9.8	9.6	6.7	15.2

Anticoagulation Prior to Elective Device Implant

As of published data from 2011, each year more than one million pacemakers and more than 400,000 implantable cardioverter-defibrillators are implanted worldwide [7]. Between 14% and 35% of those patients are on long-term oral anticoagulation. For many years, data was extrapolated from interventional procedures performed in the catheterization lab such that for procedures performed via the femoral site, the preferred target INR was less than 1.8 in order to reduce the risks of bleeding [8]. In order to reduce the risk of thromboembolic events, guidelines suggested that patients be instructed to discontinue their oral anticoagulants several days prior to procedures, and they were often bridged to the procedure using heparin [9]. More recently, data from BRUISE CONTROL suggested that bridging was associated with a higher incidence of hematoma formation [10]. This trial was specifically designed to determine whether a strategy of continued warfarin treatment at the time of pacemaker or ICD implant or generator change, in patients at moderate-to-high risk for thromboembolic events (annual predicted risk of thromboembolism of 5% or more), reduces the incidence of clinically significant device-pocket hematoma, as compared with the current standard of practice of bridging with heparin. In those patients for whom the procedure was performed on continued oral anticoagulation, a targeted INR of less than 3.0 was used for most patients, or an INR of less than 3.5 for those with mechanical valves. Significant device hematomas, defined as a hematoma requiring further surgery, resulting in prolongation of hospitalization, or requiring interruption of oral anticoagulation therapy, occurred in 3.5% of those with uninterrupted warfarin compared with 16% of those being bridged (relative risk, 0.19; 95% confidence interval (CI), 0.10–0.36; $P < 0.001$). Hematomas themselves are associated with increased risk for infection following electrophysiology procedures. Our current strategy is to perform presurgical evaluation 2 days prior to the planned procedure and to adjust warfarin dosing such that patients arrive on the day of their procedure at the lower end of their therapeutic range. Pacemaker and defibrillator implantation is then performed without interruption of oral anticoagulation. BRUISE CONTROL 2 is studying the same intervention with the direct oral anticoagulants.

Pulmonary Vein Isolation and Catheter Ablation of Atrial Fibrillation

Some electrophysiology procedures themselves carry elevated risks for periprocedural thromboembolic events. Radiofrequency catheter ablation of atrial fibrillation is one such procedure. A consensus statement from 2007 suggested discontinuation of oral anticoagulation 3–5 days prior to the planned procedure with bridging using low molecular weight heparin [11]. But in 2012, a meta-analysis that included more than 27,000 patients was performed which showed highly consistent evidence that continuing therapeutic warfarin during radiofrequency catheter ablation of atrial fibrillation reduced the risk of thromboembolic complications without increasing the risk of bleeding [12]. When major bleeding occurs, reversal of warfarin anticoagulation with fresh frozen plasma and/or prothrombin complex concentrate (Kcentra) is the standard of care. In 2014, Di Biase and colleagues published a randomized study showing that performing catheter ablation of atrial fibrillation without warfarin discontinuation reduces the occurrence of periprocedural stroke and minor bleeding complications compared to bridging with low molecular weight heparin [13].

Since then, there have been multiple studies exploring the feasibility and safety of uninterrupted use of the direct oral anticoagulants (DOAC) for catheter ablation of atrial fibrillation. Dabigatran was the first DOAC to be approved for stroke prevention in nonvalvular atrial fibrillation. The data on uninterrupted dabigatran for stroke prevention in patients undergoing catheter ablation of atrial fibrillation thus far have been inconsistent, with some early meta-analyses raising caution over increased thromboembolic and bleeding events in patients receiving dabigatran. RE-CIRCUIT [14], the largest trial (704 patients) to compare the use of a DOAC (dabigatran) with uninterrupted warfarin in the context of atrial fibrillation ablation, suggests that dabigatran outperforms warfarin. The trial showed a 5.3% reduction (1.6% vs 6.9%) in its primary endpoint of major bleeding events during ablation or in the first 2 months post-procedure. Specifically, there were fewer incidents of periprocedural tamponade and groin hematomas. It is important to note that there were no events of stroke, systemic embolism, or transient ischemic attacks in the dabigatran group.

Data on the uninterrupted use of rivaroxaban or apixaban have also promising results [15, 16]. In 2014, Lakkireddy and colleagues published results from a multicenter prospective registry which had enrolled 642 patients with paroxysmal atrial fibrillation, half of whom received uninterrupted procedural rivaroxaban and half of whom received uninterrupted warfarin while undergoing catheter ablation of atrial fibrillation. The groups were matched for age, sex, and type of atrial fibrillation. In the 30 days following the procedures, there were no significant differences between the groups in major bleeding, minor bleeding, or embolic complications. Similarly, in 2015, Di Biase and colleagues published their data from a prospective multicenter registry including 400 patients, half of whom received uninterrupted apixaban and half of whom received uninterrupted warfarin; the groups were matched for age, gender, and type of atrial fibrillation. The apixaban group received their last dose of apixaban the morning of the procedure. There were no significant differences in the outcomes between the two groups in terms of major, minor, or total bleeding complications. Twenty-nine patients in the apixaban group received magnetic resonance imaging (MRI) to assess for silent cerebral ischemia. All the MRIs were negative for new asymptomatic cerebral ischemia.

There are circumstances in which the decision is made to hold anticoagulation because the short-term risks of thromboembolism are outweighed by the procedural bleeding risks for a particular patient. When long-term anticoagulation is held, there is concern for rebound hypercoagulability. In order to mitigate these risks, we often give low-dose aspirin when holding these medications. We hold the dose the evening before and morning of the procedure. These medications are currently irreversible, and our practice is to give intravenous heparin for 24 h until the patient has declared no bleeding complication. There is some data on the safety of resumption of the oral anticoagulation immediately post-procedure [17, 18]. These studies include few patients, and it seems more conservative to observe for some period of time prior to resuming irreversible oral anticoagulants. We also believe that patients undergoing catheter ablation of atrial fibrillation, with its inherent risks of stroke, late pericardial effusion (inflammatory, as opposed to the immediate risk of procedural tamponade due to perforation), and groin complications, should be observed in the hospital overnight regardless of the anticoagulation status.

During catheter ablation of atrial fibrillation, there is inherent stroke risk from moving catheters in the left atrium. Similar risk is seen with ablation in the left ventricle. While for left ventricular procedures we aim for a target activated clotting time (ACT) of 250–300 s, for left atrial ablations anticoagulation is more aggressive with ACT targets up to 350–400 s. This is most often done through therapy with intravenous heparin. Baetz and colleagues report on ventricular tachycardia (VT) and atrial fibrillation (AF) ablation on bivalirudin a protocol that we have also used for patients with prior heparin-induced thrombocytopenia (HIT) [19]. The protocol describes bivalirudin administered as a 0.75 mg/kg intravenous bolus, followed by a 1.75 mg/kg/h infusion. Activated clotting time (ACT) was measured after the initial bolus in each patient. However, no dosage adjustment was made based on the ACT, and the infusion rate of bivalirudin remained fixed during the procedures. Anecdotally, argatroban has also been used safely.

Access sheaths for atrial ablation are venous which makes the aforementioned data on coronary angiography less applicable. However, the sheaths are quite large, ranging from a 6 or 7 French sheath for a coronary sinus catheter up to a 15 Fr FlexCath sheath (™Medtronic) for a cryoballoon. "Figure-of-eight" stitches in the groin do show a lower incidence of groin complications [20].

All patients, even those with the lowest thromboembolic risks, should be maintained on oral anticoagulation for 3 months after ablation. There is some concern for periprocedural increased risk for thromboembolic complication. Patients will often ask about discontinuing their oral anticoagulation following "successful" ablation. They should be counseled *before* the procedure that ablative therapy is meant as management, and not "cure" of atrial fibrillation, and thus recommendations for oral anticoagulation should be similar to those patients who did not undergo ablation. These recommendations are based on continued thromboembolic risks. In the 2014 American Heart Association/American College of Cardiology/Heart Rhythm Association guidelines for the management of patients with atrial fibrillation, therapy for anticoagulation using the CHA_2DS_2-VASc risk stratification scheme is a class I recommendation [5]. While the procedure is not meant as "cure," there are certainly patients who will have the procedure and never demonstrate AF again. Such a patient is then exposed to the approximately 3% per year risk of bleeding on oral anticoagulation without the similar risk for stroke. While robust data is lacking, there are practitioners that use the implantable loop recorder to monitor patients while holding anticoagulation [21]. This should be used with caution as there may be a delay in diagnosing recurrent arrhythmia. Furthermore, there are late recurrences, even occurring beyond 5 years after the initial episode. Because of continued thromboembolic risks even after ablation, the 2014 guidelines offer a class I recommendation for the clinician and patient to engage in shared decision-making with regard to anticoagulation therapy after reviewing the patient's stroke versus bleeding risk.

Anticoagulation for Cardioversion

For many years, the conventional treatment strategy for patients with atrial fibrillation who were to undergo electrical cardioversion was to prescribe warfarin for anticoagulation for 3 weeks prior to cardioversion (see Table 12.3). In 2001, the ACUTE Multicenter Study provided data to support an alternative strategy: transesophageal echocardiography could be used to guide management [22]. Using transesophageal echocardiography to evaluate the left atrium and left atrial appendage for the presence of thrombus significantly reduced the time to cardioversion. Although this leads to fewer spontaneous conversions, it also significantly reduced the number of bleeding events compared with requiring 3 months of therapeutic anticoagulation with warfarin prior to cardioversion. There was no significant increase in the rate of thromboembolic events between the two groups, although, admittedly, the rates of events were very low in both groups. If a thrombus was detected in the left atrial appendage, the study protocol called for the same 3 weeks of anticoagulation that the conventional treatment arm was receiving, followed by repeat imaging. If the repeat transesophageal echocardiogram no longer demonstrated the presence of thrombus, cardioversion was performed. All groups received continued therapeutic anticoagulation with warfarin for 4 weeks post-cardioversion.

The data from the ACUTE trial has often been applied to those patients on DOACs. That is, patients who have been on uninterrupted oral anticoagulation should be able to proceed with electrical cardioversion. There are inherent con-

Table 12.3 Recommendations for cardioversion [5]

Class I (Level A): Pharmacologic cardioversion in patients without contraindications to selected agent
Class I (Level B)
1. Anticoagulate with warfarin for 3 weeks prior to and 4 weeks after cardioversion for AF ≥48 h (or unknown duration)
2. Cardioversion can be repeated if first attempt at restoring sinus rhythm fails
Class I (Level C)
1. For patients requiring immediate cardioversion, anticoagulate as soon as possible for at least 4 weeks after
2. For patients with AF <48 h and high stroke risk, recommend anticoagulation prior to cardioversion
3. Long-term anticoagulation after cardioversion based on risk of thromboembolic events
4. Electrical cardioversion for patients who do not respond to pharmacologic attempts
5. Electrical cardioversion for patients with AF and preexcitation and hemodynamic instability
Class IIa (Level A): Amiodarone can be used for pharmacologic cardioversion
Class IIa (Level B)
1. TEE can be used to clear LA if anticoagulation can be achieved prior to and for 4 weeks after cardioversion
2. "Pill-in-the-pocket" with flecainide or propafenone can be used once it is safely demonstrated in monitored setting
Class IIa (Level C)
1. Use of direct oral anticoagulants for ≥3 weeks prior to and 4 weeks after cardioversion
2. Reasonable to repeat cardioversion if sinus rhythm can be maintained for meaningful period of time
Class IIb (Level C): Use of direct oral anticoagulant for cardioversion in patient with AF <48 h and low thromboembolic risk
Class III (Level B): Harm with use of dofetilide that is initiated on outpatient basis

cerns for such a strategy, such as the reliability of the patient with no INR to confirm therapeutic anticoagulation. Furthermore, caution should be advised toward the application of this data to patients that were not included in the trials, for example, patients with very elevated body mass indexes or the 75 mg dosing of dabigatran. Nonetheless, there are data to support the use of dabigatran, apixaban, and rivaroxaban for anticoagulation prior to and after cardioversion; the rates of stroke and systemic embolism are similar as with warfarin. In the RE-LY trial, 1938 cardioversions were performed in 1270 patients with different strategies with respect to dosing, antecedent transesophageal echo, and duration of oral anticoagulation post-cardioversion [23]. In ARISTOTLE [24], there were 743 cardioversions in 540 patients. Results were similar. The X-VeRT investigators studied rivaroxaban versus vitamin K antagonists specifically for the purpose of cardioversion [25]. The use of 3 weeks of oral anticoagulation versus antecedent transesophageal echocardiography was at the discretion of the treating physician. For those patients undergoing early cardioversion, rivaroxaban was given at least 4 h prior. Rivaroxaban was associated with a significantly shorter time to cardioversion compared with VKAs ($P < 0.001$) and proved to be an effective safe alternative to vitamin K antagonist therapy.

The authors' experience is that those patients with severe left ventricular dysfunction are most likely to show thrombus within the left atrial appendage. Perhaps this is related to stasis in the left ventricle potentiating stasis in the left atrium and magnifying risk. Often, aggressive rate control can improve left ventricular function, thereby decreasing left atrial stasis and mitigating that risk of left atrial appendage thrombus. On seeing left atrial appendage thrombus, our practice is similar to what has been laid out in the ACUTE trial: we continue anticoagulation and wait at least 3 weeks, and then we repeat a transesophageal echocardiogram and proceed with cardioversion only if no thrombus present. If thrombus persists, we delay cardioversion further and often change anticoagulation strategy. Once we have confirmed spontaneous echo contrast in the left atrial appendage, we also tend to be more aggressive with the oral anticoagulation.

One of the limitations to the randomized controlled trials that validated the DOACs as safe and effective alternatives to warfarin is that when you maintain adequate time in therapeutic range (INR of 2–3), you reduce the relative benefits of the novel agents over warfarin. Further, there is no published data comparing warfarin use with a goal INR of 2.5–3.5, with the notable exception of the documented slightly higher bleeding risk for a patient with known left atrial thrombus. Furthermore, the benefit of these agents does appear to be blunted in those patients with a high time in therapeutic range. Thus if a patient demonstrates thrombus on a DOAC or on warfarin with therapeutic INR, our strategy is vitamin K antagonist with this higher target INR. There is evidence from meta-analyses of randomized controlled studies that home monitoring of vitamin K antagonist therapy reduces thromboembolic events by 42% compared with usual monitoring. This is similar to the 33% relative risk reduction with dabigatran 150 mg BID. [26]. As the risk of bleeding significantly increases as patients go above our therapeutic range, intensifying anticoagulation should accompany this strategy if feasible.

Left Atrial Appendage Occlusion Using Watchman

Anticoagulation remains the gold standard for prevention of thromboembolic events in patients with atrial fibrillation. For some patients, however, the risks of long-term anticoagulation outweigh benefits. In these patients, occlusion of the left atrial appendage with a Watchman device can safely and effectively reduce the long-term risks of stroke. The majority of published data on anticoagulation before or after a Watchman implantation comes from the studies that lead to its approval for use, e.g., the PROTECT AF [27] trial and the PREVAIL trial [28]. In PROTECT AF, 707 patients were randomized in a 2:1 ratio to either device placement followed by warfarin and aspirin for 45 days or then dual antiplatelet therapy with clopidogrel and aspirin for 6 months, followed by aspirin indefinitely or long-term warfarin with a target INR range of 2–3. Efficacy was determined by a composite of stroke, cardiovascular death, and systemic embolism. At 18 months, the rates of stroke, cardiovascular death, and systemic embolism were similar in intervention and control groups, suggesting noninferiority of efficacy for the Watchman compared with standard of care. However, the rates of major bleeding, pericardial effusion, and device embolization were higher with device placement (7.4 events/100 patient-years vs 4.4, rate ratio 1.69, CI 1.01–3.19). To address this periprocedural safety hazard, investigators performed the PREVAIL trial. Patients were randomly assigned (in a 2:1 ratio) to undergo LAA occlusion and subsequent discontinuation of warfarin (intervention group, $n = 269$) or receive chronic warfarin therapy (control group, $n = 138$). Two efficacy and one safety co-primary endpoints were assessed. In PREVAIL, LAA occlusion was noninferior to warfarin for ischemic stroke prevention or systemic embolism greater than 7 days post-procedure. Event rates in the group receiving the Watchman device were much lower in PREVAIL than in PROTECT AF, which has been interpreted to suggest improved procedural safety. Taken together, these two studies demonstrated the safety and efficacy of the Watchman device compared to long-term warfarin. There was significant reduction in hemorrhagic stroke and major bleeds and a suggestion of mortality benefit.

For those patients maintained on oral anticoagulation, we continue it through the procedure. However, many of the patients are not appropriate candidates for long-term anticoagulation and deserve special consideration. In these patients, aspirin 81 mg daily is started prior to Watchman implantation. The Watchman device is then implanted while the patient is receiving full-dose anticoagulation, with a goal activated clotting time (ACT) of 300–350 ms. With the large cryoballoon delivery system, the access sheath used to deliver the sheath is 14 French, and in our electrophysiology laboratory, venous hemostasis is achieved via a figure-of-eight suturing method. On the day of the procedure, warfarin is added and will be continued through 45 days post-device implantation. Post-procedural transesophageal echocardiographic imaging is routinely performed to confirm successful implantation. If there is less than 5 mm leak around the device, warfarin is substituted for clopidogrel and the dosage of aspirin is increased to 300–325 mg daily. For patients with no detectable leak at the 6-month follow-up period, clopidogrel may be stopped, and the patient remains on full-dose aspirin (300–325 mg) indefinitely. For patients with peri-device leak, the seal at the left atrial appendage site should be reassessed, and both warfarin and aspirin should be continued until there is redemonstration that there is a <5 mm leak. In the PREVAIL study, 99% of patients had stopped taking warfarin by 1 year following Watchman implantation. The EWOLUTION registry, which focused on outcomes in real-life utilization of the WATCHMAN device, demonstrated similar implant success and safety outcomes at 1-year follow-up [29].

In the original studies, patients were intended to be continued on anticoagulation for 6 weeks; however, many of them required discontinuation. In our practice, we have seen patients maintained on anticoagulation using DOACs instead of warfarin prior to and after Watchman implantation, but this use is currently off label and not yet supported by published data [30, 31]. Additionally, the ASAP registry followed patients post implant on dual antiplatelet therapy (aspirin and Plavix) [32]. Of the 150 patients enrolled, there were six cases (4%) of device-related thrombus on the device face, but only one resulted in clinical sequela (an ischemic stroke). Antiplatelet therapy will be further evaluated in the ASAP-TOO study (NCT02928497), a multicenter randomized trial for left atrial appendage occlusion in patients not suitable for oral anticoagulation. That is, more data on ideal anticoagulation therapy with this new technology will be forthcoming.

Conclusion

Management of anticoagulation during EP procedures is complex. Using the risk profile of the patient and the available data allows for the safest strategy.

Key Points

- The decision to use anticoagulation prior to, during, and/or after an electrophysiology procedure is always based on balancing the risks and benefits for the individual patient and the specific procedure.
- Current data supports implantation of pacemakers and defibrillators on therapeutic anticoagulation without interruption or bridging using heparin or low molecular weight heparin.
- Given the procedural risks of thromboembolic events, electrical cardioversion and catheter ablations should be performed using effective anticoagulation prior to, during, and after the procedure.
- As electrophysiologic procedures continue to advance, so will our understanding of the optimal regimen of anticoagulation prior to, during, and after the procedures.

Self-Assessment Questions

1. A 76-year-old woman with a past medical history of hypertension, non-insulin-dependent diabetes, and coronary artery disease status post bypass surgery 9 years ago, maintained on aspirin 81 mg daily and warfarin with a goal INR of 2.0–3.0, is now scheduled for catheter ablation of atrial fibrillation. Which of the following is true?
   (a) She should be changed to a direct oral anticoagulant prior to her procedure.
   (b) She must hold her anticoagulation for at least 5 days prior to her procedure.
   (c) She must hold aspirin for 5 days prior to her procedure irrespective of her periprocedural warfarin management.
   (d) The decision to continue or hold anticoagulation pre- and post-procedure should be made based on the risks of thromboembolism compared with the risks of bleeding.
   (e) If her ablation is successful, she will no longer require anticoagulation afterward.
2. A 68-year-old gentleman reports progressive dyspnea on exertion. His baseline EKG shows

sinus bradycardia with a rate of 49 beats/min, a first-degree AV delay with a PR interval of 240 ms, and bifascicular block. An event monitor confirms sick sinus syndrome, paroxysms of atrial fibrillation ranging from seconds to hours in duration, and conversion pauses of up to 4.9 s, one of which corresponded with witnessed syncope. He has no history of significant bleeding. He is started on warfarin with a goal INR of 2.0–3.0 to reduce his risk of thromboembolic events. A pacemaker is also recommended. Which of the following is the best option for this patient based on current data?

(a) Maintain INR 2.5–3.5 for pacemaker implantation as the procedure carries high risk of thromboembolic stroke.
(b) Hold warfarin for at least 72 h prior to pacemaker implantation and bridge with aspirin 81 mg daily.
(c) Hold warfarin for at least 72 h prior to pacemaker implantation and bridge with low molecular weight heparin.
(d) Proceed with device implantation while patient is anticoagulated with warfarin and his INR is 2.0–3.0.
(e) Pacemaker implantation should be postponed until catheter ablation of atrial fibrillation can be performed first.

3. A 45-year-old firefighter with a known history of hypertension, diabetes, previous cerebral vascular event that may have been embolic, obstructive sleep apnea, and paroxysmal atrial fibrillation is maintained on rivaroxaban daily for anticoagulation. He presents to the emergency department with shortness of breath and is found to be in atrial fibrillation with rapid ventricular response to 190 beats/min. He is rate controlled with diltiazem, and he is scheduled for a transesophageal echocardiogram and possible direct current cardioversion in the morning. Which of the following is a disadvantage of rivaroxaban compared with warfarin in this setting?
   (a) In randomized controlled studies, rivaroxaban has been shown to cause more intracranial bleeding than warfarin.
   (b) In randomized controlled studies, rivaroxaban has been shown to prevent fewer strokes than warfarin.
   (c) For unreliable patients, there is no way to verify their most recent dose of rivaroxaban, whereas you can check a patient's INR to confirm adequate anticoagulation while on warfarin.
   (d) Rivaroxaban requires twice daily dosing, reducing patient adherence.
   (e) Rivaroxaban requires more frequent monitoring than does warfarin.
4. A 64-year-old woman with previous catheter ablation of her caval-tricuspid isthmus to treat atrial flutter now presents with symptomatic paroxysmal atrial fibrillation. She is started on apixaban 5 mg orally twice a day for anticoagulation, and she is started on rate control and antiarrhythmic therapies. After failing several medical options, she discusses catheter ablation of atrial fibrillation with her electrophysiologist. Which of the following statements about her procedure is *false*?
   (a) Catheter ablation of atrial fibrillation carries a procedural risk of thromboembolic events, and patients must be anticoagulated during the procedure.
   (b) Warfarin is the only reversible option for oral anticoagulation prior to and immediately after catheter ablation of atrial fibrillation.
   (c) Catheter ablation of atrial fibrillation carries a risk of pericardial effusion.
   (d) Electrophysiologists can use activated clotting times to monitor a patient's level of anticoagulation during the procedure.
   (e) Patients are recommended to continue oral anticoagulation after catheter ablation of atrial fibrillation as there remains a risk of recurrence of atrial fibrillation and an elevated risk of thromboembolic events.
   (f) Catheter ablation of atrial fibrillation is really simple. Anyone can do it.
5. A 55-year-old gentleman presents for elective transesophageal echocardiogram and direct current cardioversion of his atrial fibrillation.

He has been maintained on apixaban 5 mg BID for the past several weeks. Prior to the planned procedure, he reports that he has not taken apixaban for 2 days because he remembers being told to hold it for 2 days prior to dental work and he figured the same advice applied to these scheduled procedures. Which of the following is true?
(a) If he takes a dose of apixaban 5 mg right now, it is safe to proceed with the procedure.
(b) If you check his INR, you may still be able to perform the cardioversion.
(c) It is not safe to perform cardioversion today.
(d) Patient can take 10 mg of apixaban right now and be safely cardioverted.
(e) Apixaban should always be held or reversed prior to invasive procedures such as transesophageal echocardiogram and cardioversion.

Self-Assessment Answers

1. (d) The decision to continue or hold anticoagulation pre- and post-procedure should be made based on the risks of thromboembolism compared with the risks of bleeding.

   For any electrophysiology procedure, the decision to continue or hold anticoagulation pre- and post-procedure should always be made based on the risks of thromboembolism compared with the risks of bleeding. There is no need to change from warfarin to a direct oral anticoagulant prior to ablation. Anticoagulation can be continued without interruption prior to ablation. Holding aspirin is not necessary prior to ablation. Ablation should reduce the burden of atrial fibrillation, but standard of care is to continue anticoagulation after successful catheter ablation of atrial fibrillation.
2. (d) Proceed with device implantation while patient is anticoagulated with warfarin and his INR is 2.0–3.0.

   BRUISE CONTROL demonstrated that bridging with heparin or low molecular weight heparin increased risks of bleeding and hematoma formation compared with continuing therapeutic anticoagulation without bridging.
3. (c) For unreliable patients, there is no way to verify their most recent dose of rivaroxaban, whereas you can check a patient's INR to confirm adequate anticoagulation while on warfarin.

   In the ROCKET AF trial, rivaroxaban was found to be non-inferior to warfarin in both bleeding and stroke. There is no precise monitoring for anticoagulation while on rivaroxaban, while INR can be measured for patients on warfarin.
4. (b) Warfarin is the only reversible option for oral anticoagulation prior to and immediately after catheter ablation of atrial fibrillation.

   Choice b is the correct choice because it is the only FALSE statement. Although warfarin is reversible, dabigatran is also reversible. In late 2015, the FDA approved idarucizumab for reversal of dabigatran. Choices a, c, d, and e are all true statements. Choice f is a matter of great debate.
5. (c) It is not safe to perform cardioversion today.

   The patient has not been effectively anticoagulated while holding the apixaban. In that time, he is at increased risk of developing thrombus that can embolize with conversion to sinus rhythm.

References

1. Kannel WB, Abbott RD, Savage DD, McNamara PM. Epidemiologic features of chronic atrial fibrillation: the Framingham study. N Engl J Med. 1982;306:1018–22.
2. Lloyd-Jones DM, Wang TJ, Leip EP, et al. Lifetime risk for development of atrial fibrillation: the Framingham Heart Study. Circulation. 2004;110:1042–6.
3. Gage BF, Waterman AD, Shannon W, Boechler M, Rich MW, Radford MJ. Validation of clinical classification schemes for predicting stroke: results from the National Registry of Atrial Fibrillation. JAMA. 2001;285(22):2864–70.
4. Lane DA, Lip GY. Use of the CHA(2)DS(2)-VASc and HAS-BLED scores to aid decision making for thromboprophylaxis in nonvalvular atrial fibrillation. Circulation. 2012;126(7):860–5.
5. January CT, Wann SL, Alpert JS, Calkins H, Cleveland JC, Writing Committee Members, ACC/

AHA TaskForce Members, et al. 2014 AHA/ACC/HRS guideline for the management of patients with atrial fibrillation: executive summary: a report of the American College of Cardiology/American Heart Association Task Force on practice guidelines and the Heart Rhythm Society. Circulation. 2014;130(23):2071–104.
6. Dewilde WJ, Oirbans T, Verheugt FW, Kelder JC, De Smet BJ, Herrman JP, et al. WOEST study investigators. Use of clopidogrel with or without aspirin in patients taking oral anticoagulant therapy and undergoing percutaneous coronary intervention: an open-label, randomised, controlled trial. Lancet. 2013;381(9872):1107–15.
7. Mond HG, Proclemer A. The 11th world survey of cardiac pacing and implantable cardioverter-defibrillators: calendar year 2009 – a World Society of Arrhythmia's project. Pacing Clin Electrophysiol. 2011;34:1013–27.
8. Bashore TM, Balter S, Barac A, et al. 2012 American College of Cardiology Foundation/Society for Cardiovascular Angiography and Interventions expert consensus document on cardiac catheterization laboratory standards update: A report of the American College of Cardiology Foundation Task Force on Expert Consensus documents developed in collaboration with the Society of Thoracic Surgeons and Society for Vascular Medicine. J Am Coll Cardiol. 2012;59:2221.
9. Douketis JD, Spyropoulos AC, Spencer FA, et al. Perioperative management of antithrombotic therapy: antithrombotic therapy and prevention of thrombosis, 9th ed: American College of Chest Physicians evidence-based clinical practice guidelines. Chest. 2012;141(Suppl):e326S–50S. [Erratum, Chest. 2012; 141:1129].
10. Birnie DH, Healey JS, Wells GA, Verma A, Tang AS, Krahn AD, BRUISE CONTROL Investigators, et al. Pacemaker or defibrillator surgery without interruption of anticoagulation. N Engl J Med. 2013; 368(22):2084–93.
11. Calkins H, Brugada J, Packer DL, Cappato R, Chen SA, Crijns HJ, et al. HRS/EHRA/ECAS expert consensus statement on catheter and surgical ablation of atrial fibrillation: recommendations for personnel, policy, procedures and follow-up. A report of the Heart Rhythm Society recommendations for personnel, policy, procedures and follow-up. A report of the Heart Rhythm Society (HRS) Task Force on catheter and surgical ablation of atrial fibrillation. Heart Rhythm. 2007;4:816–61.
12. Santangeli P, Di Biase L, Horton R. Ablation of atrial fibrillation under therapeutic warfarin reduces periprocedural complications: evidence from a meta-analysis. Circ Arrhythm Electrophysiol. 2012;5:302–11.
13. Di Biase L, Burkhardt D, Santangeli P, et al. Periprocedural stroke and bleeding complications in patients undergoing catheter ablation of atrial fibrillation with different anticoagulation management: results from the COMPARE randomized trial. Circulation. 2014;129(25):2638–44.
14. Calkins H, Gerstenfeld EP, Schilling R, et al. RE-CIRCUIT study-randomized evaluation of dabigatran etexilate compared to warfarin in pulmonary vein ablation: assessment of an uninterrupted periprocedural anticoagulation strategy. Am J Cardiol. 2015;115:154–5.
15. Lakkireddy D, Reddy YM, Di Biase L, et al. Feasibility and safety of uninterrupted rivaroxaban for periprocedural anticoagulation in patients undergoing radiofrequency ablation for atrial fibrillation: results from a multicenter prospective registry. J Am Coll Cardiol. 2014;63:982–8.
16. Di Biase L, Lakkireddy D, Trivedi C, et al. Feasibility and safety of uninterrupted periprocedural apixaban administration in patients undergoing radiofrequency catheter ablation for atrial fibrillation: results from a multicenter study. Heart Rhythm. 2015;12:1162–8.
17. Bin Abdulhak AA, Khan AR, Tleyjeh IM, et al. Safety and efficacy of interrupted dabigatran for peri-procedural anticoagulation in catheter ablation of atrial fibrillation: a systematic review and meta-analysis. Europace. 2013;15:1412–20.
18. Providencia R, Albenque JP, Combes S, et al. Safety and efficacy of dabigatran versus warfarin in patients undergoing catheter ablation of atrial fibrillation: a systematic review and meta-analysis. Heart. 2014;100:324–3.
19. Baetz BE, Gerstenfeld EP, Kolansky DM, Spinler SA. Bivalirudin use during radiofrequency catheter ablation procedures in two patients with a history of heparin-induced thrombocytopenia. Pharmacotherapy. 2010;30(9):952.
20. Aytemir K, Canpolat U, Yorgun H, Evranos B, Kaya EB, Şahiner ML, Özer N. Usefulness of 'figure-of-eight' suture to achieve haemostasis after removal of 15-French caliber femoral venous sheath in patients undergoing cryoablation. Europace. 2016;18(10):1545–50.
21. Latacha MP. Using a new, smaller implantable loop recorder to aid in arrhythmia detection and anticoagulation decisions after AF ablation: one user's experience. EP Lab Digest. 2015;15(3). https://www.eplabdigest.com/articles/Using-New-Smaller-Implantable-Loop-Recorder-Aid-Arrhythmia-Detection-and-Anticoagulation. Accessed 2018-01-23
22. Klein AL, Grimm RA, Murray RD, et al. Use of transesophageal echocardiography to guide cardioversion in patients with atrial fibrillation. N Engl J Med. 2001;344(19):1411–20.
23. Nagarakanti R, Ezekowitz MD, Oldgren J, Yang S, Chernick M, Aikens TH, et al. Dabigatran versus warfarin in patients with atrial fibrillation: an analysis of patients undergoing cardioversion. Circulation. 2011;123(2):131–6.
24. Granger CB, Alexander JH, McMurray JJ, Lopes RD, Hylek EM, Hanna M, et al. Apixaban versus warfa-

rin in patients with atrial fibrillation. N Engl J Med. 2011;365:981–92.
25. Cappato R, Ezekowitz MD, Klein AL, Camm AJ, Ma CS, Le Heuzey JY, et al. Rivaroxaban vs. vitamin K antagonists for cardioversion in atrial fibrillation. Eur Heart J. 2014;35(47):3346–55.
26. Holbrook A, Schulman S, Witt DM, Vandvik PO, Fish J, Kovacs MJ, et al. Evidence-based management of anticoagulant therapy antithrombotic therapy and prevention of thrombosis, 9th ed: American College of Chest Physicians Evidence-Based Clinical Practice Guidelines. Chest. 2012;141(2 Supplement):e152S–84S.
27. Reddy VY, Sievert H, Halperin J, Doshi SK, Buchbinder M, Neuzil P, PROTECT AF Steering Committee and Investigators, et al. Percutaneous left atrial appendage closure vs warfarin for atrial fibrillation: a randomized clinical trial. JAMA. 2014;312(19):1988–98.
28. Holmes DR Jr, Kar S, Price MJ, Whisenant B, Sievert H, Doshi SK, et al. Randomized trial of LAA occlusion or is it prospective randomized evaluation of the watchman left atrial appendage closure device in patients with atrial fibrillation versus long-term warfarin therapy: the PREVAIL trial. J Am Coll Cardiol. 2014;64(1):1–12.
29. Boersma LV, Ince H, Kische S, Pokushalov E, Schmitz T, Schmidt B, EWOLUTION Investigators, et al. Efficacy and safety of left atrial appendage closure with WATCHMAN in patients with or without contraindication to oral anticoagulation: 1-year follow-up outcome data of the EWOLUTION trial. Heart Rhythm. 2017;14(9):1302–8.
30. Price MJ, Reddy VY, Valderrábano M, Halperin JL, Gibson DN, Gordon N, et al. Bleeding outcomes after left atrial appendage closure compared with long-term warfarin: a pooled, patient-level analysis of the WATCHMAN randomized trial experience. JACC Cardiovasc Interv. 2015;8(15):1925–32.
31. Enomoto Y, Gadiyaram VK, Gianni C, Horton RP, Trivedi C, Mohanty S, et al. Use of non-warfarin oral anticoagulants instead of warfarin during left atrial appendage closure with the Watchman device. Heart Rhythm. 2017;14(1):19–24.
32. Reddy VY, Möbius-Winkler S, Miller MA, Neuzil P, Schuler G, Wiebe J, et al. Left atrial appendage closure with the Watchman device in patients with a contraindication for oral anticoagulation: the ASAP study (ASA Plavix feasibility study with Watchman left atrial appendage closure technology). J Am Coll Cardiol. 2013;61(25):2551–6.

13 Anticoagulation for Cardiac Prosthetic Devices: Prosthetic Heart Valves, Left Ventricular Assist Devices, and Septal Closure Devices

Matthew T. Crim, Supriya Shore, Suegene K. Lee, and Bryan J. Wells

Clinical Vignettes

Case 1: *An 85-year-old man presenting with recent onset orthopnea and peripheral edema is found to have severe aortic stenosis. He is high risk for surgical aortic valve replacement, and in conversation with the heart team and his family, he elects to proceed with transcatheter aortic valve replacement. The procedure goes well, and he is discharged on aspirin 81 mg daily indefinitely, along with clopidogrel 75 mg daily for 6 months. Seven months later, he presents with recurrent dyspnea and is found on transthoracic echo to have elevated aortic valve pressure gradients and thickened aortic valve leaflets. He has not had a stroke or any other clinically evident thromboembolic event. He is started on therapeutic anticoagulation with warfarin, target INR 2 to 3, along with continued aspirin 81 mg daily, for subclinical leaflet thrombosis. Two months later, his dyspnea has improved, and his transthoracic echo aortic valve appearance and pressure gradients have normalized.*

Case 2: *A 52-year-old woman with a mechanical mitral valve implanted 4 years prior for mitral valve prolapse associated with severe mitral regurgitation is evaluated for subacute biliary colic. She is found to have cholelithiasis without acute cholecystitis and is advised to undergo elective laparoscopic cholecystectomy. She is maintained on warfarin with target INR 3 for her mechanical mitral valve and has had no hemorrhagic complications of anticoagulation. Her renal function is normal and her weight is 80 kg. Her warfarin is held for 4 days prior to her procedure to allow the INR to drift down below 1.5. She is started on enoxaparin 1 mg/kg q12 h, while warfarin is held to continue therapeutic anticoagulation and continues until the night before surgery. Her cholecystectomy is performed 12 h following her last dose of enoxaparin and is uncomplicated. After surgery, she resumes warfarin with therapeutic dosing of enoxaparin and continues with bridging therapy until her INR is again therapeutic.*

M. T. Crim · S. Shore · S. K. Lee · B. J. Wells (✉)
Department of Medicine, Division of Cardiology,
Emory University School of Medicine,
Atlanta, GA, USA
e-mail: suegene.lee@emory.edu; bjwells@emory.edu

J. F. Lau et al. (eds.), *Anticoagulation Therapy*, https://doi.org/10.1007/978-3-319-73709-6_13

Introduction

From the development of open heart surgery in the 1950s, dramatic technological advances have facilitated progressively complex cardiac procedures with approaches ranging from the open or minimally invasive surgical to the percutaneous endovascular [1]. Several disease spectra have treatment options that involve securing prosthetic material in, or in communication with, the heart carrying with them the risk of thromboembolic complications. In this chapter, we review the features of cardiac prosthetic devices associated with thrombosis, the indications for device use, and the evidence guiding current recommendations for management of these devices and their hematologic complications.

Spectrum of Pathology

Cardiac Anatomy

In normal anatomy, the heart is composed of four chambers that serve the pulmonary and systemic circulations in series. For each circulation, there is a collecting chamber, the atrium, to which blood is delivered from the central veins, and a pumping chamber, the ventricle. Blood passes from the atria to the ventricles across the atrioventricular valves (tricuspid and mitral) and then to the central arteries across the semilunar valves (pulmonary and aortic). Septa separate the chambers in the pulmonary and systemic circulations at the level of the atria and ventricles.

Valvular Heart Disease

Cardiac prosthetic devices are most commonly employed in the treatment of valvular heart disease. Valve dysfunction may occur with any of the four valves when structural or functional abnormalities result in regurgitation (backward flow across the valve, opposite the intended direction) or stenosis (increased resistance to blood flow in the intended direction). There is a wide array of pathology that can contribute to valve dysfunction, including congenital malformation, calcific or degenerative changes related to aging, valvular changes associated with noxious exposures (e.g., infection, inflammation, radiation, infiltration), and structural changes of the heart.

There is a complex interplay between the mechanical function of the heart chambers and valves. Structural valve disease involves a primary abnormality of the heart valve itself, while functional valve disease results from a primary abnormality in the structure or function of the associated heart chamber. Treatment of valvular heart disease with prosthetic devices can involve whole-scale replacement of the heart valve, with or without removal of the native valve, or repair of the native valve, with maintenance of the native valve structure and addition of prosthetic material.

Cardiomyopathy

A second category of disease treated with cardiac prosthetic devices is cardiomyopathy. The treatment of heart failure is guided by one of the largest canons of literature in modern medicine and includes lifestyle interventions and pharmacotherapy. For severe cases refractory to medical therapy, advanced invasive options include placement of a left ventricular assist device (LVAD) as an end in itself (destination therapy) or as a bridge to intended heart transplant. An LVAD acts in parallel with the left ventricle (LV) to provide flow to the systemic circuit. Via a cannula in the LV apex, blood is delivered to the device and then pumped through a conduit to the aorta.

There are also a variety of clinical situations that may result in acute cardiomyopathy requiring mechanical support as a bridge to recovery or more definitive long-term support options. These cases of severe acute cardiogenic shock can result from acute ischemia, including during high-risk percutaneous coronary intervention, viral or inflammatory myocarditis, stress cardiomyopathy, ventricular tachycardia, postcardiotomy shock, and other etiologies. There are several devices that offer temporary mechanical circulatory support, including the intra-aortic balloon pump, extracorporeal membrane oxygenation, TandemHeart (CardiacAssist Inc., Pittsburgh, PA), and Impella (Abiomed, Inc., Danvers, MA), among others. These devices have varying designs and mechanisms, but all serve to provide temporary support to cardiac output [2].

Occlusion Devices

The next category of cardiac prostheses disrupts undesired communication between two chambers. Defects in the atrial or ventricular septa (atrial septal defect (ASD) and ventricular septal defect (VSD), respectively) can arise from congenital abnormalities or acquired etiologies (e.g., trauma, infarct, other cardiac procedures). In normal fetal circulation, high-pressure, oxygenated blood from the mother is delivered via the umbilical vein to the fetal IVC and then right atrium and is preferentially shunted across the atrial septum through the foramen ovale to the left atrium and systemic circulation. The foramen ovale remains patent (PFO) in approximately 25% of adults and serves as a small conduit for shunting of blood between the pulmonary and systemic circulations.

The left atrial appendage (LAA) or auricle is an outpouching of the left atrium. The location and flow characteristics of the LAA result in increased risk of thrombosis, particularly in the setting of atrial arrhythmia, such as atrial fibrillation. Abnormal communication between chambers (ASD, VSD) can cause hemodynamic derangements related to the pressure and volume of flow that can eventually lead to ventricular dilation and dysfunction. A PFO or LAA can pose an increased risk of paradoxical embolism or thrombosis, respectively, in the correct clinical context. ASD, VSD, and PFO closure, and LAA occlusion, can be accomplished with surgical or endovascular approaches.

Pathophysiology of Cardiac Thrombosis

Thrombosis occurs as a result of platelet activation and initiation of the coagulation cascade via tissue factor exposure or contact activation (see Chap. 1). Cardiac thrombosis can have deleterious effects locally to the extent that normal hemodynamics and chamber or valvular function are impaired and remotely via embolization. There are significant pressure gradients across the cardiac chambers. The largest gradients are present during ventricular systole between the ventricle and atrium, separated by the atrioventricular valves, and the lowest intracardiac pressures and flow velocity occur in the atria. The complications of embolism are dictated by the downstream vascular bed—for right-sided lesions, this is the pulmonary circulation, and for left-sided lesions, the systemic (including cerebral) circulation.

The endothelial cells that line the vasculature and inner surface of the heart play a critical role in regulating coagulation. This is achieved via contributions to multiple pathways, including control of coagulation, platelet adhesion, activation and disintegration, fibrinolysis, and vasoregulation. At baseline, endothelial cells promote anticoagulant pathways through inhibition of tissue factor and thrombin and receptors that facilitate the activation of protein C. Cell surface receptors, such as the protease-activated receptor (PAR-1), mediate intracellular signaling and a cascade of events that results in the activation of antithrombotic and anti-inflammatory effects [3].

Prosthetic materials in, or in communication with, the heart must be compatible with the native mechanisms preventing thrombosis. At initial implant, the foreign surface of the prosthetic device is a nidus for thrombus formation. This is tempered by the expansion of endothelial cells that coat the device over time. The process of endothelialization underlies the management of most devices with a greater intensity of antithrombotic therapy initially before decreasing to a lesser maintenance antithrombotic regimen. Device design is critical to minimize adverse hemodynamics that would result in thrombogenic shear stresses.

Prosthetic Heart Valves

The first artificial heart valve was implanted for treatment of aortic regurgitation in 1952, by Charles Hufnagel. The valve had a "ball-in-cage" design, in which a small acrylic ball sat within a tapered cylinder, and was implanted not in the heart, but in the descending thoracic aorta [4]. Since that time, there has been tremendous innovation resulting in a broad menu of options for each valve position. Prosthetic valves can be classified by their design, material (mechanical versus bioprosthetic), and implantation approach (surgical versus endovascular). For some valvular heart disease, valve repair with prosthetic material but without implantation of a new valve is also feasible and appropriate.

History and Development

The design of prosthetic heart valves proceeded with mechanical devices modeled on Hufnagel's caged-ball valve. The first intracardiac valve implant was performed by Albert Starr in the mitral position with a caged-ball valve in 1962, followed by Dwight Harken in the aortic position in 1963. Starr worked with M Lowell Edwards, a mechanical engineer, to refine the caged-ball design to minimize thromboembolic complications. The promise of the enterprise was apparent, though the caged-ball design posed several physiologic challenges, including a large pressure gradient required to open the ball valve and central obstruction to flow with thrombogenic recirculation regions [4].

The tilting disk mechanical valve design emerged in the late 1960s, which reduced flow resistance, turbulence, regions of stagnant flow, and shear stress. The tilting disk design was modified in 1977, with the introduction of the bileaflet valve which incorporates two tilting disks to allow for central unimpeded blood flow. Contemporary mechanical valves continue to utilize this bileaflet design with the focus of continued innovation on minimizing thrombogenicity through the materials used in valve construction [4].

Along with the evolution in mechanical valve prostheses, a parallel stream advancing the use of biologic tissue valves flowed from the first allograft (human cadaveric valve) implant in the aortic position by Donald Ross in 1962. This was followed by the first report of heterograft (other animal species) valve implants from Jean-Paul Binet and colleagues in 1965. Progress with bioprosthetic valves revolved around the method of tissue preservation and design of the structural frame, pioneered by Alain Carpentier in the late 1960s. The contributions of Starr and Carpentier were recognized with the Lasker Award in 2007 [4].

While prosthetic heart valves offer the option of valvular heart disease treatment to many, the surgical approach does involve risk which may be prohibitive for some patients. The development of less invasive treatment options through an endovascular approach began in animal models in 1965, modeled on the original Hufnagel valve, with a cone-shaped device incorporating a parachute design delivered via the carotid artery to the ascending aorta, intended for the treatment of aortic regurgitation. The first endovascular valve implant in humans was performed in the pulmonary position by Philipp Bonhoeffer in 2000, followed in the aortic position by Alain Cribier in 2002 [5]. Several dedicated transcatheter mitral valves are in development, some of which have been implanted in humans, though regulatory body approval and widespread use remains on the horizon at the time of writing [6] (Fig. 13.1).

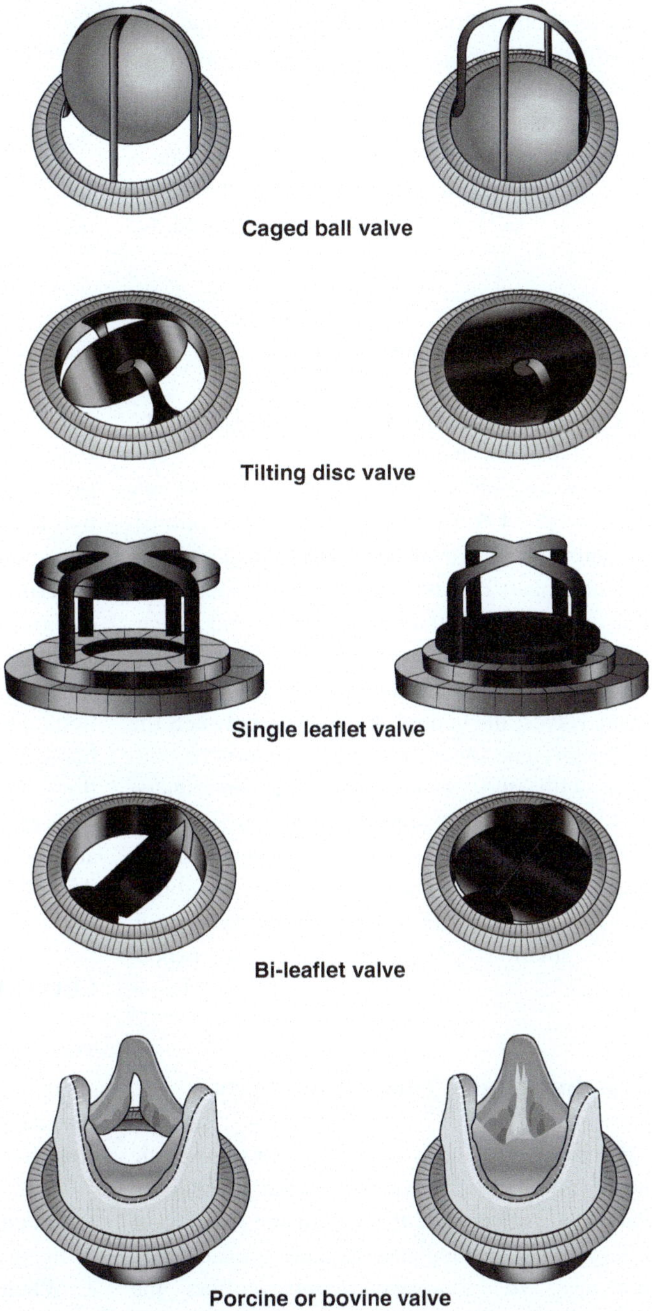

Fig. 13.1 Prosthetic valve designs. Adapted from [7]

Epidemiology of Valvular Heart Disease

The prevalence of moderate to severe valvular heart disease (regurgitation and stenosis) in the USA has been estimated at 2.5% (CI 2.2–2.7%) [8]. Mitral regurgitation is the most prevalent (1.7%), followed by aortic regurgitation (0.5%), aortic stenosis (0.4%), and mitral stenosis (0.1%). Prevalence increases significantly with age due to degenerative disease, <2% before age 65 years, 8.5% in the population aged 65–75 years, and 13.2% above age 75 years [9]. In the developing world, rheumatic heart disease remains a significant problem, with prevalence among school-age children as high as 3% in sub-Saharan Africa and South-Central Asia [10]. Data from the US National Center for Health Statistics indicates that over 102,000 heart valve procedures were performed in 2013, with a national cost over $5.2 billion (2013 dollars, adjusted for inflation) [11].

Table 13.1 Patient risk factors for thromboembolic complications with prosthetic heart valves [19–21]

Atrioventricular valve position
Multiple prosthetic valves
Prior thromboembolism
Atrial fibrillation
Mitral stenosis
Depressed left ventricular ejection fraction (<35%)

Clinical Decision-Making

For the patient with valvular heart disease, the clinical decision-making regarding optimal treatment is complex and beyond the scope of this chapter. The US and European societies publish guidelines for the evaluation and management of valvular heart disease that address in detail the diagnostic criteria of disease severity and indications for valve replacement [12–14]. Considering the choice between mechanical and bioprosthetic heart valves, the central trade-off is between the lifelong requirement for therapeutic anticoagulation with the former and the anticipated 10–20 years of valve durability prior to degeneration requiring repeat valve replacement with the latter. Thus, key considerations include (1) ability to tolerate and remain adherent with therapeutic anticoagulation and (2) anticipated life expectancy [15].

Prosthetic Valve Thrombogenicity

The risk of thrombosis associated with prosthetic heart valves varies based on features of both the valve and patient. The features of the valve most relevant are hemodynamics and construction materials. A bioprosthetic valve offers the hemodynamic function of a native valve (as long as leaflet mobility is not impaired by the structural frame), and the tissue preservation process in valve construction addresses the possibility of immune reaction to the implantation of foreign tissue.

The hemodynamics of mechanical valves differ from native valves and vary substantially based on valve design. Turbulent and stagnant flow and high shear stress increase the risk of platelet activation and thrombosis. These characteristics have been minimized through generations of valve design, though not eliminated. Valve construction materials have also been improved with exploration of metal alloys and pyrolytic carbon. Processes such as device thrombogenicity emulation employ numerical and experimental approaches to optimize valve design [16–18].

Table 13.1 lists patient characteristics known to increase the risk of thromboembolic complications [19–21]. Many of these factors impact hemodynamics by increasing low or turbulent flow. As the lower pressure and flow chambers with greater transvalvular gradients, the atria and atrioventricular valves, respectively, have greater thromboembolic potential.

Clinical Questions

There are several questions to address in the management of prosthetic heart valves relating to anticoagulation for the prevention of thromboembolic complications:

1. When is anticoagulation indicated, with what agents, and at what intensity?
2. When is antiplatelet therapy indicated, with what agents?
3. When should anticoagulation be initiated following valve replacement, and how?
4. When is bridging anticoagulation indicated during temporary cessation of warfarin therapy and with what agents?
5. When is reversal of anticoagulation necessary for hemorrhage or emergency surgery and how?

6. How to diagnose and treat prosthetic valve thrombosis?
7. How to manage anticoagulation in a pregnant woman with a prosthetic heart valve (see also Chap. 18 for a discussion of anticoagulation in pregnancy)?
8. How to manage anticoagulation in a patient with atrial fibrillation and a prosthetic heart valve (see also Chap. 11 for a discussion of anticoagulation in atrial fibrillation)?

The American Heart Association and American College of Cardiology (AHA/ACC), European Society of Cardiology and European Association for Cardio-Thoracic Surgery (ESC/EACTS), and American College of Chest Physicians (ACCP) publish guidelines addressing the management of antithrombotic therapy for prosthetic heart valves [12–14, 22]. The evidence base is limited with recommendations generally assigned a level of evidence B (R for single randomized study or NR for nonrandomized study) or C (EO for expert opinion or LD for limited data from small, retrospective, or registry studies). The guidelines largely agree, with few points of contention.

Mechanical Heart Valves

Risk of Thrombosis

The pivotal early meta-analysis defining the risk of thrombosis with mechanical heart valves was conducted by Cannegieter and colleagues in 1994. The review included 46 studies (a mix of prospective and observational) conducted from 1977 to 1992, including 13,088 patients followed for 53,647 patient-years, involving different valve designs—caged-ball, tilting disk, and bileaflet (predominantly earlier valve designs in the aortic position). With no antiplatelet or anticoagulant therapy, the incidence of valve thrombosis, major embolism, and total embolism was 1.8, 4.0, and 8.6 per 100 patient-years, respectively. This was decreased to 1.0, 1.4, and 7.5 events, respectively, with aspirin therapy, and 0.2, 1.0, and 1.8 events, respectively, with vitamin K antagonists. In multivariable regression analysis, the risk of major embolism for a valve in the mitral position was twice that of a valve in the aortic position, and the risk of major embolism was halved by vitamin K antagonists relative to antiplatelet agents alone (studies included both aspirin and dipyridamole) [19].

Based on these data, lifelong vitamin K antagonist-based anticoagulation is the cornerstone of management for mechanical heart valves (class I, level of evidence A (ACC/AHA)/B (ESC/EACTS)). This conclusion was underscored by a more recent attempt in the CAPTA trial to randomize patients with a bileaflet mechanical aortic valve to standard warfarin therapy versus dual antiplatelet therapy with aspirin and clopidogrel. This trial was stopped after enrolling only 22 patients when a patient on dual antiplatelet therapy had valve thrombosis [23]. In a recent cohort of 280 patients with mechanical heart valves (41% mitral, 44% aortic, 15% mitral and aortic) maintained on warfarin therapy that fell into a subtherapeutic INR range, 3 patients (all with mechanical mitral valves) had a thromboembolic event within 3 months of follow-up, an event rate of 4.3 per 100 person-years [24].

Warfarin Anticoagulation

Warfarin management is complex, and there is a substantial body of literature devoted to optimizing the use of warfarin in clinical practice. See Chap. 2 for a full discussion. There are also multiple references focused on warfarin management in the mechanical heart valve patient population, including use of an anticoagulation service [25–30], patient self-monitoring [31–35], telemedicine-guided therapy [36], and genetics [37–39].

INR Targets

The appropriate intensity of warfarin anticoagulation varies with the risk of thromboembolism, which is dependent on the characteristics of both

Table 13.2 Guidelines: INR targets for mechanical valves (range 0.5 above and below target) [12–14, 22]

	ACC/AHA [12, 14]	ACCP [22]	ESC/EACTS [13]
Mitral	3.0 *Class I, level of evidence (LoE) B*	3.0 *Grade 2C*	3.0 with low-risk valve (Carbomedics, Medtronic Hall, St Jude Medical, On-X bileaflet valves) 3.5 with medium risk valve (other bileaflet valves) 4.0 with high-risk valve (caged-ball and tilting-disk valves)
Aortic with patient risk factor(s)	3.0 (includes older tilting disk or caged-ball valves) *Class I, LoE B*	2.5 *Grade 1B*	3.0 with low-risk valve 3.5 with medium-risk valve 4.0 with high-risk valve
Aortic with no risk factors	2.5 (includes bileaflet and current generation single tilting disk valves) *Class I, LoE B* 1.5–2.0 with On-X valve, beginning 3 months after implant *Class IIb, LoE B-R*	2.5 *Grade 2C*	2.5 with low-risk valve 3.0 with medium-risk valve 3.5 with high-risk valve

the mechanical valve and the patient. The current anticoagulation guideline statements approach this issue differently, with the European guidelines presenting INR thresholds based on the risk profile of the valve position and design in combination with the patient risk factors, and the American guidelines presenting thresholds based primarily on valve position, with a consideration of patient risk to refine intensity for patients with mechanical aortic valves [12–14, 22] (Table 13.2).

The literature to support these recommendations has evolved from observational data to identify optimal INR ranges to multiple trials designed to narrow these targets by valve design and implant location. As valve thrombogenicity has decreased over time with improved bileaflet valve design and pyrolytic carbon construction, the studied INR targets have been steadily decreasing. The following paragraphs present a brief chronology of important studies.

An early Dutch observational study of 1608 patients with 6475 patient-years of follow-up identified an optimal INR range of 3–4 that minimized both thromboembolic and hemorrhagic complications. This cohort had a majority of aortic valves (60%) of the tilting disk design (77%). Results were consistent in subgroup analysis for patients with mitral valve replacement (30% of the cohort had mitral alone, and 10% had both aortic and mitral valve prostheses) [40].

The AREVA trial was an early French randomized comparison of target INR range 2–3 compared to 3–4.5 among 433 patients with single valve replacement (414 (96%) aortic and 19 (4%) mitral) followed for a mean of 2.2 years. There was no difference in thromboembolic complications between the two INR ranges, and there were fewer hemorrhagic events with the lower INR range (34 versus 56), though major hemorrhagic complications were not significantly different [41]. Similarly, an early Italian randomized comparison of target INR 3 versus 4 including 205 patients with a mean follow-up of 3 years found that the patients with INR 3 had fewer major hemorrhagic complications (4 versus 11 patients, $p = 0.02$), with equivalent thromboembolic events and vascular death [42].

The GELIA trial randomized 2735 patients 3 months following bileaflet design mechanical valve implant to three different target INR ranges: 3–4.5, 2.5–4, and 2–3.5. There were 6801 patient-years of follow-up; 2024 (74%) patients had aortic valve replacement only, 533 (20%) patients had mitral valve replacement only, and 158 (6%) patients had combined aortic and mitral valve replacement. There were no significant differences in either thromboembolic or hemorrhagic complications across the INR groups. Thromboembolic complications were more common with mitral valve replacement than aortic valve (1.64% per patient-year versus 0.53%), and the overall rate of severe hemorrhagic complications was 0.56% per patient-year. Among the patients that had both aortic and mitral replacement, the lower-intensity INR 2–3.5 group had increased mortality, despite equivalent rates of thromboembolic and hemorrhagic complications [43, 44].

The LOWERING-IT trial randomized 396 Italian patients with bileaflet-design mechanical aortic valve replacement, followed for a median of 5.6 years, to target INR ranges 1.5–2.5 versus 2–3. There were a significant reduction in total hemorrhagic events with the lower INR target range (6 versus 16, $p = 0.04$) and no difference in thromboembolic events [45].

The PROACT trial randomized 375 US patients with at least one thromboembolic risk factor 3 months following bileaflet-design, pyrolytic carbon construction, aortic valve replacement to INR target range 1.5–2 versus 2–3, with a mean follow-up of 3.8 years. There were no difference in thromboembolic complications and a significant reduction in both major and minor hemorrhagic events in the lower INR threshold group (1.5%/patient-year versus 3.3%, $p = 0.05$, and 1.3% versus 3.4%, $p = 0.02$, respectively). This study led to a class IIb recommendation for this lower INR threshold with the On-X aortic valve in patients with no other thromboembolic risk factors [14]. Additional PROACT studies are ongoing at the time of writing in low thromboembolic risk aortic valve replacement patients to test the comparison between antiplatelet and anticoagulant therapy and in mitral valve replacement patients to test the comparison of target INR range 2–2.5 versus 2.5–3.5 [46].

A recent meta-analysis of mechanical mitral valve replacement with current generation bileaflet designs constructed of pyrolytic carbon included 14 studies with 3595 patients followed for 12,847 patient-years. A lower-intensity INR range of 2–2.5 was compared to a higher-intensity INR of 2.5–4. The lower-intensity group had decreased major hemorrhagic complications (relative risk 0.42, 95% CI 0.3–0.6) and no difference in major thromboembolic complications [47].

The most recent studies with current generation bileaflet valves demonstrate equivalent thromboembolic event prevention with decreased hemorrhagic complications at target INR ranges as low as 1.5–2 for aortic valves and 2–2.5 for mitral valves. These ranges are lower than current guidelines and require additional study prior to widespread clinical implementation. They may inform current practice, however, in the setting of an individual patient with increased risk of hemorrhagic complications of anticoagulation that does not have a high risk of thromboembolism.

Direct Oral Anticoagulants and Mechanical Valves

The favorable efficacy and risk profile of DOACs relative to warfarin in the treatment of atrial fibrillation and venous thromboembolism, along with the convenience of no required therapeutic monitoring for dose adjustment and no vitamin K food restrictions, were met with hope that the results would translate to the anticoagulation of mechanical heart valves. A large animal study of mitral valve replacement in a porcine model with 19 animals suggested feasibility compared to warfarin in both thromboembolic and hemorrhagic complications [48].

The RE-ALIGN trial was a phase II dose validation study that intended to randomize 405 patients, either within 7 days or 3 months following the implantation of a bileaflet mechanical valve in the aortic, mitral, or both positions, to either dabigatran (150 mg twice daily (15% of patients), 220 mg twice daily (54% of patients), or 300 mg twice daily (31% of patients), based on renal function) or warfarin anticoagulation in a 2:1 ratio [49]. The trial was stopped prematurely after enrollment of 252 patients due to excess thromboembolic (9 strokes versus 0) and major hemorrhagic complications (7 events versus 2, all pericardial bleeding) [50]. As a result of this study, DOACs are contraindicated for patients with mechanical heart valves (class III, level of evidence B). This trial serves as a cautionary tale against extrapolating favorable evidence for a medication in some disease states to a different indication without direct study.

Addition of Antiplatelet Therapy

An early Canadian trial randomized 370 patients with mechanical heart valves (76%) or bioprosthetic valves and increased thromboembolic risk (atrial fibrillation or prior thromboembolism) on warfarin therapy to either aspirin 100 mg daily or placebo and followed for a mean of 2.5 years. Aspirin therapy resulted in decreased major systemic embolism and all-cause mortality (13 patients versus 33, relative risk reduction 65%, $p < 0.001$). There was no difference in major hemorrhagic complications, though aspirin use did increase hemorrhagic complications overall (71 patients versus 49, relative risk increase 55%, $p = 0.02$). In subgroup analysis, the thromboembolic and mortality benefits were present in patients with both mechanical and bioprosthetic heart valves and more prominent among patients with mechanical heart valves (major systemic embolism or death from vascular causes, mechanical 4 (3.9%) versus 20 (14.3%), bioprosthetic 2 (4.4%) versus 4 (9.1%)) [51].

This was followed by an Argentinean trial that randomized 503 patients with mechanical heart valves (66% aortic, 29% mitral, 4% both) to warfarin therapy with target INR range 2.5–3.5 and aspirin 100 mg daily versus warfarin therapy with target INR 3.5–4.5 alone and followed for a median of 23 months. There was no difference in thromboembolic or hemorrhagic complications [52]. Similarly, the LIWACAP trial randomized 198 patients with mechanical heart valves (aortic, mitral, or both) to warfarin therapy with INR goal 2.5 plus aspirin 100 mg daily for 6 months following valve replacement versus warfarin therapy with INR goal 3.7 and followed for a mean of 1.5 years. There was no difference in thromboembolic or hemorrhagic complications [53].

A French trial randomized 229 patients with mechanical mitral valve replacement on warfarin therapy with INR target range 2.5–3.5 to aspirin 200 mg daily versus no antiplatelet therapy, with 12-month follow-up. The aspirin group had decreased total thromboembolic events (including nonobstructive thrombi on transesophageal echo) (10 (9%) versus 30 (25%), $p = 0.004$), with increased major hemorrhagic complications (21 (19%) versus 10 (8%), $p = 0.02$) [54].

An early meta-analysis to address this question including 10 studies with 2199 patients showed the addition of aspirin to warfarin anticoagulation resulted in a decreased risk of thromboembolic events (odds ratio 0.41, $p < 0.001$) and increased risk of major hemorrhage (odds ratio 1.50, $p = 0.03$) [55]. An update to this meta-analysis over a decade later included 13 studies with 4122 patients, and again demonstrated that addition of aspirin to warfarin anticoagulation resulted in decreased risk of thromboembolic events (odds ratio 0.43, $p < 0.001$), along with decreased all-cause mortality (odds ratio 0.57, $p < 0.001$), with increased major hemorrhagic complications (odds ratio 1.58, $p = 0.006$) [56].

Based on these data, the American guideline statements recommend addition of low-dose aspirin to warfarin anticoagulation for patients with a mechanical heart valve, with consideration for the increased risk of hemorrhagic complications (class I, level of evidence A) [12, 22]. The European guideline statement weighs this risk-benefit consideration more heavily and emphasizes the role for aspirin therapy in patients with atherosclerotic disease or prior thromboembolism (class IIa, level of evidence C) [13].

Anticoagulation Initiation

While long-term therapeutic anticoagulation with an oral vitamin K antagonist is recommended, the mechanism for initiating this therapy in the immediate post-operative setting, with amplified risk of hemorrhagic complications, is less well defined. Several observational studies have addressed the question, as summarized below. Based on these data, the ACCP recommend use in the immediate post-operative setting of either subcutaneous unfractionated heparin (deep vein thrombosis prophylactic dosing) or low-molecular-weight heparin, over intravenous unfractionated heparin (therapeutic dosing), due to the increased risk of hemorrhagic complications with IV UFH (grade 2C) [22].

In an early French study, 208 consecutive patients following mechanical valve implantation (75% aortic, 14% mitral, 11% both) were treated around post-operative day 6 with therapeutic dosing of either subcutaneous unfractionated heparin (UFH) (first 106 patients) or low-molecular-weight heparin (LMWH) (second 102 patients) as a bridge to warfarin oral anticoagulation. Both agents were continued for a mean of 14 days, and therapeutic anticoagulation was achieved more rapidly in the LMWH group (day 2, 87% versus 9%, $p < 0.001$). There were no differences in thromboembolic or hemorrhagic complications [57].

An Indian study also assigned 538 consecutive patients to different treatment paths following mechanical valve replacement and followed for 6 months—the first 245 patients were treated with oral nicoumalone only starting on post-operative day 1, and the second 293 patients were treated with enoxaparin (dosing unclear) starting 6 h following surgery as a bridge to therapeutic oral nicoumalone anticoagulation started on post-operative day 1. There were a significant reduction in early prosthetic valve thrombosis with the addition of enoxaparin (6 (2.1%) events, all mitral versus 15 (6.1%), 10 mitral and 5 aortic, $p = 0.01$) and no difference in hemorrhagic complications [58].

In a US case-control study, 29 patients treated with therapeutic LMWH as a bridge to warfarin anticoagulation were retrospectively matched to 34 controls treated with IV UFH and followed for 90 days. There were no difference in major hemorrhagic complications and fewer thromboembolic events and deaths with LMWH (0 versus 2 and 1 versus 4, respectively) [59].

A meta-analysis compared the rates of thromboembolic and hemorrhagic complications with three post-operative anticoagulation regimens bridging to warfarin therapy: subcutaneous (SC) UFH (deep vein thrombosis prophylactic dosing) (20 studies, 3056 patients), intravenous (IV) UFH (therapeutic dosing) (7 studies, 2535 patients), and LMWH (therapeutic dosing) (3 studies, 168 patients). The rates of early post-operative thromboembolic complications were 0.9% with SC UFH, 1.1% with IV UFH, and 0.6% with LMWH. The rates of early post-operative hemorrhagic complications were 3.3% with SC UFH, 7.2% with IV UFH, and 4.8% with LMWH [60].

A more recent single-center, observational study in France assigned 1063 patients following mechanical heart valve replacement to therapeutic dose LMWH bridging therapy starting post-operative day 1 and followed for 6 weeks. Thromboembolism occurred in 11 patients (1%), and major hemorrhagic complications occurred in 44 patients (4%), mirroring the results from the earlier meta-analysis [61].

A more recent meta-analysis again compared the post-operative anticoagulation regimens of SC UFH (prophylactic dosing) (11 studies with 4222 patients), IV UFH (therapeutic dosing) (9 studies with 3313 patients), and LMWH (therapeutic dosing) (7 studies with 1999 patients). The rates of early post-operative thromboembolic complications were 2.1% with SC UFH, 1.1% with IV UFH, and 1.1% with LMWH; these were not statistically different. The rates of early post-operative hemorrhagic complications were 1.8% with SC UFH, 2.2% with IV UFH, and 5.5% with LMWH. In two studies that delayed the start of LMWH until the end of the first post-operative week, the rate of hemorrhagic complications decreased to 2%. The authors conclude that early use of full-dose LMWH is associated with increased hemorrhagic complications, and suggest delaying therapeutically dosed bridging therapy (IV UFH or LMWH) until post-operative day 4 or 5, after surgical drains are removed. The differences in the two meta-analysis findings can be partly explained by different definitions of thromboembolic and hemorrhagic events [62].

Anticoagulation Interruption and Bridging

Patients with mechanical valves may require temporary interruption of anticoagulation for emergent or elective invasive procedures or management of hemorrhagic complications. Patients may also occasionally fall below the target INR range in the course of normal follow-up. When this occurs, bridging anticoagulation with intravenous unfractionated heparin (IV UFH) or therapeutic low-molecular-weight heparin (LMWH) should be considered, weighing the risk of thromboembolism. In addition to the American and European guidelines for the management of valvular disease, this topic is also addressed in the American and European guidelines for the perioperative management of anticoagulation [12–14, 63, 64].

For surgical procedures with a low hemorrhagic risk (such as tooth extraction or cataract surgery), it is preferable to continue therapeutic oral anticoagulation without interruption; the invasive procedure may proceed with careful attention to adequate hemostasis (class I, level of evidence C). Patients with low thromboembolic risk (bileaflet-design aortic valve and no thromboembolic risk factors) do not require bridging therapy with temporary cessation of anticoagulation (class I, level of evidence C). It is reasonable to bridge all other patients with mechanical valves with therapeutic dosing of either unfractionated heparin or low-molecular-weight heparin (class IIa, level of evidence C-LD).

In an early series from the Mayo Clinic of 159 patients with mechanical heart valves undergoing 180 subsequent non-cardiac procedures with no bridging anticoagulation, there were no thromboembolic complications associated with the procedures or cessation of anticoagulation [65]. A recent retrospective US cohort included 355 patients with mechanical heart valves that underwent 547 subsequent invasive procedures. Bridging anticoagulation was used in 466 (85.2%) patients. There were no thromboembolic events and no difference in hemorrhagic complications (5.8% with bridged patients versus 1.2%, $p = 0.102$) [66].

The safety of bridging with LMWH has been demonstrated in several observational studies. An Italian multisite cohort study enrolled 1262 patients, 190 of whom had a mechanical heart valve. A standardized bridging protocol with therapeutic dosing of LMWH for high-risk patients and prophylactic dosing for low-risk patients (bileaflet-design aortic valve with no atrial fibrillation or prior thromboembolism) was prescribed. There were 5 (0.4%) total thromboembolic events, only one (0.5% of patients with a mechanical heart valve) of which occurred in a patient with a mitral valve replacement related to the valve, and 15 (1.2%) major hemorrhagic complications [67]. A US cohort compared LMWH bridging in patients with mechanical heart valves (62 episodes) to patients with non-valvular atrial fibrillation (68 episodes). There were no thromboembolic events, and the rates of major hemorrhagic complications were not different (3.2% for patients with mechanical valves versus 2.9% for patients with atrial fibrillation) [68].

There are no randomized data comparing bridging with UFH to LMWH. This question has been addressed with data from the REGIMEN multicenter registry. Among 73 patients with mechanical heart valves bridged with UFH and 172 bridged with LMWH, there was one thromboembolic event in each group. Major hemorrhagic complications were not statistically different (8.8% with UFH versus 4.2% with LMWH, $p = 0.23$). Patients treated with LMWH were more likely to be treated as outpatients or discharged from the hospital within 24 h (68.6% versus 6.8%, $p < 0.001$) [69].

It is important to note that bridging anticoagulation increases the risk of hemorrhagic complications. A meta-analysis of studies evaluating periprocedural bridging anticoagulation for patients on oral vitamin K antagonist therapy for any indication included 34 studies with 12,278 patients, 24% of whom had mechanical heart valves. The overall quality of the included studies was judged to be poor, and there was only one randomized trial. There was no difference in thromboembolic events between patients that were and were not bridged (predominantly with LMWH), though the risk of hemorrhagic complications was increased with bridging (overall bleeding in 13 studies, odds ratio 5.4, CI 3–9.7; major bleeding in 5 studies, odds ratio 3.6, CI 1.5–8.5) [70].

Similarly, an analysis of patients with atrial fibrillation enrolled in the ORBIT-AF registry evaluated the outcomes of bridging anticoagulation. Among 2200 patients (282 (13%) with mechanical heart valves), there were 2803 interruptions in oral anticoagulation; 665 (24%) were treated with bridging anticoagulation (73% LMWH). There was no difference in thromboembolic events (13 events (0.6%), overall), and there was a significant increase in major hemorrhagic complications with the use of bridging anticoagulation (18 events (3.6%) versus 20 events (1.2%), $p < 0.001$) [71]. PERIOP 2 is an ongoing Canadian randomized trial comparing bridging with therapeutic LMWH to placebo among patients with a mechanical heart valve or atrial fibrillation/flutter and elevated stroke risk that will provide additional evidence regarding this treatment strategy [72].

Reversal of Anticoagulation

Reversal of anticoagulation may become necessary in patients with mechanical heart valves on oral vitamin K antagonist therapy in the event of severe hemorrhage, emergency surgery, or excessive anticoagulation with a supratherapeutic INR. The risk of hemorrhagic complications on oral vitamin K antagonist therapy greatly increases above an INR of 6. Reversal of anticoagulation with mechanical valves is addressed in the American and European guidelines for valvular heart disease and is also specifically focused on in the French clinical practice guidelines on the management of patients on vitamin K antagonists in at-risk situations [12, 13, 73].

Options for reversal include vitamin K (oral or intravenous), fresh frozen plasma, and intravenous prothrombin complex concentrate (class IIa, level of evidence C for emergency invasive procedures, B for bleeding). There are insufficient data regarding recombinant activated factor VII in mechanical heart valves to recommend its use. The evidence for these therapies is limited, and primarily in the context of stable patients with supratherapeutic INR, the recommendations are thus based largely on expert consensus.

For patients with supratherapeutic INR and no signs of bleeding, both the American and European guidelines recommend withholding additional oral vitamin K antagonist therapy and monitoring INR. If the INR is >10, then both guidelines also recommend administration of low-dose oral vitamin K (1.25–2.5 mg). Care should be taken to avoid overcorrection of the INR and to minimize the time outside of the therapeutic INR range. Resumption of anticoagulation following a hemorrhagic event or surgery depends on the nature of the situation and should proceed as soon as it is safe.

In a study with 81 patients at 2 US centers with supratherapeutic INR and no bleeding, administration of oral vitamin K 2.5 mg brought the INR <5 without inducing resistance to further anticoagulation [74]. In another study, 102 patients with mechanical heart valves and supratherapeutic INR (4–7) were randomized to low-dose IV vitamin K or fresh frozen plasma. Six hours following reversal, the patients that received FFP had a lower INR (enrollment mean INR 4.78–2.75 versus enrollment mean INR 4.61–3.44, $p = 0.01$). No patient had an INR <2, and there was no difference in INR 1 week later. There were no adverse events (no thromboembolic complications) [75].

Bioprosthetic Heart Valves

Risk of Thrombosis

The primary advantage of bioprosthetic heart valves over mechanical prostheses is the potential for decreased intensity antithrombotic therapy over the life of the valve. The risk of thromboembolism is greatest in the post-operative period extending to 3 months, presumably related to valve endothelialization.

Heras and colleagues defined the risk of thromboembolism following bioprosthetic valve placement from 1975 to 1982 in a series of 816 patients (52% aortic, 40% mitral, 8% both) at the Mayo Clinic followed for a median of 8.6 years. The rate of thromboembolic events was 2.2% per year for aortic valve replacement, 3.1% per year for mitral valve replacement, and 1.7% per year for combined valve replacements; the rates were highest in the first 10 post-operative days and decreased further following post-operative day 90 (with mitral valves 55 events/100 patient-years in the first 10 days, 10 events/100 patient-years for post-operative days 10–90, and 2.4 events/100 patient-years for more than 90 days; with aortic valves, 41%, 3.6%, and 1.9%, respectively). The rate of hemorrhagic complications was 2.3%/year [76].

Patients were treated with varying antithrombotic regimens in this study—antiplatelet therapy (aspirin and/or dipyridamole) was prescribed in 50% of aortic valve patients, 35% of mitral valve patients, and 44% of combined valve patients, and warfarin was prescribed in 34%, 79%, and 70% of patients, respectively. In multivariable regression analysis, anticoagulation reduced the risk of thromboembolic events (coefficient −0.66, p = 0.007); patients with mitral valve replacement treated with anticoagulation had a lower rate of thromboembolic events (2.5 versus 3.9% per year, p = 0.05) [76].

Antithrombotic Therapy

The evidence underlying antithrombotic therapy in bioprosthetic valves is limited with small randomized trials and largely observational data. This has contributed to more heterogeneity in guideline recommendations and clinical practice. The AHA/ACC guidelines state that low-dose aspirin therapy (75–100 mg daily) is reasonable in all patients with a bioprosthetic valve and that 3 months of anticoagulation with a vitamin K antagonist is reasonable for mitral bioprostheses and may be reasonable for aortic bioprostheses [12, 14].

The ACCP guidelines agree with 3 months of VKA therapy for mitral bioprostheses and low-dose aspirin therapy beyond 3 months with any bioprosthetic valve but recommend only aspirin therapy for aortic bioprostheses in the first 3 months absent other indications for anticoagulation [22]. The European guidelines state that oral anticoagulation should be considered for the first 3 months with mitral bioprostheses and may be considered for the first 3 months with aortic bioprostheses, and low-dose aspirin should be considered for the first 3 months with aortic bioprostheses; they conclude that “there is no evidence to support the use of antiplatelet agents beyond 3 months” absent other indications for aspirin therapy [13] (Table 13.3).

Most studies have focused on aortic valves. The literature on mitral bioprostheses is limited to observational data. In an early retrospective, single-center, Spanish cohort of 768 patients with a mean follow-up of 32 months, there was a notably low rate of thromboembolic events (0.5% per year) with high-dose aspirin therapy (250–1000 mg daily); all events occurred in patients with atrial fibrillation [77]. A later cohort from the Mayo Clinic including 285 patients with 12 years of follow-up reported an average stroke rate of 2.5 per 100 patient-years, with the highest risk in the first post-operative month (40 strokes/100 patient-years), decreasing to 6.7

Table 13.3 Guidelines for antithrombotic therapy with bioprosthetic valves [12–14, 22]

	AHA/ACC [12, 14]	ACCP [22]	ESC/EACTS [13]
Mitral	Aspirin 75–100 mg daily *Class IIa, level of evidence (LoE) B* VKA with target INR 2.5 for 3 months *Class IIa, LoE B-NR*	VKA with target INR 2.5 for 3 months *Grade 2C* Aspirin beyond 3 months *Grade 2C*	VKA with target INR 2.5 for 3 months *Class IIa, LoE C*
Aortic	Aspirin 75–100 mg daily *Class IIa, LoE B* Vitamin K antagonist with target INR 2.5 for 3 months *Class IIb, LoE B-NR*	Aspirin 50–100 mg daily *Grade 2C*	Aspirin ≤100 mg daily for 3 months *Class IIa, LoE C* VKA with target INR 2.5 for 3 months *Class IIb, LoE C*

strokes/100 patient-years for the remainder of the first post-operative year [78].

A more contemporary cohort of patients, also at the Mayo Clinic, treated for mitral regurgitation included 1344 patients followed up to 10 years—897 (67%) underwent mitral valve repair, and 447 (33%) had mitral valve replacement, 216 (16%) with a bioprosthetic valve. The rate of any thromboembolic event with bioprosthetic mitral valve replacement was 2.8/100 patient-years and again was highest in the first post-operative month (73.5 events/100 patient-years), less in post-operative months 1–5 (4.5 events/100 patient-years), and lower after the first 6 months (1.8 events/100 patient-years). The rate of hemorrhagic complications following the first 30 days was 0.7/100 patient-years [79].

There are few, small, randomized trials comparing antithrombotic regimens following bioprosthetic aortic valve implantation. An early Canadian trial randomized 108 patients to VKA therapy with INR goal 2.5–4.0 to less intense INR goal 2.0–2.25 for 3 months following valve replacement. There was no difference in major thromboembolic events (two major events in each group), and there were fewer hemorrhagic complications with the lower INR target range (15 versus 6) [80].

This null finding was replicated in small trials comparing 3 months of VKA anticoagulation to antiplatelet therapy. A Spanish trial with 193 patients (94% aortic valves, 5% mitral valves, 1% combined valve replacement) and 6 months of follow-up compared the salicylate antiplatelet agent triflusal to VKA anticoagulation. There were no significant differences in thromboembolic (6 (6.3%) versus 3 (3.2%)) or severe hemorrhagic (3 (3.1%) versus 6 (6.3%)) complications [81]. The Spanish WoA Epic pilot trial compared warfarin (INR target range 2–3) followed by aspirin 100 mg daily to aspirin 100 mg daily alone in 75 patients with 3 months of follow-up. There were no significant differences in thromboembolic (1 (2.9%) in each group) or major hemorrhagic complications (1 (2.9%) versus 3 (8.8%)) [82].

There are a number of single-center-based cohorts. In a retrospective cohort of patients from Duke University (378 with bioprosthetic aortic valves and 370 with bioprosthetic mitral valves), 14% of patients were treated with warfarin, 68% with aspirin, and 18% with no antithrombotic therapy. There was no significant difference in thromboembolic events among patients with aortic bioprostheses. Warfarin therapy increased the risk of hemorrhagic complications (16.7%/patient-year versus 3.4% with aspirin and 3.1% with no therapy, $p = 0.03$). Among patients with mitral bioprostheses, the thromboembolic events with aspirin or no antithrombotic therapy in the first 90 days were equal to the hemorrhagic complications with warfarin use in the same time period [83].

A review of 561 patients with aortic bioprosthetic valve replacement from the Mayo Clinic that were not routinely anticoagulated and followed for 12 years showed that the risk of stroke was significantly increased with low EF (below the median 54% in the study population), older age (above the median 73 years old in the study population), preoperative atrial fibrillation, or a paced rhythm [84]. A retrospective cohort of 185 aortic valve replacements from Yale compared patients on warfarin to patients not on anticoagulation. There were no differences in stroke incidence in the post-operative periods <24 h, 24 h to 3 months, and beyond 3 months and no differences in hemorrhagic complications [85].

An Italian prospective cohort of 249 patients followed for at least 6 months (up to 16 months) compared warfarin for 3 months following bioprosthetic aortic valve implantation to aspirin alone and found no differences in thromboembolic or hemorrhagic complications [86]. Working to gain a potentially mechanistic understanding, a Canadian cohort of 56 patients with 1 year follow-up was assessed for cerebral microembolization quantified by bilateral middle cerebral artery microembolic signals at post-operative hour 4 and month 1. Patients were treated with either warfarin (target INR range 2–3) and aspirin 81 mg daily or aspirin 325 mg daily alone. There were no clinical thromboembolic events in either group, and there were no differences in cerebral microembolization at either time point [87].

More contemporary observational data are also available from several large registries. From the ACTION registry, 1118 patients with 6-month follow-up after bioprosthetic aortic valve implantation were compared by post-operative use of VKA or aspirin alone. There was no difference in thromboembolic events (14 (2.8%) with VKA versus 9 (1.5%) with aspirin), but major hemorrhagic complications were increased with VKA use (18 (3.6%) versus 8 (1.3%), $p = 0.01$) [88].

Despite these prior data showing no difference in thromboembolic events with VKA use, two large registry-based observational studies show a significant reduction in thromboembolic complications and improved mortality with warfarin use following bioprosthetic aortic valve replacement. A Danish registry including 4075 patients with a median follow up 6.6 patient-years compared patients on warfarin to those not on warfarin, excluding outcomes from the first postoperative month. At post-operative day 90, warfarin therapy was associated with significant reduction in thromboembolic events (4.0/100 patient-years versus 13.1, adjusted incidence rate ratio 2.93), hemorrhagic events (5.4/100 patient-years versus 11.9, adjusted incidence rate ratio 2.32), and cardiovascular mortality (3.8/100 patient-years versus 31.7, adjusted incidence rate ratio 7.61). The cardiovascular mortality benefit extended to the post-operative period from 3 to 6 months (2.1/100 patient-years versus 6.5, adjusted incidence rate ratio 3.51) [89].

A cohort from the Society of Thoracic Surgeons (STS) registry including 25,656 patients 65 years or older (median age 77 years) with 3 months of follow-up compared patients with bioprosthetic aortic valve replacement on aspirin alone (49%) to warfarin alone (12%) to warfarin and aspirin together (23%). The rate of thromboembolic and hemorrhagic complications with aspirin therapy alone was 1.0%, and mortality was 3.0%. Compared to aspirin alone, there was no difference with warfarin therapy alone in thromboembolic or hemorrhagic complications or mortality. However, warfarin and aspirin therapy together were associated with a decreased risk of thromboembolic events (relative risk 0.52 (CI 0.35–0.76)) and mortality (relative risk 0.80, CI 0.66–0.96), with an increased risk of hemorrhagic complications (relative risk 2.80, CI 2.18–3.60), all compared to aspirin therapy alone [90].

Direct Oral Anticoagulants and Bioprosthetic Valves

There are limited data regarding the use of DOACs in bioprosthetic valves. The potential uses include thromboprophylaxis for the first 3 post-operative months in all patients prescribed this therapy, and/or long-term use in patients with other indications for therapeutic anticoagulation, most commonly comorbid atrial fibrillation. The findings from the RE-ALIGN trial of dabigatran thromboprophylaxis in mechanical valves that noted increased thromboembolic and hemorrhagic complications compared to warfarin bear special consideration [50].

A single-center retrospective cohort from the USA including 73 patients with a bioprosthetic heart valve and atrial fibrillation followed for a mean of 17 months evaluated the outcomes of patients prescribed DOACs an average of 2.5 years post-operation from valve replacement. Most patients were also prescribed aspirin (73%). There were no strokes, one possible TIA (1.4%), and six (8.2%) major hemorrhagic complications [91]. The DAWA pilot study sought to compare the use of dabigatran at least 3 months following bioprosthetic valve replacement to warfarin for the treatment of atrial fibrillation in a phase II randomized pilot study and was terminated prematurely due to low enrollment after only 27 patients were randomized. In 90 days of follow-up, there were one TIA in the dabigatran group and one stroke and one new intracardiac thrombus by transesophageal echo in the warfarin group [92].

The largest available cohorts come from the hallmark trials of atrial fibrillation for the DOAC agents. The first two trials, RE-LY for dabigatran and ROCKET AF for rivaroxaban, excluded all patients with prosthetic heart valves [93, 94]. The latter two trials, ARISTOTLE for apixaban and ENGAGE AF-TIMI 48 for edoxaban, did enroll patients with bioprosthetic valves [95, 96]. Of the

18,201 total patients enrolled in ARISTOTLE, 4808 had at least moderate to severe valvular heart disease, and 251 had "previous valve surgery" per patient survey. Further details regarding the nature of the surgery (valve position, repair or replacement) are not available, and subgroup analysis for these patients with prior valve surgery was not presented. The results for the valvular heart disease cohort in aggregate mirrored those of the larger trial, with apixaban associated with a significant reduction of stroke or systemic embolism (hazard ratio 0.70), and equivalent outcomes to warfarin with major bleeding and mortality [97].

The ENGAGE AF-TIMI 48 trial of edoxaban in atrial fibrillation included 2824 patients with moderate to severe valvular heart disease (excluding mitral stenosis) among the total study population of 21,105. There were 191 (0.9%) patients with bioprosthetic heart valves (69% mitral, 31% aortic) followed for a median of 2.8 years. The composite outcome (stroke and systemic embolism combined with major bleeding and death) was less frequent among patients with a bioprosthetic valve with both edoxaban 60 mg daily ($n = 63$) and edoxaban 30 mg daily ($n = 58$) relative to warfarin ($n = 70$) (7.5% per year versus 15.8% per year, hazard ratio 0.46, $p = 0.03$, and 7.0% per year versus 15.8% per year, hazard ratio 0.43, $p = 0.02$, respectively). The same composite outcome in the entire valvular heart disease cohort was equivalent between edoxaban and warfarin, with a hazard ratio of 0.96, CI 0.8–1.15 [98, 99]. While these data are encouraging, more dedicated study is required before these agents become used routinely for this indication in clinical practice.

Valve Repair

In some clinical contexts, surgical repair of a valvular lesion is technically feasible and clinically preferable to valve replacement. Valve repair is most often employed with the mitral valve, and there are a wide variety of surgical techniques. Many mitral valve repairs involve the insertion of an annuloplasty ring to improve leaflet approximation and coaptation. Guideline statements regarding antithrombotic therapy for mitral valve repair are limited, reflecting the limited data available. The AHA/ACC guideline includes mitral repair with the recommendation that it is reasonable to treat with a vitamin K antagonist with goal INR 2.5 for the first 3 months following bioprosthetic mitral valve replacement (class IIa, level of evidence C), and the European guidelines agree that oral anticoagulation should be considered for the first 3 months after mitral repair (class IIa, level of evidence C) [12, 13]. The ACCP guidelines instead recommend only antiplatelet therapy for the first 3 months (grade 2C) [22] (Fig. 13.2).

The guidelines cite cohorts of mixed valve interventions to support their recommendations. A Spanish cohort of 235 patients (65 with mitral repair, 1 aortic repair, 1 tricuspid repair, and 168 bioprosthetic valves) was assigned to either 3 months of therapy with the thienopyridine antiplatelet agent ticlopidine (137 patients), warfarin (40 patients), aspirin (14 patients), or no antithrombotic therapy (18 patients) and followed for a mean of 3.2 years. The rate of thromboembolic events was 0.5%/patient-year with ticlopidine and 3%/patient-year with warfarin, and there were hemorrhagic complications with 3 ticlopidine patients and 1 warfarin patient in the first 3 months (linearized incidence 0.75%/patient-year) [101].

In the Mayo Clinic cohort of patients with mitral regurgitation described above, the 897 (67%) of 1344 patients that underwent mitral repair had a thromboembolic event rate of 2.1/100 patient-years. This rate was highest in the first post-operative month (31 events/100 patient-years), less in post-operative months 1–6 (4.2 events/100 patient-years), and lowest in the period beyond 6 months (1.6 events/patient-years). The rate of hemorrhagic complications with mitral valve repair beyond post-operative day 30 was 0.7 events/100 patient-years [79].

There have subsequently been several large observational studies published that provide additional data for consideration. In a Korean

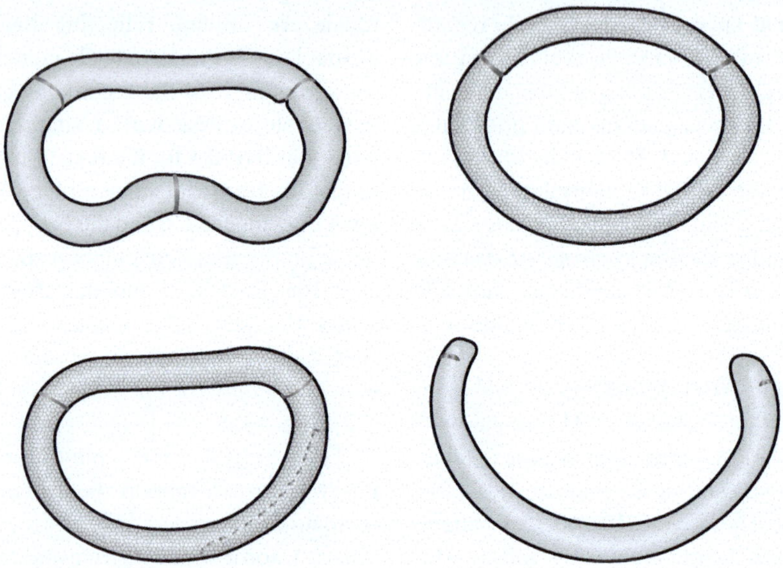

Fig. 13.2 Mitral annuloplasty rings. Adapted from [100]

cohort of 362 patients with a median follow-up 5.4 years that underwent mitral repair with concomitant maze procedure for the treatment of atrial fibrillation, 62 (17.1%) patients had late recurrence of atrial fibrillation, and 83% were free of atrial fibrillation without anti-arrhythmic drugs at 5 years. If sinus rhythm was maintained for 6 months post-operatively, warfarin was discontinued. Patients with warfarin discontinuation had four episodes of stroke/TIA (0.06%/patient-year), no difference than the patients that remained on warfarin (96 (26.5%) patients remained on warfarin beyond 6 months and 54 (14.9%) remained on warfarin through the end of follow-up) [102].

A multicenter retrospective propensity-matched cohort study of mitral repair with annuloplasty ring placement compared 858 patients on vitamin K antagonist therapy to 286 patients on antiplatelet therapy alone; none of the patients had prior atrial fibrillation. At 6 months, there was no difference in thromboembolic events (1.6 versus 2.1%), and major hemorrhagic complications were less common in the antiplatelet group (3.9 versus 0.7%, $p = 0.01$). Mortality was increased in the VKA group (2.7 versus 0.3%, $p = 0.02$), and this persisted with multivariable adjustment [103].

This signal of increased mortality with warfarin use is countered by another large observational study. In a Danish registry of 2188 patients with mitral repair followed for a median of 4.9 years, patients with VKA prescription (39%) were compared to those with no VKA prescription. VKA prescription was associated with a lower combined risk of stroke and death at 3 months (hazard ratio 0.28, $p = 0.002$), and there was no difference in hemorrhagic complications (1 versus 2%) [104].

There are limited data regarding repair of other valves. One author has published repeatedly regarding techniques for aortic valve repair utilizing pericardial tissue, either autologous or treated bovine, managed post-operatively with aspirin 100 mg daily and no anticoagulation. In one series of 91 such patients, there were no thromboembolic complications [105]. The ACCP recommends this approach (low-dose aspirin) following aortic repair (grade 2C), and the other guidelines do not address valve repair beyond the mitral valve [22]. In the absence of randomized data and the presence of inconclusive, if not conflicting, observational data, decision-making regarding the optimal antithrombotic regimens following valve repair should be influenced by guideline recommendations applied to the individual patient context.

MitraClip

The MitraClip (Abbott Vascular, Menlo Park, CA) was approved by the US FDA in 2013 for percutaneous transcatheter mitral valve repair. It is a cobalt-chromium clip covered with polypropylene fabric that grabs the anterior and posterior mitral valve leaflets, reducing the regurgitant flow by increasing the coaptation between the regurgitant valve leaflets. Per the AHA/ACC guidelines, MitraClip is indicated in patients with severely symptomatic heart failure (NYHA classes III, IV) with chronic, severe primary mitral regurgitation (MR) and who are not appropriate candidates for open surgery [12].

Currently the manufacturer does not have strict recommendations on the duration or choice of antithrombotic agents. However, animal models have shown evidence of endothelialization and fibrous encapsulation of the device by 12 weeks [106]. In the clinical trials assessing the efficacy of the MitraClip, a regimen of high-dose aspirin 325 mg daily for 6–12 months was used, as well as clopidogrel 75 mg daily for 1 month [107–109]. No device thrombosis was identified in any of these trials, although ischemic strokes have been documented [109]. While the risk of device-associated thrombosis appears to be low, the role of different antithrombotic regimens requires further study.

Plugs for Paravalvular Leak

A complication of prosthetic valve implantation that may arise in any valve position is regurgitant flow, not across the prosthetic valve orifice, but in defects at the periphery of the prosthetic valve. Paravalvular leak (PVL) is challenging to treat and may result in symptoms of heart failure as well as significant intravascular hemolysis due to the shear stress of regurgitant flow through the neo-orifice(s). While surgical repair or redo valve replacement was previously the only option for management of severe PVL, endovascular plugging of PVL offers a less invasive treatment option via a transfemoral or transapical approach for high-risk surgical patients (class IIa, level of evidence B) [12].

Operators may choose from a variety of nitinol wire mesh devices based on the anatomy of the defect including the Amplatzer septal occlusion devices (described below) or the Amplatzer Vascular Plug series (AGA Medical Corp, Plymouth, MN). The only approved device for this indication in Europe is the Occlutech Paravalvular Leak Device series (Helsingborg, Sweden) [110]. There are currently no FDA-approved devices for PVL closure in the USA so use of devices for this indication is thus off-label at the time of writing. Intra-procedural therapeutic anticoagulation is necessary, as with all procedures in the systemic circulation, typically with intravenous unfractionated heparin [111]. There are no formal recommendations for post-procedural antithrombotic therapy, though in the absence of an indication for indefinite anticoagulation, operators report use of dual antiplatelet therapy for at least 3 months, while some use routine post-procedural vitamin K antagonist therapy [110, 112].

Outcomes data from endovascular plugging of PVL are derived from case series. The technical success of the procedure ranges from 77 to 88%, while clinical success (relief of the indication for the procedure) is lower at 67–77%. Complications include obstruction of prosthetic valve leaflets (0.9% of which requires emergency valve surgery), device embolization (4%), coronary artery obstruction (either of the ostia at the aortic annulus or the left circumflex at the posterolateral mitral annulus), vascular complications (0.9–2%), stroke (1.7%), and death (1.7–2%). In the event of device embolization, the device typically migrates to the common iliac vessels; if it cannot be snared and retrieved, surgical removal is necessary [110].

Transcatheter Aortic Valve Replacement

From the first implant in 2002, use of endovascular aortic valve implantation has expanded dramatically and ushered in a new era of structural percutaneous therapy. The pivotal PARTNER trial first demonstrated the efficacy and safety of this therapy for patients with prohibitive surgical risk, and the indications have been steadily widened to include patients with progressively lower surgical risk [113]. Current American and European guidelines recommend lifelong low-dose aspirin therapy with 3–6 months of clopidogrel dual antiplatelet therapy, as used in the clinical trials (class IIb, level of evidence C), with consideration for at least 3 months of warfarin therapy with an INR goal 2.5 for patients at low risk of bleeding (class IIb, level of evidence B-NR) [12–14, 22]. There are limited data comparing these alternative regimens.

A single-center Italian study randomized 79 patients following TAVR (transcatheter aortic valve replacement) to aspirin 100 mg daily alone or aspirin 100 mg daily in addition to clopidogrel 75 mg daily for the first 3 months and found no difference in the composite endpoint (all-cause mortality, myocardial infarction, stroke, valve surgery, major bleeding) at 30 days (13% versus 15%) or 6 months (18 versus 15%) [114]. This study is to be followed with the larger POPular-TAVI trial, aiming to enroll 1000 patients to compare monotherapy with aspirin or oral anticoagulant (if the patient has a prior indication, such as atrial fibrillation or mechanical heart valve) to dual therapy with the addition of clopidogrel following TAVR [115].

Therapeutic anticoagulation during the TAVR procedure is necessary with catheters in the systemic circulation to reduce the risk of thromboembolic complications. Intravenous unfractionated heparin is the standard agent used. BRAVO-3, an international randomized controlled trial, compared intra-procedural bivalirudin to UFH in 802 patients during TAVR. There was no difference in early major hemorrhagic complications (within 48 h or prior to hospital discharge) between the agents, and bivalirudin was non-inferior (not superior) in a combined endpoint at 30 days (all-cause mortality, myocardial infarction, stroke, and major bleeding) [116].

There has been a growing appreciation for the presence and repercussions of subclinical leaflet thrombosis with TAVR. An initial report was motivated by the observation of reduced leaflet motion on chest CT in a TAVR patient enrolled in a clinical trial, noted after the patient had a stroke. An analysis of CT findings from 55 other trial patients and 132 patients from a combined registry of patients with transcatheter or bioprosthetic surgical aortic valves from two centers revealed the presence of reduced leaflet motion in 22 (40%) trial patients and 17 (13%) registry patients. Patients on warfarin were less likely to have reduced leaflet motion than patients on dual antiplatelet therapy (0 versus 55% among trial patients, $p = 0.01$; 0 versus 29% among registry patients, $p = 0.04$), and patients on warfarin were more likely to have restoration of leaflet motion on follow-up CT (11 (100%) versus 1 (10%), $p < 0.001$). Reduced leaflet motion was associated with incident stroke or TIA among registry patients (3 (18%) versus 1 (1%), $p = 0.007$), with a trend in the same direction among the trial patients that did not meet statistical significance with low numbers (2 (9%) versus 0, $p = 0.16$) [117].

Reviewing the experience with transcatheter aortic valve thrombosis, an international, multicenter consortium reported 26 (0.61%) cases among 4266 TAVR procedures. The most common clinical presentation was dyspnea (17 (65%) patients), while 8 (31%) patients were asymptomatic. Transthoracic echo demonstrated marked elevation in the mean aortic valve pressure gradient (40.5 ± 14 mmHg), thickened valve leaflets (20 patients (77%)), and in 6 (23%)

patients a thrombotic mass. Patients were treated with anticoagulation (IV UFH or LMWH with or without oral VKA), and 23 (88%) had significant decrease in aortic valve gradients within 2 months of therapy [118].

Another registry-based series in two centers (USA and Denmark) including 752 TAVR patients with universal CT imaging reported subclinical leaflet thrombosis in 101 patients (13%), along with 5 (4%) of the 138 patients with a surgically implanted bioprosthetic aortic valve ($p = 0.001$). Over the mean follow-up of 540 days, subclinical leaflet thrombosis was associated with increased rates of TIA (4.2/100 person-years versus 0.6/100 person-years, $p = 0.0005$) but not stroke (4.1/100 person-years versus 1.9/100 person-years, $p = 0.10$). Fifty-eight of the 106 patients with subclinical leaflet thrombosis had repeat CT imaging. Among this group, 100% of the 36 patients treated with 3 months of therapeutic anticoagulation (67% VKA, 33% DOAC) had restoration of normal leaflet motion, while 91% of the remaining 22 patients not treated with therapeutic anticoagulation had either persistence or progression of reduced leaflet motion ($p < 0.0001$) [119].

While investigation into this clinical entity and the optimal antithrombotic regimens to prevent clinical complications is ongoing, it is notable that post-procedural bleeding is a significant complication associated with TAVR. In a two-site registry from Spain and Canada, 316 (44%) of 720 patients had a total of 506 unplanned readmissions following TAVR over a median follow-up of 23 months. Bleeding was the cause for 36 (7.1%) readmissions, and a combined regimen of anticoagulant and antiplatelet agents was associated with early readmission within 1 month following the procedure (hazard ratio 1.62, $p = 0.014$) [120].

Prosthetic Valve Thrombosis and Embolic Complications

Thrombosis of a prosthetic heart valve is a feared complication with the associated risks of mechanical valve failure and embolic complications. Thrombosis must be distinguished from pannus formation, which is a process of fibrous tissue ingrowth, and does not rely on activation of the coagulation cascade [121]. Several imaging modalities are available to facilitate the diagnosis, including transthoracic and transesophageal echo, valve cinefluoroscopy (in the case of mechanical valves), and CT [122, 123]. The American Society of Echocardiography, in conjunction with multiple international echo societies, published recommendations for the echo evaluation of prosthetic valves [124].

Management of valve thrombosis depends on the location and characteristics of the lesion, and the options include valve surgery or fibrinolysis. Valve surgery is a much more invasive procedure, although it is associated with higher success rates and may be necessary to avert the potentially catastrophic complications of valve thrombosis. The risks of fibrinolysis include hemorrhagic complications, embolization, and recurrent thrombosis. The American and European guidelines recommend surgery for left-sided lesions associated with severe symptoms (NYHA classes III to IV) (class I, level of evidence B-NR) and state that surgery is reasonable for left-sided lesions that are large (>0.8 cm^2 in the American guidelines, >10 mm in the European guidelines) or mobile (due to greater risk of embolization) (class IIa, level of evidence B). Fibrinolytic therapy is reasonable for right-sided lesions and left-sided lesions that do not meet those criteria (class IIa, level of evidence B) [12–14, 22].

Thromboembolic complications of prosthetic heart valves may arise due to inadequate antithrombotic therapy or despite appropriate therapy. Following a thromboembolic event, the adequacy of antithrombotic management should be thoroughly assessed, along with potential alternative etiologies of thromboembolism. Balancing the risks of recurrent thromboembolic events and hemorrhagic complications of antithrombotic therapy, the American and European guidelines recommend increasing the intensity of antithrombotic therapy following a thromboembolic complication [12, 13]. If an event occurred despite warfarin anticoagulation, the INR target can be increased. If warfarin was not previously prescribed, it can be started. If low-dose aspirin was not previously prescribed, it can be started.

Pregnancy

Young women that are pregnant with prosthetic heart valves have a high risk of adverse maternal and fetal outcomes and require extensive preconception counseling and close surveillance in an experienced center. There are many features to the management of valvular heart disease in pregnancy, particularly given the significant hemodynamic changes that occur with normal pregnant physiology. This section will summarize only the management of anticoagulation for prosthetic heart valves. This subject is addressed with supporting literature in the valve guidelines from the AHA/ACC and ESC/EACTS, as well as separate guidelines focused on pregnancy from the ACCP and ESC [12, 13, 125, 126]. Anticoagulation decision-making is particularly challenging in the first trimester, due to the fetal toxicity of warfarin therapy, and near term, due to the risk of hemorrhage associated with delivery.

Vitamin K antagonist use in the first trimester is associated with fetal embryopathy and death, though this risk appears to be attenuated at daily doses of 5 mg or less. For patients with mechanical heart valves that require long-term vitamin K antagonist therapy, a decision must be made between continued warfarin therapy (if the required dose for therapeutic INR is 5 mg or less) and temporary transition to low-molecular-weight or unfractionated heparin (which do not cross the placenta and are not associated with fetal toxicity) for the duration of the first trimester.

Vitamin K antagonist therapy may then be resumed from weeks 13 to 36, along with low-dose aspirin therapy, when a transition is recommended back to heparin anticoagulation with cessation of aspirin in anticipation of delivery. An alternative regimen is the use of heparin (LMWH or UFH) throughout the entire pregnancy; therapeutic monitoring of both agents is critical, regardless of the duration of use. Women treated with LMWH past 36 weeks are recommended to transition to IV UFH prior to planned delivery to facilitate titration of anticoagulation.

Recent cohorts offer a contemporary perspective on the risks. In the global ROPAC registry, pregnancy outcomes were assessed among 212 patients with mechanical valves, 134 with bioprosthetic valves, and 2620 with no prosthetic heart valve. Maternal mortality was 1.4% among women with mechanical valves, 1.5% with bioprosthetic valves, and 0.2% with no prosthetic valve ($p = 0.03$). Valve thrombosis occurred in ten (4.7%) women with a mechanical valve (4.4% of mitral valves and 2.6% of aortic valves, $p = 1.00$); five of these episodes occurred in the first trimester while on heparin (3.6% of patients on heparin and 0% on VKA, $p = 0.17$). Maternal hemorrhagic complications occurred in 23.1% of women with mechanical valves, 5.1% with bioprosthetic valves, and 4.9% with no prosthetic valve ($p < 0.001$). Use of VKA in the first trimester compared to heparin was associated with increased miscarriage (29 versus 9%, $p < 0.001$) and late fetal death (7 versus 0.7%, $p = 0.016$) [127].

Another cohort from Australia included 136 patients with prosthetic valves. There was no maternal mortality, though there was an increase in maternal complications relative to pregnancies with no prosthetic valves: severe morbidity (139/1000 births, rate ratio 10.0, CI 6.3–15.7) and major cardiovascular events (44/1000 births, rate ratio 34.6, CI 14.6–81.6). There was also a significant increase in the fetal complications of preterm birth (183/1000 births, rate ratio 2.8, CI 1.9–4.1) and small for gestational age (193/1000, RR 2.0, CI 1.4–3.0) [128].

The outcomes with use of low-dose warfarin during the first trimester were evaluated in a systematic review and meta-analysis of 11 observational studies with 494 patients. The rate of embryopathy was 0.9% (CI 0.4–2.4%), and the rate of fetal loss was 13.4% (CI 8.4–24.7%), primarily spontaneous abortion 12.8% (CI 7.7–22.7%). There was no maternal mortality, though the rate of prosthetic valve thrombosis was 0.6% (CI 0.3–2%), total thromboembolic events 1.8% (CI 1.1–3.6%), and major maternal hemorrhagic complications 3.4% (CI 2–5.1%). A subset of patients with decreased INR target range to 1.5–2.5 for the first trimester had lower fetal loss than those with INR target range 2.5–3.5 (2.1% (CI 0.5–6.9%) versus 16.1% (CI 13.1–34.4%)) [129].

Left Ventricular Assist Devices

Introduction

The first left ventricular assist device (LVAD) was implanted by Michael DeBakey in 1966, providing short-term support after cardiac surgery for 10 days [130]. Over the last three decades, considerable changes in LVAD technology have quadrupled the average life span of end-stage heart failure (HF) patients [131]. Bleeding and thromboembolic events are the most common causes of morbidity and mortality among patients with LVADs. Accordingly, appropriate antiplatelet and anticoagulant therapies play a key role in management of LVAD patients. At present, over 1500 LVADs are implanted in patients with advanced HF in the USA each year [132]. These numbers continue to rise given the increasing incidence of HF and the limited availability of donor hearts for transplant [133, 134].

LVAD Mechanics and the Effect on Circulation

All LVADs propel blood collected from the left ventricle via an inflow cannula in the apex into the ascending aorta via an outflow cannula, hence bypassing a failing left ventricle. These devices are implanted internally but connect to a power source through an externalized percutaneous driveline. First-generation LVADs mimicked the pulsatility seen in the innate circulatory system using an oscillating membrane, and hence only antiplatelet therapy was required without the need for systemic anticoagulation to avert thrombosis within the pump (Fig. 13.3) [135]. However, these devices were not durable over the long term and are presently only used in the pediatric population due to the small patient size. Contemporary LVADs are continuous-flow devices lacking the physiologic pulsatile flow seen in the circulatory system. They can further be characterized into axial-flow devices (e.g., HeartMate II (Thoratec Corp, Pleasanton, CA)) that propel blood using the Archimedes screw principle [136] and centrifugal devices (e.g., HeartWare (Framingham, MA), HeartMate III (Thoratec Corp, Pleasanton, CA)) that use a magnetically levitated rotor [137] (Fig. 13.4).

All LVADs cause hemolysis due to shear stress. However, the degree of hemolysis is higher in axial-flow devices as the device diameter is smaller requiring the motor to spin at a high rate of 7000–12,000 revolutions per minute (RPM) to generate adequate cardiac output. In contrast, the newer centrifugal devices have a larger rotor diameter and hence spin at lower rates of 2000–3000 RPM. Furthermore, since the rotor is magnetically levitated, there is no friction creating less shear, which results in less hemolysis [140].

In addition to hemolysis, these devices are also associated with changes in components of the coagulation cascade, partly due to contact with the artificial LVAD surface. These changes include a decrease in coagulation proteins (factors XI and XII and prekallikrein) [141], activation of the fibrinolytic system [142], and platelet activation [143, 144] and occur nearly immediately after LVAD implantation. Thus, there has been an increased focus on improving hemocompatibility of LVADs in newer centrifugal devices (e.g., HeartMate III) by providing a textured surface in contact with the blood to potentially reduce risks of bleeding and thrombosis. Additionally, HF in itself causes hepatic and renal dysfunction that compromise the hemostatic system [145].

Furthermore, nearly all patients with LVADs develop acquired von Willebrand disease, a condition also well described in severe aortic stenosis [146, 147]. Secondary to the non-physiologic high shear stress, von Willebrand factor (vWF) unravels and is exposed to proteolysis by ADAMTS-13, rendering it inactive [148]. Several studies have found altered vWF multimer

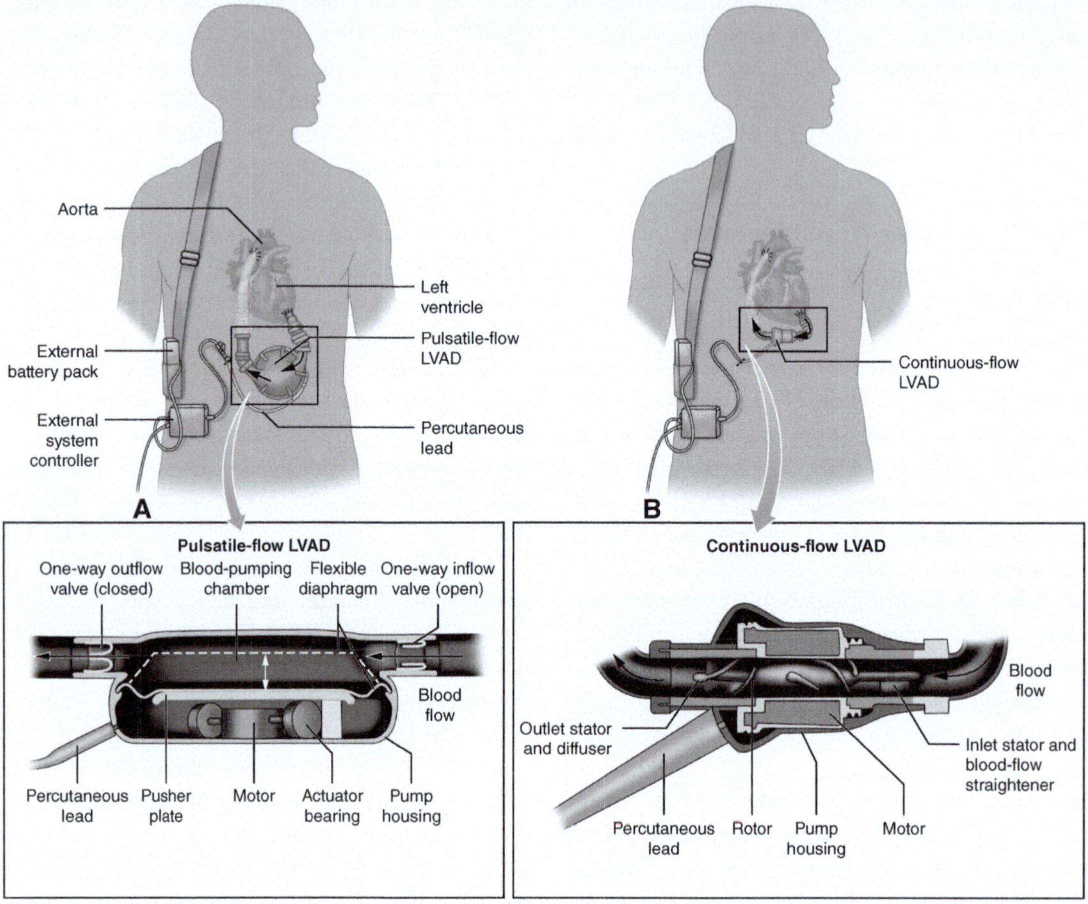

Fig. 13.3 Designs of LVADs. (**a**) Pulsatile-flow devices use positive displacement pumps to propel blood throughout the body as a healthy ventricle would do. Although pulsatile flow is seemingly more physiological, left ventricular unloading and hemodynamic improvement is comparable to that achieved with continuous-flow pumps. (**b**) Continuous-flow devices use either centrifugal or axial-flow pumps to propel blood continuously throughout the body. These devices are more reliable, have a longer functional life, and operate more quietly than pulsatile devices. Adapted from [138]

composition in patients with continuous-flow LVADs but not in pulsatile LVADs. When compiled, current evidence strongly supports the presence of acquired von Willebrand disease in continuous-flow LVADs, which is likely a key contributor to bleeding complications seen with these devices [149, 150].

Finally, to prevent thrombus formation within the pump of contemporary continuous-flow LVADs due to lack of flow pulsatility, systemic anticoagulation is required. To optimize pump hemodynamics, new continuous-flow centrifugal LVADs such as the HeartMate III have incorporated an artificial pulse mode in which the rotor speed varies the set speed by 2000 RPM to produce changes in blood flow and arterial blood pressure every 2 s [151]. Nonetheless, this does not obviate the need for systemic anticoagulation. The bleeding risk in LVAD patients is much higher due to changes in the circulatory system as highlighted above compounded with the anticoagulation requirement to prevent pump thrombosis.

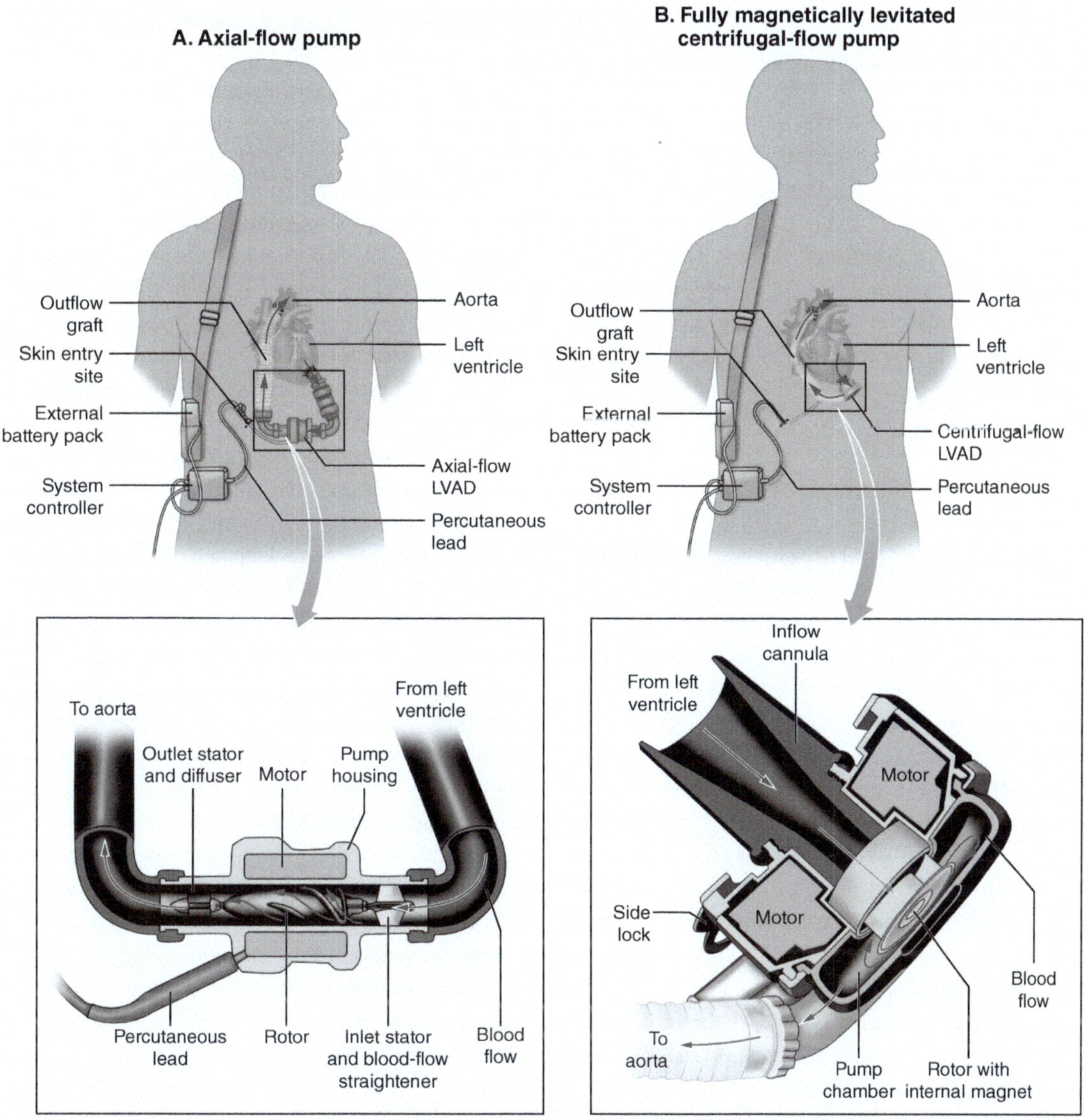

Fig. 13.4 Diagrams of axial-flow and continuous-flow pump. (**a**) Axial-flow pump: Blood enters at one end of the rotor and is driven along the axis of the rotor to the outflow of the pump. (**b**) Fully magnetically levitated centrifugal pump: Blood enters at the central axis of the rotor and is driven outward centrifugally to the outflow of the pump. Adapted from [139]

Antithrombotic Therapy Management

Aspirin and oral vitamin K antagonists form the cornerstone for anticoagulation in patients with LVADs. Initial trials with continuous-flow LVADs required aspirin with or without dipyridamole and warfarin anticoagulation to maintain a goal INR of 2.5–3.5. However, bleeding was a common adverse event with an incidence of 81% in patients with axial-flow LVADs [152]. These high bleeding rates coupled with low rates of thromboembolism have resulted in current guidelines recommending modified anticoagulation and antiplatelet strategies. At present, there exists wide variation in antithrombotic strategies across various sites. This was highlighted in the systematic review by Baumann Kreuziger and colleagues that evaluated various anticoagulant and antiplatelet strategies and their association with LVAD outcomes [153]. They noted variation in target INR goals for warfarin therapy and use of differing antiplatelet agents including aspirin, dipyridamole, and clopidogrel. In the absence of randomized trials evaluating antithrombotic strategies, the International Society for Heart and Lung Transplantation (ISHLT) provided guidance on antiplatelet and anticoagulation strategies in patients with LVADs largely based on expert consensus in 2013 [154].

Preoperative Management

Placement of an LVAD requires a median sternotomy, use of cardiopulmonary bypass, and also intraperitoneal pump placement for some LVAD models. Coagulopathy secondary to the pathophysiologic processes of HF compounded by coagulation abnormalities produced by LVAD implantation leads to bleeding being the most common perioperative adverse event. The 2013 ISHLT guidelines recommend preoperative evaluation of INR, partial thromboplastin time, and platelet count with further evaluation of baseline abnormalities unexplained by pharmacological therapy in all patients being considered for LVAD implantation. Patients with a history of thrombophilia should also have a hypercoagulable assessment prior to implantation.

Approximately 60% of patients with advanced HF are on anticoagulation for concomitant indications such as atrial fibrillation or prosthetic heart valves prior to LVAD implantation [155]. Typically, such patients are transitioned to warfarin (if they are otherwise taking a DOAC) once they are approved for a cardiac transplant or LVAD. In patients undergoing planned LVAD implantation, warfarin is stopped 5–7 days prior to surgery, and heparin is initiated due to easy reversibility. In addition, guidelines recommend cessation of thienopyridine antiplatelet agents for at least 5 days prior to surgery unless there is a compelling indication for continued use.

Perioperative Management

During surgery, guidelines recommend complete reversal of heparin once a patient is placed on cardiopulmonary bypass. After surgery, anticoagulation with heparin is recommended once hemostasis is achieved on post-operative day 1 and the target activated partial thromboplastin time is gradually prolonged over successive days. Initiation of aspirin is also recommended on post-operative day 1 if possible. Warfarin is usually initiated after removal of chest tubes once the patient can tolerate oral medications with a target INR of 2.0–3.0.

Post-operative bridging with intravenous unfractionated heparin until the target INR is achieved is currently under debate. In a study of 418 HeartMate II LVAD patients, Slaughter and colleagues retrospectively evaluated differences in thromboembolic and hemorrhagic events between patients bridged with IV UFH to goal INR as compared to those who were not. While there were no differences in thromboembolic complications, the risk of post-operative bleeding requiring transfusion from days 3 to 30 was significantly lower in the group that did not receive heparin for bridging [156]. However, in the early post-operative period, unopposed use of warfarin with its initially procoagulant effects in the first 48–72 h remains a concern. Accordingly, in the absence of randomized trials comparing perioperative anticoagulation strategies, current guidelines recommend bridging with IV UFH in the post-operative setting after hemostasis is achieved.

Long-Term Post-operative Management

Anticoagulation Therapy

Patients with LVAD should receive anticoagulation with oral vitamin K antagonists (VKA) to maintain an INR within the range specified by each device manufacturer. Current ISHLT recommendations include target INR goals (2–3) that are identical for both axial and centrifugal pumps. Data from retrospective studies examining the association between INR and bleeding and thromboembolic complications support this recommendation [157].

Management of VKA therapy in LVAD patients poses several challenges. As opposed to patients without LVADs on VKAs for other indications who have a time in therapeutic INR range of approximately 70%, patients with LVADs are in the therapeutic range only 31–51% of the time [158, 159]. Jennings and colleagues evaluated differences in the pharmacodynamic response to warfarin in patients before and after LVAD implantation and observed that 54% of patients required a change in warfarin dose after LVAD implantation in the absence of other interacting medications [160]. The median dose change was 22% (range 8–44%) with most patients needing lower doses. Whether strategies such as patient INR self-monitoring or pharmacist-directed intensive monitoring help improve time in therapeutic INR range in LVAD patients is not known.

For patients who have a subtherapeutic INR during routine testing, bridging with low-molecular-weight heparin (LMWH) is frequently used at some sites with the exception of patients who are obese or have advanced chronic renal disease. In such patients, IV UFH is administered in the inpatient setting until the patient attains the target INR.

The role of DOACs in LVADs as an alternative to VKAs remains undefined. A small case series involving seven LVAD patients from Europe showed successful use of dabigatran without an increased risk for bleeding or thrombosis in comparison to VKA [161]. A pilot, randomized open-label trial comparing dabigatran to VKA is ongoing in Austria (EudraCT number 2010-024534038). However, the concerning finding of increased risk for thromboembolic and hemorrhagic events with dabigatran in patients with mechanical heart valves in the RE-ALIGN trial necessitates definitive evidence in the form of a randomized trial to establish the safety of DOACs in patients with LVADs [50]. Until such evidence is available, LVAD patients should be routinely anticoagulated with vitamin K antagonists.

Antiplatelet Therapy

In addition to warfarin, chronic antiplatelet therapy with aspirin (dose 81–325 mg daily) is recommended. Dual antiplatelet therapy with aspirin and dipyridamole was optional in the HeartMate II trials, but its routine use is no longer recommended due to the high bleeding rates observed. Some sites use platelet function tests such as thromboelastography to assess daily antiplatelet needs until stable levels are achieved. However, there is insufficient data to support routine use of this practice at present.

LVAD Complications

Bleeding

Contemporary data suggests that nonsurgical bleeding requiring surgery or transfusion is the most common adverse effect of continuous-flow LVADs. Common sites of bleeding include epistaxis, gastrointestinal (GI) bleeds, intracranial hemorrhage, and bleeding into the thorax or mediastinum [131, 162]. Location of bleeding varies depending on the time from LVAD implantation with thoracic or mediastinal bleeds being most common immediately after surgery and gastrointestinal bleeds being most common over the longer term [163]. Retrospective cohort analysis has identified risk factors for bleeding, including female sex, older age (greater than 65 years), preoperative anemia, and ischemic cardiomyopathy [164]. Table 13.4 shows contemporary estimates of the rates of bleeding complications.

Bleeding rates are similar between axial and centrifugal continuous-flow LVADs. However, as compared to older generation pulsatile-flow LVADs, patients with contemporary LVADs have a significantly higher risk of bleeding [135, 162]. Putative explanatory factors for this difference include the need for systemic anticoagulation with newer devices, acquired von Willebrand disease, and impaired platelet function. Another synergistic factor for GI bleeds is the formation of arteriovenous malformations (AVMs) by mechanisms similar to those described in aortic stenosis. These include increased intraluminal pressures and vascular smooth muscle contraction leading to increased sympathetic tone that results in smooth muscle relaxation with arteriovenular dilation leading to AVMs [165]. Another proposed mechanism is that a reduced pulse pressure causes intestinal hypoperfusion leading to regional hypoxia, vascular dilation, and AVMs (Fig. 13.5) [162].

Management of hemorrhagic complications with LVADs involves an amalgamation of cessation of anticoagulation and reversal of VKA, transfusion, endoscopic therapies for GI bleeds (in particular for AVMs), and surgical therapies for surgical site bleeds or intracranial hemorrhages [162] (Table 13.4).

Table 13.4 The frequency of major complications in LVAD patients [149, 152, 164, 166–174]

Complication	Cumulative frequency (%)
Bleeding	
Intraoperative/post-operative bleeding [149, 152, 166]	20–30
Gastrointestinal bleeding [167–169]	16–23
CNS bleeding [170, 171]	7–11
Thrombosis	
Pump thrombosis [172, 173]	2–9
Stroke [164, 174]	4–6

Thrombosis

In contrast to bleeding complications, thrombotic complications are less common but can be more devastating. LVADs activate the coagulation system and lead to device-related thrombosis. In the REMATCH trial, the rate of cerebrovascular accident was reported at 0.19 events/patient-year [175]. With newer generation devices, the risk for thrombosis has declined secondary to improved hemocompatibility. Other sites for thrombus formation include the left ventricle secondary to the sluggish flow of end-stage heart failure. This degree of stasis is dependent partly on flow across the native aortic valve, and hence sites have increasingly incorporated LVAD programing to allow for intermittent opening of the aortic valve and optimize LVAD speeds to ensure maximal decompression of the left ventricle [176].

Pump thrombosis is among the most feared complications of LVAD therapy (Fig. 13.6). It

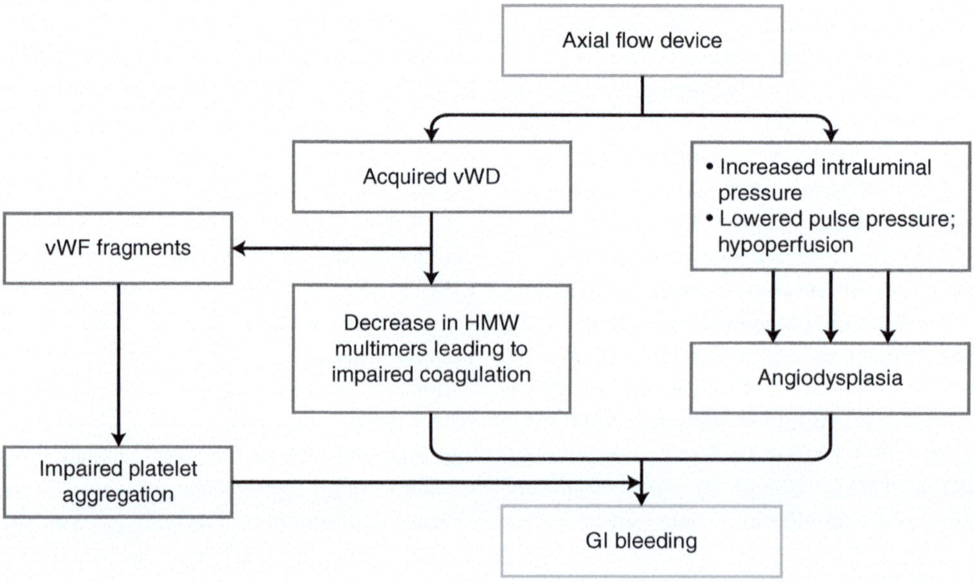

Fig. 13.5 Mechanisms implicated in gastrointestinal bleeding in patients with continuous-flow LVADs. Continuous-flow LVADs lead to increased intraluminal pressure and lowered pulse pressure, resulting in hypoperfusion of the intestines. These physiological changes result in an increased risk of developing angiodysplasia. These devices also decrease the high-molecular-weight (HMW) von Willebrand factor (vWF) multimer size because of excessive cleavage by the metalloprotease ADAMTS13. This results in an acquired form of vWF disease and inhibition of platelet aggregation. These mechanisms work synergistically to cause GI tract bleeding. Adapted from [135]

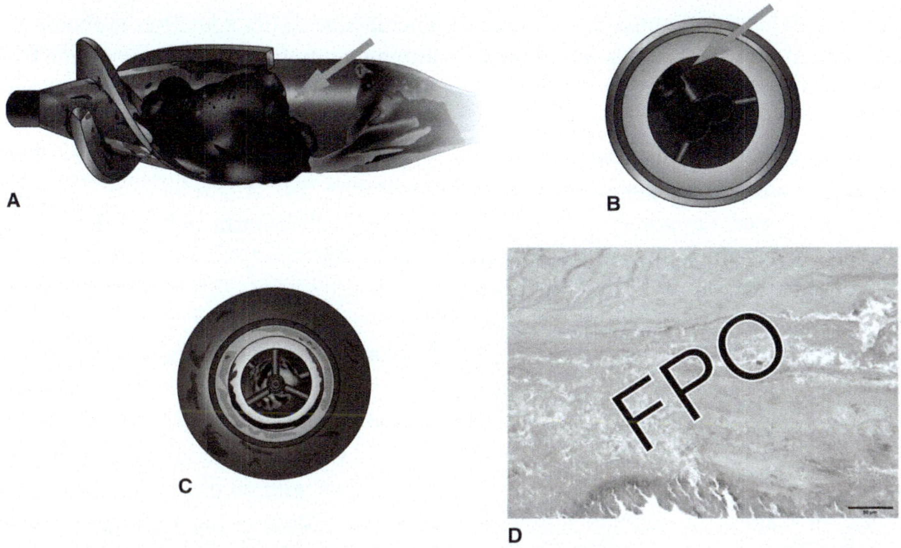

Fig. 13.6 Thrombus in continuous-flow LVAD identified during device explant. Thrombus formation on the impeller part of the HeartMate II device (arrows). These were identified during device removal postmortem (**a**) and during heart transplantation (**b**, **c**). (**d**) Photomicrograph of the excised thrombus, consisting predominately of fibrin and platelets (hematoxylin and eosin, original magnification ×200). Adapted from [177]

typically manifests as hemolysis on laboratory testing (reflected by a rising LDH), symptoms of heart failure, and/or increased pump power. Diagnosis is suggested by transthoracic echo findings of increased aortic valve opening, left ventricular dilation with inadequate decompression, and worsening mitral regurgitation. Therapy frequently involves IV UFH anticoagulation, in addition to fibrinolytics and glycoprotein IIb/IIIa inhibitors. Surgical pump exchange is the treatment of choice [176].

With improving LVAD designs, the risk for pump thrombosis seen in clinical trials is declining. The most recent MOMENTUM 3 trial compared rates of pump thrombosis and stroke with the new HeartMate III pump (magnetically levitated, centrifugal continuous-flow pump that incorporates an intrinsic artificial pulse) to the HeartMate II (axial continuous-flow pump) [139]. The rates of reoperation for pump thrombosis were lower with HeartMate III with no difference in rates of stroke, all-cause mortality, or bleeding.

LVAD Conclusion

LVADs are increasingly utilized for management of advanced HF patients. Bleeding and thrombosis are the most common causes of morbidity and mortality among LVAD patients. Implantation of the device is associated with hemolysis, acquired von Willebrand disease, and platelet dysfunction. Present generation LVADs require antiplatelet therapy with aspirin and anticoagulation with vitamin K antagonists.

Temporary Mechanical Circulatory Support

There is a wide range of devices that offer temporary mechanical circulatory support through decreased cardiac preload and afterload, increased cardiac output, and improved tissue perfusion. The construction and placement of each device vary but all involve contact with blood and alteration of normal flow with the concomitant risk of thromboembolic complications. Thus, all require therapeutic anticoagulation and there is limited evidence comparing different regimens. Given the critical status of patients requiring this nature of support, ready titration of anticoagulation is required, and intravenous heparin is the most commonly used agent [178].

Intra-aortic balloon pump counterpulsation is among the longest used temporary mechanical support devices, first employed in 1968. Placed via the femoral or axillary artery, a gas-filled balloon inflates and deflates in the proximal descending thoracic aorta in time with the cardiac cycle [179]. The need for continuous IV UFH to prevent thromboembolic complications and limb ischemia downstream of the arterial access site has been questioned in several small observational studies. In cohorts of patients following cardiac surgery (203 patients and 153 patients) managed with or without heparin, a cohort of 252 patients in the cardiac intensive care unit managed with universal heparin versus selective heparin (only if another indication was present), and a cohort of 97 patients managed with glycoprotein IIb/IIIa antagonist infusion following percutaneous coronary intervention, the rate of vascular complications was unchanged relative to standard UFH, and there were increased hemorrhagic complications with the use of heparin [180, 181].

The Impella device is an Archimedes screw-based axial-flow pump inserted via the femoral or axillary artery with a cannula that extends across the aortic valve into the left ventricle and pumps blood into the ascending aorta. The TandemHeart is an extracorporeal centrifugal pump that draws oxygenated blood from a cannula in the left atrium (via the femoral vein and across the interatrial septum) and pumps it into a cannula in the femoral artery. Both devices require continuous anticoagulation, typically with IV UFH, and institutional device-specific protocols are reported [182].

Extracorporeal membrane oxygenation is able to provide the greatest level of cardiac output support and is derived from cardiopulmonary bypass. In the case of cardiac failure, large cannulae are inserted into a large artery and vein. Deoxygenated blood is drawn from the venous system, passed through a membrane oxygenator, and pumped back to the arterial circulation. Therapeutic anticoagulation is required to avoid thromboembolic complications and ECMO circuit thrombosis. The Extracorporeal Life Support Organization publishes guidelines for anticoagulation therapy, and recommends UFH, with bivalirudin or argatroban as alternatives for patients with heparin-induced thrombocytopenia (HIT) [183].

Septal Closure Devices

Percutaneous device closure is a safe and effective endovascular alternative to surgical closure for patients with an ostium secundum atrial septal defect (ASD) or patent foramen ovale (PFO). It may also be a treatment option for some patients with ventricular septal defects, based on the anatomy and risks of surgical management. Here we discuss recommended antithrombotic regimens for FDA-approved devices for septal closure.

Amplatzer Septal Occluder

The Amplatzer (AGA Medical, Minneapolis, MN) was approved for percutaneous secundum ASD closure in 2001. It is composed of two round disks connected by a short waist, made of nitinol-titanium with polyester patches that facilitate occlusion and endothelialization. Preliminary animal studies showed that complete endothelialization of the device occurred within weeks after implantation and there was 100% defect closure at 3 months [184, 185]. However, in humans there have been varying degrees of endothelialization of this device, with reports of no endothelialization even 18 months after ASD closure [186].

Following device implantation, antiplatelet or anticoagulation therapy for 6 months is recommended. Typically, aspirin is prescribed at 81–325 mg daily, and clopidogrel 75 mg daily is sometimes added for 1 month after the procedure, depending on the discretion of the referring physician. Reported thrombus formation with the Amplatzer has been lower compared to other devices used for transcatheter closure [187–189].

The Amplatzer membranous ventricular septal defect (VSD) occluder has complete closure by 6 months on echocardiography [190, 191]. Patients in these trials were maintained on antiplatelet therapy for 6 months following device placement, as with those who received the Amplatzer for ASD repair.

Gore HELEX

The HELEX septal occluder (W.L. Gore & Associates, Flagstaff, AZ) consists of a corkscrew-type nitinol wire covered with polytetrafluoroethylene. Its unique features include its ability to conform to a non-curvilinear surface of the atrial septum, as well as a built-in method for device retrieval after placement.

In a nonrandomized, non-inferiority study of 247 patients, 98.1% of patients who received the device were reported to have defect closure at 12 months post-implantation [192]. These patients were also maintained on a single antiplatelet agent for 6 months after the procedure.

Gore Cardioform

Gore Cardioform Septal Occluder, previously known as the Gore Septal Occluder, is a device approved for repair of ASD or PFOs with a diameter up to 17 mm, and the manufacturer again recommends 6 months of antiplatelet therapy after implantation. It is a flexible, retrievable double-disk device with a petal design made of nitinol and covered by polytetrafluoroethylene. Initial studies showed 25% residual shunt in patients who underwent PFO closure and 0–11% residual shunt in patients with ASDs at 3 months [193, 194]. However, at the time of writing, larger clinical trials assessing the safety and efficacy of this device were not available.

Left Atrial Appendage Occlusion Devices

Left atrial appendage (LAA) occlusion devices were developed as an alternative to chronic anticoagulation for lowering stroke risk in patients with atrial fibrillation, as the left atrial appendage (LAA) is the source of thrombi in more than 90% of patients with non-valvular atrial fibrillation [195]. Here we discuss antithrombotic therapy in patients who receive percutaneous LAA occlusion devices.

Watchman Device

The Watchman device (Boston Scientific, Marlborough, MA) is the most studied LAA occlusion device. It is a self-expandable nitinol cage, covered by a layer of permeable polyethylene terephthalate, and is deployed in the LAA.

The device was endothelialized within 45 days in animal models, and as thrombi may form as the implant surface endothelializes, anticoagulation is necessary during this period. In the PROTECT AF trial, 707 patients were randomized in a 2:1 ratio to either device placement followed by warfarin and aspirin for 45 days or then dual antiplatelet therapy with clopidogrel and aspirin for 6 months, followed by aspirin indefinitely or long-term warfarin with a target INR range of 2–3 [196]. At 18 months, the primary efficacy event (stroke, cardiovascular death, and systemic embolism) rate was similar in intervention and control groups, consistent with non-inferiority of the device. There were more serious adverse events (major bleeding, pericardial effusion, and device embolization) with device placement (7.4 events/100 patient-years versus 4.4, rate ratio 1.69, CI 1.01–3.19).

The ASAP study assessed the efficacy and safety of the Watchman in 150 patients who had contraindications to anticoagulation (93% due to "hemorrhagic/bleeding tendencies") [197]. These patients had a $CHADS_2$ score ≥ 1 and were eligible for 6 months of treatment with a thienopyridine antiplatelet agent (clopidogrel or ticlopidine) and lifelong aspirin. At a mean follow-up of

14.4 months, there were 4 patients with all-cause stroke or systemic embolism (2.3% per year), 3 of these patients had ischemic stroke (1.7% per year), and 1 patient had a hemorrhagic stroke (0.6% per year). The rate of ischemic stroke was less than the 7.3% per year rate that would be expected per the $CHADS_2$ score. Serious adverse events related to the device occurred in 13 (8.7%) patients.

A recent meta-analysis of 19 randomized controlled trials comparing the efficacy and safety of the Watchman to medical therapy found that LAA closure devices were superior to placebo and antiplatelet therapy and similar to DOAC for preventing mortality, stroke, or systemic embolism [198]. The incidence of major bleeding was comparable between the device, placebo, antiplatelet therapy, and DOAC therapy. Again, patients included in this meta-analysis were treated with therapeutic anticoagulation for the first 45 days, dual antiplatelet therapy for 6 months, and single antiplatelet therapy indefinitely.

In consideration of a lower-intensity antithrombotic regimen, Rodriguez-Gabella and colleagues assessed the outcomes following LAA closure with single antiplatelet therapy (either aspirin 80–100 mg daily or clopidogrel 75 mg daily) indefinitely in 31 patients [199]. No stroke or systemic embolism during the mean follow-up period of 19 months was reported. The bleeding rate in this study (3.2% with major gastrointestinal bleeding) was lower than expected based on the HAS-BLED score.

Lariat Device

Another device that can be used for LAA closure is the Lariat (SentreHeart, Redwood City, CA). It consists of an occlusion balloon catheter, magnet-tipped guidewire, and a suture delivery device and requires access to both the endocardial and epicardial space. The magnetic guide placed within the LAA allows a lasso to be placed epicardially to tie off the LAA. This device was designed with the goal of a better safety profile, as the risk of device embolization and thrombus formation is averted with epicardial ligation and the absence of prosthetic endocardial component.

In 2013, Bartus and colleagues tested the efficacy and safety of the Lariat in 89 patients [200]. In this study, patients with a contraindication to warfarin remained off warfarin, whereas those with a $CHADS_2$ score of 2 or higher were continued on warfarin after their ligation. The choice of anticoagulation in patients with a $CHADS_2$ score of 1 was left to the discretion of the referring physician. If patients were not on warfarin, aspirin therapy was recommended. At 1-month and 3-month follow-up, 95% of patients had complete LAA closure. 3.5% of patients had residual LAA leak immediately following ligation, and at 1-year follow-up, 2% of patients had incomplete closure. No thromboembolic events were reported during the follow-up period.

A recent study of 98 patients who underwent successful LAA ligation with the Lariat device were evaluated for leaks, defined as the presence of flow on transesophageal echo [201]. Post-procedure, 50% of patients were discharged on antiplatelet therapy (monotherapy or dual therapy), and 35% on oral anticoagulation. Twenty-three percent of patients had various degrees of LAA leak after the Lariat, and 3% had thrombus at the site of LAA occlusion (two patients on aspirin and one patient without any antithrombotics). During a mean follow-up period of 16.1 months, five patients developed neurological thromboembolic events. Although leaks have not been associated with thromboembolic events in previous studies, the presence of a leak provides a conduit through which thrombi can pass and embolize. Currently there are no standard recommendations in place for anticoagulation after the LARIAT, but this study suggests that discontinuing anticoagulation after the LARIAT prematurely without proper surveillance may increase the risk of thromboembolic events.

Conclusions

There is a wide array of devices that place prosthetic material in, or in communication with, the heart, to address a variety of cardiovascular diseases or structural abnormalities. Antithrombotic therapy plays a key role in mitigating the thromboembolic risks of these device therapies. With accelerating technological progress, the number of new devices will continue to grow and the current devices will continue to evolve. Most evidence evaluates the use of vitamin K antagonists and aspirin in oral therapy; the role of the direct oral anticoagulants remains to be defined for many of these devices. There is a relative paucity of randomized controlled trial data to guide management, though professional society guidelines based on expert interpretation of the best available evidence and device manufacturer recommendations are available. An understanding of the underlying pathophysiology of intracardiac and device thrombosis provides a conceptual framework for these treatment recommendations.

Key Points

- Prosthetic devices are used to treat valvular heart disease, cardiomyopathy, and undesired communications between cardiac chambers. They have a risk of thromboembolic complications that is mitigated by the use of antithrombotic therapies.
- Thrombosis of a cardiac device occurs as a result of platelet activation and initiation of the coagulation cascade via tissue factor exposure or contact activation. Thrombosis can have deleterious effects locally to the extent that normal hemodynamics and chamber or valvular function are impaired and remotely via embolization. The risk of thrombosis is reduced by device endothelialization and device design to minimize thrombogenic shear stresses.
- The risk of thrombosis associated with prosthetic heart valves varies based on features of both the valve (hemodynamics and construction materials) and patient (high-risk features include atrioventricular valve position, multiple prosthetic valves, prior thromboembolism, atrial fibrillation, depressed left ventricular ejection fraction (i.e., LVEF <35%), and mitral stenosis).
- Professional society guidelines synthesize the evidence regarding management of antithrombotic therapy with prosthetic valves, including the special circumstances of initiation, interruption, reversal, pregnancy, and valve thrombosis.
- Vitamin K antagonist-based anticoagulation is the cornerstone of management for prosthetic valves. Patients with mechanical valves require life-long anticoagulation, with INR thresholds based on their valve and risk factors. Direct oral anticoagulants (DOACs) are contraindicated for patients with mechanical heart valves.
- Bleeding and thromboembolic events are the most common causes of morbidity and mortality among patients with LVADs. Aspirin and oral vitamin K antagonists play a key role in LVAD management.
- LVADs alter hemostasis in several ways, including: hemolysis, changes in components of the coagulation cascade (decreased factors XI and XII and prekallikrein), activation of the fibrinolytic system, platelet activation, and acquired von Willebrand disease.

Self-Assessment Questions

1. A 67-year-old man with ischemic cardiomyopathy (left ventricular ejection fraction 30%) underwent mechanical aortic valve replacement for aortic stenosis with a current generation bileaflet valve (low thrombotic risk) at the time of his coronary artery bypass graft surgery. He tolerated the surgery well, has an

estimated glomerular filtration rate of 60 mL/min, and is in sinus rhythm. In addition to daily low-dose aspirin, what additional agent is appropriate to reduce the risk of thromboembolic complications?
(a) Warfarin with a target INR of 3.5 (range 3–4)
(b) Clopidogrel 75 mg daily
(c) Warfarin with a target INR of 3.0 (range 2.5–3.5)
(d) Dabigatran 150 mg twice daily
(e) Warfarin with a target INR of 2.5 (range 2–3)

2. A robust 77-year-old woman 5 years status post a bioprosthetic aortic valve replacement is incidentally found to have new onset atrial fibrillation during a clinic visit for a mild ankle sprain that occurred while she was playing tennis. Her history is otherwise notable only for hypertension that is well-controlled with lisinopril; she has no past stroke, myocardial infarction, peripheral vascular disease, heart failure, or diabetes. Her renal function is normal. What is the most appropriate antithrombotic regimen for stroke risk reduction?
   (a) Aspirin 325 mg daily
   (b) Warfarin with target INR 2.5 (range 2–3)
   (c) Aspirin 81 mg daily with clopidogrel 75 mg daily
   (d) Dabigatran 150 mg twice daily
   (e) Rivaroxaban 20 mg daily
3. A 73-year-old man with severe mitral regurgitation, hypertension, diabetes, and paroxysmal atrial fibrillation undergoes mitral valve repair with annuloplasty ring placement. He has normal renal and hepatic function, has no past stroke, does not drink alcohol or use illicit drugs, and has not had hemorrhagic complications of anticoagulation. What is the best antithrombotic regimen for this patient following mitral valve repair?
   (a) Warfarin with target INR 2.5 (range 2–3) indefinitely
   (b) Warfarin with target INR 2.5 (range 2–3) for 3 months
   (c) Aspirin 325 mg daily indefinitely
   (d) Aspirin 81 mg daily for 3 months
   (e) Aspirin 81 mg daily indefinitely with clopidogrel 75 mg daily for 3 months
4. A 28-year-old woman with a mechanical mitral valve is considering pregnancy and presents for preconception counseling. A transthoracic echo demonstrates normal valve function including normal mitral valve pressure gradients. She has normal renal function, weighs 62 kg, and is maintained on warfarin with a target INR 3.0 and an average daily dose of 7.5 mg. In addition to counseling regarding the risks of pregnancy, and referral to an experienced center, what is the appropriate recommendation for anticoagulation in the first trimester?
   (a) Continue warfarin with a target INR 3.0
   (b) Transition to apixaban 5 mg twice daily
   (c) Transition to therapeutic enoxaparin with dose adjustment by peak anti-Xa
   (d) Transition to therapeutic unfractionated heparin with dose adjustment by aPTT or anti-Xa
   (e) Either C or D
5. A 47-year-old woman with nonischemic cardiomyopathy progressed to stage D heart failure and underwent left ventricular assist device implantation with a HeartMate II device as a bridge to transplant. She is maintained on warfarin anticoagulation with target INR range 2–3 and aspirin 162 mg daily. Eleven months following LVAD placement, she is admitted with symptomatic anemia and found to have a gastrointestinal bleed. What factor(s) contribute to gastrointestinal bleeding as one of the most common complications of LVAD therapy?
   (a) Acquired von Willebrand syndrome
   (b) Formation of gastrointestinal arteriovenous malformations
   (c) Therapeutic anticoagulation
   (d) Impaired platelet function
   (e) All of the above

Self-Assessment Answers

1. (c) Warfarin with a target INR of 3.0 (range 2.5–3.5)

This patient has a low thrombotic risk valve in the aortic position but has an additional risk factor of low ejection fraction (<35%). According to the guidelines, he should be prescribed warfarin with a goal INR of 3.0. Other thrombotic risk factors include atrioventricular valve position, multiple prosthetic valves, prior thromboembolism, atrial fibrillation, and mitral stenosis. Dabigatran is contraindicated with mechanical valves.

2. (b) Warfarin with target INR 2.5 (range 2–3)

   This patient has a CHADS-VASc score of 4 (age, sex, and hypertension) and would benefit from therapeutic anticoagulation for stroke risk reduction. Neither dabigatran nor rivaroxaban is approved for use with a prosthetic heart valve.

3. (a) Warfarin with target INR 2.5 (range 2–3) indefinitely

   This patient has a CHADS-VASc score of at least 3 (age, hypertension, and diabetes) and a HAS-BLED score of 2 (age and hypertension). In the setting of paroxysmal atrial fibrillation, he would benefit from indefinite therapeutic anticoagulation for stroke risk reduction.

4. (e) Either C or D

   As this patient requires a daily warfarin dose exceeding 5 mg, transition to either enoxaparin or unfractionated heparin with therapeutic dosing and dose adjustment is indicated. Apixaban is not approved for use with mechanical valves.

5. (e) All of the above

   There are multiple factors that increase the risk of gastrointestinal bleeding with a left ventricular assist device. These include acquired von Willebrand syndrome, formation of gastrointestinal arteriovenous malformations, therapeutic anticoagulation, and impaired platelet function.

References

1. Cohn LH. Fifty years of open-heart surgery. Circulation. 2003;107(17):2168–70.
2. Atkinson TM, Ohman EM, O'Neill WW, Rab T, Cigarroa JE. A practical approach to mechanical circulatory support in patients undergoing percutaneous coronary intervention: an interventional perspective. JACC Cardiovasc Interv. 2016;9(9):871–83.
3. van Hinsbergh VW. Endothelium--role in regulation of coagulation and inflammation. Semin Immunopathol. 2012;34(1):93–106.
4. Chaikof EL. The development of prosthetic heart valves--lessons in form and function. TN Engl J Med. 2007;357(14):1368–71.
5. Bourantas CV, Serruys PW. Evolution of transcatheter aortic valve replacement. Circ Res. 2014;114(6):1037–51.
6. De Backer O, Piazza N, Banai S, Lutter G, Maisano F, Herrmann HC, et al. Percutaneous transcatheter mitral valve replacement: an overview of devices in preclinical and early clinical evaluation. Circ Cardiovasc Interv. 2014;7(3):400–9.
7. ETH Zurich IoFD. Types of heart valves. Zurich, Switzerland.
8. Iung B, Vahanian A. Epidemiology of valvular heart disease in the adult. Nat Rev Cardiol. 2011;8(3):162–72.
9. Nkomo VT, Gardin JM, Skelton TN, Gottdiener JS, Scott CG, Enriquez-Sarano M. Burden of valvular heart diseases: a population-based study. Lancet. 2006;368(9540):1005–11.
10. Marijon E, Ou P, Celermajer DS, Ferreira B, Mocumbi AO, Jani D, et al. Prevalence of rheumatic heart disease detected by echocardiographic screening. N Engl J Med. 2007;357(5):470–6.
11. Statistics NCfH. In: Services UDoHaH, editor. Health, United States, 2015: with special feature on racial and ethnics health disparities. Hyattsville: National Center for Health Statistics; 2016.
12. Nishimura RA, Otto CM, Bonow RO, Carabello BA, Erwin JP, Guyton RA, et al. 2014 AHA/ACC guideline for the management of patients with valvular heart disease: a report of the American College of Cardiology/American Heart Association Task Force on Practice Guidelines. J Am Coll Cardiol. 2014;63(22):e57–185.
13. Vahanian A, Alfieri O, Andreotti F, Antunes MJ, Barón-Esquivias G, Baumgartner H, Joint Task Force on the Management of Valvular Heart Disease of the European Society of Cardiology (ESC); European Association for Cardio-Thoracic Surgery (EACTS), et al. Guidelines on the management of valvular heart disease (version 2012). Eur Heart J. 2012;33(19):2451–96.
14. Nishimura RA, Otto CM, Bonow RO, Carabello BA, Erwin JP, Fleisher LA, et al. 2017 AHA/ACC focused update of the 2014 AHA/ACC guideline for the management of patients with valvular heart disease: a report of the American College of Cardiology/American Heart Association Task Force on clinical practice guidelines. Circulation. 2017;135(25):e1159–95.
15. Pibarot P, Dumesnil JG. Prosthetic heart valves: selection of the optimal prosthesis and long-term management. Circulation. 2009;119(7):1034–48.
16. Bluestein D, Rambod E, Gharib M. Vortex shedding as a mechanism for free emboli forma-

tion in mechanical heart valves. J Biomech Eng. 2000;122(2):125–34.
17. Yang Y, Franzen SF, Olin CL. In vivo comparison of hemocompatibility of materials used in mechanical heart valves. J Heart Valve Dis. 1996;5(5):532–7.
18. Alemu Y, Girdhar G, Xenos M, Sheriff J, Jesty J, Einav S, et al. Design optimization of a mechanical heart valve for reducing valve thrombogenicity-A case study with ATS valve. ASAIO J. 2010;56(5):389–96.
19. Cannegieter SC, Rosendaal FR, Briet E. Thromboembolic and bleeding complications in patients with mechanical heart valve prostheses. Circulation. 1994;89:635–41.
20. Horstkotte D, Scharf RE, Schultheiss HP. Intracardiac thrombosis: patient-related and device-related factors. J Heart Valve Dis. 1995;4(2):114–20.
21. Butchart EG, Ionescu A, Payne N, Giddings J, Grunkemeier GL, Fraser AG. A new scoring system to determine thromboembolic risk after heart valve replacement. Circulation. 2003;108(Suppl 1):II68–74.
22. Whitlock RP, Sun JC, Fremes SE, Rubens FD, Teoh KH, American College of Chest P. Antithrombotic and thrombolytic therapy for valvular disease: antithrombotic therapy and prevention of thrombosis, 9th ed: American College of Chest Physicians Evidence-Based Clinical Practice Guidelines. Chest. 2012;141(2 Suppl):e576S–600S.
23. Schlitt A, von Bardeleben RS, Ehrlich A, Eimermacher A, Peetz D, Dahm M, et al. Clopidogrel and aspirin in the prevention of thromboembolic complications after mechanical aortic valve replacement (CAPTA). Thromb Res. 2003;109(2-3):131–5.
24. Dentali F, Pignatelli P, Malato A, Poli D, Di Minno MN, Di Gennaro L, et al. Incidence of thromboembolic complications in patients with atrial fibrillation or mechanical heart valves with a subtherapeutic international normalized ratio: a prospective multicenter cohort study. Am J Hematol. 2012;87(4):384–7.
25. Aziz F, Corder M, Wolffe J, Comerota AJ. Anticoagulation monitoring by an anticoagulation service is more cost-effective than routine physician care. J Vasc Surg. 2011;54(5):1404–7.
26. Lalonde L, Martineau J, Blais N, Montigny M, Ginsberg J, Fournier M, et al. Is long-term pharmacist-managed anticoagulation service efficient? A pragmatic randomized controlled trial. Am Heart J. 2008;156(1):148–54.
27. Chiquette E, Amato MG, Bussey HI. Comparison of an anticoagulation clinic with usual medical care: anticoagulation control, patient outcomes, and health care costs. Arch Intern Med. 1998;158(15):1641–7.
28. Witt DM, Sadler MA, Shanahan RL, Mazzoli G, Tillman DJ. Effect of a centralized clinical pharmacy anticoagulation service on the outcomes of anticoagulation therapy. Chest. 2005;127(5):1515–22.
29. Locke C, Ravnan SL, Patel R, Uchizono JA. Reduction in warfarin adverse events requiring patient hospitalization after implementation of a pharmacist-managed anticoagulation service. Pharmacotherapy. 2005;25(5):685–9.
30. Wittkowsky AK, Nutescu EA, Blackburn J, Mullins J, Hardman J, Mitchell J, et al. Outcomes of oral anticoagulant therapy managed by telephone *vs* in-office visits in an anticoagulation clinic setting. Chest. 2006;130(5):1385–9.
31. Koertke H, Zittermann A, Tenderich G, Wagner O, El-Arousy M, Krian A, et al. Low-dose oral anticoagulation in patients with mechanical heart valve prostheses: final report from the early self-management anticoagulation trial II. Eur Heart J. 2007;28(20):2479–84.
32. Matchar DB, Love SR, Jacobson AK, Edson R, Uyeda L, Phibbs CS, et al. The impact of frequency of patient self-testing of prothrombin time on time in target range within VA Cooperative Study #481: The Home INR Study (THINRS), a randomized, controlled trial. J Thromb Thrombolysis. 2015;40(1):17–25.
33. Heneghan C, Ward A, Perera R, Bankhead C, Fuller A, Stevens R, et al. Self-monitoring of oral anticoagulation: systematic review and meta-analysis of individual patient data. Lancet. 2012;379(9813):322–34.
34. Mair H, Sachweh J, Sodian R, Brenner P, Schmoeckel M, Schmitz C, et al. Long-term self-management of anticoagulation therapy after mechanical heart valve replacement in outside trial conditions. Interact Cardiovasc Thorac Surg. 2012;14(3):253–7.
35. Thompson JL, Burkhart HM, Daly RC, Dearani JA, Joyce LD, Suri RM, et al. Anticoagulation early after mechanical valve replacement: improved management with patient self-testing. J Thorac Cardiovasc Surg. 2013;146(3):599–604.
36. Koertke H, Zittermann A, Wagner O, Secer S, Sciangula A, Saggau W, et al. Telemedicine-guided, very low-dose international normalized ratio self-control in patients with mechanical heart valve implants. Eur Heart J. 2015;36(21):1297–305.
37. Wypasek E, Ciesla M, Suder B, Janik L, Sadowski J, Undas A. CYP2C9 polymorphism and unstable anticoagulation with warfarin in patients within the first 3 months following heart valve replacement. Adv Clin Exp Med. 2015;24(4):607–14.
38. Tatarunas V, Lesauskaite V, Veikutiene A, Grybauskas P, Jakuska P, Jankauskiene L, et al. The effect of CYP2C9, VKORC1 and CYP4F2 polymorphism and of clinical factors on warfarin dosage during initiation and long-term treatment after heart valve surgery. J Thromb Thrombolysis. 2014;37(2):177–85.
39. Giansante C, Fiotti N, Altamura N, Pitacco P, Consoloni L, Scardi S, et al. Oral anticoagulation and VKORC1 polymorphism in patients with a mechanical heart prosthesis: a 6-year follow-up. J Thromb Thrombolysis. 2012;34(4):506–12.

40. Cannegieter SC, Rosendaal FR, Wintzen AR, van der Meer FJ, Vandenbroucke JP, Briet E. Optimal oral anticoagulant therapy in patients with mechanical heart valves. N Engl J Med. 1995;333(1):11–7.
41. Acar J, Iung B, Boissel JP, Samama MM, Michel PL, Teppe JP, et al. AREVA: multicenter randomized comparison of low-dose versus standard-dose anticoagulation in patients with mechanical prosthetic heart valves. Circulation. 1996;94(9):2107–12.
42. Pengo V, Barbero F, Banzato A, Garelli E, Noventa F, Biasiolo A, et al. A comparison of a moderate with moderate-high intensity oral anticoagulant treatment in patients with mechanical heart valve prostheses. Thromb Haemost. 1997;77(5):839–44.
43. Hering D, Piper C, Bergemann R, Hillenbach C, Dahm M, Huth C, Horstkotte D. Thromboembolic and bleeding complications following St. Jude medical valve replacement. Chest. 2005;127:53–9.
44. Pruefer D, Dahm M, Dohmen G, Horstkotte D, Bergemann R, Oelert H. Intensity of oral anticoagulation after implantation of St. Jude medical mitral or multiple valve replacement: lessons learned from GELIA (GELIA 5). Eur Heart J Suppl. 2001;3(Suppl Q):Q39–43.
45. Torella M, Torella D, Chiodini P, Franciulli M, Romano G, De Santo L, et al. LOWERing the INtensity of oral anticoaGulant Therapy in patients with bileaflet mechanical aortic valve replacement: results from the "LOWERING-IT" trial. Am Heart J. 2010;160(1):171–8.
46. Puskas J, Gerdisch M, Nichols D, Quinn R, Anderson C, Rhenman B, et al. Reduced anticoagulation after mechanical aortic valve replacement: interim results from the prospective randomized on-X valve anticoagulation clinical trial randomized Food and Drug Administration investigational device exemption trial. J Thorac Cardiovasc Surg. 2014;147(4):1202–10. discussion 10-1
47. Xu Z, Wang ZP, Ou JS, Yin SL, Liu LJ, Zhang X. Is low anticoagulation intensity more beneficial for patients with bileaflet mechanical mitral valves? A meta-analysis. J Cardiovasc Surg. 2016;57(1):90–9.
48. Schomburg JL, Medina EM, Lahti MT, Bianco RW. Dabigatran versus warfarin after mechanical mitral valve replacement in the swine model. J Investig Surg. 2012;25(3):150–5.
49. Van de Werf F, Brueckmann M, Connolly SJ, Friedman J, Granger CB, Hartter S, et al. A comparison of dabigatran etexilate with warfarin in patients with mechanical heart valves: THE Randomized, phase II study to evaluate the safety and pharmacokinetics of oral dabigatran etexilate in patients after heart valve replacement (RE-ALIGN). Am Heart J. 2012;163(6):931–7e1.
50. Eikelboom JW, Connolly SJ, Brueckmann M, Granger CB, Kappetein AP, Mack MJ, et al. Dabigatran versus warfarin in patients with mechanical heart valves. N Engl J Med. 2013;369(13):1206–14.
51. Turpie AG, Gent M, Laupacis A, Latour Y, Gunstensen J, Basile F, et al. A comparison of aspirin with placebo in patients treated with warfarin after heart-valve replacement. N Engl J Med. 1993;329(8):524–9.
52. Meschengieser SS, Fondevila CG, Frontroth J, Santarelli MT, Lazzari MA. Low-intensity oral anticoagulation plus low-dose aspirin versus high-intensity oral anticoagulation alone: a randomized trial in patients with mechanical prosthetic heart valves. J Thorac Cardiovasc Surg. 1997;113:910–6.
53. Pengo V, Palareti G, Cucchini U, Molinatti M, Del Bono R, Baudo F, et al. Low-intensity oral anticoagulant plus low-dose aspirin during the first six months versus standard-intensity oral anticoagulant therapy after mechanical heart valve replacement: a pilot study of low-intensity warfarin and aspirin in cardiac prostheses (LIWACAP). Clin Appl Thromb Hemost. 2007;13(3):241–8.
54. Laffort P, Roudaut R, Roques X, Lafitte S, Deville C, Bonnet J, et al. Early and long-term (one-year) effects of the association of aspirin and oral anticoagulant on thrombi and morbidity after replacement of the mitral valve with the St. Jude medical prosthesis: a clinical and transesophageal echocardiographic study. J Am Coll Cardiol. 2000;35(3):739–46.
55. Massel DL, Little SH. Risks and benefits of adding anti-platelet therapy to warfarin among patients with prosthetic heart valves: a meta-analysis. JACC. 2001;37(2):569–78.
56. Massel DR, Little SH. Antiplatelet and anticoagulation for patients with prosthetic heart valves. Cochrane Database Syst Rev. 2013;7:CD003464.
57. Montalescot G, Polle V, Collet JP, Leprince P, Bellanger A, Gandjbakhch I, et al. Low molecular weight heparin after mechanical heart valve replacement. Circulation. 2000;101(10):1083–6.
58. Talwar S, Kapoor CK, Velayoudam D, Kumar AS. Anticoagulation protocol and early prosthetic valve thrombosis. Indian Heart J. 2004;56(3):225–8.
59. Fanikos J, Tsilimingras K, Kucher N, Rosen AB, Hieblinger MD, Goldhaber SZ. Comparison of efficacy, safety, and cost of low-molecular-weight heparin with continuous-infusion unfractionated heparin for initiation of anticoagulation after mechanical prosthetic valve implantation. Am J Cardiol. 2004;93:247–50.
60. Kulik A, Rubens FD, Wells PS, Kearon C, Mesana TG, van Berkom J, et al. Early postoperative anticoagulation after mechanical valve replacement: a systematic review. Ann Thorac Surg. 2006;81(2):770–81.
61. Kindo M, Gerelli S, Hoang Minh T, Zhang M, Meyer N, Announe T, et al. Exclusive low-molecular-weight heparin as bridging anticoagulant after mechanical valve replacement. Ann Thorac Surg. 2014;97(3):789–95.
62. Passaglia LG, de Barros GM, de Sousa MR. Early postoperative bridging anticoagulation after mechanical heart valve replacement: a system-

atic review and meta-analysis. J Thromb Haemost. 2015;13(9):1557–67.
63. Douketis JD, Spyropoulos AC, Spencer FA, Mayr M, Jaffer AK, Eckman MH, et al. Perioperative management of antithrombotic therapy: antithrombotic therapy and prevention of thrombosis, 9th ed: American College of Chest Physicians Evidence-Based Clinical Practice Guidelines. Chest. 2012;141(2 Suppl):e326S–50S.
64. Poldermans D, Bax JJ, Boersma E, Task Force for Preoperative Cardiac Risk A, Perioperative Cardiac Management in Non-cardiac S, European Society of C, et al. Guidelines for pre-operative cardiac risk assessment and perioperative cardiac management in non-cardiac surgery. Eur Heart J. 2009;30(22):2769–812.
65. Tinker JH, Tarhan S. Discontinuing anticoagulant therapy in surgical patients with cardiac valve prostheses. Observations in 180 operations. JAMA. 1978;239(8):738–9.
66. Delate T, Meisinger SM, Witt DM, Jenkins D, Douketis JD, Clark NP. Bridge therapy outcomes in patients with mechanical heart valves. Clin Appl Thromb Hemost. 2016;23(8):1036–41.
67. Pengo V, Cucchini U, Denas G, Erba N, Guazzaloca G, La Rosa L, et al. Standardized low-molecular-weight heparin bridging regimen in outpatients on oral anticoagulants undergoing invasive procedure or surgery: an inception cohort management study. Circulation. 2009;119(22):2920–7.
68. Bui HT, Krisnaswami A, Le CU, Chan J, Shenoy BN. Comparison of safety of subcutaneous enoxaparin as outpatient anticoagulation bridging therapy in patients with a mechanical heart valve versus patients with nonvalvular atrial fibrillation. Am J Cardiol. 2009;104(10):1429–33.
69. Spyropoulos AC, Turpie AG, Dunn AS, Kaatz S, Douketis J, Jacobson A, et al. Perioperative bridging therapy with unfractionated heparin or low-molecular-weight heparin in patients with mechanical prosthetic heart valves on long-term oral anticoagulants (from the REGIMEN Registry). Am J Cardiol. 2008;102(7):883–9.
70. Siegal D, Yudin J, Kaatz S, Douketis JD, Lim W, Spyropoulos AC. Periprocedural heparin bridging in patients receiving vitamin K antagonists: systematic review and meta-analysis of bleeding and thromboembolic rates. Circulation. 2012;126(13):1630–9.
71. Steinberg BA, Peterson ED, Kim S, Thomas L, Gersh BJ, Fonarow GC, et al. Use and outcomes associated with bridging during anticoagulation interruptions in patients with atrial fibrillation: findings from the outcomes registry for better informed treatment of atrial fibrillation (ORBIT-AF). Circulation. 2015;131(5):488–94.
72. Kovacs M. PERIOP 2 - a safety and effectiveness study of LMWH bridging therapy versus placebo bridging therapy for patients on long term warfarin and require temporary interruption of their warfarin (NCT00432796). 2007. https://clinicaltrials.gov/ct2/show/study/NCT00432796.
73. Pernod G, Godier A, Gozalo C, Tremey B, Sie P, French National Authority for H. French clinical practice guidelines on the management of patients on vitamin K antagonists in at-risk situations (overdose, risk of bleeding, and active bleeding). Thromb Res. 2010;126(3):e167–74.
74. Weibert RT, Le DT, Kayser SR, Rapaport SI. Correction of excessive anticoagulation with low-dose oral vitamin K1. Ann Intern Med. 1997;126(12):959–62.
75. Yiu KH, Siu CW, Jim MH, Tse HF, Fan K, Chau MC, et al. Comparison of the efficacy and safety profiles of intravenous vitamin K and fresh frozen plasma as treatment of warfarin-related over-anticoagulation in patients with mechanical heart valves. Am J Cardiol. 2006;97(3):409–11.
76. Heras M, Chesebro JH, Fuster V, Penny WJ, Grill DE, Bailey KR, Danielson GK, Orszulak TA, Pluth JR, Puga FJ, Schaff HV, Larsonkeller JJ. High risk of thromboemboli early after bioprosthetic cardiac valve replacement. JACC. 1995;25(5):1111–9.
77. Nunez LGA, Larrea JL, Celemin D, Oliver J. Prevention of thromboembolism using aspirin after mitral valve replacement with porcine bioprosthesis. Ann Thorac Surg. 1984;37(1):84–7.
78. Orszulak TA, Schaff HV, Pluth JR, Danielson GK, Puga FJ, Ilstrup DM, et al. The risk of stroke in the early postoperative period following mitral valve replacement. Eur J Cardiothorac Surg. 1995;9(11):615–9. discuss 20
79. Russo A, Grigioni F, Avierinos JF, Freeman WK, Suri R, Michelena H, et al. Thromboembolic complications after surgical correction of mitral regurgitation incidence, predictors, and clinical implications. J Am Coll Cardiol. 2008;51(12):1203–11.
80. Turpie AG, Gunstensen J, Hirsh J, Nelson H, Gent M. Randomised comparison of two intensities of oral anticoagulant therapy after tissue heart valve replacement. Lancet. 1988;1(8597):1242–5.
81. Aramendi JI, Mestres CA, Martinez-Leon J, Campos V, Munoz G, Navas C. Triflusal versus oral anticoagulation for primary prevention of thromboembolism after bioprosthetic valve replacement (trac): prospective, randomized, co-operative trial. Eur J Cardiothorac Surg. 2005;27(5):854–60.
82. Colli AMC, Castella M, et al. Comparing warfarin to aspirin (WoA) after aortic valve replacement with the St. Jude medical epic heart valve bioprosthesis: results of the WoA epic pilot trial. J Heart Valve Dis. 2007;16:667–71.
83. Blair KL, Hatton AC, White WD, Smith LR, Lowe JE, Wolfe WG, et al. Comparison of anticoagulation regimens after Carpentier-Edwards aortic or mitral valve replacement. Circulation. 1994;90(5 Pt 2):II214–9.
84. Orszulak TA, Schaff HV, Mullany CJ, Anderson BJ, Ilstrup DM, Puga FJ, et al. Risk of thromboembo-

lism with the aortic Carpentier-Edwards bioprosthesis. Ann Thorac Surg. 1995;59(2):462–8.
85. Moinuddeen K, Quin J, Shaw R, Dewar M, Tellides G, Kopf G, et al. Anticoagulation is unnecessary after biological aortic valve replacement. Circulation. 1998;98(19 Suppl):II95–8. discussion II8-9
86. Gherli T. Comparing warfarin with aspirin after biological aortic valve replacement: a prospective study. Circulation. 2004;110(5):496–500.
87. Al-Atassi T, Lam K, Forgie M, Boodhwani M, Rubens F, Hendry P, et al. Cerebral microembolization after bioprosthetic aortic valve replacement: comparison of warfarin plus aspirin versus aspirin only. Circulation. 2012;126(11 Suppl 1):S239–44.
88. Colli A, Verhoye JP, Heijmen R, Antunes M. Low-dose acetyl salicylic acid versus oral anticoagulation after bioprosthetic aortic valve replacement. Final report of the ACTION registry. Int J Cardiol. 2013;168(2):1229–36.
89. Mérie C, Køber L, Skov Olsen P, Andersson C, Gislason G, Skov Jensen J, Torp-Pedersen C. Association of warfarin therapy duration after bioprosthetic aortic valve replacement with risk of mortality, thromboembolic complications, and bleeding. JAMA. 2012;308(20):2118–25.
90. Brennan JM, Edwards FH, Zhao Y, O'Brien S, Booth ME, Dokholyan RS, et al. Early anticoagulation of bioprosthetic aortic valves in older patients: results from the Society of Thoracic Surgeons Adult Cardiac Surgery National Database. J Am Coll Cardiol. 2012;60(11):971–7.
91. Yadlapati A, Groh C, Malaisrie SC, Gajjar M, Kruse J, Meyers S, et al. Efficacy and safety of novel oral anticoagulants in patients with bioprosthetic valves. Clin Res Cardiol. 2016;105(3):268–72.
92. Duraes AR, de Souza RP, de Almeida NB, Albuquerque FP, de Bulhoes FV, de Souza Fernandes AM, et al. Dabigatran versus warfarin after bioprosthesis valve replacement for the management of atrial fibrillation postoperatively: DAWA Pilot Study. Drugs R D. 2016;16(2):149–54.
93. Connolly SJ, Ezekowitz MD, Yusuf S, Eikelboom J, Oldgren J, Parekh A, et al. Dabigatran versus warfarin in patients with atrial fibrillation. N Engl J Med. 2009;361(12):1139–51.
94. Patel MR, Mahaffey KW, Garg J, Pan G, Singer DE, Hacke W, et al. Rivaroxaban versus warfarin in nonvalvular atrial fibrillation. N Engl J Med. 2011;365(10):883–91.
95. Granger CB, Alexander JH, McMurray JJ, Lopes RD, Hylek EM, Hanna M, et al. Apixaban versus warfarin in patients with atrial fibrillation. N Engl J Med. 2011;365(11):981–92.
96. Giugliano RP, Ruff CT, Braunwald E, Murphy SA, Wiviott SD, Halperin JL, et al. Edoxaban versus warfarin in patients with atrial fibrillation. N Engl J Med. 2013;369(22):2093–104.
97. Avezum A, Lopes RD, Schulte PJ, Lanas F, Gersh BJ, Hanna M, et al. Apixaban in comparison with warfarin in patients with atrial fibrillation and valvular heart disease: findings from the apixaban for reduction in stroke and other thromboembolic events in atrial fibrillation (ARISTOTLE) trial. Circulation. 2015;132(8):624–32.
98. Renda G, De Caterina R, Carnicelli A, Nordio F, Mercuri M, Ruff C, et al. Outcomes in 2824 patients with valvular heart disease treated with edoxaban or warfarin in the ENGAGE AF-TIMI 48 trial. J Am Coll Cardiol. 2016;67(13_S):2194.
99. Carnicelli AP, De Caterina R, Halperin JL, Renda G, Ruff CT, Trevisan M, et al. Edoxaban for the prevention of thromboembolism in patients with atrial fibrillation and bioprosthetic valves. Circulation. 2017;135(13):1273–5.
100. Lifesciences E. Device ring photo. Scientific American; 2012.
101. Aramendi JL, Agredo J, Llorente A, Larrarte C, Pijoan J. Prevention of thromboembolism with ticlopidine shortly after valve repair or replacement with a bioprosthesis. J Heart Valve Dis. 1998;7(6):610–4.
102. Hwang SK, Yoo JS, Kim JB, Jung SH, Choo SJ, Chung CH, et al. Long-term outcomes of the Maze procedure combined with mitral valve repair: risk of thromboembolism without anticoagulation therapy. Ann Thorac Surg. 2015;100(3):840–3. discussion 3–4
103. Paparella D, Di Mauro M, Bitton Worms K, Bolotin G, Russo C, Trunfio S, et al. Antiplatelet versus oral anticoagulant therapy as antithrombotic prophylaxis after mitral valve repair. J Thorac Cardiovasc Surg. 2016;151(5):1302–8.e1.
104. Valeur N, Merie C, Hansen ML, Torp-Pedersen C, Gislason GH, Kober L. Risk of death and stroke associated with anticoagulation therapy after mitral valve repair. Heart. 2016;102(9):687–93.
105. Duran CM, Gometza B, Shahid M, Al-Halees Z. Treated bovine and autologous pericardium for aortic valve reconstruction. Ann Thorac Surg. 1998;66(6 Suppl):S166–9.
106. Luk A, Butany J, Ahn E, Fann JI, St Goar F, Thornton T, et al. Mitral repair with the Evalve MitraClip device: histopathologic findings in the porcine model. Cardiovasc Pathol. 2009;18(5):279–85.
107. Feldman T, Wasserman HS, Herrmann HC, Gray W, Block PC, Whitlow P, et al. Percutaneous mitral valve repair using the edge-to-edge technique: six-month results of the EVEREST PHASE I Clinical Trial. J Am Coll Cardiol. 2005;46(11):2134–40.
108. Mauri L, Garg P, Massaro JM, Foster E, Glower D, Mehoudar P, et al. The EVEREST II Trial: design and rationale for a randomized study of the evalve mitraclip system compared with mitral valve surgery for mitral regurgitation. Am Heart J. 2010;160(1):23–9.

109. Feldman T, Foster E, Glower DD, et al. Percutaneous repair or surgery for mitral regurgitation. N Engl J Med. 2011;364:1395–406.
110. Cruz-Gonzalez I, Rama-Merchan JC, Rodriguez-Collado J, Martin-Moreiras J, Diego-Nieto A, Barreiro-Perez M, et al. Transcatheter closure of paravalvular leaks: state of the art. Neth Hear J. 2017;25(2):116–24.
111. Rihal CS, Sorajja P, Booker JD, Hagler DJ, Cabalka AK. Principles of percutaneous paravalvular leak closure. JACC Cardiovasc Interv. 2012;5(2):121–30.
112. Cruz-Gonzalez I, Rama-Merchan JC, Arribas-Jimenez A, Rodriguez-Collado J, Martin-Moreiras J, Cascon-Bueno M, et al. Paravalvular leak closure with the Amplatzer Vascular Plug III device: immediate and short-term results. Rev Esp Cardiol. 2014;67(8):608–14.
113. Leon MB, Smith CR, Mack M, Miller DC, Moses JW, Svensson LG, et al. Transcatheter aortic-valve implantation for aortic stenosis in patients who cannot undergo surgery. N Engl J Med. 2010;363(17):1597–607.
114. Ussia GP, Scarabelli M, Mule M, Barbanti M, Sarkar K, Cammalleri V, et al. Dual antiplatelet therapy versus aspirin alone in patients undergoing transcatheter aortic valve implantation. Am J Cardiol. 2011;108(12):1772–6.
115. Nijenhuis VJ, Bennaghmouch N, Hassell M, Baan J Jr, van Kuijk JP, Agostoni P, et al. Rationale and design of POPular-TAVI: antiplatelet therapy for patients undergoing transcatheter aortic valve implantation. Am Heart J. 2016;173:77–85.
116. Dangas GD, Lefevre T, Kupatt C, Tchetche D, Schafer U, Dumonteil N, et al. Bivalirudin versus heparin anticoagulation in transcatheter aortic valve replacement: the randomized BRAVO-3 trial. J Am Coll Cardiol. 2015;66(25):2860–8.
117. Makkar RR, Fontana G, Jilaihawi H, Chakravarty T, Kofoed KF, de Backer O, et al. Possible subclinical leaflet thrombosis in bioprosthetic aortic valves. N Engl J Med. 2015;373(21):2015–24.
118. Latib A, Naganuma T, Abdel-Wahab M, Danenberg H, Cota L, Barbanti M, et al. Treatment and clinical outcomes of transcatheter heart valve thrombosis. Circ Cardiovasc Interv. 2015;8(4):e001779.
119. Chakravarty T, Sondergaard L, Friedman J, De Backer O, Berman D, Kofoed KF, et al. Subclinical leaflet thrombosis in surgical and transcatheter bioprosthetic aortic valves: an observational study. Lancet. 2017;389(10087):2383–92.
120. Nombela-Franco L, del Trigo M, Morrison-Polo G, Veiga G, Jimenez-Quevedo P, Abdul-Jawad Altisent O, et al. Incidence, causes, and predictors of early (</=30 days) and late unplanned hospital readmissions after transcatheter aortic valve replacement. JACC Cardiovasc Interv. 2015;8(13):1748–57.
121. Barbetseas J, Nagueh SF, Pitsavos C, Toutouzas PK, Quinones MA, Zoghbi WA. Differentiating thrombus from pannus formation in obstructed mechanical prosthetic valves: an evaluation of clinical, transthoracic and transesophageal echocardiographic parameters. J Am Coll Cardiol. 1998;32(5):1410–7.
122. Tong AT, Roudaut R, Ozkan M, Sagie A, Shahid MS, Pontes Junior SC, et al. Transesophageal echocardiography improves risk assessment of thrombolysis of prosthetic valve thrombosis: results of the international PRO-TEE registry. J Am Coll Cardiol. 2004;43(1):77–84.
123. Symersky P, Budde RP, de Mol BA, Prokop M. Comparison of multidetector-row computed tomography to echocardiography and fluoroscopy for evaluation of patients with mechanical prosthetic valve obstruction. Am J Cardiol. 2009;104(8):1128–34.
124. Zoghbi WA, Chambers JB, Dumesnil JG, Foster E, Gottdiener JS, Grayburn PA, et al. Recommendations for evaluation of prosthetic valves with echocardiography and doppler ultrasound: a report From the American Society of Echocardiography's Guidelines and Standards Committee and the Task Force on Prosthetic Valves, developed in conjunction with the American College of Cardiology Cardiovascular Imaging Committee, Cardiac Imaging Committee of the American Heart Association, the European Association of Echocardiography, a registered branch of the European Society of Cardiology, the Japanese Society of Echocardiography and the Canadian Society of Echocardiography, endorsed by the American College of Cardiology Foundation, American Heart Association, European Association of Echocardiography, a registered branch of the European Society of Cardiology, the Japanese Society of Echocardiography, and Canadian Society of Echocardiography. J Am Soc Echocardiogr. 2009;22(9):975–1014. quiz 82-4
125. Bates SM, Greer IA, Middeldorp S, Veenstra DL, Prabulos AM, Vandvik PO. VTE, thrombophilia, antithrombotic therapy, and pregnancy: antithrombotic therapy and prevention of thrombosis, 9th ed: American College of Chest Physicians Evidence-Based Clinical Practice Guidelines. Chest. 2012;141(2 Suppl):e691S–736S.
126. Regitz-Zagrosek V, Blomstrom Lundqvist C, Borghi C, European Society of G, Association for European Paediatric C, German Society for Gender M, et al. ESC guidelines on the management of cardiovascular diseases during pregnancy: the Task Force on the Management of Cardiovascular Diseases during Pregnancy of the European Society of Cardiology (ESC). Eur Heart J. 2011;32(24):3147–97.
127. van Hagen IM, Roos-Hesselink JW, Ruys TP, Merz WM, Goland S, Gabriel H, et al. Pregnancy in women with a mechanical heart valve: data of the European Society of Cardiology Registry

of Pregnancy and Cardiac Disease (ROPAC). Circulation. 2015;132(2):132–42.
128. Lawley CM, Lain SJ, Algert CS, Ford JB, Figtree GA, Roberts CL. Prosthetic heart valves in pregnancy: a systematic review and meta-analysis protocol. Syst Rev. 2014;3:8.
129. Hassouna A, Allam H. Limited dose warfarin throughout pregnancy in patients with mechanical heart valve prosthesis: a meta-analysis. Interact Cardiovasc Thorac Surg. 2014;18(6):797–806.
130. DeBakey ME. Left ventricular bypass pump for cardiac assistance. Clinical experience. Am J Cardiol. 1971;27(1):3–11.
131. Slaughter MS, Rogers JG, Milano CA, Russell SD, Conte JV, Feldman D, et al. Advanced heart failure treated with continuous-flow left ventricular assist device. N Engl J Med. 2009;361(23):2241–51.
132. Montori VM, Permanyer-Miralda G, Ferreira-Gonzalez I, Busse JW, Pacheco-Huergo V, Bryant D, et al. Validity of composite end points in clinical trials. BMJ. 2005;330(7491):594–6.
133. Evans RW, Manninen DL, Garrison LP Jr, Maier AM. Donor availability as the primary determinant of the future of heart transplantation. JAMA. 1986;255(14):1892–8.
134. Chen J, Normand SL, Wang Y, Krumholz HM. National and regional trends in heart failure hospitalization and mortality rates for Medicare beneficiaries, 1998-2008. JAMA. 2011;306(15):1669–78.
135. Suarez J, Patel CB, Felker GM, Becker R, Hernandez AF, Rogers JG. Mechanisms of bleeding and approach to patients with axial-flow left ventricular assist devices. Circ Heart Fail. 2011;4(6):779–84.
136. Griffith BP, Kormos RL, Borovetz HS, Litwak K, Antaki JF, Poirier VL, et al. HeartMate II left ventricular assist system: from concept to first clinical use. Ann Thorac Surg. 2001;71(3 Suppl):S116–20. discussion S4-6
137. Bourque K, Gernes DB, Loree HM, Richardson JS, Poirier VL, Barletta N, et al. HeartMate III: pump design for a centrifugal LVAD with a magnetically levitated rotor. ASAIO J. 2001;47(4):401–5.
138. Abraham WT, Smith SA. Devices in the management of advanced, chronic heart failure. Nat Rev Cardiol. 2013;10(2):98–110.
139. Mehra MR, Naka Y, Uriel N, Goldstein DJ, Cleveland JC Jr, Colombo PC, et al. A fully magnetically levitated circulatory pump for advanced heart failure. N Engl J Med. 2017;376(5):440–50.
140. Birschmann I, Dittrich M, Eller T, Wiegmann B, Reininger AJ, Budde U, et al. Ambient hemolysis and activation of coagulation is different between HeartMate II and HeartWare left ventricular assist devices. J Heart Lung Transplant. 2014;33(1):80–7.
141. Himmelreich G, Ullmann H, Riess H, Rosch R, Loebe M, Schiessler A, et al. Pathophysiologic role of contact activation in bleeding followed by thromboembolic complications after implantation of a ventricular assist device. ASAIO J. 1995;41(3):M790–4.
142. Slaughter MS, Sobieski MA, Gallagher C, Graham J, Brandise J, Stein R. Fibrinolytic activation during long-term support with the HeartMate II left ventricular assist device. ASAIO J. 2008;54(1):115–9.
143. John R, Panch S, Hrabe J, Wei P, Solovey A, Joyce L, et al. Activation of endothelial and coagulation systems in left ventricular assist device recipients. Ann Thorac Surg. 2009;88(4):1171–9.
144. Matsubayashi H, Fastenau DR, McIntyre JA. Changes in platelet activation associated with left ventricular assist system placement. J Heart Lung Transplant. 2000;19(5):462–8.
145. Jafri SM, Ozawa T, Mammen E, Levine TB, Johnson C, Goldstein S. Platelet function, thrombin and fibrinolytic activity in patients with heart failure. Eur Heart J. 1993;14(2):205–12.
146. Klovaite J, Gustafsson F, Mortensen SA, Sander K, Nielsen LB. Severely impaired von Willebrand factor-dependent platelet aggregation in patients with a continuous-flow left ventricular assist device (HeartMate II). J Am Coll Cardiol. 2009;53(23):2162–7.
147. Meyer AL, Malehsa D, Budde U, Bara C, Haverich A, Strueber M. Acquired von Willebrand syndrome in patients with a centrifugal or axial continuous flow left ventricular assist device. JACC Heart Fail. 2014;2(2):141–5.
148. Tsai HM, Sussman II, Nagel RL. Shear stress enhances the proteolysis of von Willebrand factor in normal plasma. Blood. 1994;83(8):2171–9.
149. Uriel N, Pak SW, Jorde UP, Jude B, Susen S, Vincentelli A, et al. Acquired von Willebrand syndrome after continuous-flow mechanical device support contributes to a high prevalence of bleeding during long-term support and at the time of transplantation. J Am Coll Cardiol. 2010;56(15):1207–13.
150. Crow S, Chen D, Milano C, Thomas W, Joyce L, Piacentino V 3rd, et al. Acquired von Willebrand syndrome in continuous-flow ventricular assist device recipients. Ann Thorac Surg. 2010;90(4):1263–9. discussion 9
151. Bourque K, Cotter C, Dague C, Harjes D, Dur O, Duhamel J, et al. Design rationale and preclinical evaluation of the HeartMate 3 left ventricular assist system for hemocompatibility. ASAIO J. 2016;62(4):375–83.
152. Pagani FD, Miller LW, Russell SD, Aaronson KD, John R, Boyle AJ, et al. Extended mechanical circulatory support with a continuous-flow rotary left ventricular assist device. J Am Coll Cardiol. 2009;54(4):312–21.
153. Baumann Kreuziger LM, Kim B, Wieselthaler GM. Antithrombotic therapy for left ventricular assist devices in adults: a systematic review. J Thromb Haemost. 2015;13(6):946–55.
154. Feldman D, Pamboukian SV, Teuteberg JJ, Birks E, Lietz K, Moore SA, et al. The 2013 International

Society for Heart and Lung Transplantation Guidelines for mechanical circulatory support: executive summary. J Heart Lung Transplant. 2013;32(2):157–87.
155. Gurbel PA, Tantry US. Antiplatelet and anticoagulant agents in heart failure: current status and future perspectives. JACC Heart Fail. 2014;2(1):1–14.
156. Slaughter MS, Naka Y, John R, Boyle A, Conte JV, Russell SD, et al. Post-operative heparin may not be required for transitioning patients with a HeartMate II left ventricular assist system to long-term warfarin therapy. J Heart Lung Transplant. 2010;29(6):616–24.
157. Nassif ME, LaRue SJ, Raymer DS, Novak E, Vader JM, Ewald GA, et al. Relationship between anticoagulation intensity and thrombotic or bleeding outcomes among outpatients with continuous-flow left ventricular assist devices. Circ Heart Fail. 2016;9(5):e002680.
158. Jennings D, McDonnell J, Schillig J. Assessment of long-term anticoagulation in patients with a continuous-flow left-ventricular assist device: a pilot study. J Thorac Cardiovasc Surg. 2011;142(1):e1–2.
159. Bishop MA, Streiff MB, Ensor CR, Tedford RJ, Russell SD, Ross PA. Pharmacist-managed international normalized ratio patient self-testing is associated with increased time in therapeutic range in patients with left ventricular assist devices at an academic medical center. ASAIO J. 2014;60(2):193–8.
160. Jennings DL, Brewer R, Williams C. Impact of continuous flow left ventricular assist device on the pharmacodynamic response to warfarin early after implantation. Ann Pharmacother. 2012;46(9):1266–7.
161. Terrovitis JV, Ntalianis A, Kapelios CJ, Vakrou S, Diakos N, Katsaros L, et al. Dabigatran etexilate as second-line therapy in patients with a left ventricular assist device. Hell J Cardiol. 2015;56(1):20–5.
162. Crow S, John R, Boyle A, Shumway S, Liao K, Colvin-Adams M, et al. Gastrointestinal bleeding rates in recipients of nonpulsatile and pulsatile left ventricular assist devices. The J Thorac Cardiovasc Surg. 2009;137(1):208–15.
163. Genovese EA, Dew MA, Teuteberg JJ, Simon MA, Kay J, Siegenthaler MP, et al. Incidence and patterns of adverse event onset during the first 60 days after ventricular assist device implantation. Ann Thorac Surg. 2009;88(4):1162–70.
164. Boyle AJ, Jorde UP, Sun B, Park SJ, Milano CA, Frazier OH, et al. Pre-operative risk factors of bleeding and stroke during left ventricular assist device support: an analysis of more than 900 HeartMate II outpatients. J Am Coll Cardiol. 2014;63(9):880–8.
165. Letsou GV, Shah N, Gregoric ID, Myers TJ, Delgado R, Frazier OH. Gastrointestinal bleeding from arteriovenous malformations in patients supported by the Jarvik 2000 axial-flow left ventricular assist device. J Heart Lung Transplant. 2005;24(1):105–9.
166. Pal JD, Piacentino V, Cuevas AD, Depp T, Daneshmand MA, Hernandez AF, et al. Impact of left ventricular assist device bridging on posttransplant outcomes. Ann Thorac Surg. 2009;88(5):1457–61. discussion 61
167. Singh G, Albeldawi M, Kalra SS, Mehta PP, Lopez R, Vargo JJ. Features of patients with gastrointestinal bleeding after implantation of ventricular assist devices. Clin Gastroenterol Hepatol. 2015;13(1):107–14.e1.
168. Shrode CW, Draper KV, Huang RJ, Kennedy JL, Godsey AC, Morrison CC, et al. Significantly higher rates of gastrointestinal bleeding and thromboembolic events with left ventricular assist devices. Clin Gastroenterol Hepatol. 2014;12(9):1461–7.
169. Draper KV, Huang RJ, Gerson LB. GI bleeding in patients with continuous-flow left ventricular assist devices: a systematic review and meta-analysis. Gastrointest Endosc. 2014;80(3):435–46.e1.
170. Wilson TJ, Stetler WR Jr, Al-Holou WN, Sullivan SE, Fletcher JJ. Management of intracranial hemorrhage in patients with left ventricular assist devices. J Neurosurg. 2013;118(5):1063–8.
171. Bunte MC, Blackstone EH, Thuita L, Fowler J, Joseph L, Ozaki A, et al. Major bleeding during HeartMate II support. J Am Coll Cardiol. 2013;62(23):2188–96.
172. Starling RC, Moazami N, Silvestry SC, Ewald G, Rogers JG, Milano CA, et al. Unexpected abrupt increase in left ventricular assist device thrombosis. N Engl J Med. 2014;370(1):33–40.
173. Kirklin JK, Naftel DC, Kormos RL, Pagani FD, Myers SL, Stevenson LW, et al. Interagency Registry for Mechanically Assisted Circulatory Support (INTERMACS) analysis of pump thrombosis in the HeartMate II left ventricular assist device. J Heart Lung Transplant. 2014;33(1):12–22.
174. Morgan JA, Brewer RJ, Nemeh HW, Gerlach B, Lanfear DE, Williams CT, et al. Stroke while on long-term left ventricular assist device support: incidence, outcome, and predictors. ASAIO J. 2014;60(3):284–9.
175. Rose EA, Gelijns AC, Moskowitz AJ, Heitjan DF, Stevenson LW, Dembitsky W, et al. Long-term use of a left ventricular assist device for end-stage heart failure. N Engl J Med. 2001;345(20):1435–43.
176. Eckman PM, John R. Bleeding and thrombosis in patients with continuous-flow ventricular assist devices. Circulation. 2012;125(24):3038–47.
177. Hasin T, Deo S, Maleszewski JJ, Topilsky Y, Edwards BS, Pereira NL, et al. The role of medical management for acute intravascular hemolysis in patients supported on axial flow LVAD. ASAIO J. 2014;60(1):9–14.
178. Gilotra NA, Stevens GR. Temporary mechanical circulatory support: a review of the options, indications, and outcomes. Clin Med Insights Cardiol. 2014;8(Suppl 1):75–85.
179. Ihdayhid AR, Chopra S, Rankin J. Intra-aortic balloon pump: indications, efficacy, guidelines and future directions. Curr Opin Cardiol. 2014;29(4):285–92.
180. Kogan A, Preisman S, Sternik L, Orlov B, Spiegelstein D, Hod H, et al. Heparin-free manage-

ment of intra-aortic balloon pump after cardiac surgery. J Card Surg. 2012;27(4):434–7.

181. Pucher PH, Cummings IG, Shipolini AR, McCormack DJ. Is heparin needed for patients with an intra-aortic balloon pump? Interact Cardiovasc Thorac Surg. 2012;15(1):136–9.
182. Sieg A, Mardis BA, Mardis CR, Huber MR, New JP, Meadows HB, et al. Developing an Anti-Xa-based anticoagulation protocol for patients with percutaneous ventricular assist devices. ASAIO J. 2015;61(5):502–8.
183. Raiten JM, Wong ZZ, Spelde A, Littlejohn JE, Augoustides JG, Gutsche JT. Anticoagulation and transfusion therapy in patients requiring extracorporeal membrane oxygenation. J Cardiothorac Vasc Anesth. 2017;31(3):1051–9.
184. Lock JERJ, Davis R, et al. Transcatheter closure of atrial septal defects: experimental studies. Circulation. 1989;79:1091–9.
185. Sharafuddin MJA, Gu X, Titus JL, Urness M, Cervera-Ceballos JJ, Amplatz K. Transvenous closure of secundum atrial septal defects : preliminary results with a new self-expanding nitinol prosthesis in a swine model. Circulation. 1997;95(8):2162–8.
186. Chessa M, Carminati M, Butera G, Bini RM, Drago M, Rosti L, et al. Early and late complications associated with transcatheter occlusion of secundum atrial septal defect. J Am Coll Cardiol. 2002;39(6):1061–5.
187. Anzai H, Child J, Natterson B, Krivokapich J, Fishbein MC, Chan VK, et al. Incidence of thrombus formation on the CardioSEAL and the Amplatzer interatrial closure devices. Am J Cardiol. 2004;93(4):426–31.
188. Krumsdorf U, Ostermayer S, Billinger K, Trepels T, Zadan E, Horvath K, et al. Incidence and clinical course of thrombus formation on atrial septal defect and patient foramen ovale closure devices in 1,000 consecutive patients. J Am Coll Cardiol. 2004;43(2):302–9.
189. Masura J, Gavora P, Podnar T. Long-term outcome of transcatheter secundum-type atrial septal defect closure using Amplatzer septal occluders. J Am Coll Cardiol. 2005;45(4):505–7.
190. YC F, Bass J, Amin Z, Radtke W, Cheatham JP, Hellenbrand WE, et al. Transcatheter closure of perimembranous ventricular septal defects using the new Amplatzer membranous VSD occluder: results of the U.S. phase I trial. J Am Coll Cardiol. 2006;47(2):319–25.
191. Butera G, Carminati M, Chessa M, Piazza L, Micheletti A, Negura DG, et al. Transcatheter closure of perimembranous ventricular septal defects: early and long-term results. J Am Coll Cardiol. 2007;50(12):1189–95.
192. Jones TK, Latson LA, Zahn E, Fleishman CE, Jacobson J, Vincent R, et al. Results of the U.S. multicenter pivotal study of the HELEX septal occluder for percutaneous closure of secundum atrial septal defects. J Am Coll Cardiol. 2007;49(22):2215–21.
193. Freixa X, Ibrahim R, Chan J, et al. Initial clinical experience with the GORE septal occluder for the treatment of atrial septal defects and patent foramen ovale. EuroIntervention. 2013;9(5):629–35.
194. Nyboe C, Hjortdal VE, Nielsen-Kudsk JE. First experience with the GORE (®) Septal Occluder in children and adults with atrial septal defects. Catheter Cardiovasc Interv. 2013;82(6):929–34.
195. Blackshear JLOJ. Appendage obliteration to reduce stroke in cardiac surgical patients with atrial fibrillation. Ann Thorac Surg. 1996;61(2):755–9.
196. Holmes DRRV, Turi ZG, et al. Percutaneous closure of the left atrial appendage versus warfarin therapy for prevention of stroke in patients with atrial fibrillation: a randomised non-inferiority trial. Lancet. 2009;374:534–42.
197. Reddy VY, Mobius-Winkler S, Miller MA, Neuzil P, Schuler G, Wiebe J, et al. Left atrial appendage closure with the Watchman device in patients with a contraindication for oral anticoagulation: the ASAP study (ASA Plavix Feasibility Study With Watchman Left Atrial Appendage Closure Technology). J Am Coll Cardiol. 2013;61(25):2551–6.
198. Sahay S, Nombela-Franco L, Rodes-Cabau J, Jimenez-Quevedo P, Salinas P, Biagioni C, et al. Efficacy and safety of left atrial appendage closure versus medical treatment in atrial fibrillation: a network meta-analysis from randomised trials. Heart. 2016;103(2):139–47. https://doi.org/10.1136/heartjnl-2016-309782.
199. Rodriguez-Gabella T, Nombela-Franco L, Regueiro A, Jimenez-Quevedo P, Champagne J, O'Hara G, et al. Single antiplatelet therapy following left atrial appendage closure in patients with contraindication to anticoagulation. J Am Coll Cardiol. 2016;68(17):1920–1.
200. Bartus K, Han FT, Bednarek J, Myc J, Kapelak B, Sadowski J, et al. Percutaneous left atrial appendage suture ligation using the LARIAT device in patients with atrial fibrillation: initial clinical experience. J Am Coll Cardiol. 2013;62(2):108–18.
201. Gianni C, Di Biase L, Trivedi C, Mohanty S, Gokoglan Y, Gunes MF, et al. Clinical implications of leaks following left atrial appendage ligation with the LARIAT device. JACC Cardiovasc Interv. 2016;9(10):1051–7.

14 Anticoagulation in Venous Thromboembolism

Geoffrey D. Barnes and Elizabeth T. Renner

Clinical Vignettes

Case 1: *A 55-year-old man presents to his primary care provider with 2 days of unilateral left leg swelling and pain. He has no prior medical history other than obesity and takes no medications. His primary care provider orders a compression duplex ultrasound and diagnoses him with an acute femoral-popliteal deep vein thrombosis. They discuss the various treatment options and elect to initiate apixaban therapy at 10 mg twice daily for 7 days followed by 5 mg twice daily. At his return visit in 2 months, they discuss his risk of recurrence. Given his male gender, he elects to continue use of a secondary prophylactic agent. Since he has tolerated apixaban therapy well, he chooses to continue on apixaban, but at the lower 2.5 mg twice-daily dose after he completes his initial 3 months of anticoagulation therapy.*

Case 2: *A 60-year-old woman with a history of well-controlled hypertension, diabetes mellitus, and obesity presents to the emergency department with acute-onset shortness of breath and chest pain. She is diagnosed with an acute unilateral pulmonary embolism in her left mainstem pulmonary artery. She is hemodynamically stable, but her right ventricle is enlarged on CT imaging and she has a mildly positive troponin. After extensive discussion, the patient and the physician team decide to purse catheter-directed thrombolysis. Following the procedure, she is initiated on edoxaban 60 mg daily for long-term anticoagulation therapy.*

Introduction

Venous thromboembolism (VTE) is a condition where a blood clot forms inside a vein. Disruptions to the vein's normal physiology, such as with vascular injury, venous stasis, or a state of hypercoagulability, may result in thrombus formation. A venous clot can remain stationary or can travel to the lungs. As such, VTE encompasses two main diagnoses: deep vein thrombosis (DVT) and pulmonary embolism (PE).

G. D. Barnes (✉)
Department of Internal Medicine, Division of Cardiovascular Medicine, Frankel Cardiovascular Center at the University of Michigan, Ann Arbor, MI, USA
e-mail: gbarnes@umich.edu

E. T. Renner
Anticoagulation Service, Faculty Group Practice: Pharmacy Innovations and Partnerships, University of Michigan, Ann Arbor, MI, USA
e-mail: eperrell@med.umich.edu

J. F. Lau et al. (eds.), *Anticoagulation Therapy*, https://doi.org/10.1007/978-3-319-73709-6_14

Table 14.1 Risk factors for development of venous thromboembolism [1].

• Advanced age
• Prolonged immobility
– Long-distance travel
– Casted extremity
– Recent or current hospitalization
– Recent surgery (general and orthopedic)
• Pregnancy/postpartum period
• Obesity
• Cancer (solid tumor and myeloproliferative disorders)
• Frailty and chronic medical illness
• Prior VTE
• Trauma
• Genetic thrombophilia (e.g., protein C or S deficiency)
• Acquired thrombophilia (e.g., antiphospholipid antibody syndrome)
• Prior superficial venous thrombosis
• Medical illness
– Inflammatory conditions (e.g., inflammatory bowel disorder)
– Nephrotic syndrome
– Vasculitis (e.g., Wegener's)
• Use of hormone therapy

VTE venous thromboembolism.

Table 14.2 Clinical factors associated with anticoagulation versus surveillance.

Factors favoring anticoagulation	Factors favoring surveillance for 2 weeks
High risk for clot propagation	Thrombus confined to soleus or gastrocnemius
• Positive D-dimer	High risk of bleeding
• Thrombus >5 cm length	Mild symptoms
• Thrombus in multiple veins	
• Thrombus >7 mm diameter	
• Thrombus near proximal veins	
• Lack of reversible provoking factor for thrombus	
• Active cancer	
• History of VTE	
• Inpatient status	
• Severe symptoms	

VTE venous thromboembolism.

When VTE develops as a direct consequence of a known risk factor (Table 14.1), it is considered "provoked." While many risk factors are easily reversed or self-resolved (transient risk factors), such as a recent orthopedic surgery or use of estrogen-containing medications, others may not be reversible or resolvable, e.g., permanent extremity paralysis. When a likely cause cannot be identified, the event is considered "unprovoked" or idiopathic. Determining the provoked nature of a VTE helps to predict risk of recurrence and influences medical decision-making.

VTE is a common diagnosis. The Center for Disease Control and Prevention (CDC) estimates that 900,000 people are affected every year in the United States [2, 3]. With 30-day mortality estimated at 10–30%, the importance of timely and accurate diagnosis with appropriate treatment cannot be understated. PE is especially concerning; sudden death is the presenting symptom in approximately 25% of cases. A 2002 study estimated annual direct medical costs associated with VTE at $1.5 billion [4].

Whether to Treat Patients with Isolated Distal DVT

DVT which is confined to the distal veins of the lower extremity (below the knee) resolves spontaneously without anticoagulation in about 85% of cases. A meta-analysis of randomized trials of treatment vs. surveillance for isolated distal DVT found that there was no difference in rates of PE development. Treatment with anticoagulation did reduce the finding of clot propagation, though it increased the risk for bleeding events [5]. While older studies have reported proximal extension rates between 25 and 33%, more recent and rigorous studies have reported rate less than 5% [6]. As a result, the best approach to these patients is unclear. Experts suggest that patients be evaluated for risks of clot propagation and symptom severity in determining whether patients should undergo anticoagulation treatment or serial imaging of the distal veins (Table 14.2). In patients for whom surveillance is selected, a common method is to repeat the DVT scan at 1 week and 2 weeks post-diagnosis, with initiation of anticoagulation if clot extension is detected [7].

VTE Management in the Acute Care Setting

Anticoagulation Therapy for Acute Venous Thromboembolism

Anticoagulation therapy is the cornerstone of acute VTE management. Anticoagulation should be initiated immediately for patients with confirmed VTE and no contraindication to anticoagulation therapy. If there is any potential delay in diagnostic testing, anticoagulation therapy should also be initiated for patients with moderate to high likelihood of VTE [7].

Once a diagnosis of acute VTE is established, anticoagulation therapy can be broken down into three phases (Fig. 14.1). The first (acute or initial) phase, lasting 5–10 days, requires anticoagulant therapy with rapid onset, often at higher total daily doses. This is intended to stop the active clotting process. Traditionally this has been achieved using parenteral agents, such as intravenous unfractionated heparin, subcutaneous low-molecular-weight heparin, or fondaparinux. More recently, this can also be achieved using oral rivaroxaban or apixaban.

The second (long-term) phase lasts from the time of VTE diagnosis through the first 3 months. In this phase, maintenance oral anticoagulant therapy is most commonly used to prevent recurrence, which is highest in the initial 3 months following diagnosis [7, 8]. Traditionally this has been achieved using oral vitamin K antagonists, such as warfarin. More recently, the use of dabigatran, rivaroxaban, apixaban, or edoxaban has been shown to be similarly effective to warfarin in this phase [9–13].

The third (extended) phase involves secondary prophylaxis against recurrent VTE. This phase begins 3 months following initial diagnosis of acute VTE and continues indefinitely. Potential therapeutic choices include full-dose anticoagulants, low-dose anticoagulants, antiplatelet medications, and no antithrombotic therapy (watchful waiting). Striking the balance between recurrent VTE prevention and bleeding risk with long-term therapy has been under considerable debate for years. For this reason, most guidelines and experts support a patient-physician-shared decision-making process to determine the optimal therapeutic choice for each individual patient [7, 14–16].

Thrombolysis for Acute Pulmonary Embolism

Since anticoagulant therapy aims to prevent clot propagation and VTE recurrence, not to “dissolve” an acute clot for the purpose of reperfusion, select patients may benefit from additional reperfusion therapy. For patients who present with acute PE, hemodynamic instability (massive PE), and no contraindication to thrombolytic use,

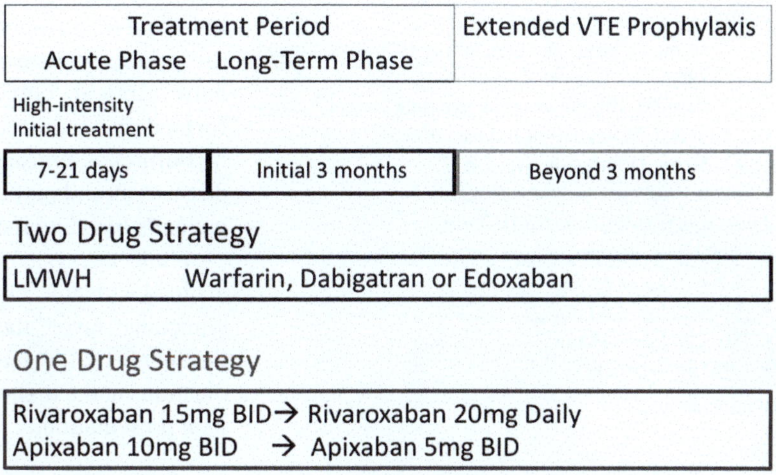

Fig. 14.1 Anticoagulation options for each phase of venous thromboembolism treatment. VTE, venous thromboembolism; BID, twice a day.

administration of intravenous thrombolytic therapy is generally recommended (Table 14.3) [14, 17, 18].

Significantly more debate exists over the role of thrombolytic therapy for patients with acute PE and stable hemodynamics but evidence of cardiac dysfunction (right ventricular enlargement and/or positive cardiac biomarkers). The best evidence comes from the PEITHO trial, where 1006 patients with acute PE, right ventricular dysfunction, and a positive troponin were randomized to heparin monotherapy or a single intravenous bolus of tenecteplase (30–50 mg weight based) plus heparin [19].

The primary outcome of all-cause death or hemodynamic decompensation was lower in the tenecteplase group than the heparin group (2.6% versus 5.6%, OR 0.44, 95% CI 0.23–0.88). However, a higher incidence of hemorrhagic or ischemic stroke and extracranial major bleeding occurred in the tenecteplase group than the heparin-only group (2.4% versus 0.2%, OR 12.10, 95% CI 1.57–93.39 and 6.3% versus 1.2%, OR 5.55, 95% CI 2.3–13.39, respectively). Subgroup analysis identified age as an important predictor of both outcomes, with patients ≤75 years of age demonstrating lower odds of death or hemodynamic decompensation (OR 0.33, 95% CI 0.13–0.85) and no statistically increased odds of extracranial major bleeding (OR 2.80, 95% CI 1.00–7.86). Thrombolysis should be given with unfractionated heparin for a target aPTT of 2.0–2.5 times the upper limit of normal or factor Xa inhibition of 0.3–0.7 IU/mL.

Table 14.3 Dosing options for systemic thrombolytics [20].

Alteplase
• Standard dose
– 10 mg IV bolus and then 90 mg IV infusion over 2 h
– Give 50–100 mg as bolus in cardiac arrest
• "Safe dose" (aka half or reduced dose)
– 50 mg IV infusion over 2 h
– 0.5 mg/kg if weight < 50 kg
Tenecteplase (weight-based IV bolus)
• <60 kg → 30 mg
• 60–<70 kg → 35 mg
• 70–<80 kg → 40 mg
• 80–<90 kg → 45 mg
• ≥90 kg → 50 mg

IV intravenous.

The optimal thrombolytic dose for acute PE patients is another topic of great debate. In an effort to reduce the risk of bleeding associated with thrombolytic therapy, a "reduced-dose" thrombolytic approach has been investigated. In two small studies randomizing patients with hemodynamic instability and "massive" or "moderate" pulmonary embolism to either full dose (100 mg) or reduced dose (50 mg) of systemic alteplase, the reduced-dose regimen appeared to be both safe and effective [21, 22]. However, these two studies lacked standardized definitions for acute PE severity and did not include mortality endpoints, limiting the generalizability of their results.

An attractive alternative to systemic thrombolysis is that of catheter-directed thrombolysis. In the ULTIMA trial, 59 patients with acute PE and evidence of right ventricular enlargement were randomized to receive intravenous unfractionated heparin plus catheter-directed, ultrasound-assisted thrombolysis (10–20 mg of alteplase) versus unfractionated heparin alone. The catheter-directed therapy arm significantly reduced right-to-left ventricular diameter ratio at 24 h of follow-up without an increased risk of bleeding [23]. While the targeted delivery of lower-dose thrombolytic medications makes this approach attractive, large-scale trials with hard clinical outcomes remain to be performed and reported.

Before administering systemic or catheter-directed thrombolytics, it is important to review a patient's bleeding risk (Table 14.4).

While all systemic thrombolytics should be avoided with any absolute contraindication, some clinicians favor the use of catheter-directed thrombolysis for patients with relative contraindications and a high-risk acute pulmonary embolism presentation.

Table 14.4 Contraindications to thrombolysis [20].

Absolute contraindications
• Active bleeding
• Previous intracranial hemorrhage
• Structural intracranial disease
• Recent ischemic stroke (≤3 months)
• Recent brain or spinal surgery (≤3 months)
• Recent head trauma (≤3 months)
• Bleeding diathesis
Relative contraindications
• Recent bleeding
• Recent surgery
• Recent invasive procedure
• Chronic anticoagulation
• Pregnancy
• Systolic blood pressure > 180 mmHg or diastolic blood pressure > 110 mmHg
• Remote ischemic stroke (>3 months)
• Traumatic cardiopulmonary resuscitation
• Pericarditis or pericardial fluid
• Age > 75
• Low body weight (<60 kg)
• Diabetic retinopathy

Thrombolysis for Acute Deep Vein Thrombosis

Patients with acute DVT are at substantial risk for developing the post-thrombotic syndrome [24]. The open vein hypothesis suggests that by removing an occlusive proximal deep vein thrombus, improved venous flow can be restored and venous hypertension avoided. This has been supported by the CaVenT study, where 209 patients with first-time acute iliofemoral DVT within 21 days were randomized to conventional therapy alone vs. conventional therapy plus catheter-directed thrombolysis with alteplase [25]. The use of catheter-directed therapy was associated with a decreased incidence of the post-thrombotic syndrome at 24 months (41.1% versus 55.6%, $p = 0.047$). Results of the larger ATTRACT trial (NCT00790335) have been presented at an international meeting, but peer-review publication is still pending. Initial data from the presentation do not support routine use of catheter-directed thrombolysis in acute DVT patients. However, there may be benefit in patients with more proximal acute DVT (e.g., iliofemoral) for the prevention of severe post-thrombotic syndrome. In the meantime, guidelines support the consideration of catheter-directed thrombolysis in select patients with acute, proximal DVT [14].

Use of Inferior Vena Cava Filters

For patients with significant clot burden in a proximal acute DVT or who could not tolerate another PE, there has been common sense support in favor of inferior vena cava (IVC) filter placement. This has been supported by a number of large, observational studies suggesting an association between IVC filter use and lower rates of mortality [26–28]. However, two large randomized trials have failed to confirm these benefits. In the PREPIC study, 400 patients with acute proximal DVT with or without PE were randomized to IVC filter or no IVC filter placement in addition to standard anticoagulation therapy [29]. After 8 years of follow-up, IVC filter use was associated with a reduced risk of PE, an increased risk of DVT, and no impact on mortality. In the PREPIC2 study, 399 patients with acute PE and DVT or superficial vein thrombus with one additional severity criterion were randomized to IVC filter or no IVC filter placement plus standard anticoagulation therapy [30]. After 6 months of follow-up, there was no difference in recurrent PE risk or mortality. Based largely on these two randomized trials, guidelines and consensus guidance documents favor the routine use of IVC filters only in patients who cannot tolerate anticoagulation therapy [14, 15, 17]. Additionally, when IVC filters are placed, all too frequently they are not removed in a timely manner (if ever), leading to high rates of complications [31].

Clinicians should be very judicious in the use of IVC filters, restricting their use primarily for high-risk patients in whom anticoagulation therapy is clearly contraindicated. Additionally, use of retrievable IVC filters with a robust filter monitoring and retrieval practice should help to reduce complications, such as fracture or migration of the filter and DVT. Table 14.5 reviews the

Table 14.5 Indications for inferior vena cava filter placement [7, 14, 18, 32, 33].

	American College of Chest Physicians [7, 14]	American College of Radiology Appropriateness Criteria [32]	Society of Interventional Radiology [33]	American Heart Association [18]
Absolute indications or high appropriateness	Acute VTE and a contraindication to anticoagulation	Chronic symptomatic PE	VTE and a contraindication to anticoagulation	Adult patients with any confirmed PE or proximal DVT with contraindications to anticoagulation or with active bleeding complications
		Free-floating iliofemoral thrombus (retrievable filter)	Failure of anticoagulation in patients with VTE	
			VTE and complications of anticoagulation	
			Recurrent PE despite adequate therapy	
			Inability to achieve/maintain adequate anticoagulation	
			Propagation/progression of DVT during therapeutic anticoagulation	
			Massive PE with residual DVT in a patient at risk for further PE	
			Free-floating iliofemoral or IVC thrombus	
			Severe cardiopulmonary disease and DVT (e.g., cor pulmonale with pulmonary hypertension)	
			Prophylaxis against VTE in patients with: • severe trauma without documented VTE • closed head injury • spinal cord injury • multiple long-bone or pelvic fractures • at high risk (e.g., immobilized or in an intensive care unit)	

Relative indications or mid-level appropriateness	Unstable patients with PE may benefit from IVC filter in conjunction with anticoagulation therapy	Acute PE with negative lower extremity Doppler ultrasound		Recurrent acute PE despite therapeutic anticoagulation
	Massive PE treated with thrombolysis/thrombectomy or chronic PE treated with thromboendarterectomy	Acute PE and/or iliofemoral DVT		Patients with acute PE and very poor cardiopulmonary reserve, including those with massive PE
	Recurrent VTE despite adequate anticoagulation and an inability to increase the intensity of anticoagulant therapy	Symptomatic chronic PE		
		Prophylaxis in high-risk patients without documented VTE (retrievable filter)		
		Phlegmasia cerulea dolens undergoing endovascular treatment		
		Free-floating iliofemoral thrombus (permanent IVC filter)		
Not indicated or not appropriate	Prophylaxis	Calf vein DVT		Routinely as an adjuvant to anticoagulation and systemic fibrinolysis in the treatment of acute PE
	In patients with VTE being treated with anticoagulation	Upper extremity DVT		

VTE venous thromboembolism, *PE* pulmonary embolism, *DVT* deep vein thrombosis, *IVC* inferior vena cava.

absolute and relative indications for IVC filter placement based on various society guidelines and appropriateness criteria.

VTE Outpatient Therapy: The First 3 Months

Patients with VTE who are clinically stable may be treated as outpatients [14]. Outpatient treatment regimens vary in duration, complexity, route of administration, and cost. Selection of an appropriate regimen is based on patient-specific clinical factors and individual preferences.

Parenteral Versus Oral Therapy

Heparin, typically used in the acute care setting around the time of the initial VTE diagnosis, is undesirable as long-term therapy, even when administered subcutaneously. It requires frequent laboratory monitoring and multiple daily injections and is associated with long-term side effects including osteoporosis. Subcutaneous low-molecular-weight heparin (LMWH) is less burdensome on patients because it can be administered once daily, does not require routine laboratory monitoring, and is less likely to result in heparin-induced thrombocytopenia or osteoporosis. However, most VTE patients without cancer are treated with oral regimens given their convenience and strong efficacy data.

Oral Anticoagulants

Warfarin, first approved for use in humans in 1954, was the only oral anticoagulant available in the United States until the advent of the direct oral anticoagulants (DOACs) in recent years (Table 14.6). Four DOACs have gained approval, with more agents likely in the near future.

Warfarin inhibits vitamin K epoxide reductase (VKOR), which in turn prevents the liver from recycling vitamin K into an active functional form. Functional vitamin K is necessary for the formation of active clotting factors II, VII, IX, and X. Patients on warfarin, therefore, have reduced functional levels of these vitamin K-dependent clotting factors.

DOACs work by one of two mechanisms of action. Dabigatran binds directly to factor II (thrombin). This prevents thrombin from exhibiting its procoagulant effects, which include generation of fibrin, activation of upstream clotting factors, and platelet activation. Rivaroxaban, apixaban, and edoxaban are factor Xa inhibitors. These drugs bind specifically to activated factor X (Xa) and prevent its normal biologic activity, most notably generation of thrombin.

Though the available oral anticoagulant drugs work by different mechanisms of action, they produce similar clinical results. All currently available DOACs have been proven non-inferior to warfarin for reduction of recurrent VTE [9–13, 34]. Rates of major bleeding are largely similar between DOACs and warfarin. Apixaban was found to have statistically lower rates of major bleeding compared to warfarin for management of acute venous thromboembolism. Edoxaban was found to have a statistically significant reduction in any bleeding, driven largely by a reduction in clinically relevant nonmajor bleeding. A summary of clinical trial data can be found in Table 14.7.

Warfarin for VTE

Most patients should start at a warfarin dose of 5 mg daily. Warfarin should be started as soon as possible after diagnosis (preferably on the day of diagnosis) along with a parenteral anticoagulant. Because of the long effective half-life of the drug and the clotting factors which it inhibits, it takes several days to reach full effectiveness. It is imperative that patients remain on a parenteral anticoagulant until the INR is above 2.0. In addition, since warfarin temporarily induces a prothrombotic state by inhibiting the body's vitamin K-dependent anticoagulants, protein C and protein S, parenteral anticoagulation should continue for at least 5 days of overlap with warfarin, even if the INR becomes therapeutic before 5 days has elapsed. It is reasonable to discontinue the paren-

Table 14.6 Oral anticoagulant medications.

Chemical name	Brand name	Drug class	Dose and regimen	Adjustment for renal dysfunction	Use in hepatic impairment	Other dose considerations
Warfarin	Coumadin®, Jantoven®	Vitamin K antagonist	5 mg once daily for most patients initially and then adjusted to target an INR 2.0–3.0	None	Use caution	Starting dose may be reduced to 2.5 mg daily in patients who are elderly, are frail, have severe kidney or liver disease, are those on certain interacting medications, or are those with multiple comorbidities
Dabigatran	Pradaxa®	Direct thrombin inhibitor	150 mg twice daily, after 5–10 days of parenteral anticoagulation	Not for use with CrCl ≤30 ml/min		Not for use if creatinine clearance ≤50 ml/min with concomitant P-glycoprotein inhibitors. Avoid use in patients on concomitant P-glycoprotein inducers
Rivaroxaban	Xarelto®	Factor Xa inhibitor	15 mg twice daily for 21 days and then 20 mg once daily thereafter	Not for use with CrCl <30 ml/min	Avoid use in Childs-Pugh class B–C	Avoid use in patients taking strong dual CYP3A4/P-glycoprotein inhibitors or inducers. Avoid use in patients on moderate dual inhibitors if creatinine clearance <80 ml/min
Apixaban	Eliquis®	Factor Xa inhibitor	10 mg twice daily for 7 days and then 5 mg twice daily thereafter	Not tested in patients with serum creatinine >2.5 mg/dL or CrCl <25 ml/min	Avoid use in Childs-Pugh class B–C	Reduce dose to 5 mg twice daily for 7 days and then 2.5 mg twice daily thereafter for patients on dual CYP3A4/P-glycoprotein inhibitors. Avoid use in patients on strong dual inducers

(continued)

Table 14.6 (continued)

Chemical name	Brand name	Drug class	Dose and regimen	Adjustment for renal dysfunction	Use in hepatic impairment	Other dose considerations
Edoxaban	Savaysa®	Factor Xa inhibitor	60 mg once daily, after 5–10 days of parenteral anticoagulation	Reduce dose to 30 mg once daily if CrCl 15–50 ml/min. Do not use if CrCl <15 ml/min or if CrCl >95 ml/min	Avoid use in Childs-Pugh class B–C	Reduce dose to 30 mg daily for body weight ≤60 kg or for patients on P-glycoprotein inhibitors. Avoid use with P-glycoprotein inducers

INR international normalized ratio, *CrCl* creatinine clearance.

teral agent in the event that the INR becomes supratherapeutic (greater than 3.0) before 5 days of overlap have been achieved [7].

Warfarin treatment for VTE requires frequent (at least weekly) INR monitoring in the first weeks of therapy. Trained anticoagulation care providers, including nurses, physicians, or pharmacists, should assist the patient with serial warfarin dose adjustments to target stable INR values between 2.0 and 3.0.

Though diagnosis-specific and drug-specific education should be given to all patients being treated for VTE, the patient education required for warfarin is more extensive than for DOACs because of the effects of patient lifestyle on warfarin dosing and INR stability. See Table 14.8 for a summary of education items which should be discussed with patients being treated for VTE with an anticoagulant drug.

DOACs for VTE

The use of dabigatran or edoxaban for VTE requires a 5–10-day run-in with a parenteral anticoagulant. Unlike with warfarin, these two treatment phases are non-overlapping. Patients commonly use enoxaparin for 5 days and then begin dabigatran or edoxaban treatment on day 6. For patients who are diagnosed during a hospitalization or whose acute care involves heparin or LMWH treatment during the first 5–10 days after diagnosis, this may not be a barrier. However, when treatment as an outpatient is preferred, this requirement increases drug cost to the patient and complexity of the treatment regimen and necessitates further education for subcutaneous injection technique.

Rivaroxaban and apixaban may be started alone, without the need for parenteral therapy. However, both of these agents require a change in dose after the first several days on therapy. Patients should be thoroughly educated on the need for dose and schedule changes.

The lack of routine INR monitoring and other bloodwork makes for a less complex treatment plan for patients and lowers workload on the healthcare provider. Clinicians are reminded, however, that in clinical trials which proved safety and efficacy of DOACs, patients maintained regular contact with anticoagulation care providers to assess medication adherence and address concerns. Studies have found an association between improved medication adherence and close contact with an anticoagulation care provider. However, these studies have been underpowered to detect differences in clinical outcomes of interest such as rates of recurrent VTE or bleeding.

Table 14.7 Clinical trials of oral anticoagulants for acute VTE treatment.

Clinical trial	Included patients	Study design	Treatment duration	*n*	Treatment groups	Percent of time in therapeutic range for warfarin group	Primary efficacy outcome	Rate of primary outcome	Rate of major bleeding
Re-cover [9]	Acute symptomatic proximal LE DVT or PE	Double-blind, double-dummy RCT	6 months	2564	Dabigatran 150 mg BID after 5–10 days of parenteral anticoagulation vs. adjusted-dose warfarin targeting INR 2.0–3.0	60%	Composite of symptomatic VTE or death associated with VTE	Dabigatran 2.4% Warfarin 2.1% HR 1.10 (0.65–1.84)	Dabigatran 1.6% Warfarin 1.9% HR 0.82 (0.45–1.48)
Re-cover II [34]	Acute symptomatic proximal LE DVT or PE	Double-blind, double-dummy RCT	6 months	2568	Dabigatran 150 mg BID after 5–10 days of parenteral anticoagulation vs. adjusted-dose warfarin targeting INR 2.0–3.0	57%	Composite of symptomatic VTE or death associated with VTE	Dabigatran 2.3% Warfarin 2.2% HR 1.08 (0.64–1.8)	Dabigatran 1.2% Warfarin 1.7% HR 0.69 (0.36–1.32%)
Einstein DVT [10]	Acute symptomatic proximal DVT without PE	Open-label RCT	Provider choice of 3, 6, or 12 months	3449	Rivaroxaban 15 mg BID × 21 days, followed by 20 mg daily vs. enoxaparin transitioned to adjusted-dose warfarin targeting INR 2.0–3.0	58%	Recurrent symptomatic VTE	Rivaroxaban 2.1% Warfarin 3.0% HR 0.68 (0.44–1.04)	Rivaroxaban 0.8% Warfarin 1.2% HR 0.65 (0.33–1.30)
Einstein PE [11]	Acute symptomatic PE with or without DVT	Open-label RCT	Provider choice of 3, 6, or 12 months	4832	Rivaroxaban 15 mg BID × 21 days, followed by 20 mg daily vs. enoxaparin transitioned to adjusted-dose warfarin targeting INR 2.0–3.0	63%	Recurrent symptomatic VTE	Rivaroxaban 2.1% Warfarin 1.8% HR 1.12 (0.75–1.68)	Rivaroxaban 1.1% Warfarin 2.2% HR 0.49 (0.31–0.79)
Amplify [12]	Acute symptomatic proximal DVT or PE	Double-blind, double-dummy RCT	6 months	5395	Apixaban 10 mg BID × 10 days, followed by 5 mg BID thereafter vs. enoxaparin transitioned to adjusted-dose warfarin targeting INR 2.0–3.0	61%	Composite of symptomatic VTE or death associated with VTE	Apixaban 2.3% Warfarin 2.7% HR 0.84 (0.60–1.18)	Apixaban 0.6% Warfarin 1.8% HR 0.31 (0.17–0.55)

(continued)

Table 14.7 (continued)

Clinical trial	Included patients	Study design	Treatment duration	*n*	Treatment groups	Percent of time in therapeutic range for warfarin group	Primary efficacy outcome	Rate of primary outcome	Rate of major bleeding
Hokusai-VTE [13]	Acute symptomatic DVT of popliteal, femoral or iliac veins, or acute symptomatic PE	Double-blind, double-dummy RCT	Provider choice of 3–12 months	8240	Edoxaban 60 mg daily (or 30 mg daily if creatinine clearance 30–50 ml/min or body weight < 60 kg) vs. adjusted-dose warfarin targeting INR 2.0–3.0	64%	Composite of recurrent symptomatic VTE or VTE-related death	Edoxaban 3.2% Warfarin 3.5% HR 0.89 (0.7–1.13)	Edoxaban 1.4% Warfarin 1.6% HR 0.81 (0.59–1.21)

LE lower extremity, *DVT* deep vein thrombosis, *PE* pulmonary embolism, *BID* twice a day, *VTE* venous thromboembolism, *HR* hazard ratio, *INR* international normalized ratio, *RCT* randomized controlled trial.

Table 14.8 Education topics for patients with VTE on oral anticoagulation.

For patients on ANY anticoagulant	Signs and symptoms of worsening or recurrent thrombosis
	Signs and symptoms of bleeding
	Potential for heavier menstrual bleeding, if applicable
	Expected duration of therapy
	Advise anticoagulation care provider if changes in medications
	Advise anticoagulation care provider of upcoming procedures or surgeries
	Avoidance of OTC medications which increase bleeding risk (i.e., NSAIDs)
	Avoidance of behaviors that increase the risk of bleeding (i.e., contact sports or other activities with risks of falling or suffering a blow to the head)
	Moderation of alcohol consumption
	What to do in case of a missed dose
	When to seek emergency care
For patients on any DOAC	Importance of medication adherence
For patients on dabigatran	Storage of capsules in original container, not pill boxes
	Importance of not breaking or opening capsules
For patients on rivaroxaban	Administration with food
For patients on warfarin	INR monitoring
	Consistency with intake of dietary vitamin K
	Awareness of hidden sources of vitamin K (nutritional shakes/ supplements, vitamins)
	Awareness of factors which effect INR (exercise, alcohol, tobacco, stress, changes in prescription and non-prescription medicines)
	Importance of consistent strength and manufacturer of warfarin tablets (notify anticoagulation provider if tablets change in color or shape)
	Pregnancy avoidance, if female

OTC over the counter, *NSAID* non-steroidal anti-inflammatory drug, *DOAC* direct oral anticoagulant, *INR* international normalized ratio.

Table 14.9 Clinical characteristics which favor treatment with warfarin over DOACs.

• Severe renal dysfunction (CrCl < 30 ml/min)
• Severe liver dysfunction (e.g., elevated baseline INR)
• Concomitant use of a medication with a known significant drug-drug interaction with DOACs
• Obesity (body weight over 100 kg)
• Need for dual antiplatelet therapy
• Concern for medication nonadherence
• Concern for medication nonadherence

DOAC direct oral anticoagulant, *CrCl* creatinine clearance, *INR* international normalized ratio.

Oral Drug Selection

The most recent iteration of the American College of Chest Physicians (ACCP) guidelines suggests preference for DOAC treatment over use of warfarin for most patients (Grade 2B) [14]. It is important to note that the strength of this recommendation is weak and based primarily on a perceived increase in convenience for patients and providers. Providers should recognize that there are groups of patients for whom warfarin remains the preferred treatment (Table 14.9).

Patients may be good candidates for either warfarin or DOAC therapy and should be actively involved in treatment decisions. Lack of involvement in the medical decision-making process has been cited as a driver for medication nonadherence which occurs at a rate estimated as high as 50% in the general population [35]. Other factors driving medication nonadherence include high drug costs and complex medication regimens. Patients should be asked about their motivations and preferences for drug therapy (Table 14.10). Insurance coverage for the selected medication should be secured before the patient is sent home. There are a variety of financial assistance mechanisms available for DOAC drugs for eligible patients (Table 14.11). These programs are subject to change over time, so the individual manufacturers' websites are the best resource for up-to-date information.

Table 14.10 Patient motivating factors and associated oral anticoagulants.

Patient motivation	Warfarin	Dabigatran	Rivaroxaban	Apixaban	Edoxaban
Avoid injections			x	x	
Medicare part D patients with coverage gap or "donut hole"	x				
Once-daily dosing	x		x		x
History of GERD symptoms	x		x	x	x
Desire for a "reversal agent"	x	x			
Take medication without regard to food or other medicines	x	x		x	x

GERD gastroesophageal reflux disease.

Table 14.11 Financial assistance mechanisms for direct oral anticoagulant medications.

	Eligible patients	Excluded patients	Pros	Cons
Free trial	Any patient new to the medication in question	None	Get a patient started on a DOAC right away while medication coverage/prior authorization/therapy decisions are made	Only helps for the first month
Co-pay reduction	Patients with commercial medication insurance	State or federal sponsored programs (Medicare/ Medicaid)	Remove high commercial co-pays as a barrier to DOAC therapy	Benefits are limited to the commercially insured (adults of working age)
Patient assistance program	Patients without medication insurance and who meet income requirements	Patients with coverage or who fail to meet low-income requirements	Provide free access to medication for underserved and indigent populations	Income requirements are restrictive. Application requires significant documentation and processing time

DOAC direct oral anticoagulant.

VTE in Cancer

Patients with cancer-associated VTE are at a markedly increased risk for VTE. For patients with a cancer-associated VTE, the 1-year risk of recurrence approaches 20% without appropriate treatment [36].

In cancer-associated VTE, use of LMWH is generally preferred over oral anticoagulants. The CLOT and CATCH trials collectively randomized over 1500 patients with cancer-associated VTE to receive either warfarin therapy or LMWH to prevent VTE recurrence [37, 38]. In the CLOT trial, dalteparin was compared to warfarin, while in the CATCH trial, tinzaparin was compared to warfarin. Neither trial used enoxaparin, although it is the most commonly used LMWH in the United States. A recent meta-analysis demonstrated 40% relative risk reduction in VTE recurrence with LMWH therapy as compared to warfarin therapy [39]. Two additional benefits of LMWH therapy include a non-oral route of administration for patients with fluctuating nutrition status or inability to tolerate oral medications and a shorter half-life for simpler therapy interruptions in case of procedures or surgeries. There is a lack of comparative data at this time for LMWH versus DOACs in this population, and thus LMWH remains the treatment of choice. Until more data is available, warfarin remains the treatment of choice in cancer patients who are either unable to tolerate or who refuse treatment with LMWH. Please refer to Chap. 20 for a more in-depth analysis of anticoagulation strategies in the patient with cancer.

VTE Outpatient Therapy: Extended Prophylaxis

Duration of Anticoagulation after VTE

Total duration of anticoagulation should be determined by examining an individual patient's risk of recurrent VTE after therapy discontinuation and risk of bleeding while on therapy. The literature has reported a wide range for VTE recurrence rates, particularly for patients with a first unprovoked VTE [36, 40–44]. Several models exist to quantify risk of VTE recurrence (Table 14.12) [45–47]. The Men Continue and HERDOO2 score has recently been validated in a prospective cohort, while the Vienna score was externally validated in a retrospective cohort [48, 49].

Table 14.12 Risk scores for recurrent venous thromboembolism.

	Men Continue and HERDOO2	Vienna risk model	DASH
Gender	X	X	X
D-dimer	X	X	X
Post-thrombotic syndrome	X		
Obesity	X		
Age			X
Location of DVT/PE		X	
Provoked?			X

DVT deep vein thrombosis, *PE* pulmonary embolism.

Figure 14.2 represents a simplified decision tree for patients with a first VTE, based on the most recent update to treatment guidelines by ACCP.

The ACCP guideline authors only suggest a 3-month time-limited anticoagulation regimen due to a lack of evidence to support other fixed durations of therapy (e.g., 6 or 12 months) [14].

Risk of VTE recurrence in patients with active cancer has been described as high as 21% in the first year off anticoagulation [36]. For this reason, patients with cancer should remain anticoagulated at least until their cancer is in remission and off therapy. As previously discussed, cancer patients have improved efficacy when LMWH is utilized, as compared to warfarin.

The optimal length of therapy for patients with a non-cancer-associated unprovoked first VTE is an area of significant debate, since risk of recurrence may be difficult to quantify. For these patients, assessing bleed risk may help inform the decision. However, bleed risk is most often assessed qualitatively as most quantitative scores have modest clinical predictive ability and can be cumbersome to calculate. One convenient bleeding risk score that has been tested in VTE populations is the RIETE score (Table 14.13) [50]. Additionally, patient preference and individual risk of VTE recurrence should also be considered.

Warfarin for Extended VTE Treatment

Warfarin has been used for continuation of VTE treatment and prevention of recurrent VTE for decades. Some investigators have suggested reducing intensity of anticoagulation in this treatment phase. While lower-intensity warfarin (INR goal 1.5–2.0) has been shown to lower risk of recurrent VTE compared to placebo, it remains inferior to warfarin at standard treatment intensity (INR goal 2.0–3.0) [51, 52]. Thus, the standard goal range remains the preferred treatment intensity throughout the course of therapy.

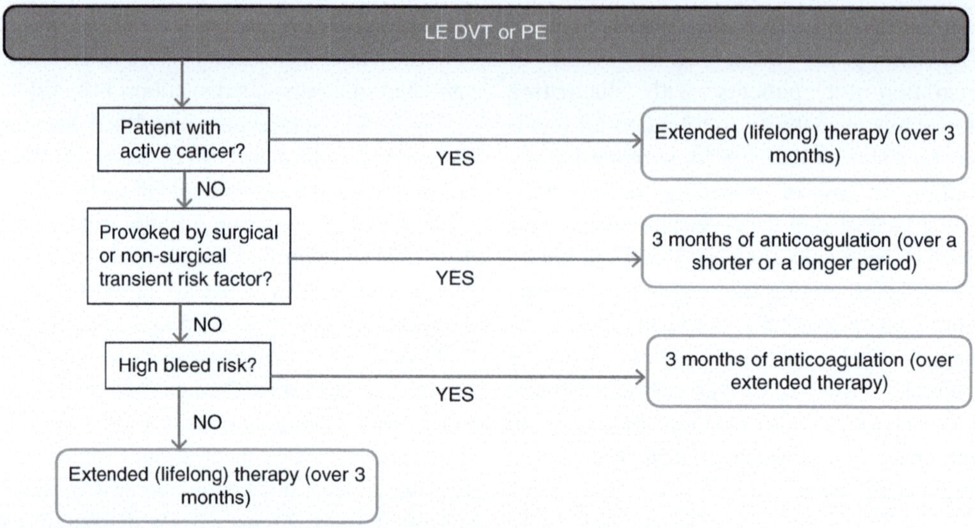

Fig. 14.2 Simplified decision tree for venous thromboembolism treatment length.

Table 14.13 RIETE score.

Condition	Points	Total points	Major bleeding (%)	Risk level
Recent major bleeding (<15 days prior to VTE)	2	0	0.1	Low
Creatinine >1.2 mg/dL	1.5	1	1.4	Moderate
Anemia (Hgb <13 g/dL in men or <12 g/dL in women)	1.5	1.5–2	2.2	
Cancer		2.5–3	4.4	
Clinically overt pulmonary embolism	1	3.5–4	4.2	
Age > 75 years	1	4.5–5	4.9	High
Total points		5.5–6	11	
		>6	20	

VTE venous thromboembolism, *Hgb* hemoglobin.

DOACs for Extended VTE Treatment

See Table 14.14 for a summary of DOAC trials in extended VTE treatment. Only dabigatran was tested in comparison with warfarin for extended secondary VTE treatment. As in the acute VTE studies of dabigatran vs. warfarin, dabigatran was found non-inferior to warfarin and exhibited a similar rate of major bleeding beyond the initial 6 months of therapy [53]. Dabigatran, rivaroxaban, and apixaban have all been compared to placebo in patients for whom there was consideration for both continuation and discontinuation of therapy [10, 53, 54]. All three drugs significantly reduced the rates of recurrent VTE as compared to placebo. Reassuringly, all three drugs also exhibited very low rates of major bleeding. At this time, there is no published data on edoxaban in extended treatment of VTE.

In the AMPLIFY-EXT trial comparing apixaban at two doses (2.5 mg and 5 mg twice daily) versus placebo for secondary VTE prevention, apixaban was superior to placebo for preventing VTE recurrence, but with no statistically increased risk of clinically relevant and major bleeding [54]. Statistical comparisons of major

Table 14.14 Clinical trials of oral anticoagulants for extended VTE treatment.

Study	Included patients	Study design	Treatment duration	*n*	Treatment groups	Percent of time in therapeutic range for warfarin group	Primary efficacy outcome	Rate of primary outcome	Rate of major bleeding
Re-MEDY [53]	Previously enrolled in RE-COVER or RE-COVER II and at increased risk of VTE after 3–12 months of therapy	Double-blind, double-dummy RCT	6–36 months	2866	Dabigatran 150 mg BID vs. adjusted-dose warfarin targeting INR 2.0–3.0	65%	Composite of symptomatic VTE or death associated with VTE	Dabigatran 1.8% Warfarin 1.3% HR 1.44 (0.78–2.64)	Dabigatran 0.9% Warfarin 1.8% HR 0.52 (0.27–1.02)
Re-SONATE [53]	Previously enrolled in RE-COVER or RE-COVER II and considered for therapy discontinuation after 6–18 months of therapy	Double-blind RCT	6 months	1353	Dabigatran 150 mg BID vs. placebo	n/a	Composite of symptomatic VTE or death associated with VTE	Dabigatran 0.4% Placebo 5.6% HR 0.08 (0.02–0.25)	Dabigatran 0.3% Placebo 0%
EINSTEIN-extension [10]	Patients with acute VTE who had received 6–12 months of therapy with VKA (from Einstein trials or not) or rivaroxaban (from Einstein trials)	Open-label RCT	6 or 12 months	1197	Rivaroxaban 20 mg daily vs. placebo	n/a	Recurrent symptomatic VTE	Rivaroxaban 1.3% Placebo 7.1% HR 0.18 (0.09–0.39)	Rivaroxaban 0.7% Placebo 0%

(continued)

Table 14.14 (continued)

Study	Included patients	Study design	Treatment duration	*n*	Treatment groups	Percent of time in therapeutic range for warfarin group	Primary efficacy outcome	Rate of primary outcome	Rate of major bleeding
Amplify-Ext [54]	Patients with acute VTE who had received 6–12 months of therapy (did not have to be previously enrolled in AMPLIFY)	Double-blind, double-dummy RCT	12 months	2486	Apixaban 2.5 mg BID, apixaban 5 mg BID, or placebo	n/a	Symptomatic recurrent VTE or death	Apixaban 5 mg BID 4.2%	Apixaban 5 mg BID 0.1%
								Apixaban 2.5 mg BID 3.8%	Apixaban 2.5 mg BID 0.2%
								Placebo 11.6%	Placebo 0.5%
								HR 0.36 (0.25–0.53) for 5 mg BID	HR 0.25 (0.03–2.24) apixaban 5 mg BID vs. placebo
								HR 0.33 (0.22–0.48) for 2.5 mg BID	HR 0.49 (0.09–2.64) apixaban 2.5 mg BID vs. placebo
									HR 1.93 (0.18–21.25) apixaban 5 mg BID vs. 2.5 mg BID

Einstein choice [55]	Patients with acute VTE who had received 6–12 months of oral anticoagulant therapy	Double-blind RCT	Up to 12 months	3365	Rivaroxaban 20 mg daily, rivaroxaban 10 mg daily, or aspirin 100 mg daily	n/a	Symptomatic recurrent fatal or nonfatal VTE	Rivaroxaban 20 mg daily 1.5%	Rivaroxaban 20 mg daily 0.5%
								Rivaroxaban 10 mg daily 1.2%	Rivaroxaban 10 mg daily 0.4%
								Aspirin 100 mg daily 4.4%	Aspirin 100 mg daily 0.3%
								HR 0.34 (0.20–0.59) for 20 mg daily	HR 2.01 (0.50–8.04) rivaroxaban 20 mg daily vs. aspirin 100 mg daily
								HR 0.26 (0.14–0.47) for 10 mg daily	HR 1.64 (0.39–6.84) rivaroxaban 10 mg daily vs. aspirin 100 mg daily
									HR 1.23 (0.37–4.03) rivaroxaban 20 mg daily vs. 10 mg daily

VTE venous thromboembolism, *RTC* randomized controlled trial, *BID* twice a day, *INR* international normalized ratio, *HR* hazard ratio, *VKA* vitamin K antagonist.

bleeding rates were not calculated in the EINSTEIN-Extension trial and RE-SONATE trials due to few events. Finally, the EINSTEIN CHOICE study compared rivaroxaban at two doses (10 mg and 20 mg once daily) vs. low-dose aspirin (100 mg) for secondary VTE prevention [55]. Rivaroxaban was shown to be superior to aspirin for the prevention of recurrent VTE with similar rates of major and clinically relevant nonmajor bleeding. Importantly, approximately 60% of the patients enrolled in EINSTEIN CHOICE were categorized as having a provoked VTE event.

Choice of Oral Anticoagulant in Extended Treatment Phase

Since all of the available oral anticoagulants are effective in the first months of therapy, and no significant red flags have been raised in extended therapy clinical trials, it seems reasonable for patients to remain on the same anticoagulant that they used in the initial treatment period. However, if there is a compelling reason to change anticoagulants, this can be done.

Discontinuation of Anticoagulation

Patients who have discontinued anticoagulant treatment after an acute VTE should be aware of their increased risk for future events. They should be counseled to monitor for signs and symptoms of DVT or PE recurrence. Patients should be aware of future situations which might put them at even higher risk, such as those that induce vascular injury (i.e., surgery), contribute to blood pooling (i.e., long-distance travel or immobility), or increase coagulability (i.e., use of hormone replacements or with diagnosis of cancer). Some clinicians assess blood tests for D-dimer or factor VIII levels, while others test for residual venous obstruction on duplex ultrasound to help determine if anticoagulant discontinuation is appropriate [56–59]. None of these have been incorporated into the ACCP guidelines [14].

Aspirin for Extended VTE Prophylaxis

Patients who do not continue anticoagulation long term may benefit from use of low-dose aspirin. The WARFASA and ASPIRE trials investigated use of aspirin 100 mg compared to placebo in patients who'd been treated for VTE with anticoagulation [60, 61]. These trials indicate that while aspirin is not as effective as anticoagulants in reducing thrombotic risk, there is probably a small decrease in the risk of recurrent VTE compared to placebo (Fig. 14.3).

Risk of bleeding with low-dose aspirin is overall low and comparable to placebo in the two trials. In addition, patients treated with aspirin do not incur the high cost associated with DOACs

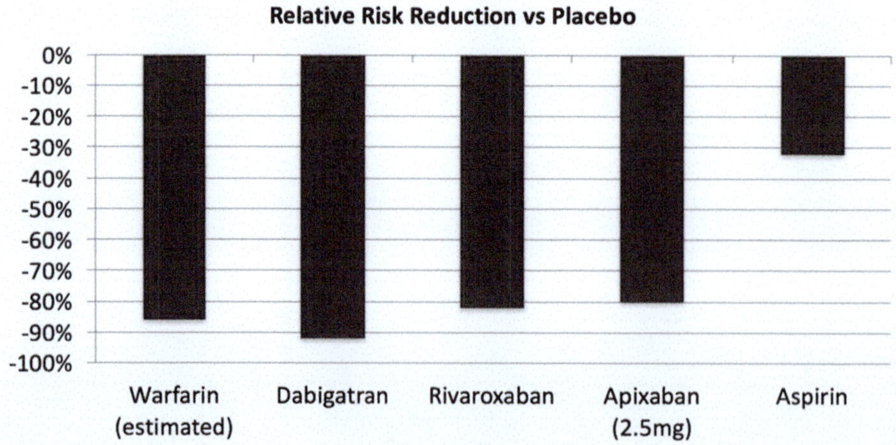

Fig. 14.3 Relative risk reduction for venous thromboembolism recurrence.

nor the necessity for INR monitoring and diet modification associated with warfarin.

Catheter-Associated VTE

Patients who develop upper extremity DVT frequently do so in the setting of an indwelling venous catheter or a pacemaker/implanted defibrillator. Patients with peripherally inserted central catheters (PICC) are at increased risk of catheter-associated DVT development as compared to patients with other central venous catheters [62]. That risk increases with increasing PICC diameter (gauge) and comorbid cancer diagnosis [63]. To address this concern, a recent set of appropriateness guidelines have been established for use of various intravenous catheters [64]. In particular, PICC lines are favored over alternative infusion methods when the expected duration of use is 6 days or greater and the smallest possible diameter PICC (usually single lumen) is preferred to reduce catheter-associated DVT risk.

When a catheter-associated VTE occurs, anticoagulation is usually first-line therapy. In fact, anticoagulation alone (without catheter removal) is adequate therapy for most patients who require the use of their indwelling venous catheter [15]. Thrombolytic therapy is also not recommended for routine use, but may be beneficial if significant venous congestive symptoms persist despite adequate anticoagulation [14]. Anticoagulation therapy should be administered for at least 3 months or as long as the venous catheter remains in place [15, 64]. Once the catheter is no longer needed, it can safely be removed. If a new catheter is required, preference should be given to the contralateral side with the smallest-sized catheter possible [64].

Venous Thrombosis in Unusual Sites

While VTE most commonly occur in the veins of the extremities or the pulmonary arteries, thrombosis can occur in other venous beds. In particular, venous thrombosis can occur in the cerebral veins, the abdominal and pelvic veins, or in the retinal veins. Given the rarer occurrence, evidence-based treatment strategies are less well developed.

Cerebral Vein Thrombosis

Cerebral vein thrombus most commonly affects young women, often presenting with headache, seizure, or focal neurologic deficit [65]. Mortality rates approach 10% over 10 years of follow-up with a similar percentage of patients experiencing residual disability [66]. Even in the presence of intracerebral bleeding at the time of diagnosis, heparin anticoagulation (either unfractionated or low-molecular-weight) should be administered acutely [65]. Oral anticoagulation should be initiated once the patient is stabilized and continued for at least 3 months. Select patients with unprovoked cerebral vein thrombosis or who have a concurrent thrombophilia should receive 6–12 months of anticoagulation therapy, with consideration of lifelong treatment.

Splanchnic Vein Thrombosis

The splanchnic veins drain blood from the various abdominal organs, including the liver, bowel, and spleen. The term "splanchnic vein thrombosis" encompasses Budd-Chiari syndrome (thrombosis of the suprahepatic vein), portal vein thrombosis, mesenteric vein thrombosis, and splenic vein thrombosis. These patients experience a substantial mortality risk, approximately 10 per 100 patient-years [67]. Patients most commonly present with abdominal pain and frequently have underlying disorders that predispose them to thrombosis in this unusual site. In particular, hematologic disorders, use of hormonal therapies, intraabdominal surgery, pancreatitis, and cancer are known risk factors. Anticoagulation therapy should be administered for a minimum of 3 months in all patients with splanchnic vein thrombosis [65]. For patients with pro-thrombotic risk factors, including comorbid cirrhosis, myeloproliferative neoplasm, and autoimmune disorders, extended anticoagulation is reasonable.

Retinal Vein Thrombosis

Retinal vein thrombosis is the second most common vascular disorder in the retina after diabetic retinopathy. It most commonly presents with sudden, unilateral, painless loss of vision and macular edema. The most concerning complication is permanent visual loss, which occurs in up to 80% of patients who initially present with poor visual acuity (<20/200) [68]. There is no strong data to support the routine use of anticoagulant or antiplatelet therapy in patients with acute retinal vein occlusion [65]. However, anticoagulant therapy with low-molecular-weight heparin can be considered for patients with severe thrombophilias (e.g., antiphospholipid antibody syndrome). In these cases, short courses (1–3 months) of anticoagulation are reasonable unless evidence of other thrombotic events has occurred.

Superficial Vein Thrombosis

Superficial vein thrombosis (SVT), commonly the greater saphenous in the lower extremity, results in symptoms similar to those of deep vein thrombosis. The thrombus often develops in a varicose vein. Factors which contribute to risk of SVT are similar to those of DVT and include long-distance travel, malignancy, chronic venous insufficiency, and various thrombophilias. There is a high rate of coexistence of DVT in patients presenting with SVT. About 10% of patients with SVT of 5 cm or more are also found to have proximal DVT, 13% of patients have a distal DVT, and 4% have a symptomatic PE [69]. For this reason, patients found to have proximal SVT should be evaluated for presence of DVT and treated according to VTE guidance as appropriate.

The goal of SVT treatment is to treat symptoms and reduce the risk of clot progression to the deep veins. Patients with SVT without evidence of DVT or PE have the option of no treatment, treatment with oral or topical NSAID for symptom relief, or anticoagulation. Most studies of SVT patients who take anticoagulation use a low or intermediate dose of anticoagulant, such as enoxaparin 40 mg daily. The largest study of anticoagulation for SVT is the CALISTO trial which investigated prophylactic dose fondaparinux (2.5 mg daily) vs. placebo in about 3000 patients [70]. This trial showed a reduction in rate of VTE and recurrence of SVT with 45 days of prophylactic fondaparinux, without an increase in risk of major bleeding. Patients taking placebo had about a 3.3% chance of developing VTE. With fondaparinux, that risk decreased to about 0.6%. Factors that increase the chance of progression from SVT to VTE are listed in Table 14.15.

Table 14.15 Factors associated with increased risk of superficial vein thrombosis progression to venous thromboembolism.

- Involvement of greater saphenous vein
- Clot extension to within 10 cm from saphenofemoral junction
- Involvement of veins above the knee
- Previous history of superficial vein thrombosis or venous thromboembolism

In light of evidence from CALISTO, authors of the ACCP VTE guidelines suggest treatment with fondaparinux 2.5 mg daily for 45 days in patients who have SVT of 5 cm or more [14]. Prophylactic dose LMWH is an alternative to fondaparinux. While many clinicians are considering the use of DOACs for SVT patients, robust data is lacking at this time.

VTE Prevention in Medical Inpatients

VTE is a common occurrence for patients hospitalized for medical illnesses, such as pneumonia, stroke, and heart failure. In fact, the risk of VTE remained significantly elevated for at least 4–6 weeks and continues to rise over 6 months [71]. Based on the recently completed APEX study, the FDA has approved use of the factor Xa inhibitor betrixaban for adult patients hospitalized for acute medical illness [72]. In this study, patients were randomized to receive either LMWH for 10 ± 4 days or betrixaban 80 mg for 35–42 days (after an initial loading dose of

160 mg). In an attempt to enrich the population for VTE, the primary study outcome was to be assessed in a population of patients hospitalized for acute medical illness either at older age (age ≥ 75) or with an elevated D-dimer on hospital admission. Secondary analysis included VTE risk in the overall population (age ≥ 40 and irrespective of D-dimer level). While the difference in VTE risk did not achieve statistical significance in the high-risk population, the risk of VTE (symptomatic or asymptomatic) was 5.3% in the betrixaban group and 7.0% in the enoxaparin group (RR 0.76, 95% CI 0.63–0.92) in the overall population. Additionally, there was no difference in the rate of major bleeding between the two groups (0.7% versus 0.6%, RR 1.19, 95% CI 0.67–2.12). However, there was a higher burden of major plus clinically relevant nonmajor bleeding in the betrixaban group (3.1% versus 1.6%, RR 1.97, 95% CI 1.44–2.68). FDA approval for betrixaban is based on the analysis of the overall population, making routine use of D-dimer testing unnecessary for use in this clinical situation.

While betrixaban is the first oral anticoagulant to be FDA approved for prevention of VTE in hospitalized medical patients, it faces numbers challenges to widespread use. First, many clinicians will need to learn about this new DOAC and its unique properties (e.g., very low renal clearance, longer half-life). Additionally, health systems will have to decide which patients are at sufficient VTE risk to necessitate extended prophylaxis. For those patients felt to benefit from extended betrixaban therapy, a mechanism is likely needed to ensure safe hospital-to-home transitions for this medication. This must address medication cost, hand off to a primary care or other provider, and ensure appropriate length of treatment.

Ongoing Studies

A number of important ongoing studies may help to better define the care of patients with VTE. As noted above, the ATTRACT trial (NCT00790335) has been presented but not yet published. When that trial is published in peer review, it should help to define the potential benefit of catheter-directed thrombolysis for patients with acute, proximal DVT to prevent the post-thrombotic syndrome. Ongoing studies exploring the role of direct oral anticoagulants for the management of cancer-associated VTE are eagerly anticipated (NCT02583191, NCT02048865, and NCT02073682).

Key Points

- VTE is highly prevalent and potentially dangerous.
- While warfarin has been the mainstay of therapy for decades, DOACs are now considered first line for many patients with VTE due to their efficacy and safety profile along with easier route of administration.
- LMWH is first-line therapy for patients who develop cancer-associated VTE.
- Longer courses of anticoagulation or antithrombotic therapy are now recommended for many patients with unprovoked or recurrent VTE.
- Thrombolytic therapy has a limited role for select patients with acute DVT and PE.

Self-Assessment Questions

1. A 60-year-old man with normal renal function whose only medication is Lisinopril 10 mg daily is diagnosed with an acute left leg deep vein thrombosis in the emergency department. Which of the following is an appropriate initial anticoagulation regimen?
   (a) Warfarin 5 mg daily
   (b) Enoxaparin 40 mg daily and warfarin 5 mg daily
   (c) Dabigatran 150 mg twice a day
   (d) Rivaroxaban 20 mg once daily
   (e) Apixaban 10 mg twice a day

2. A 66-year-old woman with baseline renal insufficiency (creatinine 1.4, estimated creatinine clearance 45 mL/min) whose only medication is over-the-counter loratadine is diagnosed with an acute right leg deep vein thrombosis by her primary care provider. Which of the following is an appropriate initial anticoagulation regimen?
   (a) Warfarin 10 mg daily
   (b) Enoxaparin 40 mg daily and warfarin 5 mg daily
   (c) Dabigatran 75 mg twice a day
   (d) Rivaroxaban 15 mg twice a day
   (e) Apixaban 2.5 mg twice a day
3. A 55-year-old woman with stage 3 breast cancer is diagnosed with a right leg deep vein thrombosis. She is currently undergoing chemotherapy. Which of the following is the most preferred initial anticoagulation regimen?
   (a) Warfarin
   (b) Enoxaparin
   (c) Dabigatran
   (d) Edoxaban
   (e) Aspirin
4. Which of the following laboratory tests have been shown to predict the risk of recurrent venous thromboembolism in multiple studies?
   (a) Troponin
   (b) Brain natriuretic peptide (BNP)
   (c) C-reactive protein
   (d) D-dimer
   (e) Total cholesterol
5. Which of the following is an absolute contraindication to the use of systemic thrombolytic agents for treatment of acute pulmonary embolism?
   (a) Age > 75
   (b) Recent arthroscopic knee surgery (6 weeks ago)
   (c) Recent ischemic stroke (8 weeks ago)
   (d) Pregnant (second trimester)
   (e) Diabetic retinopathy
6. Which of the following patient characteristics is *not* a reason to choose warfarin over a direct oral anticoagulant?
   (a) Severe renal dysfunction
   (b) Frequent travel
   (c) Obesity (body weight over 100 kg)
   (d) Need for dual antiplatelet therapy
   (e) Concern for medication nonadherence

Self-Assessment Answers

1. (e) Apixaban 10 mg twice a day

   Acute treatment for DVT should be warfarin + unfractionated heparin or LMWH, unfractionated heparin or LMWH for 5–10 days prior to dabigatran or edoxaban therapy, apixaban 10 mg twice a day for 7 days, or rivaroxaban 15 mg twice a day for 21 days.
2. (d) Rivaroxaban 15 mg twice a day

   Although many DOAC medication doses are reduced for patients with moderate renal insufficiency when used for stroke prevention in atrial fibrillation, there is no dose reduction when using these medications for acute VTE treatment. Additionally, warfarin should be administered with treatment (not prophylactic) doses of LMWH for acute VTE treatment.
3. (b) Enoxaparin

   Enoxaparin (or another LMWH) is first-line therapy for patients with cancer-associated VTE.
4. (d) D-dimer

   The D-dimer test can be used to predict recurrence of VTE. It has been used in conjunction with other clinical variables in a number of risk prediction models, such as Men and HERDOO2.
5. (c) Recent ischemic stroke (8 weeks ago)

   Recent ischemic stroke is an absolute contraindication to the use of systemic thrombolysis. Each of the other answer choices is a relative contraindication.
6. (b) Frequent travel

   Warfarin may be preferable to DOAC therapy in patients with severe renal dysfunction due to the renal clearance of most DOAC medications, extremes of body weight due to concerns with DOAC drug levels and distribution at high/low body weights, and concomitant use with dual antiplatelet therapy as there are currently limited data supporting safety and efficacy with full-dose DOAC therapies, and patients who may have nonadherence issues since the DOAC medications have a short half-life and cannot be easily monitored. Patients with frequent travel may find DOAC medication preferable to warfarin as there is no regular laboratory monitoring or dietary restriction with these medications.

References

1. Goldhaber SZ. Risk factors for venous thromboembolism. J Am Coll Cardiol. 2010;56(1):1–7.
2. The Surgeon General's Call to Action to Prevent Deep Vein Thrombosis and Pulmonary Embolism. Rockville (MD). 2008. https://www.ncbi.nlm.nih.gov/pubmed/20669525.
3. Writing Group M, Mozaffarian D, Benjamin EJ, et al. Heart disease and stroke statistics-2016 update: a report from the American Heart Association. Circulation. 2016;133(4):e38–360.
4. Spyropoulos AC, Hurley JS, Ciesla GN, de Lissovoy G. Management of acute proximal deep vein thrombosis: pharmacoeconomic evaluation of outpatient treatment with enoxaparin vs inpatient treatment with unfractionated heparin. Chest. 2002;122(1):108–14.
5. De Martino RR, Wallaert JB, Rossi AP, Zbehlik AJ, Suckow B, Walsh DB. A meta-analysis of anticoagulation for calf deep venous thrombosis. J Vasc Surg. 2012;56(1):228–37. e221; discussion 236-227.
6. Palareti G. How I treat isolated distal deep vein thrombosis (IDDVT). Blood. 2014;123(12):1802–9.
7. Kearon C, Akl EA, Comerota AJ, et al. Antithrombotic therapy for VTE disease: antithrombotic therapy and prevention of thrombosis, 9th ed: American College of Chest Physicians Evidence-Based Clinical Practice Guidelines. Chest. 2012;141(2 Suppl):e419S–94S.
8. Brandjes DP, Heijboer H, Buller HR, de Rijk M, Jagt H, ten Cate JW. Acenocoumarol and heparin compared with acenocoumarol alone in the initial treatment of proximal-vein thrombosis. N Engl J Med. 1992;327(21):1485–9.
9. Schulman S, Kearon C, Kakkar AK, et al. Dabigatran versus warfarin in the treatment of acute venous thromboembolism. N Engl J Med. 2009;361(24):2342–52.
10. Bauersachs R, Berkowitz SD, Brenner B, et al. Oral rivaroxaban for symptomatic venous thromboembolism. N Engl J Med. 2010;363(26):2499–510.
11. Buller HR, Prins MH, Lensin AW, et al. Oral rivaroxaban for the treatment of symptomatic pulmonary embolism. N Engl J Med. 2012;366(14):1287–97.
12. Agnelli G, Buller HR, Cohen A, et al. Oral apixaban for the treatment of acute venous thromboembolism. N Engl J Med. 2013;369(9):799–808.
13. Hokusai VTEI, Buller HR, Decousus H, et al. Edoxaban versus warfarin for the treatment of symptomatic venous thromboembolism. N Engl J Med. 2013;369(15):1406–15.
14. Kearon C, Akl EA, Ornelas J, et al. Antithrombotic therapy for VTE disease: CHEST guideline and expert panel report. Chest. 2016;149(2):315–52.
15. Streiff MB, Agnelli G, Connors JM, et al. Guidance for the treatment of deep vein thrombosis and pulmonary embolism. J Thromb Thrombolysis. 2016; 41(1):32–67.
16. Barnes GD, Kanthi Y, Froehlich JB. Venous thromboembolism: predicting recurrence and the need for extended anticoagulation. Vasc Med. 2015;20(2): 143–52.
17. Konstantinides SV, Torbicki A, Agnelli G, et al. 2014 ESC guidelines on the diagnosis and management of acute pulmonary embolism. Eur Heart J. 2014;35(43):3033–69, 3069a-3069k.
18. Jaff MR, McMurtry MS, Archer SL, et al. Management of massive and submassive pulmonary embolism, iliofemoral deep vein thrombosis, and chronic thromboembolic pulmonary hypertension: a scientific statement from the American Heart Association. Circulation. 2011;123(16):1788–830.
19. Meyer G, Vicaut E, Danays T, et al. Fibrinolysis for patients with intermediate-risk pulmonary embolism. N Engl J Med. 2014;370(15):1402–11.
20. Bartel B. Systemic thrombolysis for acute pulmonary embolism. Hosp Pract. 2015;43(1):22–7.
21. Wang C, Zhai Z, Yang Y, et al. Efficacy and safety of low dose recombinant tissue-type plasminogen activator for the treatment of acute pulmonary thromboembolism: a randomized, multicenter, controlled trial. Chest. 2010;137(2):254–62.
22. Sharifi M, Bay C, Skrocki L, Rahimi F, Mehdipour M, Investigators M. Moderate pulmonary embolism treated with thrombolysis (from the "MOPETT" trial). Am J Cardiol. 2013;111(2):273–7.
23. Kucher N, Boekstegers P, Muller OJ, et al. Randomized, controlled trial of ultrasound-assisted catheter-directed thrombolysis for acute intermediate-risk pulmonary embolism. Circulation. 2014;129(4):479–86.
24. Kahn SR, Comerota AJ, Cushman M, et al. The postthrombotic syndrome: evidence-based prevention, diagnosis, and treatment strategies: a scientific statement from the American Heart Association. Circulation. 2014;130(18):1636–61.
25. Enden T, Haig Y, Klow NE, et al. Long-term outcome after additional catheter-directed thrombolysis versus standard treatment for acute iliofemoral deep vein thrombosis (the CaVenT study): a randomised controlled trial. Lancet. 2012;379(9810): 31–8.
26. Stein PD, Matta F, Keyes DC, Willyerd GL. Impact of vena cava filters on in-hospital case fatality rate from pulmonary embolism. Am J Med. 2012; 125(5):478–84.

27. Stein PD, Matta F, Sabra MJ. Case fatality rate with vena cava filters in hospitalized stable patients with cancer and pulmonary embolism. Am J Med. 2013;126(9):819–24.
28. Stein PD, Matta F. Vena cava filters in unstable elderly patients with acute pulmonary embolism. Am J Med. 2014;127(3):222–5.
29. Group PS. Eight-year follow-up of patients with permanent vena cava filters in the prevention of pulmonary embolism: the PREPIC (prevention du Risque d'Embolie Pulmonaire par interruption cave) randomized study. Circulation. 2005;112(3):416–22.
30. Mismetti P, Laporte S, Pellerin O, et al. Effect of a retrievable inferior vena cava filter plus anticoagulation vs anticoagulation alone on risk of recurrent pulmonary embolism: a randomized clinical trial. JAMA. 2015;313(16):1627–35.
31. Weinberg I, Abtahian F, Debiasi R, et al. Effect of delayed inferior vena cava filter retrieval after early initiation of anticoagulation. Am J Cardiol. 2014;113(2):389–94.
32. Kinney TB, Aryafar H, Ray Jr CE, et al. ACR Appropriateness Criteria radiologic management of inferior vena cava filters. Expert panel on interventional radiology. 2012. https://guidelines.gov/summaries/summary/43868. Accessed 1 Dec 2016.
33. Caplin DM, Nikolic B, Kalva SP, et al. Quality improvement guidelines for the performance of inferior vena cava filter placement for the prevention of pulmonary embolism. J Vasc Interv Radiol. 2011;22(11):1499–506.
34. Schulman S, Kakkar AK, Goldhaber SZ, et al. Treatment of acute venous thromboembolism with dabigatran or warfarin and pooled analysis. Circulation. 2014;129(7):764–72.
35. Brown MT, Bussell JK. Medication adherence: WHO cares? Mayo Clin Proc. 2011;86(4):304–14.
36. Prandoni P, Lensing AW, Piccioli A, et al. Recurrent venous thromboembolism and bleeding complications during anticoagulant treatment in patients with cancer and venous thrombosis. Blood. 2002;100(10):3484–8.
37. Lee AY, Levine MN, Baker RI, et al. Low-molecular-weight heparin versus a coumarin for the prevention of recurrent venous thromboembolism in patients with cancer. N Engl J Med. 2003;349(2):146–53.
38. Lee AY, Kamphuisen PW, Meyer G, et al. Tinzaparin vs warfarin for treatment of acute venous thromboembolism in patients with active cancer: a randomized clinical trial. JAMA. 2015;314(7):677–86.
39. Posch F, Konigsbrugge O, Zielinski C, Pabinger I, Ay C. Treatment of venous thromboembolism in patients with cancer: a network meta-analysis comparing efficacy and safety of anticoagulants. Thromb Res. 2015;136(3):582–9.
40. Prandoni P, Lensing AW, Cogo A, et al. The long-term clinical course of acute deep venous thrombosis. Ann Intern Med. 1996;125(1):1–7.
41. Baglin T, Luddington R, Brown K, Baglin C. Incidence of recurrent venous thromboembolism in relation to clinical and thrombophilic risk factors: prospective cohort study. Lancet. 2003;362(9383):523–6.
42. Kyrle PA, Minar E, Bialonczyk C, Hirschl M, Weltermann A, Eichinger S. The risk of recurrent venous thromboembolism in men and women. N Engl J Med. 2004;350(25):2558–63.
43. Kovacs MJ, Kahn SR, Wells PS, et al. Patients with a first symptomatic unprovoked deep vein thrombosis are at higher risk of recurrent venous thromboembolism than patients with a first unprovoked pulmonary embolism. J Thromb Haemost. 2010;8(9):1926–32.
44. Streiff MB. Predicting the risk of recurrent venous thromboembolism (VTE). J Thromb Thrombolysis. 2015;39(3):353–66.
45. Rodger MA, Kahn SR, Wells PS, et al. Identifying unprovoked thromboembolism patients at low risk for recurrence who can discontinue anticoagulant therapy. CMAJ. 2008;179(5):417–26.
46. Eichinger S, Heinze G, Jandeck LM, Kyrle PA. Risk assessment of recurrence in patients with unprovoked deep vein thrombosis or pulmonary embolism: the Vienna prediction model. Circulation. 2010;121(14):1630–6.
47. Tosetto A, Iorio A, Marcucci M, et al. Predicting disease recurrence in patients with previous unprovoked venous thromboembolism: a proposed prediction score (DASH). J Thromb Haemost. 2012;10(6):1019–25.
48. Rodger MA, Scarvelis D, Kahn SR, et al. Long-term risk of venous thrombosis after stopping anticoagulants for a first unprovoked event: a multi-national cohort. Thromb Res. 2016;143:152–8.
49. Marcucci M, Iorio A, Douketis JD, et al. Risk of recurrence after a first unprovoked venous thromboembolism: external validation of the Vienna prediction model with pooled individual patient data. J Thromb Haemost. 2015;13:775–81.
50. Ruiz-Gimenez N, Suarez C, Gonzalez R, et al. Predictive variables for major bleeding events in patients presenting with documented acute venous thromboembolism. Findings from the RIETE registry. Thromb Haemost. 2008;100(1):26–31.
51. Kearon C, Ginsberg JS, Kovacs MJ, et al. Comparison of low-intensity warfarin therapy with conventional-intensity warfarin therapy for long-term prevention of recurrent venous thromboembolism. N Engl J Med. 2003;349(7):631–9.
52. Ridker PM, Goldhaber SZ, Danielson E, et al. Long-term, low-intensity warfarin therapy for the prevention of recurrent venous thromboembolism. N Engl J Med. 2003;348(15):1425–34.
53. Schulman S, Kearon C, Kakkar AK, et al. Extended use of dabigatran, warfarin, or placebo in venous thromboembolism. N Engl J Med. 2013;368(8):709–18.
54. Agnelli G, Buller HR, Cohen A, et al. Apixaban for extended treatment of venous thromboembolism. N Engl J Med. 2013;368(8):699–708.
55. Weitz JI, Lensing WA, Prins MH, Bauersachs R, Beyer-Westendorf J, Bounameaux H, et al. Rivaroxaban or aspirin for extended treatment of venous thromboembolism. N Engl J Med. 2017;376:1211–22.

56. Carrier M, Rodger MA, Wells PS, Righini M, LEG G. Residual vein obstruction to predict the risk of recurrent venous thromboembolism in patients with deep vein thrombosis: a systematic review and meta-analysis. J Thromb Haemost. 2011;9(6):1119–25.
57. Cosmi B, Legnani C, Cini M, Guazzaloca G, Palareti G. D-dimer and residual vein obstruction as risk factors for recurrence during and after anticoagulation withdrawal in patients with a first episode of provoked deep-vein thrombosis. Thromb Haemost. 2011;105(5):837–45.
58. Kearon C, Spencer FA, O'Keeffe D, et al. D-dimer testing to select patients with a first unprovoked venous thromboembolism who can stop anticoagulant therapy: a cohort study. Ann Intern Med. 2015;162(1):27–34.
59. Timp JF, Lijfering WM, Flinterman LE, et al. Predictive value of factor VIII levels for recurrent venous thrombosis: results from the MEGA follow-up study. J Thromb Haemost. 2015;13(10):1823–32.
60. Becattini C, Agnelli G, Schenone A, et al. Aspirin for preventing the recurrence of venous thromboembolism. N Engl J Med. 2012;366(21):1959–67.
61. Brighton TA, Eikelboom JW, Mann K, et al. Low-dose aspirin for preventing recurrent venous thromboembolism. N Engl J Med. 2012;367(21): 1979–87.
62. Chopra V, Anand S, Hickner A, et al. Risk of venous thromboembolism associated with peripherally inserted central catheters: a systematic review and meta-analysis. Lancet. 2013;382(9889):311–25.
63. Chopra V, Ratz D, Kuhn L, Lopus T, Lee A, Krein S. Peripherally inserted central catheter-related deep vein thrombosis: contemporary patterns and predictors. J Thromb Haemost. 2014;12(6):847–54.
64. Chopra V, Flanders SA, Saint S, et al. The Michigan appropriateness guide for intravenous catheters (MAGIC): results from a multispecialty panel using the RAND/UCLA appropriateness method. Ann Intern Med. 2015;163(6 Suppl):S1–40.
65. Ageno W, Beyer-Westendorf J, Garcia DA, Lazo-Langner A, McBane RD, Paciaroni M. Guidance for the management of venous thrombosis in unusual sites. J Thromb Thrombolysis. 2016;41(1):129–43.
66. Dentali F, Gianni M, Crowther MA, Ageno W. Natural history of cerebral vein thrombosis: a systematic review. Blood. 2006;108(4):1129–34.
67. Ageno W, Riva N, Schulman S, et al. Long-term clinical outcomes of splanchnic vein thrombosis: results of an international registry. JAMA Intern Med. 2015;175(9):1474–80.
68. Group CVOS. Natural history and clinical management of central retinal vein occlusion. The central vein occlusion study group. Arch Ophthalmol. 1997;115(4):486–91.
69. Decousus H, Quere I, Presles E, et al. Superficial venous thrombosis and venous thromboembolism: a large, prospective epidemiologic study. Ann Intern Med. 2010;152(4):218–24.
70. Decousus H, Prandoni P, Mismetti P, et al. Fondaparinux for the treatment of superficial-vein thrombosis in the legs. N Engl J Med. 2010;363(13): 1222–32.
71. Amin AN, Varker H, Princic N, Lin J, Thompson S, Johnston S. Duration of venous thromboembolism risk across a continuum in medically ill hospitalized patients. J Hosp Med. 2012;7:231–8.
72. Cohen AT, Harrington RA, Goldhaber SZ, Hull RD, Wiens BL, Gold A, et al. Extended thromboprophylaxis with betrixaban in acutely ill medical patients. N Engl J Med. 2016;375:534–44.

Thrombophilic States

15

Adriana Guigova and Tony Philip

Clinical Vignette

Mrs. Smith is a 30-year-old African American woman who is referred by her obstetrician for further evaluation of a hypercoagulable state in the setting of unprovoked recurrent venous thromboembolism. Mrs. Smith's pertinent medical history includes an unprovoked right lower extremity deep vein thrombosis (DVT) 2 years ago as well as a history of late pregnancy losses. She denies tobacco use or oral contraceptive use.

On examination she has left lower extremity swelling, minimal erythema, and tenderness to palpation which has much improved since the initiation of warfarin 1 week ago for an acute left femoral DVT. Her blood work prior to initiation of warfarin is notable for an aPTT of 50 s, an INR of 1.2, an elevated D-dimer at 4000 ng/mL, and a normal fibrinogen. Given her age, ethnicity, the nature of her clot, and pertinent laboratory findings, the hematologist considered which selected genetic and acquired hypercoagulable testing would be most appropriate.

Pathophysiology of Venous Thromboembolism

Three principal mechanisms have been identified that contribute to the development of venous thromboembolism: 1. reduced blood flow leading to stasis, 2. inherent blood hypercoagulability, and 3. vascular wall abnormalities/damage. These factors have been termed "Virchow's triad" in honor of Rudolf Virchow, the nineteenth century Austrian pathologist who first theorized that pulmonary embolism was due to an embolic event and not in situ thrombosis. Thrombus formation represents the end result of a disturbance of the normal hemostatic balance that exists between the procoagulant coagulation proteins (e.g., factor VIII, factor X, prothrombin, fibrinogen) and the endogenous anticoagulant proteins (e.g., antithrombin, protein C, protein S) and the fibrinolytic system. Hypercoagulability can result from excessive procoagulant activity (e.g., factor V Leiden, elevated factor VIII levels) or insufficient anticoagulant activity (e.g., antithrombin deficiency) [1].

In the classic "waterfall" or "cascade" model, coagulation is divided into three separate pathways, intrinsic, extrinsic, and common. While it is now known that this classic model does not accurately reflect coagulation in vivo, this model is

A. Guigova · T. Philip (✉)
Division of Hematology/Oncology, Department of Medicine, Zucker School of Medicine at Hofstra/Northwell, Northwell Health,
Lake Success, NY, USA
e-mail: aguigova@northwell.edu; tphilip@northwell.edu

J. F. Lau et al. (eds.), *Anticoagulation Therapy*, https://doi.org/10.1007/978-3-319-73709-6_15

still useful clinically for the interpretation of basic coagulation tests. Coagulation is initiated when factor VIIa binds to tissue factor that is exposed on the subendothelium at sites of vascular injury. The tissue factor-factor VIIa complex activates factor IX and X on the phospholipid-rich surface of activated platelets. In the absence of factor Va, factor Xa inefficiently activates a small amount of prothrombin to form thrombin. Thrombin initiates a critical positive feedback loop activating the critical cofactors VIII and V as well as factor XI. The result is the formation of the tenase complex (factors VIIIa and IXa) and, subsequently, the prothrombinase complex (factor Va and Xa) which lead to thrombin generation followed by fibrin formation as well as factor XI, VIII, and V activation and platelet and factor XIII activation. Ultimately, this series of coordinated chemical reactions leads to the formation of covalently cross-linked fibrin clots which in conjunction with activated platelets form an effective hemostatic plug at the site of vascular injury (Fig. 15.1).

Unopposed, these procoagulant forces would result in pathologic thrombus formation and vascular occlusion. Endogenous anticoagulant proteins and the fibrinolytic system maintain hemostatic balance by opposing the action of the procoagulant proteins. The most important endogenous anticoagulant proteins are antithrombin, protein C, and protein S. Antithrombin functions as an anticoagulant by forming an inhibitory complex with its serine protease targets (factor IIa [thrombin] and factor Xa as well as factors XIIa, XIa, IXa, and kallikrein) that is removed from the circulation by the liver. Antithrombin's activity is accelerated several thousandfold by endogenous and exogenous glycosaminoglycans such as heparins which underlies the anticoagulant activity of unfractionated and low-molecular-weight heparin. In an example of the human body's ingenious design, protein C is activated by thrombin bound to thrombomodulin, a thrombin receptor protein expressed on the surface of intact endothelium. Activated protein C in conjunction with its cofactor protein S inactivates factors Va and VIIIa on platelet and endothelial cell surfaces down regulating thrombin generation. When this balance between positive and negative regulators of the coagulation cascade is disturbed, then thrombosis or bleeding occurs.

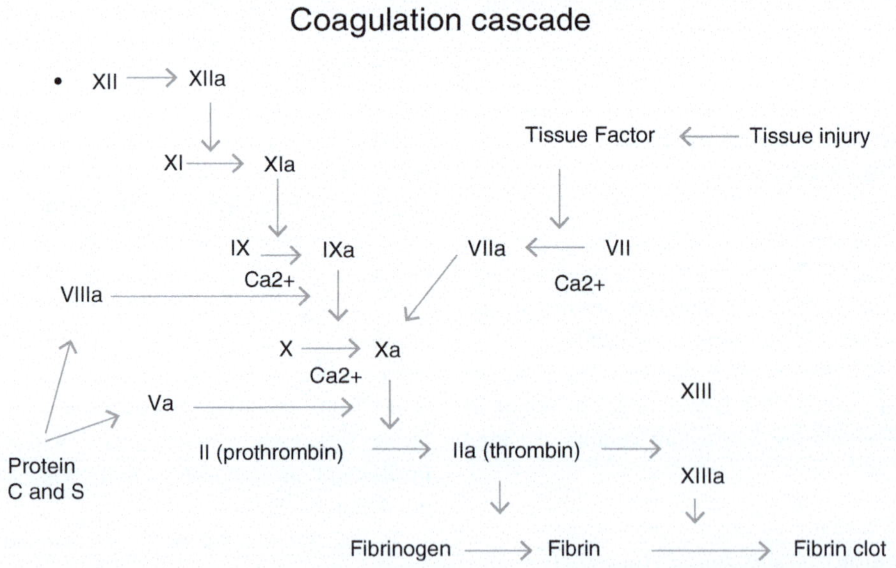

Fig. 15.1 The coagulation cascade is a physiologically complex step-by-step process that happens in vivo when blood vessel injury occurs. The intrinsic pathway is initiated upon contact between blood and exposed negatively charged surfaces, while the extrinsic pathway begins upon vascular injury which leads to exposure of tissue factor (TF). Both pathways then converge to convert factor X to Xa. Active factor Xa then activates prothrombin to thrombin so that it can convert fibrinogen to fibrin leading to the formation of fibrin clot

Inherited Thrombophilia

Factor V Leiden

Factor V Leiden (FVL), the most common inherited thrombophilia, results from a G1691A point mutation in the factor V gene that leads to an arginine to glutamine substitution at position 506 of the factor V protein. This mutation disrupts the site where activated protein C cleaves and inactivates the activated form of factor V leading to the phenotype of "activated protein C resistance." Activated protein C also cleaves factor V which functions as a cofactor in the inactivation of factor VIIIa. Consequently, these changes prolong the half-lives of factors Va and VIIIa thereby increasing thrombin generation. It has been hypothesized that centuries ago when the FVL mutation first arose, carriers may have had an evolutionary advantage over non-carriers by virtue of a lower risk for fatal postpartum hemorrhage among women carrying the mutation. This hypothesis is supported by the observation that hemophilia patients who are heterozygous for FVL have a less severe bleeding phenotype [2].

The FVL mutation is inherited in an autosomal dominant fashion. It is important to note that FVL is not the only cause of activated protein C resistance. It can also be acquired and lead to increased risk of thrombosis. FVL is more common in Caucasians where it affects approximately 5% of the population and is less common in Hispanic Americans (2%) and African Americans (1.2%). The activated protein C resistance assay is the best screening test for FVL. Confirmatory genetic testing is performed for positive results. FVL can be inherited in a heterozygous or homozygous fashion. FVL heterozygotes are at a fourfold greater risk for initial venous thromboembolism (VTE) (odds ratio [OR] 4.2; 95% CI 3.4–53), while homozygotes are at 11-fold greater risk (OR 11.5; 95% CI 6.8–19.3) as compared to the general population [3]. The risk of recurrence is modestly increased for FVL heterozygotes (OR 1.4; 95% CI 1.1–1.8) [4]. When combined with other congenital and acquired risk factors, FVL is associated with a synergistic increase in risk for initial VTE. FVL heterozygotes who use combined estrogen-progesterone-containing oral contraceptives are 35-fold more likely to develop VTE than FVL-negative nonusers. The odds ratio for VTE is 20 for compound heterozygotes for both the FVL and G20210A prothrombin gene mutations. FVL is associated with a greater risk for DVT than PE. FVL does not appear to be associated with a significant increased risk of arterial thromboembolism [5, 6].

Prothrombin 20210 Gene Mutation

The prothrombin gene G20210A mutation (PGM) is inherited in autosomal dominant fashion. This point mutation in the 3' untranslated region of the factor II gene increases the efficiency of mRNA translation or the stability of the mRNA transcript leading to a 30% increase in circulating prothrombin protein levels. Most patients are heterozygous for the mutation with very few being homozygous. The PGM is the second most common inherited risk factor for venous thrombosis. It is primarily seen in Caucasians where its prevalence varies from 1–6% with an average of 2%. PGM is identified by genetic testing [7]. The risk of thrombosis in heterozygotes for the PGM is three- to fourfold that of the general population. The risk of thrombosis is higher in homozygous PGM; however, there are insufficient data to generate a reliable estimate. It remains unclear whether the PGM is associated with an increased risk of recurrent VTE. PGM is predominantly a risk factor for venous thromboembolism, and it is associated with venous thrombosis in unusual sites. Interestingly, the PGM has been associated with an increased risk of ischemic stroke in patients younger than 50 years of age with no history of diabetes, hypertension, or hyperlipidemia. In one study, up to 15% of these patients had the PGM, therefore testing for the PGM should be considered in patients with this clinical presentation. PGM has also been associated with an increased risk of myocardial infarction, especially in setting of smoking [8–10].

Protein C Deficiency

Protein C deficiency is present in a small minority of patients with VTE (<5%). Its prevalence is about 1.2% in the general population, and it has no racial predisposition [1, 11, 12]. Protein C is a vitamin K-dependent protein zymogen that is produced in the liver and is converted to activated protein C by thrombin bound to thrombomodulin expressed on intact endothelial cells. Activated protein C in a complex with cofactor protein S inactivates factors Va and VIIIa. Protein C deficiency is inherited in autosomal dominant fashion and increases the risk of predominantly venous thromboembolism by five- to tenfold.

There are two types of protein C deficiency. Type I protein C deficiency is characterized by mutations that result in reduced protein C synthesis, while type II protein C deficiency is due to mutations that result in the production of dysfunctional protein C molecules with reduced protein function. Type I deficiency is most commonly caused by missense or nonsense mutations that lead to low protein C activity and antigen levels. Type II deficiency is caused by mutations that affect the amino acid sequence of protein C leading to a dysfunctional protein characterized by low protein C activity but normal protein C antigen levels. Patients with protein C deficiency typically have protein C activity levels approximately 50% of normal. Protein C deficiency is characterized by considerable phenotypic variation between carriers with similar levels leading experts to believe that there are additional factors that lead to thromboembolism in symptomatic patients [1, 11, 13, 14].

The protein C activity (functional) assay is the most specific and sensitive test for the diagnosis of protein C deficiency since it is reduced in patients with either type I or type II protein C deficiency. A prothrombin time (PT) should always be checked when protein C activity is measured to ensure that vitamin K deficiency (or vitamin K antagonist therapy) is not present as these conditions would lead to false-positive test results. In patients with a low protein C activity, a protein C antigen test can be performed to determine whether type I or II deficiency is present. In patients with type I protein C deficiency, both protein C activity and antigen level will be low, while patients with type II protein C deficiency will have a low protein C activity but a normal antigen level. Since there are over 150 different mutations that can result in protein C deficiency, a DNA-based assay is impractical at present for diagnosis [1, 11, 13].

Acquired protein C deficiency is commonly seen in patients with acute thrombosis, vitamin K antagonist therapy, and liver disease. The range of normal protein C levels in the general population varies significantly. Because it is common to have transiently low values particularly in association with acute thrombosis, it is important to check the assay in the absence of active thromboembolism or vitamin K antagonist therapy. In the absence of an acquired cause, a protein C level below 55% is very likely to be consistent with true deficiency, whereas levels from 55 to 65% can be also due to normal variation in the general population [4]. Protein C deficiency is associated with a five- to tenfold increased risk of VTE compared to the general population. The risk of recurrent VTE is also higher with 37% of patients suffering a recurrent event within 5 years of discontinuation of anticoagulation [14]. It is unclear whether protein C deficiency increases the risk of arterial thromboembolism [15].

Protein S Deficiency

Protein S deficiency is inherited in an autosomal dominant fashion. It is due to a mutation in the PROS1 gene located on chromosome 3, and the majority of patients are heterozygous. Protein S is a vitamin K-dependent protein, and it is synthesized by hepatocytes, endothelial cells, and megakaryocytes. Protein S exists in two different forms, as an unbound (or free) protein and in a complex with complement factor C4b-binding protein. In normal plasma, about 60% of protein S is complex bound and 40% is free. Free protein S is a cofactor of activated protein C that inactivates factors Va and VIIIa [16].

There are three types of protein S deficiency. Type I protein S deficiency is a quantitative deficiency state where both the total and free protein S antigen levels are decreased resulting in reduced protein S activity. The total protein S antigen is approximately 50% of normal, and free protein S antigen can be as low as 15% of normal. In type II protein S deficiency, there is a qualitative defect that leads to production of a dysfunctional protein leading to low protein S activity but normal free and total protein S antigen levels. It is rare. Type III protein S deficiency results from mutations that disrupt the equilibrium between free and bound protein S resulting in disproportionate reductions in free protein S reflected in low free protein S antigen levels but normal levels of total protein S antigen. Since free protein S is the principal form responsible for its anticoagulant activity, protein S activity is also reduced. The majority of known protein S mutations lead to type I or type III protein S deficiency (Table 15.1) [1, 8, 13, 17–20].

Protein S activity assays are notoriously sensitive to pre-analytical variables. Therefore, many experts recommend using the free protein S antigen level to screen for protein S deficiency. The protein S activity assay has the advantage of being a sensitive screening test that will identify all three types of protein S deficiency. However, if the protein S activity results are abnormal, it is important to confirm them with repeat testing and use free and total protein S antigen levels to determine the subtype of protein S deficiency. In patients with type I protein S deficiency, the protein S activity level and the protein S total and free antigen levels are low. In type II protein S deficiency, the activity level is low but the total and free protein S antigen levels are normal. In type III protein S deficiency, the protein S activity and the free protein S antigen are low, but the total antigen is normal, reflecting a mutation that shifts the balance of protein S preferentially toward the less active form of protein S bound to C4b-binding protein (Table 15.1). Falsely low protein S activity can be seen with high factor VIII levels, the FVL mutation, or in the presence of a lupus anticoagulant. Protein S levels are low in the setting of estrogen therapy, pregnancy, liver disease, nephrotic syndrome, DIC, inflammatory disorders, and therapy with vitamin K antagonists [21].

In studies of symptomatic probands and their families, protein S deficiency has been associated with a 31-fold increased risk of VTE compared to unaffected family members. The cumulative risk of recurrent VTE after discontinuation of anticoagulation was 40% at 5 years in this family study [22]. In contrast, the MEGA population-based case-control study of patients with a first episode of VTE found that only very low free protein S antigen levels (<33 U/dL) were associated with an increased risk of VTE. Only eight patients (0.4% of the total patient population) were in this subgroup. These data emphasize that protein S deficiency is a rare cause of VTE in unselected patients with VTE [23]. Protein S deficiency is an uncommon finding in young patients with stroke [24]. A prospective cohort study found no association between protein S deficiency and stroke [1, 14, 18, 25].

Antithrombin Deficiency

Antithrombin (AT) is a proteinase inhibitor that binds and inhibits the activated serine proteases factors IIa (thrombin), Xa, IXa, XIa, and XIIa. It is inherited in an autosomal dominant fashion, and more than 130 different genetic mutations have been identified. Antithrombin deficiency is a rare inherited thrombophilia that affects 0.02–0.2% of the general population. There are two types of AT deficiency: type I, which is characterized by a reduction in AT activity and antigen levels, and type II, which results in abnormal AT

Table 15.1 Protein S deficiency and the results of protein S testing

Protein S assay	Free PS antigen	Total PS antigen	PS activity
Type I = quantitative	Decreased	Decreased	Decreased
Type II = qualitative	Normal	Normal	Decreased
Type III = quantitative	Decreased	Normal	Decreased

activity despite normal antigen levels (due to a mutation that interferes with function but not production).

Type I AT deficiency is caused by small or large deletions, insertions, or single base substitutions. These mutations lead to reduced synthesis of AT protein causing roughly equivalent reductions in AT activity and antigen. Type II deficiency is caused by mutations in the coding sequence of the protein that result in production of normal amounts of a dysfunctional AT protein. Mutations can affect the thrombin-binding region at the carboxy-terminal end of the protein, the heparin-binding region on the amino-terminal end, and general pleotropic defects. The majority of deficiencies that are identified are type II defects, particularly heparin-binding defects. Type II AT deficiency due to heparin-binding defects is not considered to be highly thrombogenic [1, 13, 14, 18].

When testing for AT deficiency, a functional assay is preferred as it allows for identification of quantitative (type I AT deficiency) and qualitative defects (type II AT deficiency). If the AT activity assay is abnormal, then an AT antigen assay can be performed to determine if the patient has type I or type II AT deficiency. In patients with type II AT deficiency, mutations can affect the thrombin- or heparin-binding sites. AT activity assays performed in the absence or presence of heparin can be used to determine if the mutation affects the thrombin- or heparin-binding site. The normal range for the AT activity assay is 80–120%. In patients with heterozygous AT deficiency, activity and/or antigen levels are typically in the range of 40–60%. Homozygous AT deficiency is thought to be incompatible with survival [26, 27].

One can see acquired AT deficiency in patients with sepsis, DIC, acute thrombosis, heparin therapy, liver disease, nephrotic syndrome, L-asparaginase chemotherapy, and acute fatty liver of pregnancy [1, 13, 18–20].

AT deficiency is associated with a high risk of VTE. In a large retrospective family cohort study, the annual risk of VTE was 1.8%. However, it is important to note the type of mutation that is present, particularly in patients with type II AT deficiency. Among patients with heparin-binding site defects, the prevalence of VTE is only 6%, whereas the prevalence of VTE is 58% among patients with thrombin-binding site defects. There is a risk of recurrent thrombosis in setting of no anticoagulation as high as 10–17% per year [1, 13, 14, 18]. Venous thromboembolism is the most common clinical manifestation of AT deficiency. Arterial thrombosis occurs less often.

Factor VIII

As far back as 1995, elevated factor VIII levels were identified as a risk factor for venous thromboembolism. In the Leiden Thrombophilia Study, Koster and colleagues [28] noted that factor VIII concentrations >150 international units/dL were associated with nearly a fivefold risk of VTE (adjusted odds ratio of 4.8 [95% Cl 2.3–10.0]). Nearly 25% of unselected thrombosis patients had elevated factor VIII levels making this one of the more common thrombophilic conditions. Several years later [29], Kraaijenhagen and colleagues confirmed this association and noted that 33% of thrombosis patients had factor VIII activity above 175%. In the Austrian Study of Recurrent Venous Thromboembolism (AUREC), Kyrle and colleagues [30] found that elevated factor VIII levels were also a risk factor for recurrent VTE. The relative risk of recurrent venous thrombosis was 1.08 (95% confidence interval, 1.04–1.12; $P < 0.001$) for each 10 IU/dL increase in the factor VIII level. Compared to patients with lower levels, patients with factor VIII levels above the 90th percentile were nearly sevenfold more likely to suffer recurrent VTE (adjusted relative risk 6.7 [95% CI 3.0–14.8]). It is important to note, however, that factor VIII levels can vary substantially in the presence of systemic inflammatory disorders, older age, liver disease, and non-ABO blood group O. Therefore, the clinical utility of factor VIII levels in patients with thrombosis remains controversial so patients should be evaluated on an individual basis to determine if factor VIII testing is worthwhile.

Dysfibrinogenemia

Dysfibrinogenemia is an inherited thrombophilia due to a mutation in the gene for one of fibrinogen's polypeptide chains that leads to a qualitative defect. The hereditary dysfibrinogenemias represent a group of abnormalities that can range from being completely asymptomatic to clinically significant thrombosis, bleeding, or both bleeding and thrombosis. Normally, fibrinopeptides are released from fibrinogen by thrombin proteolysis leading to the formation of fibrin monomers. Fibrin monomers then polymerize to form a fibrin polymer that is held together by hydrostatic bonds. Factor XIIIa (a transglutaminase that is activated by thrombin) then catalyzes the formation of covalent bonds between fibrin monomers leading to a stabilized fibrin clot. The clearance of fibrin clot is controlled via plasmin-dependent proteolysis. Patients with dysfibrinogenemia have inherited defects which impair fibrin polymer formation or dissolution that can lead to bleeding or thrombosis.

Hereditary thrombotic dysfibrinogenemia is rare cause of venous and less commonly arterial thromboembolism with a prevalence of 0.8% among patients with venous thromboembolism. Patients typically present with venous thromboembolism in the late 20s to early 30s with a mean age of presentation of 27 years. Approximately 30% of patients with dysfibrinogenemia suffer thrombotic events before age 50 [13, 14].

The best screening tests for dysfibrinogenemia are the thrombin time (prolonged by heparin) or the reptilase time (unaffected by heparin in the sample) or a functional fibrinogen assay such as the Clauss fibrinogen assay. In the presence of reduced functional fibrinogen levels, the thrombin time and the reptilase time will be prolonged and the functional fibrinogen level will be below the normal range (often below 100 mg/dL). To confirm the presence of dysfibrinogenemia, a fibrinogen antigen test (which measures the amount of fibrinogen protein but not its function) should be sent. In patients with dysfibrinogenemia, the fibrinogen antigen will be normal or low (patients with low fibrinogen antigens most accurately labeled as hypodysfibrinogenemia) but significantly higher than the functional fibrinogen test results. Precise molecular diagnosis is only available in select research laboratories. Since the PT is prolonged by reductions in fibrinogen, it is important to correlate the PT/international normalized ratio (INR) with chromogenic factor X activity assays or factor X activity assays (INR of 2–3 should correlate with factor X activity of 20–40%) to ensure that patients on warfarin are actually therapeutic when their INR is 2–3. Failure to recognize this characteristic abnormality has resulted in recurrent thromboembolism in some patients with dysfibrinogenemia.

Homocysteine and MTHFR

Severe hyperhomocysteinemia (homocysteine levels >200 μmol/L) is generally caused by the congenital metabolic disorder, homocystinuria, which is characterized by homozygous mutations in the cystathionine beta-synthetase gene which converts homocysteine to cysteine via the transsulfuration pathway (see Fig. 15.2). Associated abnormalities in patients with homocystinuria include marfanoid body habitus, severe myopia, ectopia lentis, intellectual disability, and recurrent arterial or venous thrombotic events. Homocysteine is also metabolized to methionine by methionine synthetase, a reaction that requires vitamin B12 as a cofactor as well as 5-methyltetrahydrofolate. The methylenetetrahydrofolate reductase (MTHFR) enzyme is required for regeneration of 5-methyltetrahydrofolate from 5,10-*N*-methylenetetrahydrofolate. Consequently, vitamin B12 and folate deficiency are associated with hyperhomocysteinemia to a variable degree and therefore these deficiency states should be excluded in patients diagnosed with hyperhomocysteinemia. Thermolabile mutations in the MTHFR gene (C677T or A1298C) are common genetic changes that are associated with mild to moderate hyperhomocysteinemia. The heterozygous C677T mutation is present in about 35% of the general population, and 12% are homozygous, mostly Caucasian. Heterozygous A1298C is present in 9–20% of most ethnic populations. Elevated homocysteine levels can be found in homozygous C677T mutation or heterozygous

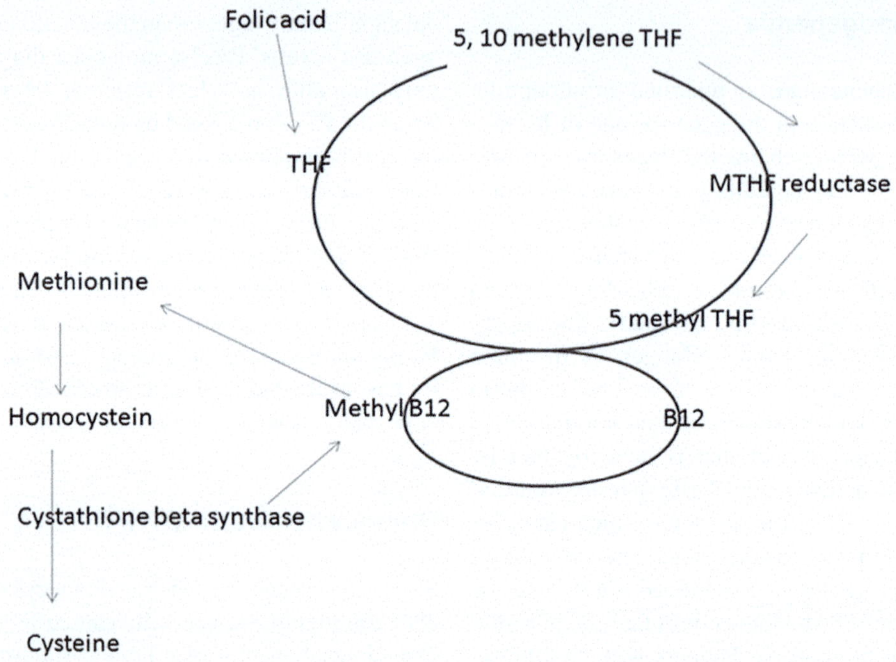

Fig. 15.2 Homocystinuria results from the accumulation of homocysteine and its metabolites when there is a disruption of any of the three pathways (deficiency in the cystathionine beta-synthase enzyme, defective methylcobalamin synthesis, or abnormality in MTHFR) involved in methionine metabolism. Methylenetetrahydrofolate reductase (MTHFR), tetrahydrofolate (THF)

C677T plus A1298C mutations. Mild to moderate hyperhomocysteinemia has been identified as an independent risk factor for arterial and venous thromboembolism [14, 17, 31].

It is not clear if homocysteine levels alone are the pathogenic factor in the thrombotic predisposition noted in patients with mild to moderate hyperhomocysteinemia. In the HOPE-2 placebo-controlled randomized clinical trial which randomly assigned 5522 patients to folate, vitamin B12, and pyridoxine or placebo, the VTE incidence was the same in both arms. Consequently, elevated homocysteine levels may not be the cause of thrombosis but rather a marker of increased risk for thrombotic events [32].

Therefore, there is no indication to screen for MTHFR mutations or treat mild-moderate hyperhomocysteinemia as lowering homocysteine levels does not affect the risk of thromboembolism [11]. One important exception would be in young patients suspected to have homocystinuria in whom treatment of high levels of homocysteine is recommended [11].

Acquired Thrombophilia

Antiphospholipid Antibody Syndrome

Antiphospholipid antibodies are acquired antibodies that target phospholipids and phospholipid-binding proteins. These proteins include beta-2 glycoprotein 1 and prothrombin. Antiphospholipid antibody syndrome is typically associated with venous or arterial thrombosis as well as pregnancy loss. In order to fulfill criteria for the antiphospholipid antibody syndrome (APS), the patient must have clinical manifestations (objectively confirmed venous or arterial thrombosis, one or more late fetal losses [second or third trimester], or three or more first-trimester losses) and consistently positive laboratory tests separated by at least 12 weeks [33]. Laboratory criteria include 1. elevated IgG or IgM anti-beta-2 glycoprotein 1 antibodies (greater than 99th percentile), 2. elevated IgG or IgM cardiolipin antibodies (greater than 99th percentile or 40 GPL or MPL units, respectively), and 3. presence of a lupus inhibitor (abnormal phospholipid-dependent coagulation test such as the dilute Russell viper venom time). False-positive lupus inhibitor test results can be seen in the presence of vitamin K antagonist therapy and oral direct factor Xa inhibitors such as apixaban, edoxaban, or rivaroxaban. Antibody tests that have not been established to be associated with clinical manifestations and therefore do not fulfill criteria for APS include elevated IgA cardiolipin or anti-beta-2 glycoprotein 1 antibodies, anti-phosphatidylserine antibodies, anti-phosphatidylethanolamine antibodies, and anti-phosphatidylinositol antibodies [1, 12, 14, 34, 35].

Table 15.2 APS diagnostic criteria summary [1, 14, 34, 35]

- Laboratory criteria
  - Lupus anticoagulant
  - Elevated cardiolipin antibody levels (IgG or IgM) High titer: >40 gpl/mpl or 99th percentile
  - Beta-2 glycoprotein 1 antibodies (IgG or IgM) 99th percentile

Abnormal tests confirmed on 2 or more occasions, >12 weeks apart

- Clinical criteria
  - Vascular thrombosis/microvascular thrombosis
  - Pregnancy morbidity
  - Clinical manifestations include immune thrombocytopenia and livedo reticularis

Antiphospholipid antibodies are frequently found in patients with systemic lupus erythematosus (SLE). The antibodies can be identified in as many as 50% of SLE patients and 40% of SLE patients fulfill criteria for APS. In the general population, the prevalence of antiphospholipid antibodies is 1–5% [18, 36]. Antiphospholipid antibodies can also be found in conjunction with infections such as syphilis; however these antibodies are generally transient and not typically associated with thromboembolism.

It is important to recognize that lupus inhibitors can influence the results of PT testing depending upon the reagent used to perform the test. Therefore, PT/INR results should be correlated with a chromogenic factor X activity assay (therapeutic range 20–40% factor X activity correlates with an INR of 2–3 in the absence of a lupus inhibitor) to ensure that the standard INR range of 2–3 represents a therapeutic level of warfarin. In patients with lupus inhibitors that influence the INR, the therapeutic range should be chosen based upon the chromogenic factor X activity therapeutic range. Once the appropriate INR range is identified, then periodic correlations of the INR with the chromogenic factor X activity should be performed because the titer of lupus inhibitors can change over time. If the INR does not appear to be influenced by the lupus inhibitor, then the INR can be used to manage warfarin therapy without periodic chromogenic factor X activity assays. If the laboratory changes its PT/INR reagent, another correlation between the INR with the new reagent and a chromogenic factor X activity assays should be performed to ensure the new reagent is not significantly influenced by the patient's lupus inhibitor. In many instances, lupus inhibitors significantly influence point of care INR results so venipuncture samples should be used to monitor the INR in these patients.

Unlike many thrombophilic conditions, APS is associated with arterial and venous thromboembolism. Among APS laboratory tests, lupus inhibitors are associated with a highest risk of thromboembolism followed by beta 2 glycoprotein I antibodies and then cardiolipin antibodies. IgG beta 2 glycoprotein antibodies and cardiolipin antibodies are associated with greater risk than IgM antibodies. Patients with triple positivity (lupus inhibitors as well as cardiolipin and beta-2 glycoprotein 1 antibodies) appear to have the highest risk of thromboembolism. APS patients are thought to be at high risk for recurrent thromboembolism, so lifelong anticoagulation is recommended (Table 15.2).

Myeloproliferative Neoplasms

Essential thrombocythemia (ET) and polycythemia vera (PV) are two myeloproliferative neoplasms that are commonly associated with venous and/or arterial thromboembolism. They are both associated with a high risk for thrombosis. Arterial thrombosis is more common than venous thrombosis. ET and PV are often associated with gain-of-function mutations in JAK2. JAK2 is a tyrosine kinase involved in JAK-STAT intracellular signaling pathway associated with growth factor receptors. The most common JAK2 mutation is the JAK2 V617F mutation that results from the substitution of valine for phenylalanine at codon 617. This mutation is found in 97% of patients with PV and in 50% of patient with ET, where it is heterozygous. A few patients (3%) with PV have exon 12 mutations in JAK2 [37].

PV is a disease primarily of adults with a median age at diagnosis of 60 years. The incidence of PV has been estimated to be 1.9/100,000 per year. The incidence of PV is higher in men (2.8 cases per 100,000) than in women (1.3 cases/100,000 per year) [38]. The thrombotic risk in polycythemia vera (PV) is thought to be predominantly due to hyperviscosity associated with the elevated red cell mass [11]. The risk of thrombosis is significantly reduced by phlebotomy to a goal hematocrit below 45% in men and 42% in women. The chance of developing arterial thrombosis is about 16% and venous thrombosis is about 7% in patients with polycythemia vera. Bleeding associated with PV is typically seen in patients with extreme thrombocytosis (platelet counts in excess of 1,000,000/μL) which can cause acquired type 2 von Willebrand disease due to accelerated clearance of high molecular weight multimers by the increased numbers of abnormal platelets. Platelet cytoreduction can reverse the bleeding diathesis.

The diagnosis of PV is characterized by a constellation of clinical symptoms and signs and laboratory abnormalities. Early diagnosis is essential to avoid preventable morbidity and mortality due to thromboembolism. Common clinical symptoms and signs include headache, dizziness, visual disturbances, aquagenic pruritus (especially after hot showers), early satiety due to splenomegaly, and a ruddy or plethoric complexion or complications such as thrombosis (particularly in unusual locations such as hepatic or portal veins or cerebral venous sinuses) or bleeding. Some patients will complain of burning dysesthesias in the dorsum of the hands or feet associated with warmth and erythema.

Laboratory findings of PV often include panmyelosis manifested as leukocytosis, thrombocytosis, and erythrocytosis. Erythrocytosis is also commonly seen in other disorders associated with tissue hypoxia including smoking, sleep apnea, severe pulmonary disease, congenital cyanotic heart disease, and high-affinity hemoglobinopathies. Exogenous androgen use and rare disorders of erythropoietin synthesis such as Chuvash polycythemia and erythropoietin-secreting tumors (e.g., renal cell carcinoma, hepatocellular carcinoma, hemangioblastoma) should also be considered in select cases.

Absolute erythrocytosis is likely to be present in women when the hemoglobin concentration exceeds 16.5 g/dL and in men when the hemoglobin concentration exceeds 18.5 g/dL [11]. Leukocytosis and thrombocytosis can be seen in inflammatory or infectious disorders as well as other myeloproliferative neoplasms such as ET and chronic myeloid leukemia. PV is often (but not always) associated with a reduction in erythropoietin since red cell production is erythropoietin-independent. The diagnosis of PV is typically confirmed by the presence of the JAK2 V617F mutation which is present in 97% of patients with PV. The remainders have mutations in JAK2 exon 12. For most patients with PV, the constellation of panmyelosis with or without splenomegaly, aquagenic pruritus, erythromelalgia, or plethora in conjunction with the JAK2 mutation confirms the diagnosis.

If available, nuclear medicine red cell volume and plasma volume studies provide useful confirmatory evidence of absolute erythrocytosis characteristic of PV. Red cell volume/plasma volume studies use dilutions of radiolabeled red cells and albumin to directly measure the red cell and plasma volume. These are very useful diagnostic tests that can facilitate identification of different causes of erythrocytosis. Red cell volume/plasma volume studies can differentiate between relative erythrocytosis (increase in hematocrit and hemoglobin due to reduction in the plasma volume) and absolute erythrocytosis (as the term suggests an absolute increase in the red cell volume). PV is characterized by an increased red cell volume and normal or elevated plasma volume. In contrast, secondary causes of absolute erythrocytosis (hypoxia due to smoking or sleep apnea, excess erythropoietin production due to tumors or congenital disorders such as Chuvash polycythemia or erythropoietin signaling, or receptor defects or androgen excess) are characterized by reductions in plasma volume in the presence of an elevated red cell volume. Relative erythrocytosis (e.g., dehydration) is characterized by a normal red cell volume and reduced plasma volume. The incidence of essential thrombocythemia (ET) in the United States is approximately 2.5 cases/100,000 population per year; this means approximately 6000 people are diagnosed each year as having ET. The median age at diagnosis is 60 years although 20% of cases are diagnosed before 40 years of age. ET occurs more frequently in women by a ratio of 2:1. Presenting symptoms vary largely but include headache, lightheadedness, syncope, atypical chest pain, acral paresthesia, livedo reticularis, burning pain of the hands or feet associated with erythema and warmth, or a complete absence of symptoms. Thrombotic events can include stroke, retinal artery or venous occlusions, coronary artery ischemia, deep vein thrombosis/pulmonary embolism, and hepatic or portal vein thrombosis. In an international multicenter study of 891 ET patients, the rate of fatal and nonfatal thrombotic events was 1.9 per 100 patient years [39]. Risk factors for arterial thrombosis included age >60, a history of previous thrombosis, the presence of cardiovascular risk factors, a white blood cell count >11,000/μL, and the presence of the JAK2 V617F mutation. Male gender was associated with venous thrombosis. The rate of major bleeding in ET occurs at a rate of 0.79% of patients per year. Risk factors for bleeding include leukocytosis, previous hemorrhage, and aspirin therapy [40]. Extreme thrombocytosis (platelet counts exceeding 1,000,000/μL) can also be associated with acquired type 2 von Willebrand disease in patients with ET and increase the risk of bleeding similar to patients with PV.

Paroxysmal Nocturnal Hemoglobinuria (PNH)

PNH is characterized by acquired mutations in the PIGA gene whose protein product is responsible for the synthesis of glycosylphosphatidylinositol anchors that link proteins such as CD59 and CD55 to the surface of red cells, white cells, and platelets. CD59 and CD55 are complement defense proteins that prevent hemolysis and activation of platelets. Clinical manifestations of PNH include intra- and extravascular hemolysis, recurrent thrombosis, and bone marrow failure. The risk of thrombosis is greater for patients with larger PNH clone sizes particularly in patients with PNH clones exceeding 50%. Venous thrombosis exceeds arterial thrombosis in PNH patients and unusual sites of thrombosis are not uncommon including hepatic, portal, mesenteric, and cerebral vein thrombosis [17]. Rapid diagnosis can be made via flow cytometry detecting deficiencies of glycosylphosphatidylinositol-linked proteins in red cells and neutrophils. Although the exact mechanism of thrombosis in PNH is unclear, hemolysis appears to play an important role as the risk of thrombosis is reduced by over 90% with eculizumab, the humanized monoclonal antibody against C5a [41].

Cancer

Cancer is associated with a four- to sevenfold increased risk of thromboembolism. Thrombosis is the second leading cause of death among cancer patients after the cancer itself. Cancer patients are at increased risk for venous and arterial thromboembolism. The risk varies with the stage and type of cancer. The risk of thromboembolism is highest among patients with pancreatic cancer followed by brain tumors, gastric cancer, renal cell cancer, and ovarian cancer. Multiple mechanisms have been identified as contributing to the thrombophilic state associated with cancer including tissue factor expression by the cancer cells and host monocytes, activation of factor X by a cancer procoagulant enzyme, endothelial-tumor cell interactions, and platelet activation [11]. More information on cancer and thromboembolism can be found in Chap. 20.

Pregnancy

Venous thromboembolism is a common complication of pregnancy affecting 0.76–1.72 per 1000 pregnancies. This rate is four times greater than the risk of thromboembolism in nonpregnant women of similar age and ethnicity. The risk is greatest in the immediate postpartum period and gradually declines to baseline by 12 weeks postpartum [42]. The risk of VTE is higher during the third trimester compared to the first and second trimesters [43].

Multiple hemostatic changes occur during pregnancy that contribute to its associated hypercoagulable state including reductions in protein S activity (due to reductions in free protein S) and fibrinolytic activity (due to increases in plasminogen activator inhibitor 1) and increases in factors II, VII, VIII, and X as well as fibrinogen and von Willebrand factor. Anatomic changes also contribute to the increased risk of VTE. The gravid uterus preferentially compresses the left iliac vein leading to a 50% reduction in venous flow velocity by week 25–29 of gestation that lasts until about 6 weeks post-delivery. A systematic review found that 88% of deep vein thrombosis involves the left leg in pregnant patients as a consequence of these anatomic changes [44]. Due to their proximal location, it can be difficult to identify deep vein thrombosis in some pregnant patients. Therefore, additional imaging should be considered in patients with negative duplex ultrasound studies who are thought to have a high pretest probability of thrombosis. Patients can present with abdominal pain, back pain, and swelling of the leg or be completely asymptomatic. Risk factors for VTE in pregnancy include inherited thrombophilia, heart disease, African American race, sickle cell disease, lupus, smoking, obesity, and maternal age greater than 35 [13, 14, 18, 45] (see Chap. 18).

Medication-Associated Thrombophilia: Oral Contraceptive Pills, Hormonal Therapy, Bevacizumab, and Lenalidomide/Thalidomide

Combined estrogen-progestin oral contraceptive pills (OCP) are associated with a three- to fourfold increased risk of VTE that synergizes with other risk factors including obesity, smoking, and hereditary thrombophilia. In setting of hereditary thrombophilia, the risk of thrombosis can be as high as 30- to 50-fold the risk in the general population. The absolute per patient risk of VTE is small such that guidelines do not recommend thrombophilia testing prior to starting OCP. However, if there is strong family history of VTE (i.e., first-degree relatives) or previously identified hereditary thrombophilia, then alternative non-thrombogenic approaches to contraception such as copper wire intrauterine devices, low-dose progesterone intrauterine devices, low-dose oral progesterone, or barrier methods should be considered [46].

It is well documented that the use of selective estrogen receptor modulators such as tamoxifen and raloxifene increase the risk of venous thrombosis. The risk of venous thromboembolism is increased two- to threefold in women taking tamoxifen and increased further when the treatment course of tamoxifen is extended from 5 to 10 years. Similar to OCP, the risk of VTE is accentuated in patients with hereditary thrombophilia on tamoxifen. In patients with a history of VTE, the use of an aromatase inhibitor instead of tamoxifen should be considered. In patients with hereditary thrombophilia and no previous history of VTE, the use of tamoxifen or alternative approaches to endocrine ablation should be made on a case-by-case basis considering the efficacy of the alternative treatment options and the history of VTE in the patient's family.

Immunomodulatory agents such as thalidomide, lenalidomide, and pomalidomide are associated with a modest increased risk of VTE that is significantly increased when used in conjunction with high-dose dexamethasone or combination chemotherapy. Consequently, low-molecular-weight heparin (LMWH) thromboprophylaxis is recommended for patients on these highly thrombogenic regimens. Many newer myeloma regimens use lower doses of dexamethasone or include bortezomib which are associated with lower risks of VTE such that aspirin thromboprophylaxis is more commonly used at present [47].

Bevacizumab is a monoclonal antibody targeting vascular endothelial growth factor (VEGF) that inhibits binding of the normal VEGF ligand to its receptor. A patient-level meta-analysis of randomized controlled clinical trials of bevacizumab found no increased risk of VTE [48]. However, bevacizumab was associated with a 1.4-fold increase in arterial thromboembolism [49]. A trial level meta-analysis of VEGF receptor tyrosine kinase inhibitors (sunitinib, sorafenib, pazopanib, vandetanib, and axitinib) also noted no excess risk of VTE [50]. In contrast, epidermal growth factor receptor antagonist monoclonal antibodies but not tyrosine kinase inhibitors have been associated with an increased risk of VTE [51, 52].

Anatomic/Mechanical Compression

May-Thurner syndrome is characterized by compression of the left common iliac vein between the overlying right common iliac artery and the underlying vertebral body. It is a common anatomic variant in the general population which has been associated with unprovoked left iliofemoral deep vein thrombosis. May-Thurner is most commonly seen in women between the ages of 20 and 50. In patients in whom this anatomic vascular compression is not relieved, recurrent thrombosis can occur even in the presence of therapeutic anticoagulation. Therefore, catheter-directed thrombolysis, venous angioplasty, and intravascular stenting should be considered in patients with May-Thurner syndrome.

Venous thoracic outlet syndrome is another mechanical cause for thrombosis that is important to consider in patients with unprovoked proximal upper extremity deep vein thrombosis. It is caused by compression of the subclavian vein by one or more structures at the costoclavicular junction, such as a cervical first rib, clavicle, subclavius muscle, or anterior scalene muscle. Similar to May-Thurner syndrome, surgical treatment to relieve the anatomic compression in addition to thrombolysis/thrombectomy and subsequent anticoagulation is thought to be necessary for successful treatment. Effort related thrombosis, also known as Paget-Schroetter syndrome, can occur when there is microtrauma to the subclavian vein due to repetitive arm movements as seen for example with overhead physical activities or vigorous upper extremity exercises.

Duplex ultrasound of the subclavian vein with the arm in neutral and stress positions (which trigger compression of the thoracic outlet) is the diagnostic test of choice. Contrast venography remains the gold standard for diagnosis. Treatment of Paget-Schroetter syndrome should include exclusion of the thoracic outlet syndrome as many of these patients have acquired thoracic outlet compression. If vascular compression is noted, surgical therapy followed by anticoagulation is warranted. Since patients with thoracic outlet syndrome and May-Thurner syndrome have anatomic triggers, limited duration anticoagulation (at least 3 months) is usually sufficient once the anatomic risk factors are eliminated. Thrombophilia testing is generally not recommended as it has not been demonstrated to significantly influence therapeutic outcomes in these patients [53].

When Testing Should Be Done

In the current environment of dramatic escalations in health care spending it is essential that laboratory and radiology testing be performed in cost-conscious manner. Thrombophilia testing has yet to be demonstrated to contribute significantly to decision-making regarding anticoagulation therapy. Therefore, thrombophilia testing should only be performed in select individuals. Patients with unprovoked VTE in whom indefinite anticoagulation is planned are unlikely to benefit from thrombophilia testing. Similar reasoning can be applied to patients with VTE associated with potent situational triggers such as major surgery or trauma. We believe that thrombophilia testing is unnecessary in patients with a first episode of provoked VTE, patients 50 years of age or older with a first episode of spontaneous VTE, and patients with active malignancy, inflammatory bowel disease, myeloproliferative neoplasms, heparin-induced thrombocytopenia with thrombosis, or retinal vein thrombosis including that in the setting of preeclampsia. Clinically significant inherited thrombophilia such as antithrombin deficiency is more likely to present early in life, so thrombophilia testing should be focused on patients 45 years of age or less, especially in patients with first-degree relatives with a history of thromboembolism or complications of therapy such as warfarin skin necrosis.

Antiphospholipid antibody syndrome (APS) is more common in patients with systemic lupus erythematosus or a history of recurrent miscarriages, so testing for this entity should focus on these patient subgroups. APS is also associated with arterial thromboembolism so testing should be considered in select patients. Testing for inherited thrombophilia disorders is not warranted in patients with arterial thrombosis, since hereditary thrombophilia does not appear to increase the risk of arterial thromboembolism. In patients with hepatic, portal, or mesenteric vein thrombosis, investigation for paroxysmal nocturnal hemoglobinuria or a myeloproliferative neoplasm (e.g., polycythemia vera or essential thrombocythemia) should be considered. Likewise, recurrent ipsilateral proximal upper extremity or lower extremity deep vein thrombosis in the absence of central venous catheters should prompt investigation for thoracic outlet syndrome and May-Thurner syndrome [10, 54].

When considering which thrombophilia tests to send, it is important to consider which vascular territories are primarily affected by the various thrombophilic states. Venous clots tend to be fibrin-rich while arterial thrombi are platelet-rich. Therefore, most of the thrombophilic states which influence fibrin formation predispose primarily to venous thromboembolism. Antiphospholipid antibodies precipitate both fibrin formation and platelet activation so they are commonly associated with both venous and arterial thromboembolism (Table 15.3).

If you determine that thrombophilia testing is clinically useful in a particular patient, it is essential to conduct testing in a setting that will not lead to false-positive results or at a minimum to be aware of the influence of clinical conditions on test results. Acute thrombosis and anticoagulants can affect the results of thrombophilia testing. Therefore, if testing is conducted in a setting of acute thrombosis, it is important to recognize that the results of some thrombophilia tests may be affected. Ideally, tests should be performed a minimum of 2 weeks following discontinuation of anticoagulation. Although not all tests are affected by acute thrombosis or anticoagulants, this approach avoids unnecessary repeated testing (Tables 15.4 and 15.5).

Table 15.3 Thrombophilic states and sites of thrombosis [17]

Thrombophilic state	Primary vascular territory of thrombosis
Factor V Leiden	Venous
Prothrombin gene mutation	Venous
Antithrombin deficiency	Venous
Protein C and S deficiency	Venous
Lupus anticoagulant	Venous or arterial

Table 15.4 The impact of clinical events or interventions on thrombophilia test results [20]

Event	Altered result
Acute thrombosis	Decreased antithrombin, protein C, and protein S
Heparin	Decreased antithrombin, false detection of lupus anticoagulant (with heparin concentrations >1 unit/mL)
Warfarin	Decreased protein S, protein C, false detection of lupus anticoagulant
Direct thrombin inhibitor (argatroban, dabigatran)	Increased antithrombin, protein S, and protein C
Factor Xa inhibitor (fondaparinux, rivaroxaban, apixaban)	Increased antithrombin

Table 15.5 Effects of anticoagulants on thrombophilic tests [20]

Thrombophilic state	Acute thrombosis	Heparin	Warfarin
Antithrombin deficiency	Can be lowered	Lowered	Rarely increased
Lupus anticoagulant	Not changed	Not changed	Occasionally false-positive
Factor V Leiden	Not changed	Not changed	Not changed
Protein C	Can be lowered	Not changed	Cannot be measured
Protein S	Can be lowered	Not changed	Cannot be measured
Prothrombin gene mutation	Not changed	Not changed	Not changed

Summary

Thrombophilia testing has become increasingly utilized in the hospital as well as the outpatient setting. However, it is important to emphasize that such testing is indicated in only few specific clinical scenarios. In the majority of clinical situations, it is not cost-effective and may lead to unintended patient harm. In summary, patients can be divided into five categories (Table 15.6) where hypercoagulable testing should/should not be considered: 1. provoked venous thromboembolism, 2. unprovoked venous thromboembolism, 3. in relatives of patients with thrombosis, 4. in female relatives of patients with thrombosis considering estrogen use, and 5. in female relatives of patients with thrombosis who are considering pregnancy [55].

Timing of thrombophilia testing is critical in order to not perform unnecessary tests. Do not perform thrombophilia testing at the time of VTE diagnosis or during the initial 3-month course of anticoagulant therapy. Testing should be performed only after anticoagulation has been held.

Key Points

- Factor V Leiden is the most common inherited thrombophilia, which is inherited in autosomal dominant fashion.
- Antithrombin deficiency can be seen in patients with sepsis, DIC, acute thrombosis, heparin therapy, liver disease, nephrotic syndrome, L-asparaginase chemotherapy, and acute fatty liver of pregnancy.
- It is unclear if homocysteine levels alone are pathogenic in patients with hyperhomocysteinemia. Elevated homocysteine levels may not be the cause of thrombosis but rather a marker of increased risk for thrombotic events.
- Antiphospholipid antibody syndrome is associated with arterial and venous thromboembolism.
- Thrombosis is the second leading cause of death among cancer patients after the cancer itself.
- Risk of thrombosis is greatest in the immediate postpartum period and gradually declines to baseline by 12 weeks postpartum.

Self-Assessment Questions

1. A 60-year-old woman with history of hepatitis C-associated cirrhosis presents to the ED with the acute onset of shortness of breath, presyncope, and palpitations. On imaging, she is noted to have a saddle pulmonary embolus. Her history is notable for estrogen supplementation for hot flashes, no prior episodes of thromboembolism, and no family history of thrombosis. She is initially started on a heparin drip with plans to bridge to warfarin. Several days later, her hypercoagulable workup reveals protein S deficiency. What is the most likely cause of her low protein S level?
   (a) Estrogen supplementation
   (b) Cirrhosis
   (c) Warfarin
   (d) All of the above
2. A 30-year-old woman presents to your hematology office for a second opinion. Her history

Table 15.6 Patient categories

Provoked venous thrombosis	Thrombophilia testing does not need to be performed
Unprovoked venous thrombosis	Thrombophilia testing in patients following an episode of unprovoked VTE is not necessary. Indefinite anticoagulation is the preferred approach to therapy. If a patient with unprovoked VTE wishes to stop anticoagulation, thrombophilia test results in most cases do not influence therapeutic decision-making (exceptions: antiphospholipid syndrome, antithrombin, protein C or S deficiency)
In relatives of patients with thrombosis	Thrombophilia testing in asymptomatic family members of patients with VTE or hereditary thrombophilia should not be routinely performed
Female relatives of patients with thrombosis considering estrogen use	If a woman contemplating estrogen use has a first-degree relative with VTE and known hereditary thrombophilia, testing for that thrombophilic defect would change the decision to use estrogen. However, family history of VTE in a first-degree relative predicts an excess risk of thrombosis with estrogen use, even when thrombophilia testing is negative
In female relatives of patients with thrombosis who are considering pregnancy	If a woman contemplating pregnancy has a first-degree relative with VTE and a known hereditary thrombophilia, test for that thrombophilia if the result would change VTE prophylaxis decisions. Women with a personal history of unprovoked, estrogen-associated or pregnancy-associated VTE already carry an indication for prophylaxis and are unlikely to benefit from thrombophilia testing. Women with multiple family members affected by VTE are more likely to carry a higher risk thrombophilia such as AT deficiency which may impact prophylaxis decisions

dates back to the age of 20 when she had an unprovoked pulmonary embolism. She was treated with warfarin for 1 year. Since completing her warfarin, approximately 6 years ago, she has had four spontaneous abortions all prior to 10 weeks. Each time a hypercoagulable workup has been done by a hematologist.

The following results are available:

- Protein C, protein S, antithrombin III, and homocysteine levels all normal
- Negative mutations for factor V Leiden and the prothrombin gene mutation
- Lupus anticoagulant tested 12 weeks apart negative
- IgG and IgM anticardiolipin antibodies negative 12 weeks apart
- What is the next step in her management?
  - (a) She does not have a hypercoagulable state and should continue trying to get pregnant.
  - (b) Malignancy workup needed.
  - (c) Check MTHFR and homocysteine levels.
  - (d) Check IgA anticardiolipin antibodies.
  - (e) Check beta-2 glycoprotein antibodies.

3. Which of the following is the most common thrombophilic condition?
   - (a) Polycythemia vera
   - (b) Factor V Leiden mutation
   - (c) Antiphospholipid antibody syndrome
   - (d) Heparin-induced thrombocytopenia
4. A 34-year-old woman who is a known heterozygote for both factor V Leiden and the prothrombin gene mutation is 12 weeks pregnant. She has a prior history of lower extremity DVT diagnosed several years ago and had been treated with warfarin at the time. Her family history is positive for older sister who suffered an unprovoked DVT. What recommendation would you make regarding anticoagulation at this time?
   - (a) No need for anticoagulation
   - (b) Anticoagulate with enoxaparin only during pregnancy
   - (c) Anticoagulate with warfarin during pregnancy
   - (d) Anticoagulate with enoxaparin only after delivery
   - (e) Anticoagulate with enoxaparin during pregnancy and 12 weeks after delivery
5. A 40-year-old man suffers multiple long bone lower extremity fractures in a car accident. A day after prolonged surgery he is noted to have a lower extremity DVT. He has no per-

sonal or family history of blood clots. He is started on enoxaparin and bridged to warfarin. Which tests are needed to be sent now in order to determine etiology of blood clot?
(a) Antithrombin III
(b) Protein C
(c) Protein S
(d) FVL
(e) None

Self-Assessment Answers

1. (d) All of the above

   Protein S deficiency can be the cause of thrombosis, but it is important to rule out more common causes for protein S deficiency that can be found during a hypercoaguable workup. Estrogen use, liver dysfunction, and warfarin use are all known causes of protein S deficiency.
2. (e) Check beta-2 glycoprotein antibodies

   To make the diagnosis of antiphospholipid antibody syndrome, clinical criteria, i.e., pregnancy morbidity or vascular thrombosis, are needed along with a positive lupus anticoagulant, anticardiolipin antibody, or beta-2 glycoprotein.
3. (b) Factor V Leiden mutation

   Factor V Leiden is the most common inherited thrombophilia in Caucasians where it affects approximately 5% of the population and is less common in Hispanic Americans (2%) and African Americans (1.2%).
4. (e) Anticoagulate with enoxaparin during pregnancy and 12 weeks after delivery

   Risk of thrombosis is increased in pregnancy with the greatest risk in the immediate postpartum period and gradually declining to baseline by 12 weeks postpartum. Additionally in patients with a family history of DVT and inherited thrombophilia, the risk is even higher and should be considered for thromboprophylaxis during and after pregnancy.
5. (e) None

   No additional workup is needed in patients with a known risk factor, i.e., long bone fractures and immobility and no prior personal or family history of thrombosis.

References

1. Beutler E, Licktman M, Coller B, Kipps T, Seligsohn U. Chapter 127 hereditary thrombophilia. In: Goodnight SH, Griffin JH, editors. Williams hematology. 6th ed. New York: McGraw Hill; 2000.
2. Thorelli E, Kaufman RJ, Dahlbäck B. Cleavage of factor V at Arg 506 by activated protein C and the expression of anticoagulant activity of factor V. Blood. 1999;93(8):2552.
3. Simone B, De Stefano V, Leoncini E, Zacho J, Martinelli I, Emmerich J, Rossi E, et al. Risk of venous thromboembolism associated with single and combined effects of Factor V Leiden, Prothrombin 20210A and Methylenetetrahydrofolate reductase C677T: a meta-analysis involving over 11,000 cases and 21,000 controls. Eur J Epidemiol. 2013;28(8):621–47.
4. Segal JB, Brotman DJ, Necochea AJ, Emadi A, Samal L, Wilson LM, et al. Predictive value of factor V Leiden and prothrombin G20210A in adults with venous thromboembolism and in family members of those with a mutation: a systematic review. JAMA. 2009;301(23):2472–85.
5. Rosendaal FR, Koster T, Vandenbroucke JP, Reitsma PH. High risk of thrombosis in patients homozygous for factor V Leiden (activated protein C resistance). Blood. 1995;85(6):1504.
6. Middeldorp S, Meinardi JR, Koopman MM, van Pampus EC, Hamulyák K, van Der Meer J, et al. A prospective study of asymptomatic carriers of the factor V Leiden mutation to determine the incidence of venous thromboembolism. Ann Intern Med. 2001;135(5):322.
7. Leroyer C, Mercier B, Oger E, Chenu E, Abgrall JF, Férec C, Mottier D. Prevalence of 20210 A allele of the prothrombin gene in venous thromboembolism patients. Thromb Haemost. 1998;80(1):49.
8. Meeks SL, Abshire TC. Abnormalities of prothrombin: a review of the pathophysiology, diagnosis, and treatment. Haemophilia. 2008;14(6):1159–63.
9. De Stefano V, Martinelli I, Mannucci PM, Paciaroni K, Rossi E, Chiusolo P, et al. The risk of recurrent venous thromboembolism among heterozygous carriers of the G20210A prothrombin gene mutation. Br J Haematol. 2001;113(3):630.
10. Margaglione M, Brancaccio V, Giuliani N, D'Andrea G, Cappucci G, Iannaccone L, et al. Increased risk for venous thrombosis in carriers of the prothrombin G-->A20210 gene variant. Ann Intern Med. 1998; 129(2):89.
11. Hillman R, Ault K, Leporrier M, Rinder H. Thrombophilia. In: Hematology in clinical practice. 5th ed. New York: McGraw Hill Education; 2010.
12. Mannucci PM, Vigano S. Deficiencies of protein C, an inhibitor of blood coagulation. Lancet. 1982;2(8296):463.
13. Weingarz L, Schwonberg J, Schindewolf M, Hecking C, Wolf Z, Erbe M, et al. Prevalence of thrombophilia according to age at the first manifestation of venous

thromboembolism: results from the MAISTHRO registry. Br J Haematol. 2013;163(5):655–65.
14. Baglin T, Gray E, Greaves M, Hunt BJ, Keeling D, Machin S, British Committee for Standards in Haematology, et al. Clinical guidelines for testing for heritable thrombophilia. Br J Haematol. 2010;149(2):209.
15. MacCallum PK, Cooper JA, Martin J, Howarth DJ, Meade TW, Miller GJ. Associations of protein C and protein S with serum lipid concentrations. Br J Haematol. 1998;102(2):609.
16. Amiral J, Grosley B, Boyer-Neumann C, Marfaing-Koka A, Peynaud-Debayle E, Wolf M, Meyer D. New direct assay of free protein S antigen using two distinct monoclonal antibodies specific for the free form. Blood Coagul Fibrinolysis. 1994;5(2):179.
17. Khan S, Dickerman JD. Hereditary thrombophilia. Thromb J. 2006;4:15.
18. Garcia D, Middeldorp S, Sharathkumar AA. American Society of Hematology self assessment program 5th ed. Thrombosis and thrombophilia.
19. Lowe GD. Virchow's triad revisited: abnormal flow. Pathophysiol Haemost Thromb. 2003;33(5-6):455.
20. Malcolm L, Brigden M. The hypercoagulable state. Postgrad Med. 1997;101(5):249–67.
21. Al-Mugeiren MM, Abdel Gader AG, Al-Meshari AA, Al-Rasheed SA, Al-Jurayyan NA, Al Hawasy MN. Normal levels of the natural anticoagulants (proteins C&S and antithrombin III) and the fibrinolytic factors (tPA and PAI) in Arab children. Ann Saudi Med. 1996;16(5):501–4.
22. Lijfering WM, Brouwer JL, Veeger NJ, Bank I, Coppens M, Middeldorp S, et al. Blood. 2009;113(21):5314–22.
23. Pintao MC, Ribeiro DD, Bezemer ID, Garcia AA, de Visser MC, Doggen CJ, et al. Blood. 2013;122(18):3210–9.
24. Munts AG, van Genderen PJ, Dippel DW, van Kooten F, Koudstaal PJ. Coagulation disorders in young adults with acute cerebral ischaemia. J Neurol. 1998;245(1):21.
25. Ken-Dror G, Cooper JA, Humphries SE, Drenos F, Ireland HA. Free protein S level as a risk factor for coronary heart disease and stroke in a prospective cohort study of healthy United Kingdom men. Am J Epidemiol. 2011;174(8):958–68.
26. Fitches AC, Appleby R, Lane DA, De Stefano V, Leone G, Olds RJ. Impaired cotranslational processing as a mechanism for type I antithrombin deficiency. Blood. 1998;92(12):4671.
27. Hultin MB, McKay J, Abildgaard U. Antithrombin Oslo: type Ib classification of the first reported antithrombin-deficient family, with a review of hereditary antithrombin variants. Thromb Haemost. 1988;59(3):468.
28. Koster T, Blann AD, Briet E, Vandenbroucke JP, Rosendaal FR. Role of clotting factor VIII in effect of von Willebrand factor on occurrence of deep-vein thrombosis. Lancet. 1995;345:152–5.
29. Kraaijenhagen RA, in't Anker PS, Koopman MM, et al. High plasma concentration of factor VIIIc is a major risk factor for venous thromboembolism. Thromb Haemost. 2000;83:5–9.
30. Kyrle PA, Minar E, Hirschl M, et al. High plasma levels of factor VIII and risk of recurrent thromboembolism. N Engl J Med. 2000;343:457–62.
31. Bruce A, Massicotte MP. Thrombophilia screening: whom to test? Blood. 2012;120:1353–5.
32. The Heart Outcomes Prevention Evaluation (HOPE) 2 Investigators. Homocysteine lowering with folic acid and B vitamins in vascular disease. N Engl J Med. 2006;354:1567–77.
33. Miyakis S, Lockshin MD, Atsumi T, Branch DW, Brey RL, Cervera R, et al. International consensus statement on an update of the classification criteria for definite antiphospholipid syndrome (APS). J Thromb Haemost. 2006;4(2):295.
34. Pengo V, Tripodi A, Reber G, Rand JH, Ortel TL, Galli M, De Groot PG, Subcommittee on Lupus Anticoagulant/Antiphospholipid Antibody of the Scientific and Standardisation Committee of the International Society on Thrombosis and Haemostasis. Update of the guidelines for lupus anticoagulant detection. Subcommittee on Lupus Anticoagulant/Antiphospholipid Antibody of the Scientific and Standardisation Committee of the International Society on Thrombosis and Haemostasis. J Thromb Haemost. 2009;7(10):1737.
35. Giannakopoulos B, Passam F, Ioannou Y, Krilis SA. How we diagnose the antiphospholipid syndrome. How we diagnose the antiphospholipid syndrome. Blood. 2009;113(5):985.
36. Love PE, Santoro SA. Antiphospholipid antibodies: anticardiolipin and the lupus anticoagulant in systemic lupus erythematosus (SLE) and in non-SLE disorders. Prevalence and clinical significance. Ann Intern Med. 1990;112(9):682.
37. Scott LM, Beer PA, Bench AJ, Erber WN, Green AR. Prevalence of JAK2 V617F and exon 12 mutations in polycythaemia vera. Br J Haematol. 2007;139(3):511.
38. Anía BJ, Suman VJ, Sobell JL, Codd MB, Silverstein MN, Melton LJ. Trends in the incidence of polycythemia vera among Olmsted County, Minnesota residents, 1935-1989. Am J Hematol. 1994;47(2):89.
39. Carobbio A, Thiele J, Passamonti F, Rumi E, Ruggeri M, Rodeghiero F, et al. Risk factors for arterial and venous thrombosis in WHO-defined essential thrombocythemia: an international study of 891 patients. Blood. 2011;117(22):5857.
40. G F, Carobbio A, Thiele J, Passamonti F, Rumi E, Ruggeri M, et al. Incidence and risk factors for bleeding in 1104 patients with essential thrombocythemia or prefibrotic myelofibrosis diagnosed according to the 2008 WHO criteria. Leukemia. 2012;26(4):716–9.
41. Hill A, Kelly RJ, Hillmen P. Thrombosis in paroxysmal nocturnal hemoglobinuria. Blood. 2013;121(25):4985–96. quiz 5105

42. Kamel H, Navi BB, Sriram N, Hovsepian DA, Devereux RB, Elkind MSV. Risk of thrombotic event after the 6-week postpartum period. N Engl J Med. 2014;370:1307–15.
43. Sultan AA, West J, Tata LJ, Fleming KM, Nelson-Piercy C, Grainge MJ. Risk of first venous thromboembolism in and around pregnancy: a population-based cohort study. Br J Haematol. 2012;156(3):366–73.
44. Chan WS, Spencer FA, Ginsberg JS. Anatomic distribution of deep vein thrombosis in pregnancy. CMAJ. 2010;182(7):657–60.
45. Gerhardt A, Scharf RE, Zotz RB. Effect of hemostatic risk factors on the individual probability of thrombosis during pregnancy and the puerperium. Thromb Haemost. 2003;90(1):77.
46. Peragallo Urrutia R, Coeytaux RR, McBroom AJ, Gierisch JM, Havrilesky LJ, Moorman PG, et al. Risk of acute thromboembolic events with oral contraceptive use: a systematic review and meta-analysis. Obstet Gynecol. 2013;122(2 Pt 1):380–9.
47. Palumbo A, Rajkumar SV, Dimopoulos MA, Richardson PG, San Miguel J, Barlogie B, et al. International Myeloma Working Group prevention of thalidomide- and lenalidomide-associated thrombosis in myeloma. Leukemia. 2008;22(2):414.
48. Hurwitz HI, Saltz LB, Van Cutsem E, Cassidy J, Wiedemann J, Sirzén F, et al. Venous thromboembolic events with chemotherapy plus bevacizumab: a pooled analysis of patients in randomized phase II and III studies. J Clin Oncol. 2011;29(13):1757–64.
49. Ranpura V, Hapani S, Chuang J, Wu S. Risk of cardiac ischemia and arterial thromboembolic events with the angiogenesis inhibitor bevacizumab in cancer patients: a meta-analysis of randomized controlled trials. Acta Oncol. 2010;49(3):287–97.
50. Sonpavde G, Je Y, Schutz F, Galsky MD, Paluri R, et al. Venus thromboembolic events with vascular endothelial growth factor receptor tyrosine kinase inhibitors: a systematic review and meta-analysis of randomized clinical trials. Crit Rev Oncol Hematol. 2013;87:80–9.
51. Petrelli F, Cabiddu M, Borgonovo K, Barni S. Risk of venous and arterial thromboembolic events associated with anti-EGFR agents: a meta-analysis of randomized clinical trial. Ann Oncol. 2012;23:1672–9.
52. Nalluri SR, Chu D, Keresztes R, Zhu X, Wu S. Risk of venous thromboembolism with the angiogenesis inhibitor bevacizumab in cancer patients: a meta-analysis. JAMA. 2008;300(19):2277–85.
53. Schneider DB, Dimuzio PJ, Martin ND, Gordon RL, Wilson MW, Laberge JM, et al. Combination treatment of venous thoracic outlet syndrome: open surgical decompression and intraoperative angioplasty. J Vasc Surg. 2004;40(4):599–603.
54. Bertina RM. Genetic approach to thrombophilia. Thromb Haemost. 2001;86(1):92.
55. Bates SM, Jaeschke R, Stevens SM, Goodacre S, Wells PS, Stevenson MD, Kearon C, Schunemann HJ, Crowther M, Pauker SG, Makdissi R, Guyatt GH. Diagnosis of DVT: antithrombotic therapy and prevention of thrombosis, 9th ed. American College of Chest Physicians evidence-based clinical practice guidelines. Chest. 2012;141(2 Suppl):e351S–418S.

16 Thrombophilia Testing

Teresa L. Carman

Clinical Vignettes

Case 1: *A 65-year-old woman is admitted to the medicine service with gallstone pancreatitis. She has not had similar symptoms in the past. She has been otherwise well. She is morbidly obese with a BMI of 43. She has underlying hypertension, diabetes without associated complications, osteoarthritis, and hyperlipidemia. She has not had prior surgeries. She is a nonsmoker. She is treated conservatively with nasogastric suction for ileus and kept NPO. "Routine" thromboprophylaxis is ordered with sequential compression devices (SCDs) and enoxaparin 40 mg subcutaneously daily. On hospital day 4, she is experiencing left leg swelling and calf pain. Duplex ultrasound demonstrates popliteal, posterior tibial, and soleal vein deep vein thrombosis. She is started on unfractionated heparin. The medicine service is concerned that she developed thrombosis despite prophylaxis and asks what additional testing should be considered?*

Case 2: *A 28-year-old woman, G1P1001, presents with a 2-week history of left leg pain. She has mild ankle swelling. She denies a preceding history of trauma or injury. She has not had any recent illness, hospitalizations, or surgeries. Her only medication is a combination estrogen/progesterone contraceptive (OCP) which was prescribed for dysmenorrhea related to endometriosis. There is no history of thrombosis in immediate family members, but several second-degree relatives have experienced thrombosis related to cancer and one related to pregnancy. BMI is 27. She is clinically well without signs or symptoms of pulmonary embolism. You would like to treat her with a direct oral anticoagulant (DOAC). Is thrombophilia testing warranted?*

T. L. Carman (✉)
Division of Cardiovascular Medicine, University Hospitals Cleveland Medical Center, Cleveland, OH, USA

Department of Medicine, Case Western Reserve University School of Medicine, Cleveland, OH, USA
e-mail: teresa.carman@uhhospitals.org

J. F. Lau et al. (eds.), *Anticoagulation Therapy*, https://doi.org/10.1007/978-3-319-73709-6_16

Introduction

When called to see patients with arterial or venous thromboembolism (VTE), clinicians are frequently asked as part of the consultative question "What tests should we order?" There seems to be an underlying supposition that the answer or diagnosis underlying thrombotic events will be found using laboratory testing. In reality, etiologies contributing to thromboembolism are multifactorial. Both venous and arterial thromboembolism should be viewed as a complex interaction between environmental, inherited, or acquired thrombophilic predispositions, as well as endogenous or patient-specific factors. The combination of these factors influence or predispose an individual to thromboembolism. While the goal is to provide patients with the best understanding of their medical condition, rarely does thrombophilia testing alone solve the puzzle or fully explain the clinical presentation.

Random thrombophilia testing is not warranted, and testing just to see what may be found is equally ill-advised. Indeed, as part of the "Choosing Wisely" campaign the American Society of Hematology (ASH) recommends against thrombophilia testing in adults with venous thromboembolism associated with a major transient risk factor such as surgery, trauma, or prolonged immobilization. This recommendation recognizes that thrombophilia testing is costly and in the setting of a transient risk factor should not influence the management. The ASH recommendations further recognize that when VTE occurs in association with pregnancy, hormone therapy, or if there is a strong family history with a major transient risk factor, the role of thrombophilia testing is complex [1]. Proper management requires an understanding of the laboratory complexities as well as the potential implications of identifying a genetic condition that may not influence care. Therefore, essentially all thrombophilia testing should include shared-decision making with the patient.

Once the decision has been made to pursue testing, it should be recognized that laboratory testing may be affected by many patient-related, therapy-related, and laboratory-related factors. Understanding the timing and role or goals of thrombophilia testing will help the practitioner provide the best care. Prior to ordering any laboratory testing, one should consider the potential impact of testing [2]. Will testing influence the choice of anticoagulation, the duration of therapy, or provide additional information to the patient or clinician that may influence patient management?

In addition, it is important to understand the limits of thrombophilia testing. By far, acutely acquired conditions such as hospitalization and comorbid illness along with other coexisting predispositions, i.e., pregnancy, indwelling medical devices, and medications that influence thrombosis, have a greater impact on both venous and arterial thromboembolism than inherited or acquired thrombophilia [3]. In addition, it is likely that we have yet to understand or identify all potential thrombophilic conditions. Most epidemiologic studies suggest approximately 50% of idiopathic thrombosis is influenced, and not caused, by the known thrombophilias [4]. Identification and correction or elimination of acquired causes when possible will likely have the largest impact on patient outcomes.

It is also becoming evident that more emphasis should be placed on the phenotype of the thrombotic presentation as opposed to the genotype identified during testing. A strong family history of thrombosis even in the absence of an identified defect should be recognized as a significant thrombotic risk. As a general rule, in patients with an idiopathic event in whom long-term therapy is anticipated and in asymptomatic patients with a strong family history or women with a strong family history of thrombosis who are contemplating using hormonal therapy or pregnancy, testing is not warranted unless it would impact therapy.

Case 1 Discussion

In most clinical series, clinical conditions which increase the risk for thrombosis outweigh the thrombophilic conditions. These clinical risks are frequently underappreciated with respect to their contribution to thrombosis and clinical outcomes. The impact on increased risk for acquired thrombosis from clinical prothrombotic conditions is not just an additive but exponentially increases thrombosis risk when more than one condition is present. It is well recognized that despite improvements in prophylaxis, there has been little impact on the incidence of VTE. From a recent study conducted in Olmstead County, Minnesota, after adjusting for age and gender, VTE risk was essentially unchanged between 1988 and 2010. However, the prevalence of obesity, cancer, surgery, and leg paresis was increasing and, along with nursing home confinement, accounted for 79% of VTE [5]. Advanced age is one of the most important risks for thrombosis. Thromboembolism is uncommon in children and teens. After adolescence, the incidence increases through each decade of life with an annual incidence of approximately 1/100 over the age of 80. Men have a higher incidence of VTE compared to women [6]. Clinical conditions associated with increased VTE risk are numerous. Table 16.1 illustrates many of the clinical conditions associated with VTE.

As noted above, thrombophilia testing is not warranted in patients with situational thrombotic events. In addition, there is little role for testing for inherited thrombophilia in patients over the age of 50. In this situation, it is unlikely that additional thrombophilia testing will change the current therapy or duration of therapy. Evaluation to assure the SCDs were applied as requested and enoxaparin was given as direct is prudent. While hospital day 4 is early for the development of heparin-induced thrombocytopenia, a review of the platelet counts is required. In addition, recommendations for outpatient age- and gender-appropriate cancer screening should be made.

Case 2 Discussion

Testing for most thrombophilia should not be done in the acute setting. If testing is deemed appropriate, then attention to the timing of testing should be considered. Anticoagulants, acute thrombosis with associated acute-phase reactants, and hormonal states including pregnancy or exogenous hormone therapy can influence test results, frequently resulting in false positives. The only two classes of testing which are not overtly influenced by acute venous thromboembolism and the administration of anticoagulation are (1) antibody testing, such as anticardiolipin antibodies and β2-glycoprotein-1 antibodies, and (2) genetic testing done for Factor V Leiden (FVL) and prothrombin (G20210A) gene mutation (PTG). Testing for the natural anticoagulant deficiencies and factor VIII (FVIII) should not be performed during the acute presentation as many of these may be influenced by the acute thromboembolism. Depending on the assay and the chosen anticoagulants, lupus anticoagulant testing may be performed, but this should be confirmed within the local laboratory (Table 16.2).

This event would indeed be considered a situational event—related to the use of the combination oral contraceptive. Given the prior successful pregnancy and the lack of first-degree relatives

Table 16.1 Clinical conditions associated with venous thromboembolism

Advancing age
Cancer and chemotherapy—including myeloproliferative disorders and multiple myeloma
Chronic obstructive pulmonary disease
Congestive heart failure
Hormonal therapy—including testosterone and selective estrogen receptor modifiers
Immobilization
Indwelling devices—including venous access and pacemakers
Inflammatory states
Sepsis/SIRS
Inflammatory bowel disease/Crohn's disease
Pancreatitis
Vasculitis
Lupus and other inflammatory arthropathies
Any infectious or inflammatory condition
Liver disease
Major surgery—including orthopedic, abdominal, or neurosurgery
Nephrotic syndrome
Neurologic disease/injury
Obesity
Pregnancy and peripartum
Stroke
Trauma—including spinal cord injury

with thrombosis, many practitioners would defer testing. The intention should be to treat her with anticoagulation for a minimum of 3 months for a single situational event. Future hormonal therapy (especially estrogen-containing) should be avoided. Consideration should be given toward aggressive prophylaxis in other high-risk settings including additional pregnancies.

Prior to any testing, the patient and providers should engage in a discussion regarding thrombophilia testing and the potential impact of the results. Would positive testing influence her care? Would positive testing create undo anxiety for her or other family members without impacting outcomes? Is there a potential for influencing other aspects of her care including her future ability to obtain life insurance, disability, or long-term care insurance? If testing is deemed appropriate, one must consider whether a "full" thrombophilia panel (Table 16.2) is warranted or if limited testing would suffice.

Natural Anticoagulant Thrombophilias

Antithrombin (AT), protein C (PC), and protein S (PS) deficiency are loss of function defects. Many different genetic mutations that influence the loss of function phenotype have been identified for each of these proteins making genetic testing impractical. Therefore, testing for AT, PC, and PS deficiency is performed using functional or activity assays and antigen assays.

The defects associated with AT, PC, and PS deficiency may relate to a qualitative defect in the protein or a quantitative defect (Table 16.3). With a "type I" deficiency—there is insufficient quantity of a normally functioning protein—a quantitative defect. In a qualitative defect, there is a normal amount of a nonfunctioning protein—hence a functional deficiency. This is called a "type II" deficiency. In general, functional or activity assays are employed initially for screening for all three defects. Functional assays determine the activity of the protein in plasma and thus will identify if there is a type I (quantitative) deficiency or type II (qualitative) deficiency. Antigen assays are used only to distinguish between type I and type II deficiency.

Antithrombin is a serine protease synthesized in the liver. It is a natural anticoagulant responsible for the clearance of activated serine proteases within the coagulation cascade. The activity of AT is augmented by the administration of heparin, low-molecular-weight heparin (LMWH) or fondaparinux. While it is the least common thrombophilia, AT deficiency was the first thrombophilia to be identified. It is present in 0.02–0.17% of the population and in up to 1% of patients with VTE. The inheritance is autosomal dominant with variable penetrance. AT is considered a "high-risk" thrombophilia with up to 50-fold increased risk for thrombosis in some series. Thrombosis typically occurs between ages 20 and 40 and almost always before age 50 [2, 7]. Screening is done using a functional (activity) assay. Patients with type I deficiency have decreased activity and antigen levels—usually less than 70%. Type II deficiency demonstrates decreased activity on functional testing but quantitatively normal antigen levels.

Acquired causes of antithrombin deficiency are common. Liver disease, active thrombosis, recent surgery, DIC, malnutrition, proteinuria/nephrotic syndrome, active heparin, or heparin-like product administration, and L-asparaginase therapy can cause acquired antithrombin deficiency. Repeat testing to confirm a suspected antithrombin deficiency to demonstrate reproducible results is warranted [7]. The presence of heparin may interfere with functional testing—depending on which available testing method is in use. In addition, since the administration of heparin may lower AT levels, functional testing is best done off anticoagulants.

PC and PS are vitamin K-dependent natural anticoagulants synthesized in the liver. PC deficiency occurs in 0.14–0.5% of the general population. Inheritance is autosomal dominant, and spontaneous mutations have been noted. Heterozygous PC deficiency is associated with a 7- to 11-fold increased risk for thrombosis. Up to 3% of individuals with VTE may be identified as having heterozygous PC deficiency [2, 8]. Homozygous PC deficiency is uncommon and

Table 16.2 Thrombophilia laboratory tests and the expected influence from anticoagulants and acute illness

Thrombophilia assay	Testing on heparin	Testing on LMWH[a]	Testing on warfarin	Testing on DTI[b]	Testing on Xa inhibitor[c]	Acute illness/ thrombosis
Antithrombin activity	Potentially decreased	Potentially decreased	Decreased	Falsely increased	No effect	Decreased
Antithrombin antigen	Potentially decreased	Potentially decreased	No effect	No effect	No effect	Decreased
Protein C activity	No effect	Falsely increased[d]	Decreased	Falsely increased	Falsely increased	Decreased
Protein C antigen	No effect	No effect	Decreased	No effect	No effect	Decreased
Protein S activity	Falsely increased[d]	Falsely increased[d]	Decreased	Falsely increased	No effect	Decreased
Protein S free and total antigen	No effect	No effect	Decreased	No effect	No effect	Decreased
Activated protein C resistance	No effect	No effect	No effect	Not able to be performed	No effect	No effect
Factor V Leiden	No effect	No effect	No effect	No effect	No effect	No effect
Prothrombin gene mutation	No effect	No effect	No effect	No effect	No effect	No effect
Factor VIII activity	Potentially decreased	Potentially decreased	No effect	Potentially decreased	Potentially decreased	Potentially increased
Factor IX antigen	No effect	No effect	Decreased	No effect	No effect	No effect
Factor XI antigen	No effect	No effect	No effect	No effect	No effect	No effect
Anticardiolipin antibodies	No effect	No effect	No effect	No effect	No effect	No effect
β2-Glycoprotein-1 antibodies	No effect	No effect	No effect	No effect	No effect	No effect
Lupus anticoagulant	Potential false positive	Potential false positive	Potential false positive	False positive	Potential false positive	No effect
Homocysteine[e]	No effect	No effect	No effect	No effect	No effect	No effect

[a]*LMWH* low-molecular-weight heparin, i.e., enoxaparin or dalteparin
[b]*DTI* direct thrombin inhibitor, i.e., argatroban, bivalirudin, or dabigatran
[c]Rivaroxaban, apixaban, or edoxaban
[d]At high concentrations
[e]Testing should be conducted on a fasting specimen

Table 16.3 Laboratory findings in natural anticoagulant type I (quantitative) defect versus type II (qualitative) defect

Natural anticoagulant	Defect	Antigen	Activity
Protein C	Type I	Decreased	Decreased
	Type II	Normal	Decreased
Protein S	Type I	Decreased	Decreased
	Type II	Normal	Decreased
Antithrombin	Type I	Decreased	Decreased
	Type II	Normal	Decreased

may present with purpura fulminans or disseminated intravascular coagulation (DIC) in the neonatal period. Similar to AT, initial screening for PC deficiency should be done using a functional (activity) assay. If this is low, then additional antigen (immunoassay) testing is warranted to determine the deficiency subtype—type I or type II [2, 8].

It is important to have knowledge of the type of testing being performed in local laboratories. Activity assays are performed using either spectrophotometric or clot-based assays. Spectrophotometric methods are more commonly employed. Both assays suffer from limitations in testing. Clot-based assays may result in falsely elevated PC levels in patients with lupus anticoagulants and in the setting of anticoagulants including heparin, direct thrombin inhibitors (DTI), or the direct oral anticoagulants. In these settings, one must either defer testing or use a chromogenic assay. Falsely low PC levels may occur in the setting of conditions that shorten clotting times—including elevated FVIII, elevated PS, or FVL [9].

Acquired causes of PC deficiency are far more common than inherited PC deficiency. Acquired PC deficiency may be the result of decreased hepatic synthesis associated with warfarin therapy, liver dysfunction or malnutrition/vitamin K deficiency or L-asparaginase therapy, and decreased protein synthesis. Acquired PC deficiency also occurs in the setting of increased clearance or consumption during acute medical illness, inflammatory states including elevated FVIII levels, recent thrombosis, DIC, and trauma [9]. If PC deficiency is suspected, confirmation testing with repeated assays off anticoagulation is advocated. In addition, confirmation testing in first-degree relatives may be helpful [8].

PS, unlike AT or PC, circulates in both a free form (approximately 40%) and bound to C4b-binding protein (approximately 60%). True PS deficiency is present in 0.03–0.1% of the general population and up to 2% of patients with VTE [2]. Inherited PS deficiency is also autosomal dominant. It is important to recognize that low protein S levels may be found in up to 13% of the general population. Similar to PC and AT, acquired causes for PS deficiency outnumber inherited deficiencies. Decreased hepatic synthesis in liver disease or nutritional deficiencies as well as increased consumption during acute thrombosis or DIC may result in PS deficiency. In addition, because PS circulates bound to C4b-binding protein—any illness or condition that alters the C4b-binding protein concentrations may result in acquired PS deficiency. Examples include acute or chronic inflammation and increased estrogen states associated with OCPs, hormone replacement, or pregnancy since these exposures all increase C4b-binding protein synthesis [10].

Similar to AT and PC deficiency, PS deficiency should be initially evaluated using an activity assay (typically clot based) and further characterized by type using antigen assays. In suspected PS deficiency, however, antigen assays should include both total and free PS. Type I PS deficiency is a quantitative defect; activity level and both the free and total amount of PS are decreased. Type II PS deficiency is a qualitative defect—the activity level is low with normal free and total antigen levels. Type III PS deficiency is a qualitative defect; activity levels are low with a normal total protein S but reduced free (circulating or functional) PS due to mutations in protein S which influence its interaction with C4b-binding protein. Similar to PC testing, PS clot-based functional testing is limited by laboratory as well as patient-related conditions that may result in false-positive results. Because the functional PS assay testing has many limitations, and since the qualitative (type II) defect is rare, some authorities recommend free PS antigen testing as the best approach for evaluating protein S deficiency. Both free and total PS are measured by immunologic assay and suffer from fewer methodologic limitations. Testing must be performed at appropriate times, since the number of environmental and clinical factors affects the free and total PS levels. Patients should be off all vitamin K antagonists for at least 3–4 weeks. Patient should not be tested within 3 months of pregnancy or use of estrogen preparations. In addition, patient should be in a state of "wellness" free from inflammatory or other systemic illness. Abnormal results require confirmation with repeated testing at 4–6 weeks [10].

Gain of Function Thrombophilias

There are three notable gain of function thrombophilic defects: Factor V Leiden, prothrombin gene G20210A mutation (PTG), and factor VIII (FVIII) excess. When indicated, FVL and PTG can be evaluated using genetic analysis. These assays are not affected by common clinical conditions or anticoagulants. Activated protein C resistance (APC-r) was identified in thrombophilic families in the 1993 by Björn Dahlbäck [11]. He noted that some individuals' aPTT clotting times did not prolong when activated protein C was added which he labeled as "activated protein C resistance." Subsequently he and others noted that the APC-r phenotype was due to a mutation in factor V. In the FVL genotype, there is an amino acid substitution (R506Q) at an arginine cleavage site which renders the activated factor V (FVa) protein resistant to cleavage and inactivation by activated protein C—hence activated protein C resistance [11, 12].

FVL is the most common prothrombotic mutation in Caucasian populations. Inheritance is autosomal dominant. Heterozygous FVL occurs in up to 10% of some populations. Homozygosity is estimated to occur in 1 in 5000 individuals. FVL may be identified in up to 20% of individuals with a first thrombosis and up to 50% of patients with a positive family history in first-degree relatives. The heterozygous FVL gene defect is associated with a three- to sevenfold increased risk for thrombosis and a lifetime risk estimated at 10%. This risk is multiplicatively increased in the setting of additional risk factors including pregnancy, surgery, estrogen therapy, and advanced age [11, 12].

Testing for ACP-r helps screen for FVL. The ACP-r assay is an activated partial thromboplastin time (aPTT) ratio test. In normal individuals, the ratio should be >2.0, and in individuals with FVL, it is <2.0. Similar to other clotting-based assays, this can be influenced by exogenous factors including pregnancy, estrogen therapy, acute-phase reactants, factor deficiencies, disseminated intravascular coagulopathy, lupus anticoagulants, and anticoagulation therapy. The second-generation assays which dilute the patient plasma sample in factor V-deficient pooled plasma and include polybrene to bind heparin mitigate some of these interferences [11]. Genetic testing for FVL does not suffer from these limitations.

In contrast, FVL genetic testing in the absence of APC-r testing can lead to misdiagnosis in the setting of liver (FVL positive or negative donor liver) or bone marrow transplantation (FVL positive or negative donor marrow) since genetic testing is performed on peripheral blood white blood cell DNA. Therefore, it is ideal to send both plasma-based APC-r testing and FVL DNA testing in combination to avoid misdiagnosis [11, 12]. In addition, APC-r testing will pick up other defects in the factor V gene that will not be identified by FVL DNA testing including Factor V Hong Kong, Factor V Cambridge, and Factor V Liverpool although the contribution of these rare defects to thrombophilic risk is less well characterized. A complex haplotype of the factor V gene has also been identified, the factor V HR2 haplotype. This is increasingly part of some thrombophilia testing; however, the contribution of this haplotype to a prothrombotic phenotype remains to be clarified [13].

Prothrombin G20210A gene defect is a gain in function defect in the 3′ untranslated region of the prothrombin gene that results in an approximately 30% increase in plasma prothrombin levels. There is no screening assay for PTG. Genetic testing is required to identify this gene mutation. PTG is inherited in an autosomal dominant fashion. The prevalence is approximately 2–3% of the general population and up to 6% of patient with VTE. Heterozygous carriers have a three- to fourfold increased risk for VTE; in homozygous carriers, the risk is up to 30-fold [2]. The risk for recurrent VTE is low in heterozygotes at approximately 1.4-fold.

Cohort and case-controlled studies have identified elevated factor VIII levels >150 IU/dL as a risk factor for VTE with approximately a fivefold increased risk compared to levels <100 IU/dL. There are data suggesting elevated FVIII is not only a risk for initial VTE but also recurrent episodes [14]. Despite the association with both arterial and venous thrombosis, no clear mechanism has been identified. It has been proposed that FVIII may play a role in the thrombin amplification process. FVIII has high binding affinity for von Willebrand factor (vWF), and approximately 96% circulates in a bound form. Both FVIII and vWF increase during the acute-phase response. In addition, advancing age, female gender, exercise, stress, pregnancy, cancer, inflammation, infection, trauma, and surgery can also increase both FVIII and vWF. Since most studies that have evaluated FVIII excess do so in relation to acute thrombosis, it may be difficult to determine whether the increased risk related to FVIII is an inherited thrombophilia, represents an acquired prothrombotic thrombophilia, or is a prevalent acute-phase response [15]. If FVIII testing is deemed appropriate, it should only be undertaken 3–6 months after the inciting event *and* after therapy has been completed. In addition, the patient should be well without associated evidence of an inflammatory state. Some labs perform concomitant C-reactive protein (CRP) testing to help ensure the value of the result. Testing may be done using functional clotting assays, chromogenic assays, or enzyme-linked immunosorbent assays [9].

Elevated factor IX (FIX) and factor XI (FXI) have also been variable associated with venous thromboembolism [16]. Elevated FXI has also been associated with ischemic stroke [17]. The Longitudinal Investigation of Thromboembolism Etiology (LITE) cohort demonstrated increased risk for venous thromboembolism in participants with higher FIX and FXI levels at baseline. In addition, the odds ratio (OR) for venous thromboembolism increased with increasing quintiles; OR for FIX was 1.4, and for FXI was 2.0 for the 5th compared to the 1st quintile. However, after adjusting for other traits, including age, gender, race, BMI, diabetes, and FVIII, the OR for FIX was no longer significant at 1.0, while OR for FXI remained elevated at 1.6 [16].

Dysfibrinogenemia is another less common cause of thrombosis. Indeed, the phenotype associated with dysfibrinogenemia may range from bleeding to thrombosis. Typically, thrombosis in the setting of dysfibrinogenemia occurs in a younger age group. However, the prevalence of dysfibrinogenemia in patients with VTE is low, and routine testing is not warranted. Patients with dysfibrinogenemia may have a baseline prolonged prothrombin time making INR management difficult. Use of low-molecular-weight heparin for anticoagulation management has been recommended [18]. Warfarin monitoring using factor X activity assays or chromogenic factor X assays is also an option for patients who prefer oral anticoagulants. Direct oral anticoagulants are likely to be effective as well although clinical experience is limited given the rarity of this thrombophilia.

Antiphospholipid Antibodies

Antiphospholipid antibody syndrome (APS) is an acquired thrombophilic disorder associated with arterial and venous thrombosis as well as obstetrical complications in the setting of persistently positive antiphospholipid antibody testing. APS may be primary—occurring in the absence of known associated comorbid conditions or secondary occurring in the setting of other autoimmune disorders such as systemic lupus erythematosus.

The Sapporo criteria are international diagnostic criteria used to identify APS that include clinical and pathologic findings [19]. The diagnosis of APS requires one clinical and one pathologic criteria from Table 16.4.

APS antibodies are directed against plasma proteins which have affinity for and bind to anionic phospholipids. Current recommendations and testing includes lupus anticoagulant (LA), anticardiolipin antibody (ACA), and β2-glycoprotein-1 antibody (β2GP-1). However, general consensus suggests that β2GP-1 antibodies are the most clinically relevant [20]. Only IgG or IgM ACA at a titer >40 and β2GP-1 either IgG or IgM titers >99th percentile are included in the Sapporo diagnostic criteria. The role of IgA ACA and β2GP-1 or low or moderate titer ACA or β2GP-1 is unclear. In addition, testing for other antiphospholipid antibodies such as antiphosphatidylserine and antiphosphatidylethanolamine is not recommended [21]. One important defining criterion for APS is the need for the LA, ACA, or β2GP-1 antibodies to be persistently positive over time. Specifically, additional testing for confirmation is required at least 12 weeks (and not more than 5 years) after the initial testing [19].

As defined by the International Society on Thrombosis and Haemostasis (ISTH), LA testing is a three-step process. Step 1 is a screening test that demonstrates prolongation of a phospholipid-based clotting assay. The typical screening tests include a sensitive aPTT, dilute Russell viper venom time (DRVVT), or kaolin clotting time.

Step 2 is a mixing test that confirms the presence of an inhibitor and the absence of factor deficiency. Mixing studies are performed by adding normal plasma to the patient plasma in a 1:1 ratio and assessing clotting time. In the presence of a factor deficiency, clotting times will normalize, while with a LA the clotting time remains prolonged. Step 3 is confirmation that the inhibitor is phospholipid dependent. This is typically done by a platelet neutralization procedure or using an aPTT that contains hexagonal phospholipids. The demonstration of a shortening of the clotting time with the addition of excess phospholipid confirms phospholipid dependence (Table 16.5) [22]. In general, LA testing should be deferred in the setting of anticoagulation. False-positive results are not uncommon. DOACs and DTIs interfere with testing, and a false-positive test is likely. The effect from warfarin is highly variable. Although many commercial tests now include a heparinase or neutralizer and testing may be done while on heparin or LMWH, testing according to local laboratory standards is advised [21].

Table 16.4 Sapporo criteria for antiphospholipid antibody syndrome (Adapted from [19])

Clinical criteria (must have at least one)
Thrombosis—including one or more objectively confirmed arterial, venous, or small vessel thrombosis. Superficial thrombosis is excluded
Pregnancy morbidity—fetal demise in one or more normal fetus after 10 weeks gestation, one or more premature births of a normal pregnancy before 34 weeks gestation and associated with severe preeclampsia or eclampsia, or three or more unexplained, consecutive spontaneous abortions before 10 weeks gestation with maternal and chromosomal abnormalities excluded
Pathologic criteria—must have at least one positive[a]
Lupus anticoagulant—positive testing using a phospholipid-dependent clotting assay with evidence of phospholipid dependence
Anticardiolipin antibody—medium- or high-titer IgG (>40 GPL) or IgM (>40 MPL) anticardiolipin antibody ELISA (or >99th percentile)
Anti-β2-glycoprotein-1 antibody—IgG or IgM β2-glycoprotein-1 antibody ELISA titer >99th percentile

[a]Confirmation of a persistent antiphospholipid antibody requires a second positive confirmation test at least 12 weeks after initial testing

ACA and β2GP-1 testing is typically performed using enzyme-linked immunosorbent assays (ELISA). Testing can be done for all immunoglobulin subclasses: IgA, IgG, and IgM. However as previously noted the Sapporo criteria only include recognition of high-titer IgG and IgM subtypes [19].

The pathogenesis and thrombosis related to antiphospholipid antibodies are complex, and many different anionic phospholipids have been identified as targets for binding. Most antiphospholipid antibodies are directed against phospholipid-binding proteins on the surface of endothelial cells, monocytes, and platelets. In some models these have been shown to induce cellular activation and procoagulant activity. In addition, complement activation has been proposed as a mechanism for some of the activity including pregnancy-related placental issues [20, 23]. It is important to note that not all identified antiphospholipid antibodies are thrombogenic; in one study up to 8% of healthy blood donors tested positive for antiphospholipid antibodies [24]. In addition, they can be found transiently in association with infections and viral illness—the clinical significance of these transient antibodies remains unknown.

There are a number of thrombophilic defects where there is less certainty regarding their clinical impact. These include defects of the fibrino-

Table 16.5 Recommended three-step process for determining the presence of a lupus anticoagulant

Step 1
Screening test—sensitive aPTT, dRVVT, or KCT
Demonstrates prolongation of a phospholipid-dependent coagulation assay
Step 2
Confirm the inhibitor—1:1 mixing study
Excludes factor deficiency and acquired factor inhibitors
Step 3
Confirms phospholipid dependence—PNP or aPTT that contains hexagonal phospholipids or dRVVT with addition of purified phospholipid reagent (dRVVT; confirm step)

PTT activated partial thromboplastin time, *dRVVT* dilute Russell Viper venom time, *KCT* kaolin clotting time, *PNP* platelet neutralization procedure

lytic pathway (plasminogen, plasminogen activator inhibitor-1(PAI-1)), and thrombin-activatable fibrinolysis inhibitor (TAFI), lipoprotein (a), and homocysteine metabolism including the methylenetetrahydrofolate reductase (MTHFR) defects. These are not typically included in thrombophilia panels but may be tested individually in certain circumstances. Of all of these lesser considered thrombophilias, homocysteine is the most frequently recognized and tested.

Homocysteine is an amino acid that is a common intermediary in many metabolic reactions. Hyperhomocysteinemia has been identified as a risk factor for premature atherosclerosis and is likely a mild risk factor for both arterial and venous thrombosis. Elevated homocysteine levels associated with hyperhomocysteinemia may come from both inherited and acquired conditions. Acquired causes of hyperhomocysteinemia include advancing age, B vitamin deficiency, and renal disease. Methylenetetrahydrofolate reductase (MTHFR) is an enzyme that is important in the metabolism of homocysteine. There are two common point mutations (C677T and A1298C) that may cause a mild to moderate increase in homocysteine levels. Cystathionine β-synthase is another enzyme intermediary in homocysteine metabolism. Cystathionine β-synthase deficiency is typically associated with a more severe form of hyperhomocysteinemia known as homocystinuria that is associated with premature atherosclerosis, venous and arterial thromboembolism, intellectual developmental disabilities, and dislocated ocular lenses.

Homocysteine testing should be done fasting, using a plasma, not serum, sample. Alternatively, a normal non-fasting plasma level essentially excludes hyperhomocysteinemia. It is clear that while hyperhomocysteinemia is associated with thrombosis, the MTHFR genetic variants are not and as such should not be tested when evaluating thrombophilia [25, 26]. Hyperhomocysteinemia can be treated using folate with or without the addition of vitamin B6 and vitamin B12. However, it should be noted that in trials of cardiovascular disease and venous thromboembolism, homocysteine reduction using dietary supplementation did not appear to have an effect of clinical outcomes. Thus, the role of homocysteine testing and of hyperhomocysteinemia in atherosclerosis and venous thromboembolism remains ill-defined [26].

Conclusions

Current laboratory capabilities allow for testing of many known thrombophilias. However, unless testing is done with appropriate clinical timing, usually in the absence of anticoagulants, false-positive results may impede our opportunity to provide our patients with appropriate clinical recommendations. It is imperative that we understand the limitations of testing and the many patient-related, therapy-related, and laboratory-related factors that may impact results.

Key Points

- Thrombophilia laboratory testing is affected by many patient-related, laboratory-related, and treatment-related variables. When performed, testing should only be done when the results will directly impact patient care.
- Anticoagulation may impact thrombophilia testing. As such, the timing of the testing is very important.
- Positive antithrombin activity, protein C activity, protein S activity, or antiphospholipid antibody testing requires additional confirmatory testing/evaluation.
- Decisions regarding the pursuit of testing should take into account patient preferences.

Self-Assessment Questions

1. A 67-year-old woman undergoes otherwise uneventful knee arthroplasty. Approximately 4 weeks after surgery, she presents with pain and swelling of the left leg. Duplex ultrasound is positive for a femoral and popliteal vein

thrombosis. She is obese but in otherwise good health. She denies a personal history of venous thromboembolism, but her daughter had pulmonary embolism following the delivery of her 3rd child. She is planning to have the other knee replaced in the near future. After discussing the role of thrombophilia testing, what would you recommend?
   (a) Given the positive family history, full testing is warranted prior to the additional surgery.
   (b) Given the positive family history, genetic testing for Factor V Leiden and prothrombin gene G20210A is required.
   (c) No testing is warranted since this is a situational event.
   (d) She should avoid any other surgeries because of increased venous thromboembolism risk.
2. A 26-year-old woman developed a left leg deep vein thrombosis after a spontaneous abortion at 12 weeks gestation. She is currently on rivaroxaban (Xarelto®) 20 mg daily. Which of the following test results may be inaccurate if check while on the current therapy?
   (a) Antiphosphatidylserine antibodies
   (b) Anticardiolipin antibodies
   (c) β2-glycoprotein-1 antibodies
   (d) Lupus anticoagulant panel
3. Which of the following autosomal dominant genetic traits may be tested to assist with venous thromboembolism risk stratification?
   (a) Prothrombin gene G20210A
   (b) Protein C
   (c) Protein S
   (d) Antithrombin
4. A 36-year-old woman presents to you for a second opinion. She is G3P3 without prior obstetrical complications. She recently developed a calf vein DVT after arthroscopic surgery. She was on a combined estrogen/progestin contraceptive at the time of surgery. The primary care physician did a thrombophilia work-up that demonstrated heterozygous Factor V Leiden, heterozygous MTHFR A1298C with normal plasma homocysteine, and elevated protein C activity at 210%. How should you counsel her regarding these findings?
   (a) She will require indefinite anticoagulation therapy given all of these abnormalities.
   (b) Reassure her that she can complete her duration of therapy for a situational DVT and then stop anticoagulation.
   (c) Continue her anticoagulation indefinitely and advise additional family members get tested for the identified thrombophilias.
   (d) She should avoid the use of estrogen-containing therapies, extend the duration of therapy for an additional 6–12 months, and then consider prolonged secondary prophylaxis with aspirin.
5. A 56-year-old man developed a right iliofemoral deep vein thrombosis and pulmonary embolism after traveling to Israel. He has completed 6 months of anticoagulation and is currently on warfarin. The most recent INR is 2.6. Thrombophilia testing was ordered prior to stopping anticoagulation. Which of the following laboratory tests require additional testing for confirmation?
   (a) Activated protein C resistance (APC-r) ratio 2.1
   (b) Anticardiolipin antibody IgG of 65 GPL
   (c) Antithrombin activity 145% (lab normal 80–120%)
   (d) Heterozygous prothrombin gene G20210A mutation

Self-Assessment Answers

1. (c) No testing is warranted since this is a situational event.

   Given her age and the acquired risks for VTE including obesity and a recent surgery, additional testing is not warranted. Despite the positive family history, identification of Factor V Leiden or prothrombin gene mutation will not impact her current therapy or duration of anticoagulation. Both she and her surgeon must approach any additional procedures with the knowledge that she has an increased risk for thromboembolism. Aggressive and extended venous thromboembolism would be warranted in the periprocedural setting. No additional testing would impact her current plan of care or future recommendations for perioperative management.

2. (d) Lupus anticoagulant panel

   Given the association between the pregnancy loss and deep vein thrombosis, testing for antiphospholipid antibodies is prudent. There is currently no recommendation for testing antiphosphatidylserine antibodies. Both anticardiolipin antibodies and β2-glycoprotein-1 antibodies are tested using ELISA assay. The anti-Xa anticoagulants will not affect this testing. Lupus anticoagulant testing is performed using clot-based assays. The anti-Xa anticoagulants will generate a false positive, and testing should be avoided.

3. (a) Prothrombin gene G20210A

   While protein C, protein S, and antithrombin deficiency all demonstrate an autosomal dominant inheritance, they are associated with many different genetic abnormalities. Therefore, genetic testing is not warranted. Testing for the natural anticoagulant deficiencies is performed using activity and antigen-based assays. Factor V Leiden and prothrombin gene G20210A mutations are identified using genetic testing.

4. (b) Reassure her that she can complete her duration of therapy for a situational DVT and then stop anticoagulation.

   The only relevant thrombophilia identified is the heterozygous FVL. In the setting of oral contraceptives and surgery this likely was an additional trigger. MTHFR has not been validated as a DVT risk, and elevated levels of protein C activity are inconsequential. Family members should only be advised testing if the information regarding the FVL will change a medical therapy or affect future family planning. There is no data regarding the prolongation of therapy for heterozygous FVL, and this would be unnecessary. Aspirin has been evaluated for extended secondary prophylaxis only in patients with idiopathic DVT. Whether it is warranted in this setting is unknown.

5. (b) Anticardiolipin antibody IgG of 65 GPL

   APC-r >1.9 is normal and excludes the presence of FVL. No additional testing is warranted. Elevated levels of protein C, protein S, or antithrombin do not require additional testing. Genetic testing for prothrombin gene mutation is not affected by anticoagulation and will not change during therapy. Positive anticardiolipin antibodies required confirmatory testing. To diagnose antiphospholipid antibody syndrome, it requires a confirmed thrombotic event and persistently positive antiphospholipid antibody testing done at interval >12 weeks apart.

References

1. American Society of Hematology. Ten Things Physicians and Patients Should Question. http://www.choosingwisely.org/societies/american-society-of-hematology/.
2. Mannucci PM, Franchini M. Classic thrombophilic gene variants. Thromb Haemost. 2015;114:885–9.
3. Heit JA. Epidemiology of venous thromboembolism. Nat Rev Cardiol. 2015;12(8):464–74.
4. Morange PE, Tregouet DA. Current knowledge on the genetics of incident venous thromboembolism. J Thromb Haemost. 2013;11(suppl 1):111–21.
5. Heit JA, Ashrani A, Crusan DJ, McBane RD, Petterson TM, Bailey KR. Reasons for the persistent incidence of venous thromboembolism. Thromb Haemost. 2017;117(2):390–400.
6. Heit JA, Spencer FA, White RH. The epidemiology of venous thromboembolism. J Thromb Thrombolysis. 2016;41:3–14.
7. Khor B, Van Cott EM. Laboratory testing for antithrombin deficiency. Am J Hematol. 2010;85:947–50.
8. Khor B, Van Cott EM. Laboratory tests for protein C deficiency. Am J Hematol. 2010;85:440–2.
9. Eby C. Laboratory aspects of Thrombophilia testing. In: Kotte-Marchant K, editor. An algorithmic approach to hemostasis testing. Northfield: College of American Pathologists (CAP); 2008.
10. Marlar RA, Gausman JN. Protein S abnormalities: a diagnostic nightmare. Am J Hematol. 2011;86:418–21.
11. Van Cott EM, Khor B, Zehnder JL. Factor V Leiden. Am J Hematol. 2016;91:46–9.
12. Kadauke S, Khor B, Van Cott EM. Activated protein C resistance testing for factor V Leiden. Am J Hematol. 2014;89:1147–50.
13. Castaman G, Faioni EM, Tosetto A, Bernardi F. The factor V HR2 haplotype and the risk of venous thrombosis: a meta-analysis. Haematologica. 2003;88:1182–9.
14. Cosmi B, Legnani C, Cini M, Favaretto E, Palareti G. D-dimer and factor FVIII are independent risk factors for recurrence after anticoagulation withdrawal

for a first idiopathic deep vein thrombosis. Thromb Res. 2008;122:610–7.
15. Jenkins VP, Rawley O, Smith OP, O'Donnell JS. Elevated factor VIII levels and risk of venous thrombosis. Br J Haematol. 2012;157:653–66.
16. Cushman M, O'Meara ES, Folsom AR, Heckbert SR. Coagulation facotes IX through XIII and the risk of future venous thrombosis: the longitudinal investigation of thromboembolism etiology. Blood. 2009;114:2878–83.
17. Key NS. Epidemiology and clinical data linking factors XI and XII to thrombosis. Hematology Am Soc Hematol Educ Program. 2014;2104(1):66–70.
18. Casini A, Neerman-Arbex M, Ariens RA, De Moerloose P. Dysfibrinogenemia: from molecular anomalies to clinical manifestations and management. J Thromb Haemost. 2015;13:909–19.
19. Miyakis S, Lockshin MD, Atsumi T, Branch DW, Brey RL, Cervera R, et al. International consensus statement on an update of the classification criteria for definite antiphospholipid antibody syndrome (APS). J Thromb Haemost. 2006;4:295–306.
20. Salmon JE, de Groot PG. Pathogenic role of antiphospholipid antibodies. Lupus. 2008;17:405–11.
21. Chaturvedi S, McCrae KR. The antiphospholipid syndrome still an enigma. Hematology Am Soc Hematol Educ Program. 2015;2015:53–60.
22. Giannakopoulos B, Passam F, Ioannou Y, Krillis SA. How we diagnosis the antiphospholipid syndrome. Blood. 2009;113:985–94.
23. Giannakopoulos B, Passam F, Soheila R, Krillis SA. Current concepts on the pathogenesis of the antiphospholipid syndrome. Blood. 2007;109:422–30.
24. MaIntyre JA, Wagenknech DR, Waxman DW. Frequency and specificities if antiphospholipid antibodies (aPL) in volunteer blood donors. Immunobiology. 2003;207:59–63.
25. Franchini M, Martinelli I, Mannucci PM. Uncertain thrombophilia markers. Thromb Haemost. 2016;115: 25–30.
26. Eldibany MM, Caprini JA. Hyperhomocysteinemia and thrombosis: an overview. Arch Pathol Lab Med. 2007;131:872.

Heparin-Induced Thrombocytopenia

17

Emily Downs, Svetlana Goldman, Surabhi Palkimas, and Aditya M. Sharma

Clinical Vignette

A 43-year-old woman with history of hypothyroidism, morbid obesity, and gastroesophageal reflux presented to the cardiac surgery clinic with worsening dyspnea and echocardiographic findings of severe mitral and tricuspid regurgitation. She underwent successful mitral valve replacement with a bioprosthetic valve and tricuspid valve annuloplasty. She was discharged on warfarin to provide anticoagulation for the first 3–6 months, which was the time anticipated for the bioprosthetic mitral valve to fully endothelialize. Her international normalized ratio (INR) was 2.0 at the time of discharge on postoperative day 6. She presented 1 week later on postoperative day 12 with bilateral lower extremity edema and skin changes, which appeared to be ecchymosis on the dorsum of both feet (see Fig. 17.1) as well as platelet count of 50k/μL. Her platelet count was 200k/μL on postoperative day 6. Unfortunately, she had not taken any medications after discharge from the hospital. She was admitted to the hospital from the clinic. Given the concern for heparin-induced thrombocytopenia (HIT), she was treated with argatroban. Transesophageal echocardiogram (TEE) demonstrated extensive left atrial thrombus with a mobile component near the mitral valve. She was found to have positive laboratory assays for HIT including a positive HIT ELISA with an optical density (O.D.) of 2.422 and a positive serotonin release assay (SRA) with 92% release in the presence of low-dose (0.1 IU/mL) heparin. After her platelet count reached 162k/μL,

E. Downs
Department of Surgery, Division of Thoracic and Cardiovascular Surgery, University of Virginia Medical Center, University of Virginia, Charlottesville, VA, USA
e-mail: ead6m@hscmail.mcc.virginia.edu

S. Goldman · S. Palkimas
Department of Pharmacy, University of Virginia Medical Center, University of Virginia, Charlottesville, VA, USA
e-mail: sg2ac@virginia.edu; sp5dj@virginia.edu

A. M. Sharma (✉)
Department of Medicine, Cardiovascular Medicine Division, Heart and Vascular Center, University of Virginia Medical Center, University of Virginia, Charlottesville, VA, USA
e-mail: asharma@virginia.edu

J. F. Lau et al. (eds.), *Anticoagulation Therapy*, https://doi.org/10.1007/978-3-319-73709-6_17

she was bridged to warfarin therapy. She was discharged to home on warfarin with assistance to ensure she could consistently have her INR checked.

Pertinent questions related to this patient's care (which will be clarified over the course of this chapter) include:

- *What is the risk of HIT after cardiac surgery?*
- *Was the time course of her presentation typical?*
- *What is the appropriate evaluation process to diagnose HIT?*
- *What are the acute and long-term treatment strategies for HIT?*

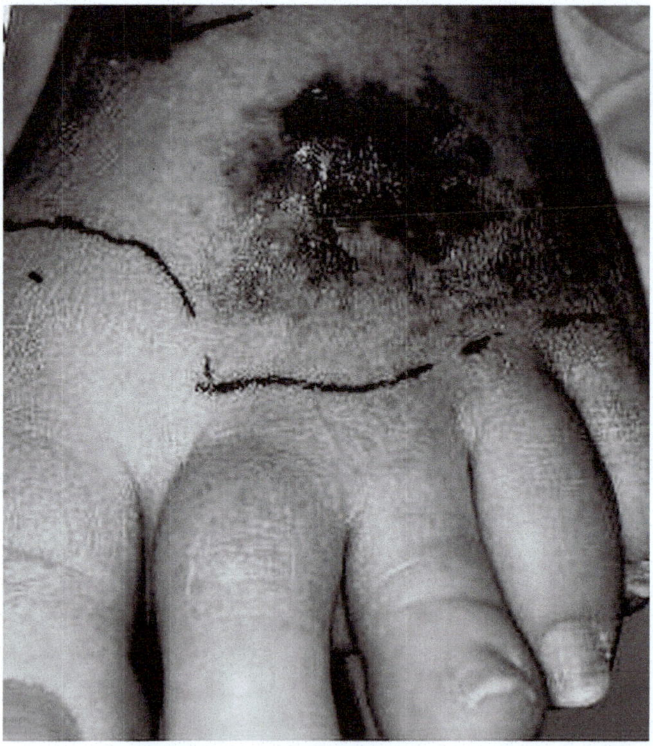

Fig. 17.1 A 43-year-old female with thrombocytopenia and ecchymosis on the dorsum of both feet

Introduction

HIT is an uncommon condition with grave consequences. It is a clinicopathological diagnosis which can often be complex; however, delayed diagnosis and inadequate or inappropriate treatment can lead to life- and limb-threatening outcomes. This chapter will describe the syndrome of HIT (and HITT) as it is now known, including its history, pathophysiology, diagnostic process with the current testing paradigm, and updated treatment options for HIT.

Historical Context

Heparin was discovered nearly 100 years ago and came into use as an anticoagulant in the 1930s [1,

2]. In 1957, Weisman presented a series of cases of paradoxical thrombosis in the setting of heparin therapy at the fifth Scientific Meeting of the International Society of Angiology [3]. The first patient in the series, a 62-year-old woman, was being treated for deep vein thrombosis (DVT) when she developed a femoral arterial occlusion requiring thrombectomy. A few days later, she developed a distal aortic occlusion while on heparin. This and other cases of arterial thrombosis during heparin treatment raised the question of heparin's role as a prothrombotic factor in some patients. The clots were described as "pale, soft, salmon-colored" and occurred roughly 10 days after initiating heparin treatment [3]. At this point in time, routine platelet count monitoring was not typically performed. In 1969, Natelson identified the association of heparin with thrombocytopenia in a subset of patients with a drop in platelet count and a rise in fibrinogen level [4]. In 1973, Rhodes and colleagues described essentially the syndrome we know as HIT today, documenting two patients with severe thrombocytopenia along with myocardial infarction, heparin resistance, and a rebound in the platelet count upon cessation of heparin therapy [5]. They noted the recurrence of thrombocytopenia when challenged with heparin several months later, and further investigation demonstrated a possible immune basis for the constellation of clinical findings, a circulating heparin-dependent platelet-activating substance. Further case reports in the 1970s continued to describe thrombocytopenia and thrombosis in the setting of heparin therapy [6–10]. In 1992, the immune basis of HIT was confirmed when Amiral and colleagues identified platelet factor 4 (PF4) complexed to heparin as the target for HIT antibodies [11]. This discovery paved the way for the development of laboratory assays to confirm the diagnosis of HIT.

Definition

HIT is defined as an immune-mediated condition associated with the occurrence of thrombocytopenia with or without thrombosis characteristically occurring 5–10 days after heparin initiation and the accompanying finding of platelet-activating HIT antibodies [12]. Clinicians may use a variation of this definition to diagnose HIT, especially in the context of specific scenarios such as recent heparin use. The following sections will further define this entity which is truly a clinicopathological diagnosis.

Nomenclature

The terminology surrounding HIT has varied over the past several decades and is worth mentioning to aid in the interpretation of the literature. There exists a nonimmune reaction to heparin due to platelet aggregation which induces a modest transient decrease in platelets that rarely declines below 100k/μL. This entity has been called HIT type I or heparin-associated thrombocytopenia in the past. More recently it has been suggested that this clinical occurrence should be referred to as nonimmune heparin-associated thrombocytopenia. The diagnosis of HIT, previously called HIT type II or immune-mediated HIT, is most commonly known as simply HIT in the modern literature [13].

Pathophysiology

HIT is a result of platelet-activating immune complexes generated by IgG molecules which recognize heparin bound to platelet factor 4 (PF4). When heparin, a negatively charged particle, is administered, it has a high affinity for positively charged platelet factor 4 (PF4) released from platelet alpha-granules and found on some cell surfaces. In the process of forming heparin/PF4 complexes, PF4 undergoes a conformational change which exposes new epitopes that can stimulate the immune system to generate antibodies to this complex (anti-heparin/PF4 antibodies, or "HIT antibodies") [14]. It takes approximately 5 days from initial heparin exposure for these antibodies to form. It remains unclear why some patients form these antibodies and others do not. Once these antibodies form, they bind to the heparin/PF4 complexes, and the Fc component binds to Fc receptors on platelets. This event causes platelet activation, platelet alpha- and delta-granule release, aggregation, and platelet microparticle formation resulting in thrombin generation and consumptive thrombocytopenia leading to venous and arterial thrombosis. Anti-heparin/PF4 antibodies also bind to monocytes and endothelial cells, which leads to tissue factor expression and further thrombin generation [12]. Since it takes approximately 5 days for these antibodies to form after initial heparin exposure (regardless of whether heparin treatment continues), the typical clinical presentation of HIT is 5–10 days after heparin exposure. In most patients, these antibodies disappear in roughly 50–85 days. If patients have had heparin exposure within the past 90 days and particularly within the last 30 days, circulating antibodies have the potential to cause the same reaction within a very short time after a new heparin exposure [12]. Figure 17.2 provides a summary of this pathophysiology.

It has been known for some time that not all patients who develop HIT antibodies develop the clinical HIT syndrome. Cardiovascular surgery patients develop HIT antibodies at a particularly high rate; anywhere from 20 to 61% of patients develop HIT antibodies, but only 1–3% of patients develop clinical HIT [14, 15]. Research is beginning to clarify the circumstances required for HIT antibodies to cause clinical HIT. Nazi and colleagues developed a unique assay to examine serum containing HIT antibodies, both from patients who developed clinical HIT and those who did not. Their work suggests that these antibodies do not always lead to platelet activation (and thus cannot cause clinical HIT) and that the antibodies must be present in a sufficient threshold level in order to cause HIT [16]. Rollin and colleagues identified that patients with FCGR2A 131RR genotype had greater risk of thrombosis with HIT compared to others due to defective platelet activation control [17]. These observations begin to explain why some patients form HIT antibodies but do not develop HIT, but further work is necessary to assess patient risk in a prospective fashion.

Incidence

The incidence of HIT ranges from 0.1% to approximately 5% and varies widely by patient population and the type of heparin treatment used. Two consistent observations are reported in clinical studies: (1) surgical patients develop HIT more commonly than medical patients, and (2) treatment with unfractionated heparin (UFH) is associated with a tenfold higher frequency of HIT than low-molecular-weight heparin (LMWH). Among surgical populations, cardiac surgery patients are at particularly high risk of HIT with rates from 1 to 3%. Postoperative patients receiving unfractionated heparin have 1–5% incidence of HIT compared to <1% in those receiving low-molecular-weight heparin (LMWH). HIT incidence can be as high as 11% in patients undergoing cardiac transplantation [14, 15]. Medical patients with cancer have a relatively high rate of HIT at roughly 1%, while obstetric patients have very low rates at <0.1%. Frequency of HIT is as high as 3.2% in newly initiated dialysis patients [14].

Clinical Characteristics

HIT can present in variety of manners including venous or arterial thrombosis, cutaneous changes, as well as other serious manifestations which are listed below and also summarized in Table 17.1.

Thrombosis

Unlike many other procoagulant states, HIT predisposes patients to both venous and arterial thrombosis. Venous thrombosis is more common, with rates of DVT or pulmonary embolism (PE) reported from 17 to 55% [15]. Greinacher and colleagues described a multi-institutional cohort of over 400 patients, all of whom had positive functional assays for HIT, and found at least one thromboembolic complication in 55% of patients. Of the thromboembolic complications, the site was venous in 71% of patients, with arterial

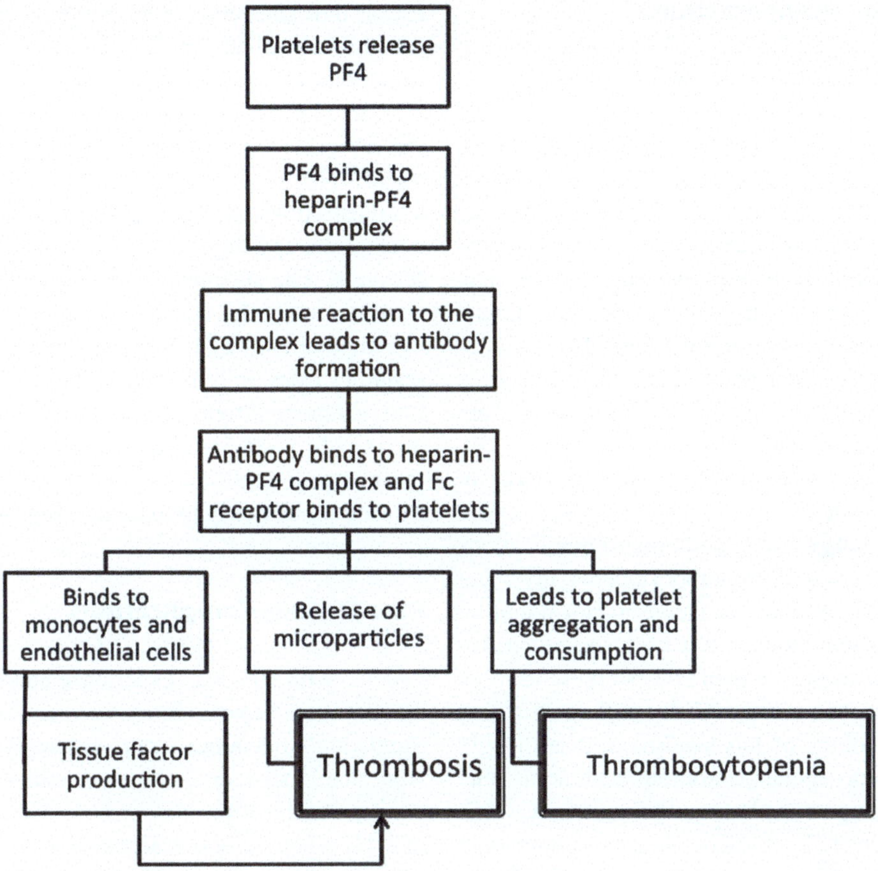

Fig. 17.2 Pathophysiology of heparin-induced thrombocytopenia

Table 17.1 Complications of HIT

Thrombosis			
Arterial	Venous	Cutaneous manifestations	Rare, serious complications
• Myocardial infarction	• DVT	• Skin necrosis at heparin injection site(s)	• Anaphylactoid reaction
• Stroke	• PE	• Warfarin-induced skin necrosis	• Adrenal hemorrhage and insufficiency
• Limb ischemia, amputation	• Venous limb gangrene		

thrombosis in 29% [18]. In the overall population, venous thromboembolism predominated, with a ratio of 2.4:1. However, in cardiovascular surgery patients, arterial thromboemboli were much more common with a ratio of 1:8.5. Of the venous thromboemboli, 44.5% were proximal or distal DVTs, and 23.8% were PEs. On the arterial side, limb arterial thromboses predominated, accounting for 16.4% of thromboembolic events, while stroke and myocardial infarction (MI) were much less common. The authors note that this is the opposite distribution of arterial thrombotic events seen in the non-HIT setting [18]. Other researchers have observed that many arterial and venous thromboses in HIT appear to be related to recent venous or arterial catheterization at the site that later develops thrombosis; the catheter-associated vessel injury may predispose to HIT-related thrombosis once the pathologic changes of HIT have occurred [19].

Cutaneous Manifestations

Cutaneous manifestations of HIT may occur in some patients. One such manifestation is skin necrosis at the site of heparin injection, hypothesized to occur as a result of localized platelet activation and microvascular thromboses at the injection site. These lesions initially appear as erythematous plaques or patches that may progress to frank necrosis. Over the clinical course of HIT, these lesions can also occur at cutaneous sites distant from the local injection. Approximately 10–20% of patients with HIT are reported to develop this manifestation [20]. Importantly, this complication may occur prior to thrombocytopenia or without thrombocytopenia occurring but portends additional complications from HIT even if thrombocytopenia does not develop [20]. Another cutaneous manifestation of HIT is warfarin-induced skin necrosis, which also occurs outside the realm of HIT but presents more readily in patients with HIT due to the underlying pathophysiology of this syndrome. It is thought that the procoagulant, thrombin-generating state of HIT coupled with acquired protein C deficiency induced by warfarin therapy combines to promote warfarin-induced skin necrosis. These lesions are classically seen over the trunk, abdomen, or breasts. The risk is elevated if patients are initiated on warfarin when the platelet count remains less than 150×10^9/L or if therapeutic anticoagulation with a non-heparin, non-warfarin agent has not been achieved [21].

Limb Gangrene

Venous limb gangrene is a related complication of HIT occurring in conjunction with warfarin therapy. This complication is characterized by limb ischemia in the presence of a pre-existing DVT and intact distal pulses. This complication tends to occur more often in patients with supratherapeutic INRs, perhaps reflecting particularly intense suppression of protein C levels in the setting of ongoing thrombin generation characteristic of HIT. However, this relationship between higher INR and venous limb gangrene is not consistently borne out [15, 22]. Since limb loss due to venous limb gangrene is a very real risk of HIT, in addition to limb ischemia due to arterial thromboses, there exist specific treatment recommendations regarding the timing of warfarin administration and overlapping parenteral anticoagulant therapy in an effort to prevent this complication. The specifics of these guidelines will be discussed in the Treatment section.

Amputation is a dreaded complication of HIT resulting from limb arterial occlusion or venous limb gangrene. Studies report an amputation rate of roughly 9–11% in HIT patients with severe thrombotic complications [14]. Amputation contributes significantly to the morbidity of HIT.

Rare Serious Complications

Patients with HIT may experience anaphylactoid reactions to heparin in certain circumstances. Singla and colleagues report a case of a patient who manifested erythematous skin lesions at enoxaparin injection sites without other evidence of HIT; when he was readmitted with unilateral lower leg edema, he was administered a bolus of UFH to treat a presumed DVT and rapidly developed anaphylaxis and cardiac arrest [20, 23]. This is a much less common but severe complication of HIT. The authors point out that while not all skin reactions to heparin are linked to HIT (indeed, some are better characterized as delayed-type hypersensitivity), these skin manifestations should prompt clinicians to pause prior to administering therapeutic heparin [20, 23].

Bilateral adrenal hemorrhage is another rare serious complication of HIT that can present insidiously as adrenal insufficiency. A case report and literature review by Rosenberger and colleagues discusses a postoperative patient with thrombocytopenia and suspected HIT who developed hemodynamic collapse on postoperative day 11 [24]. A CT scan to evaluate for possible etiologies of shock demonstrated bilateral adrenal enlargement consistent with hemorrhage and laboratory evaluation confirmed adrenal insufficiency. The literature review yielded 18 similar cases with thrombocytopenia characteristic of HIT and adrenal insufficiency presenting within a few days of the platelet count nadir. In most cases, patients were evaluated thoroughly for an etiology of shock with sepsis high on the differential, and usually a combination of laboratory findings and CT results led to the correct diagnosis. However, in three cases, the adrenal findings were not noted until autopsy. This rare complication of HIT should be kept in mind when patients develop unusual symptoms, including altered mentation, emesis, dizziness, or signs such as hypotension or hyponatremia [24].

Evaluation and Diagnosis

Clinical Findings and Scoring Systems

The process of diagnosing HIT begins with recognizing the clinical symptoms and signs that may reflect the presence of HIT. These include thrombocytopenia in a patient with ongoing or recent heparin use (specifically, a drop of more than 50% and typically with a nadir between 40,000 and 80,000/mm^3), as well as new venous or arterial thrombotic events. Since many clinical conditions can cause thrombocytopenia or thrombosis, one must maintain HIT on the differential diagnosis to ensure it is promptly identified. With HIT in mind as a potential diagnosis, clinicians should then use one of the available pretest probability models to assess the individual patient's risk of having HIT. These scoring systems vary slightly from one another and use clinical and laboratory data to predict patients' risk for HIT ranging from low to high. These clinical risk profiles may assist with management decisions prior to the return of laboratory results and can also guide whether to obtain laboratory assays and discontinue heparin.

The most popular and well-validated scoring system is the 4T score (Fig. 17.3). This pretest probability model was developed from scoring systems previously used to test diagnostic assays, and cutoffs were designated as low, intermediate, or high. The 4Ts themselves are thrombocytopenia, timing of platelet count fall, thrombosis or other sequelae, and other causes of thrombocytopenia. Each category can be awarded 0–2 points for a maximum score of 8 [15, 25]. The 4T score is relatively quick to calculate with some knowledge of the patient's clinical situation as well as their platelet count and platelet count trend over recent days. The creators of this score note that it has a high negative predictive value, such that a low score of 0–3 is associated with a very low rate of HIT. However, many of the patients who are noted to have an intermediate to high score do not in fact have HIT, creating a relatively low positive predictive value. This phenomenon is seen with other risk scoring systems for HIT as well and highlights the fact that a patient's clinical scenario and laboratory results must be taken together in making decisions regarding anticoagulation treatment for HIT.

The HIT Expert Probability (HEP) score (Table 17.2) is a newer and less extensively validated pretest probability model than the 4T score, and its development was based on broad expert opinion. Initial examination of this scoring system indicates that it is associated with improved interobserver agreement compared to the 4T score, as well as greater sensitivity and specificity. The scoring process is more complex than the 4T score, with eight categories which contribute varying points to the score, and some categories have as many as seven options. For screening purposes, the authors reported that a score of 2 or greater provides 100% sensitivity and 60% specificity, while a score of 5 or greater optimized sensitivity and specificity with values of 86% and 88%, respectively. Positive predictive value at the screening level was 29%, and at the higher optimized level of 5 points, it was 55%. While this tool was developed using a more detailed modeling process than the 4T score, it also has limitations in that a relatively small population used for validation as well as the possibility of clinicians having insufficient clinical data to apply the score in each and every available category [26].

Subsequent validation and comparison of the 4T score and HEP score have not been able to establish superiority of either model. Joseph and

	Score = 2	Score = 1	Score = 0
Thrombocytopenia Compare the highest platelet count within the sequence of declining platelet counts with the lowest count to determine the % of platelet fall. **(Select only 1 option)**	o > 50% platelet fall AND nadir of ≥ 20 AND no surgery within preceding 3 days	o > 50% platelet fall BUT surgery within preceding 3 days OR o any combination of platelet fall and nadir that does not fit criteria for Score 2 or Score 0 (eg, 30-50% platelet fall or nadir 10-19)	o < 30% platelet fall o any platelet fall with nadir < 10
Timing (of platelet count fall or thrombosis*) Day 0 = first day of most recent heparin exposure **(Select only 1 option)**	o platelet fall day 5-10 after start of heparin o platelet fall within 1 day of start of heparin AND exposure to heparin within past 5-30 days	o consistent with platelet fall days 5-10 but not clear (eg, missing counts) o platelet fall within 1 day of start of heparin AND exposure to heparin in past 31-100 days o platelet fall after day 10	o platelet fall ≤ day 4 without exposure to heparin in past 100 days
Thrombosis (or other clinical sequelae) **(Select only 1 option)**	o confirmed new thrombosis (venous or arterial) o skin necrosis at injection site o anaphylactoid reaction to IV heparin bolus o adrenal hemorrhage	o recurrent venous thrombosis in a patient receiving therapeutic anticoagulants o suspected thrombosis (awaiting confirmation with imaging) o erythematous skin lesions at heparin injection sites	o thrombosis suspected
oTher cause for Thrombocytopenia** **(Select only 1 option)**	o no alternative explanation for platelet fall is evident	**Possible other cause is evident:** o sepsis without proven microbial source o thrombocytopenia associated with initiation of ventilator o other	**Probable other cause present:** o within 72 h of surgery o confirmed bacteremia/ fungemia o chemotherapy or radiation within past 20 days o DIC due to non-HIT cause o posttransfusion purpura (PTP) o platelet count < 20 AND given a drug implicated in causing D-ITP (see list) o non-necrotizing skin lesions at LMWH injection site (presumes DTH) o other

Drugs implicated in drug-induced immune thrombocytopenia (D-ITP)

Relatively Common: glycoprotein IIb/IIIa antagonists (abciximab, eptifibatide, tirofiban); quinine, quinidine, sulfa antibiotics, carbamazepine, vancomycin
Less Common: actinomycin, amitriptyline, amoxicillin/piperacillin/nafcillin, cephalosporins (cefazolin, ceftazidime, ceftriaxone), celecoxib, ciprofloxacin, esomeprazole, fexofenadine, fentanyl, fucidic acid, furosemide, gold salts, levofloxacin, metronidazole, naproxen, oxaliplatin, phenytoin, propranolol, propoxyphene, ranitidine, rifampin, suramin, trimethoprim. Note: This is a partial list.

Fig. 17.3 The "4T score" for diagnosis of heparin-induced thrombocytopenia [15]. Reprinted from CHEST, Vol. 141/Issue 2 Suppl, Linkins LA, Dans AL, Moores LK, Bona R, Davidson BL, Schulman S, Crowther M, Treatment and prevention of heparin-induced thrombocytopenia: antithrombotic therapy and prevention of thrombosis 9th ed: American College of Chest Physicians Evidence-based Clinical Practice Guidelines, pages e495s–e530s, © 2012, with permission from Elsevier

colleagues identified area under the receiver operating curves for each score as 0.74 for 4T and 0.73 for HEP, not significantly different. In their population, a 4T score >3 (intermediate or high risk) had a 93% sensitivity and 35% specificity, while a HEP score of 2 or greater was 100% sensitive and 16% specific [27, 28].

A third risk score, developed by Louet and colleagues (Table 17.3), was designed specifically for use in cardiac surgery patients [29]. It is fairly straightforward to calculate and incorporate knowledge of the unique circumstances of cardiac surgery and recent cardiopulmonary bypass. This will be discussed in more detail in the HIT in Cardiac Surgery section of this chapter.

The principal value of these three scoring systems is that they are able to identify patients at low risk for HIT, who do not warrant laboratory testing or initiation of alternative forms of anticoagulation. The converse of this capability is a limited ability to accurately predict who actually has HIT. For all of these scores, patients scored at intermediate to high risk of HIT only occasionally have positive laboratory assay results (e.g., 24–61% for the 4T score). The scores do provide a useful first step in evaluating the patient, and even the

Table 17.2 HIT Expert Probability score [26]

Typical-onset HIT		Alternative scoring for suspected rapid-onset HIT (applies to listed components, otherwise use left column)	
Component	Score	Component	Score
Magnitude of fall in platelet count			
< 30%	-1		
30-50%	1		
> 50%	3		
Timing of platelet count fall (relative to heparin exposure)		Timing of platelet count fall (relative to re-exposure)	
< 4 days	-2	< 48 hours	2
4 days	2	> 48 hours	-1
5-10 days	3		
11-14 days	2		
> 14 days	-1		
Nadir platelet count			
≤ 20 k/μL	-2		
> 20 k/μL	2		
Thrombosis (select one)		Thrombosis (select one)	
New VTE or ATE ≥4 days after heparin exposure	3	New VTE or ATE after heparin exposure	3
Progression of pre-existing VTE or ATE while receiving heparin	2	Progression of pre-existing VTE or ATE while receiving heparin	2
Skin necrosis at subcutaneous heparin injection sites	3		
Acute systemic reaction after IV heparin bolus	2		
Bleeding, petechiae, or extensive bruising	-1		
Other causes of thrombocytopenia (select all that apply)			
• Presence of chronic thrombocytopenia	-1		
• Newly initiated medication causing thrombycytopenia	-2		
• Severe infection	-2		
• Severe DIC (fibrinogen < 100mg/dL,D-dimer> 50μg/mL)	-2		
• Indwelling intra-arterial device (IABP, VAD, ECMO)	-2		
• Cardiopulmonary bypass within previous 96 hours	-1		
• No other apparent cause	3		

Score components are colored based on relative contribution, with findings that imply more likelihood of HIT colored in progressively darker red and clinical parameters that lead away from a diagnosis of HIT colored in progressively darker green

Table 17.3 Diagnostic score for HIT in patients with thrombocytopenia after CPB [29]

Variables	Score
Platelet count time course (see inset panel at right)	
Pattern A	2
Pattern B	1
Time from CPB to index date	
≥5 days	2
<5 days	0
CPB duration	
≤118 min	1
>118 min	0
Classification	Total score
High probability of HIT	≥2
Low probability of HIT	<2

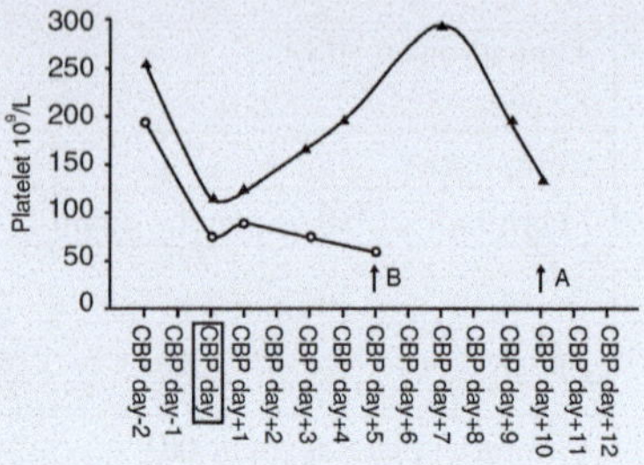

Reprinted with permission from Lillo-Le Louët A, Boutouyrie P, Alhenc-Gelas M, Le Beller C, Gautier I, Aiach M, et al. Diagnostic score for heparin-induced thrombocytopenia after cardiopulmonary bypass, Journal of Thrombosis and Haemostasis, Vol 2, No. 11, pages 1882–1888, © 2004, with permission from John Wiley and Sons

more extensive HEP is estimated to take less than 5 min to calculate. These risk scores may become more useful with additional validation in the future and for the moment do provide valuable information to the clinical team.

Laboratory Evaluation

The challenge of using laboratory assays for detection of HIT is applying them to appropriate patients to ensure that diagnosis is made promptly when present and that false-positive results are minimized. There exist several practical challenges in using laboratory assays for the diagnosis of HIT including the limited availability of the tests at various institutions and the potential delay in returning results if a center is only able to perform the assay a limited number of times per week. This is an important issue since HIT patients have a high incidence of thrombosis in the first few days and inadequate anticoagulant therapy while awaiting test results may lead to disastrous thrombotic consequences. Hence, it is useful to risk stratify patients using one of the clinical pretest probability scores as these can help a clinician decide whether to pursue empiric non-heparin anticoagulation until laboratory assay results return.

The two major categories of HIT laboratory assays include immunoassays and functional assays. Immunoassays detect the presence of antibodies to PF4/heparin complexes, while functional assays measure the ability of antibodies to activate donor platelets (a hallmark of the pathogenesis of HIT). Immunoassays are very sensitive but cannot differentiate between antibodies which can and cannot cause clinical HIT. For this reason, immunoassays are recommended for the initial diagnosis of HIT, while functional assays are used to confirm the diagnosis in most algorithms [30].

Enzyme-linked immunosorbent assays (ELISAs) were the initial laboratory assay developed for the detection of HIT antibodies. Patient serum is added to sample wells containing immobilized PF4. After washing away non-specific antibody binding with sample buffer, a secondary antihuman Fc antibody is added which is linked to an enzyme that produces a colored product when incubated in the presence of its target substrate. The test is semiquantitative in that the intensity, or optical density, of the colored product is correlated with the concentration of bound HIT antibodies [30]. Evaluation of ELISA tests and modern variations has confirmed that these tests are highly sensitive for HIT, but their specificity is approximately 85% which means that a nontrivial proportion of patients who test positive have antibodies which will not result in clinical HIT. In patients with a low pretest probability for HIT but a positive ELISA result, additional confirmation with a functional assay is necessary [15].

Several techniques have been developed in an attempt to augment the specificity of ELISAs for HIT. Some researchers have sought to leverage the semiquantitative nature of the polyspecific ELISA and establish thresholds of optical density at which positive results correlate with true positive HIT as verified by a functional assay. One study demonstrated that positive SRA results correlated with relatively high OD values, beyond the cutoff typically used to distinguish between a positive and negative assay result. They noted that a weak-positive EIA-IgG result between 0.40 and 1.00 OD units correlated with a positive SRA in approximately 5% of patients, while a very strong positive OD >2.00 units correlated with a ~90% probability of a positive SRA. This led the authors to suggest that altering the OD cutoff might adversely affect the sensitivity of the test but that reporting the OD itself could help clinicians to better gauge the true risk of HIT based upon this initial laboratory test result [31]. The original ELISAs for HIT detect polyspecific antibodies (i.e., IgA and IgM in addition to IgG). Newer versions of the test have tried to increase its specificity by measuring only IgG antibodies which are implicated as the primary pathogenic antibodies in clinical HIT. While this appears to be logical, some studies have not been able to demonstrate that IgG-specific tests can universally provide improved specificity for HIT over polyspecific ELISAs [30].

Other variations on ELISA technique focus on creating a technique that provides a more rapid turnaround without specialized technicians. These approaches include particle gel immunoassays (PaGIA) and lateral flow assays, which have some benefits but are only able to report positive/negative results without more specialized titration studies. Chemiluminescent assays and latex agglutination assays have an added benefit of being performed on an automated basis so that they can be run 24 h a day [30]. In general, these tests vary in diagnostic performance such that the choice of one test over another depends upon numerous factors from ease of use to cost.

Functional assays for HIT are much more specific and are typically used as a confirmatory test when an ELISA or variant thereof indicates the presence of PF4/heparin antibodies. Functional assays incubate patient serum with ostensibly pathogenic antibodies with donor platelets which are either prepared as washed platelets or as platelet-rich plasma. The washed platelet technique is preferred due to the potential interference of antibodies in the donor serum/plasma. These assays demonstrate that the patient's HIT antibody can cause platelet activation, the hallmark pathophysiology of HIT, in vitro, making these tests highly specific for HIT [30]. However, functional assays are challenging to use for several reasons: donor blood is required, the tests are labor-intensive, and radiation is required for the serotonin release assay.

Research is ongoing to develop more accessible diagnostic tools. Meanwhile, many hospitals must send blood specimens out to reference labs to obtain a functional assay, which unfortunately can delay diagnostic evaluations.

Platelet Count Monitoring for Patients Receiving Prophylactic Heparin or LMWH

Platelet count monitoring is recommended for patients with a risk of HIT >1%. It can be a challenge to ensure that monitoring is actually performed, and no studies have been done to demonstrate that the benefits of platelet count monitoring outweigh the disadvantages (including cessation of indicated heparin therapy while evaluating for HIT). The American College of Chest Physicians (ACCP) guidelines recommend platelet count monitoring every 2–3 days from day 4 to 14 after initial heparin exposure in those patients with a risk of HIT that is >1% [15]. Some authors advocate testing on days 5, 7, and 9 after initial heparin exposure or after surgery if heparin was also given before surgery reflecting the finding that most patients manifest HIT within this time frame. This captures the peak platelet count after surgery, roughly day 5–7, which may be higher than the presurgery baseline and facilitate capture of a meaningful 50% decrease in platelet count [12].

Treatment

Initial Management

Initial treatment of HIT consists of prompt discontinuation of all forms of heparin including low-molecular-weight heparin, heparin flushes, and heparin-coated catheters [12, 15]. LMWHs possess high cross-reactivity with heparin antibodies in vitro and should be avoided in the treatment of HIT. Prospective cohort studies with historical controls have demonstrated that discontinuing heparin alone is not adequate to prevent thrombosis and complications of HIT [15]. Untreated patients were found to have a 5–10% daily risk of thrombosis up to 2 days after stopping heparin and a 30-day cumulative risk of new thromboembolism of up to 50% [32]. Therefore, following cessation of heparin, a therapeutic dose of an alternative anticoagulant should be initiated to prevent thrombotic complications. In patients with a low clinical probability of HIT (low 4T score), clinicians can consider continuing heparin with daily monitoring of platelets. For those with an intermediate or high probability of HIT, all heparin should be discontinued, and treatment with an alternative anticoagulant is recommended [32].

The drugs of choice for treatment of HIT include anticoagulants that quickly inhibit thrombin and lack cross-reactivity with heparin/PF4 antibodies. The anticoagulants that have been utilized for treatment of HIT include the direct thrombin inhibitors (DTIs) argatroban (FDA approved), lepirudin (FDA approved, no longer available), bivalirudin (off-label), and desirudin (off-label) and the indirect factor Xa inhibitors danaparoid (off-label, not available in the USA) and fondaparinux (off-label). The only agent that is currently available and FDA approved is argatroban which requires continuous IV infusion and laboratory monitoring with the aPTT. Several off-label agents have come into greater use due to their own unique advantages. Bivalirudin is approved for use in PCI and cardiac surgery so is sometimes used in these settings when HIT is diagnosed or suspected but is not approved for HIT treatment specifically. Desirudin and fondaparinux are appealing as both can be administered subcutaneously with straightforward dosing regimens. There are no high-quality prospective head-to-head trials between these alternative agents, so treatment selection should be based on drug availability, unique patient characteristics including renal and hepatic function, bleeding risk, the presence of thrombotic complications, and the need for invasive procedures. The drug properties outlined in Table 17.4 can help guide clinicians in choosing the most appropriate agent. We suggest a treatment algorithm noted in Fig. 17.4.

Following initial treatment with a parenteral thrombin or factor Xa inhibitor, patients will need to be transitioned to a vitamin K antagonist (VKA) for long-term anticoagulation. Warfarin is contraindicated as initial monotherapy for HIT since rapid initiation of warfarin in patients with HIT may produce a prothrombotic state due to declining levels of the natural anticoagulant, protein C [15]. This can lead to serious adverse events including warfarin-induced skin necrosis and venous limb gangrene [22]. Patient characteristics that lead to development of venous limb gangrene include recent discontinuation of the parenteral anticoagulant, a supra-therapeutic INR due to a rapid and excessive reduction in factor VII that coincides with severe drop in protein C, and a platelet count $<150 \times 10^9$/L [22]. ACCP guidelines recommend against starting a VKA until platelets have substantially recovered (at least to 150×10^9/L) over starting VKA at lower platelet counts and suggest starting warfarin at lower doses, such as 5 mg daily. When starting a VKA, it is imperative to bridge therapy with an alternative anticoagulant for a minimum of 5 days and until the INR is therapeutic for two consecutive days. Furthermore, in patients where

Table 17.4 Drug properties

Drug name	Mechanism	Admin	Monitoring	Dosing	Onset of action	Clearance (half-life)	Drug-induced antibodies	Antidote	Dialyzable	Effect on INR	Pregnancy
Argatroban (Acova)	Direct thrombin inhibitor	IV	aPTT Goal: 1.5–3 times patient's baseline or 60–90 s ACT (for PCI use, goal 300–450 s)	2 mcg/kg/min Hepatic dysfunction: see table in argatroban section	Immediate	Hepatobiliary (40–50 min)	None	None	20%	Significantly prolongs	Category B
Bivalirudin (Angiomax) Note: off-label for treatment of HIT Approved for PCI/cardiac surgery w/ HIT	Direct thrombin Inhibitor	IV	aPTT ACT or ECT (high doses) Goal: 1.5–2.5 × patient's baseline or 60–90 s	0.15 mg/kg/h Renal dysfunction: See table in bivalirudin section	Immediate	Enzymatic (80%) Renal (20%) (25 min)	Low Incidence Potentially cross-reactive with anti-lepirudin Ab	None	25%	Moderately prolongs	Category B
Lepirudin (Refludan) Note: discontinued May 2012	Direct thrombin inhibitor Recombinant hirudin	IV, SC	aPTT Goal: 1.5–2.5 × patient's baseline (initial check 4 h after starting) ECT (high doses)	Initial bolus: 0.2 mg/kg*reserved for life-threatening or limb-threatening thrombosis Followed by 0.15 mg/kg/h Renal dysfunction: see table in lepirudin section	Immediate	Renal (80 min)	40–60% anti-lepirudin antibodies *avoid reexposure to lepirudin	None	High-flux dialyzers	Slightly prolongs (dose dependent)	Category B

(continued)

Table 17.4 (continued)

Drug name	Mechanism	Admin	Monitoring	Dosing	Onset of action	Clearance (half-life)	Drug-induced antibodies	Antidote	Dialyzable	Effect on INR	Pregnancy
Desirudin (Iprivask)	Direct thrombin inhibitor	SC, IV	Not necessary (plasma levels correlate with aPTT)	15 or 30 mg SC every 12 h-studied in PREVENT-HIT (optimal dose for HIT not established)		Renal (2 h)	Low incidence Antibodies induced by lepirudin 100% cross-reactivity	None	Cleared via dialysis using special membranes	Slightly prolongs	Category C
Fondaparinux (Arixtra) Note: off-label for treatment of HIT	Indirect factor Xa inhibitor	SC	Not necessary; may consider anti-Xa levels in obese patients	<50 kg: 5 mg once daily 50–100 kg: 7.5 mg once daily >100 kg: 10 mg once daily	~2–3 h	Renal (17–20 h)	May cause HIT (very rare)	None	20%	None	Category B

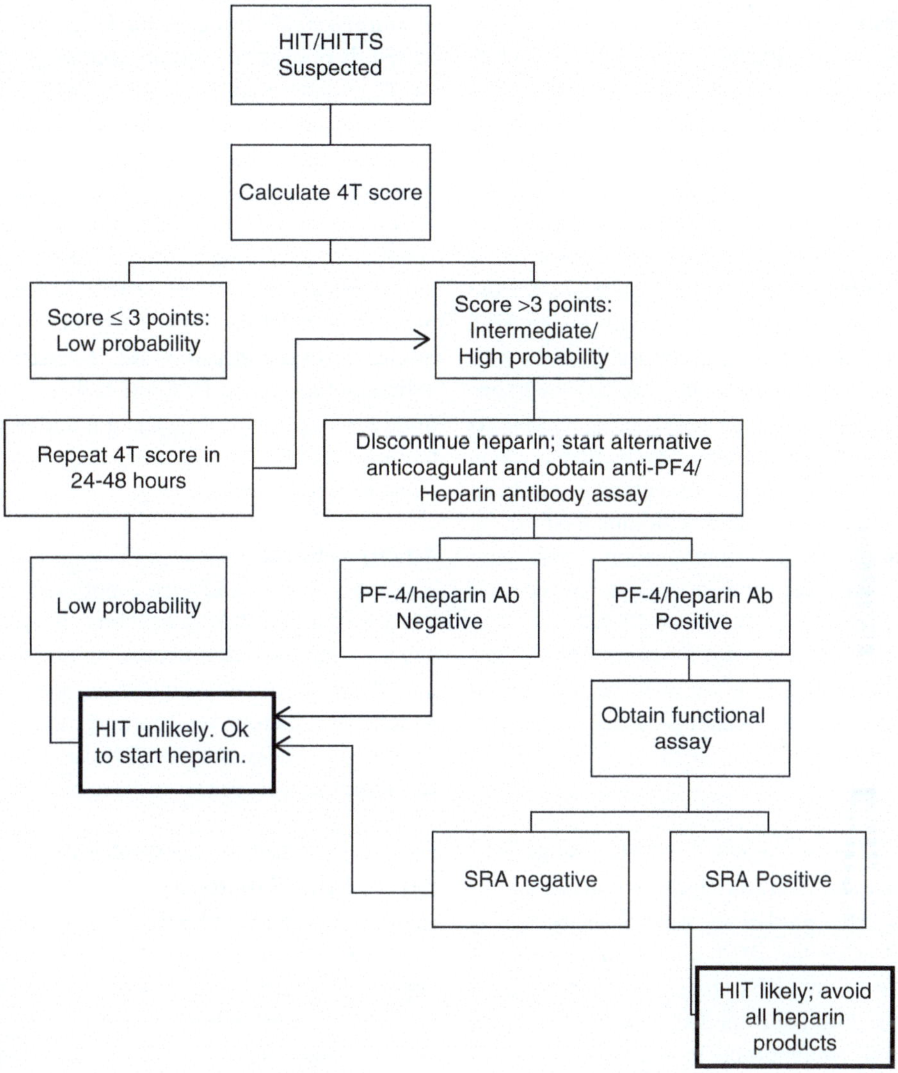

Fig. 17.4 Treatment algorithm for HIT/HITT

a VKA has been started prior to diagnosis with HIT, reversing therapy with vitamin K is recommended to replenish protein C levels [15].

Rationale for Treating HIT as well as HITT

Due to the high risk of thrombotic events in patients with isolated HIT, it is important to treat both HIT without thrombosis and HITT. Studies have shown that 17–55% of patients with isolated HIT develop thromboembolism in the absence of an alternative anticoagulant.

Pharmacologic Agents

The following descriptions provide information regarding the agents most often used in the treatment of HIT, and summary data is provided in Table 17.4.

Argatroban

Argatroban is a synthetic direct highly selective thrombin inhibitor derived from the amino acid L-arginine that reversibly binds to the active site of free and clot-associated thrombin. It inhibits all thrombin-mediated procoagulant activities including fibrin formation and the activation of coagulation factors V, VIII, and XIII and activation of protein C and platelets. It is FDA approved for the prevention and treatment of thrombosis in HIT patients and as an anticoagulant for patients with HIT undergoing percutaneous coronary intervention (PCI). When administered as a continuous infusion, argatroban produces anticoagulant effects immediately, and a steady-state effect is achieved within 1–3 h. It is metabolized through the liver via hydroxylation and aromatization, primarily excreted in the feces (~65%; 14% unchanged) and has a relatively short half-life of 40–50 min in the presence of normal hepatic function. These pharmacokinetic properties allow it to be a preferred agent for patients with renal insufficiency but have normal or preserved liver function.

Dosing

HIT: The standard regimen is an intravenous infusion of 2 mcg/kg body weight/min without an initial bolus. After initiation, argatroban therapy is monitored using the aPTT with a target range of 1.5–3 times the initial baseline value (not to exceed 100 s) with dose adjustments (dose not to exceed 10 mcg/body weight/min) as necessary to maintain a steady-state aPTT. Argatroban's half-life increases substantially (~180 min) in patients with hepatic dysfunction; therefore an initial dose of 0.5 mcg/kg body weight/min is typically recommended in these patients. Due to potentially decreased clearance, the American College of Chest Physicians Evidence-Based Clinical Practice Guidelines and the British Guidelines recommend initial doses between 0.5 and 1.2 mcg/kg body weight/min for patients with hepatic congestion, heart failure, multi-organ failure, or severe anasarca or after cardiac surgery.

Patients Undergoing PCI

An initial argatroban bolus of 350 mcg/kg followed by an infusion of 25 mcg/kg/min is recommended. The activated clotting time (ACT) is monitored 5–10 min after the bolus dose is completed. It is suggested to proceed with PCI if the ACT is greater than 300 s. If the ACT is less than 300 s, an additional bolus dose of 150 mcg/kg should be administered along with an increase in the infusion to 30 mcg/kg/min. If the ACT is greater than 450 s, the infusion should be decreased to 15 mcg/kg/min. The ACT is maintained between 300 and 450 s and should be monitored 5–10 min after each additional bolus or change in the infusion rate. If patients require anticoagulation post-PCI, argatroban can be continued at a rate of 2 mcg/kg/min and adjusted to maintain an aPTT 1.5–3 times the initial baseline value (not to exceed 100 s).

Adverse Effects

The most common adverse event associated with the use of argatroban is bleeding. It can occur at any site, and the risk is dependent on the intensity and duration of anticoagulation and individual patient risk factors for bleeding. Other adverse effects such as chest pain, hypotension, nausea, fever, and allergic reactions have been reported.

Lepirudin (No Longer Available, Discontinued in 2012)

Lepirudin is a recombinant form of hirudin, the natural anticoagulant isolated from the leech that is approved for the treatment of HIT. It is a direct irreversible thrombin inhibitor that acts on both free and clot-bound thrombin. This drug undergoes primarily renal elimination with approximately 48% of the intravenous dose excreted in the urine. The terminal half-life in healthy volunteers is about 1.3 h in the presence of normal renal function.

Dosing

Initial dosing recommendations based on the package insert advise an intravenous bolus dose of 0.4 mg/kg body weight (up to 110 kg-maximum dose of 44 mg) followed by a continuous infusion of 0.15 mg/kg/h (maximum dose based on 110 kg infusion of 16.5 mg/h). Further analysis of the clinical trials that led to approval of lepirudin demonstrated a higher risk of hemorrhage without increased clinical efficacy for doses exceeding 0.07 mg/kg/h [33]. Therefore, the most recent clinical guidelines recommend lower doses than the

Table 17.5 Lepirudin dosing recommendations based on renal function [15]

No bolus dose	
In patients with limb- or life-threatening thrombosis: initial IV bolus of 0.2 mg/kg	
Serum creatinine (mg/dL)	Continuous infusion dosing (mg/kg/h)
<1.0	0.10
1.0–1.6	0.05
1.6–4.5	0.01
>4.5	0.005

package insert recommendations [15, 32]. A bolus dose of 0.2 mg/kg is reserved for patients with life- or limb-threatening thrombosis; otherwise it is recommended to omit bolus dosing. Dose adjustments are required for renal insufficiency, and reduced continuous infusion rates are outlined in Table 17.5.

Monitoring

A baseline aPTT should be obtained prior to initiation, and patients with aPTT ratios greater than 2.5 should not be started on lepirudin. Subsequent aPTTs should be drawn 4 h after starting therapy and after each dose adjustment with a goal target aPTT ratio of 1.5–2.5 times the patient baseline.

Adverse Effects/Clinical Considerations

The most common adverse effect is bleeding, especially when this agent is used in combination with thrombolytic agents. Other adverse effects seen in clinical trials include fever, abnormal liver function tests, pneumonia, and allergic skin reactions [34, 35].

Up to 50% of patients may form anti-hirudin antibodies which bind to the drug and form large complexes that cannot be renally excreted prolonging the half-life and requiring subsequent dose reductions [36, 37]. Anaphylaxis can occur in up to 0.16%, usually after bolus dosing and more likely after reexposure [38]. In patients with prior exposure to lepirudin, bolus doses should be avoided or alternative anticoagulants should be utilized to reduce this risk.

Data and Clinical Trials

Lepirudin gained approval for treatment of HIT based on three prospective observational studies (HAT-1, HAT-2, and HAT-3) comparing this agent to untreated historical controls [35, 39, 40]. Randomized controlled trials were not possible at the time, since no other anticoagulants were approved for HIT treatment. Historical controls received care consisting of stopping heparin alone or discontinuing heparin and starting a vitamin K antagonist. Results of these studies examined the combined end point of new thromboembolic complications, limb amputations, and death and revealed improved outcomes with lepirudin compared to controls (29.7% versus 52.1%) [41]. Pooled analysis of these studies demonstrated that the rate of new thromboembolic events was significantly lower in lepirudin-treated patients (11.9 versus 32.1%) but there was no significant difference in rates of death or limb amputation. Clinical benefit was offset by increased rates of bleeding rates affecting 17.6% of patients receiving lepirudin compared to 5.8% among controls.

Lepirudin was discontinued in 2012; however it possesses similar properties to other currently available products such as desirudin, another recombinant hirudin, providing clinicians information that can help guide therapy for similar medications [32].

Desirudin

Desirudin is a highly selective direct thrombin inhibitor, offering the advantage of being the only thrombin inhibitor administered as a fixed dose subcutaneous injection [42]. It is approved for DVT prophylaxis following hip replacement surgery and has been shown to be more effective than unfractionated heparin and low-molecular-weight heparin in this setting [43, 44].

Dosing

Dosing has not been established in HIT, but the doses utilized in the PREVENT-HIT trial were 15 or 30 mg SC every 12 h. The lower dose of 15 mg every 12 h was given to patients without evidence for thrombosis, while the higher 30 mg dose was reserved for patients with clinical evidence of thrombosis [45].

Renal Impairment

Package insert recommendations for DVT prophylaxis in hip replacement recommend to reduce the dose to 5 mg every 12 h for patients with moderate renal insufficiency (defined as a creatinine clearance of 31–60 mL/min) and to 1.7 mg given every 12 h in patients with severe renal impairment (defined as creatinine clearance of ≤31 mL/min). These dosing recommendations are based on increases in total drug exposure (AUC) following single IV doses of desirudin. However, peak plasma concentration (Cmax) is a better predictor of maximal aPTT effect and bleeding risk, and Cmax is much lower following SC administration.

Monitoring

Although monitoring is not necessary, plasma levels correlate with the aPTT, and it is recommended to target an aPTT less than two times the patient's baseline value.

Clinical Considerations

Although there are limited data on the use of this agent in HIT, this drug possesses characteristics that can make it an appealing option including a fixed subcutaneous dose and minimal effect on INR, allowing for simpler administration and smoother transition to oral anticoagulant therapy.

Data and Clinical Trials

PREVENT-HIT was an open-label head-to-head trial of desirudin against argatroban [45]. Although limited to a small number of patients (16 patients total), this study had promising results with no new thrombotic events, deaths, or major bleeding in the desirudin group and a lower cost of treatment with desirudin compared to argatroban ($1688 versus $8250).

An observational multicenter registry in Europe in patients undergoing major orthopedic surgery examined a subset of patients with HIT (n = 51). Those patients with clinical HIT (14 patients) did not have any reported deaths or thrombotic events and only one major bleeding event. For patients that had a history of HIT (47 patients), 1 patient developed a DVT and 6 patients had major bleeding. While this demonstrates more promising results with low rates of thrombotic events and bleeding, it is limited due to the observational nature of the study [46]. Another observational study examined the use of desirudin in patients undergoing CABG who were positive for heparin antibodies but had no clinical evidence of HIT. No major bleeding or cases of HIT were reported after surgery [47].

Bivalirudin (for PCI or Cardiac Surgery; Off-Label HIT Treatment)

Bivalirudin is a reversible direct thrombin inhibitor, which is effective on both free and clot-bound thrombin. It is approved for use in the settings of PCI or cardiac surgery and otherwise is off-label. While this drug is not FDA approved solely for the treatment of HIT, it has been extensively studied in percutaneous coronary intervention (PCI) where it is approved for use with or without HIT [48]. In fact, the most recent CHEST guidelines recommend bivalirudin over argatroban for patients with HIT who are undergoing PCI [15]. This medication has been used successfully in patients undergoing cardiac surgery with and without cardiopulmonary bypass [49, 50].

Potential advantages of bivalirudin include its short half-life (25 min) and clearance through both enzymatic (80%) and renal (20%) pathways, offering advantages in certain patient populations such as those with renal or hepatic dysfunction and those who require urgent invasive procedures [51]. Furthermore, this medication has low immunogenicity and minimal interference with the PT/INR allowing for easier transition to oral therapy.

Dosing

HIT: The recommended initial dose for patients with HIT is 0.05–0.1 mg/kg/h with further adjustments upward or downward by 10–20% increments based on an aPTT target of 1.5–2.5 times the patient's baseline [52, 53]. No initial bolus is necessary. Patients with moderate to severe renal impairment exhibit a 20% reduction in drug clearance, and the typically short half-life can be extended to 1 h in severe renal disease (estimated creatinine clearance 10–29 mL/min) and 3.5 h in

Table 17.6 Bivalirudin for PCI in HIT and HITT: renal dose adjustment [53]

CrCl (ml/min)	Bolus dose (mg/kg)	Infusion dose (mg/kg/h)
>90	0.75	1.75
30–59	0.75	1.75
<30	0.75	1
Hemodialysis	0.75	0.25

end-stage renal disease. Bivalirudin has been studied in patients with renal impairment with specific dosage reductions outlined in Table 17.6 [53–55].

Patients Undergoing Urgent PCI

The recommended dose for patients undergoing urgent PCI is a 0.75 mg/kg intravenous bolus followed by a 1.7 5 mg/kg/h continuous infusion for the remainder of the procedure. This infusion can be continued for up to 4 h after the procedure. Then an infusion rate of 0.2 mg/kg/h can be maintained for up to 20 h, if necessary.

Monitoring

Bivalirudin is monitored using the aPTT with a recommended target range aPTT of 1.5–2.5 times the patient baseline. An aPTT should be obtained 2 h following initiation and any dose changes. During cardiac surgery the ACT is used to monitor bivalirudin. While on cardiopulmonary bypass, the ACT is maintained at 2.5 times the baseline value. An ACT of 200 s is inadequate anticoagulation to establish correct receipt of the drug.

Clinical Considerations

If used for extracorporeal circulation, it is important to avoid stasis of blood in the extracorporeal circuit, because thrombin rapidly cleaves bivalirudin which can precipitate clotting [56].

Renal Impairment

One small retrospective study examined safety, efficacy, and dosing requirements of bivalirudin in 37 patients with suspected or confirmed HIT [57]. The results showed a 3% new thrombosis rate and a 5% clinically significant bleeding rate. In addition patients were categorized into three groups based on renal function (CrCl >60 ml/min, CrCl 30–60 ml/min, and CrCl <30 ml/min or on renal replacement therapy) to determine necessary dosing adjustments. The authors concluded that dose adjustments are required in patients with moderate and severe renal dysfunction. See Table 17.7 for specific dosing recommendations.

Table 17.7 Bivalirudin dosing recommendations for treatment of HIT/HITT in patients with renal impairment [57]

Renal function	Dose/rate
CrCl >60 ml/min	0.15 mg/kg/h
CrCl 30–60 ml/min	0.08–0.1 mg/kg/h
CrCl <30 ml/min or CRRT	0.03–0.05 mg/kg/h

Data and Clinical Trials

Most evidence for the use of bivalirudin for patients with HIT and HITT is limited to case series [15]. One retrospective review examined patients with HIT treated with bivalirudin (24 patients), argatroban (13 patients), and lepirudin (5 patients) with primary outcome to assess the time to reach the desired aPTT [58]. Patients receiving bivalirudin achieved faster therapeutic anticoagulation than either argatroban or lepirudin (8.5 versus 14 and 24 h, respectively), although this was not statistically significant ($p = 0.124$). Argatroban had a longer treatment duration and lepirudin had lower bleeding rates. A composite measure of clinical outcomes (DVT, nonfatal MI, nonfatal stroke, limb amputation, and all-cause mortality) was similar among all three groups.

In addition, a more recent and larger retrospective study comparing bivalirudin (92 patients) and argatroban (46 patients) also found similar rates of achieving therapeutic anticoagulation, preventing new thromboembolic events, and bleeding events [59]. Data from these small retrospective reviews supports the potential use of bivalirudin for the treatment of HIT and showcases some of the advantages of this agent.

Recently, a larger retrospective single center study (461 patients) demonstrated bivalirudin as an effective and safe alternative for the treatment of HIT [53]. Results revealed a new thrombosis rate of 4.6% and a HIT-related death rate of 1.7%

with no patients requiring amputation after initiation of bivalirudin. Furthermore, other small single center studies have suggested that bivalirudin tends to reach a therapeutic aPTT quicker, maintain therapeutic levels more consistently, and achieve similar outcomes compared with argatroban [60, 61].

For patients undergoing PCI, there is a larger body of evidence supporting the use of bivalirudin including an analysis of five large randomized controlled trials including over 19,000 patients [62]. This meta-analysis demonstrated a similar risk of ischemic events as the control group but a lower risk of bleeding. In a smaller prospective cohort study of 52 patients, bivalirudin showed a high procedural success rate (98%) and low risk of major bleeding (2%) [63].

Fondaparinux

Fondaparinux is a synthetic pentasaccharide that selectively binds to antithrombin (ATIII) and specifically inhibits activated factor X (Xa). The neutralization of factor Xa interrupts the blood coagulation cascade, consequently inhibiting thrombin formation. Fondaparinux does not inactivate thrombin and has no known effect on platelet function, fibrinolytic activity, or bleeding time [64]. Fondaparinux has been approved for use in acute treatment of DVT and PE and for DVT prophylaxis as a weight-based, once-daily subcutaneous injection. Fondaparinux has a half-life of 17–21 h in patients with normal renal function.

Dosing

Dosing of fondaparinux in the management of HIT has not been established, but the American College of Chest Physicians (ACCP) recommends using standard therapeutic VTE treatment dosing. For patients who weigh <50 kg, 5 mg subcutaneous daily; for those who weigh 50–100 kg, 7.5 mg subcutaneous daily; and for those who weigh >100 kg, 10 mg subcutaneous daily [15].

Renal Impairment

The major route of elimination for fondaparinux is urinary excretion of unchanged drug. In patients receiving fondaparinux prophylaxis following elective hip surgery or hip fracture surgery, the total clearance of fondaparinux is approximately 25% lower in mild renal impairment (CrCl 50–80 ml/min), approximately 40% lower in moderate renal impairment (CrCl 30–50 ml/min), and approximately 55% lower in severe renal impairment (<30 ml/min) compared to patients with normal renal clearance [64]. Additionally, the incidence of major bleeding in patients treated with fondaparinux by renal function status for surgical prophylaxis and treatment of DVT and PE was increased with an increasing degree of renal impairment [64]. Based on these observations, the use of fondaparinux in patients with severe renal impairment is contradicted, and caution is advised for its use in patients with moderate renal impairment.

Monitoring

Fondaparinux does not require therapeutic monitoring in the general population as the bioavailability after injection is fairly high and dose response is predictable. However, given the issues described previously with respect to renal function and urinary excretion of the drug, creatinine clearance should be assessed periodically to ensure that the drug dosing remains appropriate. Some authors describe anti-Xa monitoring in select populations, including obese patients and in pediatrics. Anti-Xa levels have not been correlated with the effectiveness of therapy or with bleeding complications but may be of use to adjust dosing in these populations [65].

Adverse Effects

The primary adverse effect of fondaparinux is bleeding, which is increased in renal impairment and in patients weighing less than 50 kg. The manufacturer recommends against use of fondaparinux for perioperative prophylaxis of DVT in patients with body weight less than 50 kg, but the lowest dose (5 mg SC daily) can be used for DVT/PE with attention to patient-specific bleeding risks [64].

Clinical Considerations

Since fondaparinux does not cross-react with HIT antibodies, is widely available, is easy to administer, is and cost-effective, it is increasingly being used off-label for the management of patients with HIT [66, 67].

Data and Clinical Trials

Limited data is available with respect to fondaparinux for HIT treatment. One recent retrospective cohort study by Kang and colleagues examined outcomes in patients who had been treated with argatroban, danaparoid, or fondaparinux in the setting of a HIT diagnosis. Using propensity score matching, the authors found the rates of thrombosis and bleeding complications were comparable to argatroban and danaparoid [68].

Special Circumstances and Preferred Agents

Dialysis

According to the most recent ACCP guidelines, argatroban is the preferred direct thrombin inhibitor in patients with renal insufficiency, since this drug does not rely on renal clearance and its dialytic clearance by high flux membranes is considered clinically insignificant. Argatroban is preferred over danaparoid due to positive prospective data, while danaparoid has more data supporting its use in hemodialysis, although most patients studied did not have HIT. One small prospective study of 30 patients with HIT undergoing continuous renal replacement therapy and another analysis of 47 patients demonstrated low rates of thrombosis (0–4%) and major bleeding (0–6%) while on argatroban [69, 70].

Citrate has been used as a substitute for heparin during renal replacement therapy; it acts as a regional anticoagulant by chelating ionized calcium. However, it requires special dialysates and monitoring for metabolic disturbances. While it has not been studied in patients with acute HIT, it can be used as an alternative to heparin in patients with a history of HIT [15].

Cardiac Surgery

In general, heparin remains the drug of choice for intraoperative anticoagulation during cardiac surgery due to its rapid onset of action, short half-life, and reversibility with protamine. Since the HIT immune response declines over time with functional assays typically becoming negative approximately 50 days after stopping heparin and immunologic assays turning negative by 100 days, these assays can be performed to help guide clinicians whether heparin can be utilized intraoperatively or an alternative anticoagulant is safer [71].

Bivalirudin is the preferred alternative agent for use in patients with acute or subacute HIT who require urgent cardiac surgery. Prospective and randomized trials have demonstrated a high procedural success rate (defined as an absence of death, Q-wave-MI, repeat operation for coronary revascularization, or stroke) with the use of bivalirudin in both on-pump and off-pump surgery [72]. Stasis in the CPB circuit must be minimized when bivalirudin is administered due to potential for cleavage of bivalirudin by thrombin, resulting in potential clotting. Another strategy involves use of preoperative plasmapheresis followed by conventional heparin on CPB and postoperative bivalirudin for the prevention of thrombosis. This is detailed in the upcoming section describing the particulars of HIT in cardiac surgery.

Urgent PCI

Bivalirudin is the preferred agent for patients with acute or subacute HIT undergoing urgent PCI. As outlined in the bivalirudin drug section, this medication possesses unique advantages for patients undergoing invasive procedures including a short half-life and elimination through nonrenal pathways. The ATBAT prospective trial evaluated the safety and efficacy of bivalirudin in patients with either a history of HIT or new diagnosis [63]. Procedural success (<50% stenosis) and clinical success (without death, emergency bypass surgery, or myocardial infarction) were achieved in 98% and 96% of patients, respectively. Furthermore, a large meta-analysis of over 19,000 patients supported bivalirudin's efficacy during PCI [62]. Dosing for use in PCI is referenced in the Drug section above.

Pregnancy

The incidence of HIT in pregnancy is very low, as illustrated by a meta-analysis of over 2000 pregnant patients receiving treatment with LMWH where no instances of HIT occurred [73]. Nonetheless, if HIT is confirmed, all forms of heparin should be discontinued, and an alternative anticoagulant should be initiated. Guidelines recommend danaparoid over other non-heparin anticoagulants for pregnant patients. Danaparoid use was reviewed in a retrospective case series (30 women with acute HIT) with results highlighting a 90.4% live birth rate and maternal adverse events including two post-cesarean deaths, three major bleeds, three thromboembolic events, and ten recurrent rashes [74]. In this case series, there was no evidence of anti-Xa levels in umbilical cord blood samples from six infants.

However, danaparoid is not available in the USA. Data for argatroban and fondaparinux are limited to case reports. Fondaparinux may be preferred since this can be administered subcutaneously, while argatroban is limited to intravenous administration. One small prospective cohort study of women with hypersensitivity while receiving LMWH (10 patients, 12 pregnancies) examined fondaparinux 2.5 mg BID until the start of labor [75]. (Dosing was chosen due to lack of available 7.5 mg therapeutic injection in the Netherlands where the study was performed; please see Table 17.4 for appropriate weight-based dosing in the general population.) None of the 13 infants had any congenital abnormalities, and no major bleeding occurred. Similar results were seen in a retrospective case series of 29 women who received fondaparinux 2.5 mg daily [76]. One concern regarding the use of fondaparinux in pregnancy is that this medication does cross the placenta. While the concentration of fondaparinux in umbilical cord blood was lower than that required for therapeutic anticoagulation, potential adverse effects cannot be ruled out [77].

Transitioning to Outpatient Therapy

Warfarin

As mentioned previously, patients with acute HIT are at risk for venous limb gangrene if warfarin is initiated without adequate overlap with a parenteral anticoagulant due to the rapid decline in protein C. The following precautions are recommended to avoid these complications:

1. For patients that are receiving a vitamin K antagonist (VKA) at the time HIT is diagnosed, VKA should be stopped and vitamin K should be administered for reversal.
2. VKA should not be started until the platelet count has recovered to a stable level (at least 150×10^9/L).
3. Avoid large loading doses of warfarin (i.e., >5 mg) and ensure overlap of VKA with a parenteral anticoagulant for 5 days or more and until the INR has reached the goal range.
4. Ensure a minimum of 5 days of overlap for parenteral anticoagulation with warfarin, as 5 days is the accepted minimum time needed for warfarin to decrease prothrombin levels to those associated with effective anticoagulation.

Other challenges unique to transitioning patients to oral VKA are the INR prolonging effects of parenteral agents. Argatroban significantly prolongs the INR; therefore, when transitioning patients to warfarin, specific validated algorithms should be used to avoid under-anticoagulation and increasing thromboembolic risk. In an analysis of patients transitioning from argatroban to warfarin, 21% had a subtherapeutic INR 4 h following cessation of argatroban despite an INR of >3.0 while receiving argatroban with warfarin [78]. Thus, most recommendations suggest ensuring that the INR is >4 before argatroban is discontinued. See Table 17.8 for additional details regarding the transition from argatroban to warfarin.

Table 17.8 Transitioning from argatroban to warfarin [79]

Argatroban dose	Management using INR monitoring	Alternative when CFX assay is available
≤2 mcg/kg/min	• Stop argatroban when INR on combined argatroban and warfarin is >4	• Titrate argatroban based on aPTT values
	• Repeat INR in 4–6 h • If INR is <2, restart argatroban at 10% increased dose	• Overlap warfarin and argatroban at least 5 days (ideally CFX measurements are more accurate under these conditions)
		• Discontinue argatroban when CFX result is <45%
	• Repeat procedure until INR ≥2 is reached	• Can consider obtaining a confirmatory INR at least 4–6 h after cessation of argatroban. INR may remain elevated due to poor argatroban clearance in patients with hepatic insufficiency or critical illness in general
>2 mcg/kg/min	• Reduce argatroban dose to 2 mcg/kg/min	
	• Repeat INR in 4–6 h	
	• Stop argatroban when INR on combined argatroban and warfarin is >4	
	• Repeat INR in 4–6 h	
	• If INR is <2, restart argatroban at 10% increased dose	
	• Repeat procedure until INR ≥2 is reached	

Some centers have reported the use of a chromogenic factor X activity assay (CFX) as an alternative to monitoring INR. CFX activity is minimally affected by argatroban and so can be used to monitor warfarin therapy while argatroban infusion is ongoing. CFX assays measure the enzymatic activity of factor X as a percentage of normal. A chromogenic factor X activity of 20–45% correlates with an INR of approximately 2.0–3.5. This assay may be particularly useful in critically ill patients, as argatroban's clearance may be delayed and the INR may appear therapeutic after stopping argatroban when in fact the patient is not yet therapeutic on warfarin [80]. This alternative is possible for centers that can perform CFX assays with rapid return of results (hours rather than days).

One advantage of danaparoid is that it does not influence the INR, eliminating some of the complications outlined above when transitioning from argatroban to warfarin. Fondaparinux also shares this advantage, and some experts have suggested an approach of switching from a DTI (e.g., argatroban, lepirudin, bivalirudin) to fondaparinux for patients with normal renal function once the platelets have recovered [81]. See Table 17.9 for a description of this process. Successful use of this approach has been highlighted in case reports [82, 83].

Table 17.9 Alternative mode of transitioning to warfarin (DTI to fondaparinux to warfarin)

Step 1	Once platelet count has recovered (>150 × 10^9/L) and patient has normal renal function (CrCl >30 ml/min)
	Discontinue DTI and immediately initiate weight based fondaparinux:
	<50 kg: 5 mg subcutaneously once daily
	50–100 kg: 7.5 mg subcutaneously once daily
	>100 kg: 10 mg subcutaneously once daily
Step 2	Continue daily warfarin and fondaparinux, ensuring a total overlap of either DTI or fondaparinux to warfarin for a minimum of 5 days and until INR >2 for two consecutive days
Step 3	Once target INR goal maintained for 2 days then discontinue fondaparinux and continue daily warfarin adjusting per INR

Direct Oral Anticoagulants (DOACs)

The use of DTIs or indirect factor Xa inhibitors for transitioning to warfarin therapy involves increased monitoring and cost along with the inconvenient route of administration. Furthermore, continuation of warfarin therapy thereafter requires routine INR monitoring, periodic warfarin dose adjustments, and consistency with foods containing vitamin K. These limitations have led to interest in utilizing direct oral anticoagulants (DOACs) such as dabigatran, rivaroxaban, or apixaban in patients with HIT. These agents do not interact with anti-PF4/heparin antibodies or cause platelet activation mediated by the anti-PF4/heparin complex [84].

A retrospective analysis of 12 adult patients with SRA positive, confirmed HIT was recently conducted. All patients were initially treated with a DTI until platelet counts recovered (between 50–150 × 10^9/L), which is when patients were transitioned to either apixaban ($n = 10$) or rivaroxaban ($n = 2$) [85]. Major bleeding was observed in two patients, one patient had a gastrointestinal bleed in the setting of known varices while on clopidogrel for coronary disease and the other patient with a recent diagnosis of malignancy developed hemoptysis. No recurrent thrombosis was observed in these patients. Another study retrospectively identified 22 patients with HIT that were followed prospectively for development of outcomes [86]. These patients initially received argatroban (0.3–0.5 mcg/kg/min) which was dose-adjusted to maintain an aPTT between 50 and 90 s for approximately 32 h. Patients were transitioned to dabigatran (n = 6), apixaban (n = 5), or rivaroxaban (n = 11) 2 h after discontinuation of argatroban. No bleeding, limb loss, recurrent VTE, or death was reported. Five patients developed DVTs, but none of them developed arterial thrombosis. Finally, Linkins and colleagues performed a multicenter, single-arm cohort study examining the role of rivaroxaban as a primary treatment for HIT. They dealt with enrollment challenges but were able to treat 12 HIT-positive (4T score of 4 or greater plus positive SRA) with rivaroxaban and demonstrated good preliminary results. One patient had extension of known upper extremity DVT while on treatment, and one required bilateral lower extremity amputations for worsening ischemia from acute on chronic arterial disease present at the time that anticoagulation with rivaroxaban was initiated. No major bleeding episodes were observed, and no other new or recurrent thrombosis was seen [87]. These small case series suggest that DOACs may be a safe alternative for outpatient management of patients with HIT where routine monitoring, dietary restrictions, and dose adjustments are not required. Further larger studies are needed to understand the efficacy of these agents in patients with HIT.

Duration of Therapy

HIT (4 weeks) Versus HITT (3 months)

Since HIT is considered a reversible provoking risk factor for thrombosis, it is generally recommended to continue anticoagulation therapy for 3 months in patients with HITT. In patients with isolated HIT, guidelines recommend continuing anticoagulation with an alternative anticoagulant or warfarin for 4 weeks due to the increased risk of thrombosis for 2–4 weeks after treatment for HIT is started [15].

Things to Avoid in Therapy

Premature Initiation of Warfarin Therapy

Warfarin is contraindicated as initial monotherapy for HIT since rapid initiation of warfarin in patients with HIT may produce a prothrombotic state due to declining levels of the natural anticoagulant, protein C [15]. As discussed in the initial treatment section above, guidelines recommend against starting a VKA until platelets have substantially recovered (at least 150 × 10^9/L) over starting VKA at lower platelet counts.

LMWH Cross-Reactivity

LMWHs possess high cross-reactivity with heparin antibodies in vitro and, therefore, should be avoided in the treatment of HIT.

Platelet Transfusion

Despite profound thrombocytopenia in HIT, bleeding is uncommon. However, sometimes patients with HIT may require invasive procedures when platelet transfusions are administered. Small case series have suggested that platelet transfusions may exacerbate HIT, potentially increasing the risk of thromboembolism [15]. However, two case series of 41 patients did not demonstrate an increased risk of thrombotic complications [88, 89]. Since evidence is quite limited, it is still unclear whether platelet transfusions are safe in this population. Guidelines recommend only giving platelet transfusions in the event of bleeding or during performance of an invasive procedure with high bleeding risk [15].

IVC Filters

IVC filters are traditionally indicated in the setting of acute venous thromboembolism associated with a contraindication to anticoagulation. In fact, the bleeding risk related to HIT itself is low, and anticoagulation with alternative agents is preferred over IVC filter placement which does not address the hypercoagulable state of HIT and does not protect against arterial events. Reports have detailed progression to venous limb gangrene in the setting of HIT with IVC filter placement [90]. A retrospective study identified that 9 of 10 patients who received IVC filters had new thrombosis [91]. Caution should be exercised in patients who are felt to be at risk of bleeding for reasons other than the thrombocytopenia related to HIT itself, which should resolve with heparin cessation and initiation of an alternative anticoagulant.

HIT in Cardiac Surgery Patients

Heparin-induced thrombocytopenia after cardiac surgery is a particularly vexing problem. Patients undergoing cardiopulmonary bypass (CPB) are almost universally exposed to heparin, as well as the effects of CPB itself and several other clinical factors which may predispose to thrombocytopenia. When a diminished platelet count is observed, clinicians have a low threshold to evaluate for HIT as the complications associated with this condition may be deadly. This is especially true in the cardiovascular surgery population, where arterial thrombosis predominates over venous [18].

Risk Assessment

Cardiac surgery patients present a unique challenge in the diagnosis and management of HIT. First, most risk scores do not take into account the typical pattern of platelet count change after CPB. Patients almost universally suffer an acute drop in platelet count immediately following surgery due to the consumption of platelets during cardiopulmonary bypass, and this fall can be difficult to distinguish from a platelet count decrease associated with HIT. Additionally, one of the four "T's" in the 4T score is the presence of other causes of thrombocytopenia, which cardiac surgery patients qualify for in the form of CPB. This means that three parameters of the 4T score (degree of thrombocytopenia, timing of thrombocytopenia, and presence of other causes of thrombocytopenia—i.e., CPB) are affected by the process of cardiac surgery itself [25]. In an attempt to account for the unique setting of cardiac surgery with respect to HIT risk; Louet and colleagues have developed a risk score (see Table 17.3) specific to the cardiac surgery population. It utilizes (1) platelet fall patterns which take into account the initial drop seen after CPB, (2) the time from CPB to "index date" (or date HIT is first suspected), and (3) the duration of cardiopulmonary bypass. The platelet fall patterns are presented pictorially and in text, with the highest-risk pattern demonstrating a biphasic form with platelet rebound after CPB followed by a second drop in line with the expected time of HIT antibody formation. The less likely platelet pattern is one in which platelet count remains low after CPB, without a second drop attributable to HIT. The time from CPB to "index date" when HIT is first suspected separated patients undergoing HIT evaluation before or after postoperative day 5. Patients in whom HIT is suspected sooner are more likely to have other reasons for thrombocytopenia, while those being scrutinized for HIT more than 5 days after surgery were more likely to have HIT. In fact, despite many patients having recently received heparin for cardiac catheterization or for acute coronary syndrome, these preoperative exposures rarely lead to preformed antibodies or rapid onset HIT in the first few days after CPB [92]. Finally, a duration of CPB of less than 118 min was more associated with HIT [29]. These parameters attempt to tease out the confounding factors that can affect platelet count following cardiac surgery to create a more realistic risk assessment in this population. However, like many risk scores for this condition, this score has a low positive predictive value as it is focused on the parameters that make HIT less likely—which contributes to creating a high negative predictive value. It does provide some assistance in identifying patients who are at low risk of HIT, minimizing the number of patients who would be advised to receive therapeutic anticoagulation while awaiting laboratory confirmation of HIT [93].

Cardiac surgery patients are more likely than many other populations exposed to heparin to develop HIT antibodies, and many more patients develop these antibodies than go on to develop clinical HIT. This is described in the Iceberg Model of HIT, which indicates that substantially more patients develop HIT antibodies and even positive functional assays than those who develop clinical HIT. Further, the fraction of patients who develop clinical HIT with respect to those with HIT antibodies varies by medical and surgical populations. This is pertinent to clinicians caring for either medical or surgical patients, as it affects the diagnosis and treatment process [94].

As discussed previously, thrombotic events in HIT are predominantly venous, with the exception of HIT associated with cardiovascular procedures (including cardiac surgery with CPB) where arterial events predominate. This is likely related to the use of intravascular devices (cannulae, invasive monitoring lines, etc.) as well as underlying cardiovascular pathology in the form of atherosclerosis. The tendency toward arterial thromboembolic events produces significant morbidity for cardiac surgery patients with HIT, and mortality in this population is as high as 28% [92].

Treatment

Treatment of HIT in cardiac surgery patients is much the same as in other populations. Cessation of all heparin products, therapeutic anticoagulation with non-heparin parenteral agents, and the initiation of oral warfarin after platelet recovery are all standard measures. Challenges arise when cardiac surgery patients with HIT or a history of HIT require cardiopulmonary bypass. This issue can be divided into three phases: acute, subacute, and late. If CPB is required during acute HIT, then bivalirudin is the preferred agent. During subacute HIT, where thrombocytopenia is improved but circulating HIT antibodies remain, our preference is to delay CPB if at all possible to allow resolution of the antibodies. If this is impossible, bivalirudin is the drug of choice. If a patient has a history of HIT but more than 100 days previously, and no HIT antibodies are detected in the bloodstream, then limited use of heparin only for CPB can be considered with close monitoring postoperatively for development of clinical HIT/HITT. However, both preoperative and postoperative heparin should be avoided to limit the potential for new antibody formation [92]. Welsby and colleagues reported their experience in a series of 11 patients undergoing complex cardiac surgery with recent HITT and ongoing presence of HIT antibodies. They utilized plasmapheresis intraoperatively, followed by standard dosing of heparin for cardiopulmonary bypass and bivalirudin postoperatively when systemic anticoagulation was indicated (i.e., for patients receiving left ventricular assist devices or mechanical valve). They did not have any patients with evidence of clinical HIT postoperatively [95]. This experience suggests an alternative to the irreversible direct thrombin inhibitors for patients requiring CPB with recent HITT history; however, this technique has not been widely studied and the appropriate perioperative monitoring strategy and anticoagulation regimen have not been well defined.

Management of Patients with Prior History of HIT

Often patients with a prior history of HIT on chronic anticoagulation for other reasons may need bridging when a temporary discontinuation of anticoagulation is necessary. In such instances, the ACCP recommends that bridging can be pursued with fondaparinux in individuals without active antibodies. The use of fondaparinux for bridging is complicated by its long elimination half-life (17–21 h). If a high bleeding risk procedure is planned, the use of an IV DTI for bridging or simple discontinuation of anticoagulation without bridging anticoagulation should be considered. If HIT antibodies are present, then argatroban or bivalirudin is recommended [15].

Conclusions

HIT is a complex clinical entity that requires a high index of suspicion in susceptible patients, awareness of risk factors, knowledge of the available pretest probability scoring systems and laboratory assays (as well as knowledge of the available assays at one's own institution), and knowledgeable pharmacy assistance with alternative anticoagulants and dosing. Specific populations, including patients on dialysis and cardiac surgery patients, require additional consideration. With appropriate attention to the evidence and guidelines, these patients can avoid devastating consequences of this high-risk clinical entity.

Key Point

- The goal of therapy is to reduce thrombosis risk by decreasing thrombin generation and platelet activation.

Self-Assessment Questions

1. A patient recovering from coronary artery bypass grafting on postoperative day 5 has a platelet count which has dropped to 60 k/uL. He has been receiving subcutaneous heparin for DVT prophylaxis. His mediastinal tubes have not had high output, and he has no risk factors for gastrointestinal or other bleeding. His pretest probability of HIT is judged to be moderate. What is the appropriate management for this patient?
   (a) Stop all heparin administration, including flushes.
   (b) Initiate therapeutic anticoagulation with bivalirudin.
   (c) Send PF4 antibody assay and serotonin release assay if PF4 is positive.
   (d) All of the above.
2. Which of the following agents is not FDA approved for the treatment of acute HIT?
   (a) Lepirudin
   (b) Argatroban
   (c) Bivalrudin
3. Which of the following agents is preferred for the treatment of HIT in patients with severe renal insufficiency?
   (a) Argatroban
   (b) Apixaban
   (c) Danaparoid
   (d) Lepirudin
4. A 40-year-old woman was admitted to the ICU 10 days ago. She was diagnosed with HITTS and has been treated with argatroban for 6 days maintained in the therapeutic aPTT range. She was started on warfarin therapy yesterday. Her renal function is stable with a CrCl of 55 ml/min, and her platelet count is 110×10^9/L. Her weight is 112 kg. The team wants to discharge the patient today and consults you for assistance in bridging this patient from argatroban to warfarin. What would you recommend?
   (a) Discontinue argatroban and immediately begin fondaparinux 7.5 mg overlapping with warfarin until INR has been in therapeutic range for at least 2 days and a total of 5 days.

   (b) Discontinue argatroban and immediately begin fondaparinux 10 mg overlapping with warfarin until INR has been in therapeutic range for at least 2 days and a total of 5 days.
   (c) Recommend holding discharge since the patient has not received argatroban and warfarin therapy for a minimum of 5 days.
5. In instances where HIT/HITTS is recognized after initiating warfarin and INR is 1.9, is it important to discontinue warfarin and administer vitamin K and why?
   (a) Yes because this approach allows practitioners to see the true prolongation of the INR due to DTI therapy alone
   (b) Yes because this therapy change is necessary to prevent venous limb gangrene
   (c) No because this therapy change is only necessary when INR is in therapeutic range
6. The team calls for recommendations regarding stopping the bivalirudin infusion for a planned surgical procedure in 2 days. The patient is a 50-year-old male with a CrCl of 55 ml/min. Which would you recommend?
   (a) Discontinue bivalirudin today; consider giving recombinant factor VII 1 mg × 1 dose.
   (b) Discontinue bivalirudin today; consider giving recombinant factor VII 1 mg × 1 and plasmapheresis.
   (c) Discontinue bivalirudin 3–5 h prior to the procedure.

Self-Assessment Answers

1. (d) All of the above

   If there is concern for HIT, all heparin and heparin-containing products (such as flushes) should be stopped. Further, if the patient is at moderate to high risk for HIT based on clinical risk score, alternative therapeutic anticoagulation should be initiated (barring any contraindications) while awaiting laboratory assay confirmation of HIT. The Heparin-PF4 ELISA is used as the initial laboratory assay at most centers with functional assays used to confirm HIT, although this may differ depending on the individual hospital's available assays.
2. (c) Bivalrudin

   Although bivalrudin is often used in the treatment of HIT especially in the setting of percutaneous coronary interventions, it is not FDA approved for the treatment of HIT.
3. (a) Argatroban

   According to the most recent CHEST guidelines, argatroban is the preferred direct thrombin inhibitor in patients with renal insufficiency and HIT, since this drug does not rely significantly upon renal clearance and dialytic clearance. Argatroban is preferred over danaparoid due to positive prospective data, while danaparoid has more data supporting its use in hemodialysis, although most patients in this study did not have HIT.
4. (b) Discontinue argatroban and immediately begin fondaparinux 10 mg overlapping with warfarin until INR has been in therapeutic range for at least 2 days and a total of 5 days.

   Argatroban significantly prolongs the INR, which makes bridging to warfarin therapy challenging. An alternative approach to bridge these patients is to transition with fondaparinux once platelet count has recovered or is above 100×10^9/L. Fondaparinux is a weight-based agent, so MP would need 10 mg subQ daily. It is important to continue fondaparinux overlap with warfarin until INR is greater than two for 2 days and a total of 5 days to avoid an increased risk for recurrent thromboembolism.
5. (b) Yes because this therapy change is necessary to prevent venous limb gangrene

   This approach is necessary to prevent venous limb gangrene due to declining levels of the natural anticoagulant, protein C. Additionally, the vitamin K prevents confounders in the management of alternative parenteral anticoagulants.
6. (c) Discontinue bivalirudin 3–5 h prior to the procedure.

   Bivalirudin has a short half-life (approximately 25 min). In patients with renal dysfunction the half-life can be prolonged. Therefore, discontinuing bivalirudin 3–5 h prior to the procedure is sufficient to restore normal hemostasis. There is no antidote available for bivalirudin. Administration of recombinant human factor VII can increase the risk of thrombosis. Plasmapheresis has not been shown to remove bivalirudin and would require placement of an additional central venous line which can increase the patient's risk for bleeding.

References

1. Howell WH, Holt E. Two new factors in blood coagulation – hepatin and pro-antithrombin. Am J Phys. 1916;47:328–41.
2. Crafood C. Preliminary report on postoperative treatment with heparin as a preventive of thrombosis. Acta Chir Scand. 1936;79:407–26.
3. Weismann R, Tobin R. Arterial embolism occurring during systemic heparin therapy. AMA Arch Surg. 1958;76(2):219–25, 227.
4. Natelson EA, Lynch EC, Alfrey CP, Gross JB. Heparin-induced thrombocytopenia. An unexpected response to treatment of consumption coagulopathy. Ann Intern Med. 1969;71(6):1121–5.
5. Rhodes GR, Dixon RH, Silver D. Heparin induced thrombocytopenia with thrombotic and hemorrhagic manifestations. Surg Gynecol Obstet. 1973;136(3):409–16.
6. Kelton JG, Warkentin TE. Heparin-induced thrombocytopenia: a historical perspective. Blood. 2008;112(7):2607–16.
7. Babcock RB, Dumper CW, Scharfman WB. Heparin-induced immune thrombocytopenia. N Engl J Med. 1976;295(5):237–41.
8. Green D, Harris K, Reynolds N, Roberts M, Patterson R. Heparin immune thrombocytopenia: evidence for a heparin-platelet complex as the antigenic determinant. J Lab Clin Med. 1978;91(1):167–75.
9. Nelson JC, Lerner RG, Goldstein R, Cagin NA. Heparin-induced thrombocytopenia. Arch Intern Med. 1978;138(4):548–52.
10. Trowbridge AA, Caraveo J, Green JB, Amaral B, Stone MJ. Heparin-related immune thrombocytopenia. Studies of antibody-heparin specificity. Am J Med. 1978;65(2):277–83.
11. Amiral J, Bridey F, Dreyfus M, Vissoc AM, Fressinaud E, Wolf M, et al. Platelet factor 4 complexed to heparin is the target for antibodies generated in heparin-induced thrombocytopenia. Thromb Haemost. 1992;68(1):95–6.
12. Greinacher A. Heparin-induced thrombocytopenia. N Engl J Med. 2015;373(3):252–61.
13. Franchini M, Chong B, Jang I-K, Hursting H, Warkentin T, Warkentin T, et al. Heparin-induced thrombocytopenia: an update. Thromb J. 2005;3(1):14.
14. Jang IK, Hursting MJ. When heparins promote thrombosis review of heparin-induced thrombocytopenia. Circulation. 2005;111(20):2671–83.
15. Linkins L-A, Dans AL, Moores LK, Bona R, Davidson BL, Schulman S, et al. Treatment and prevention of heparin-induced thrombocytopenia. Chest. 2012;141(2):e495S–530S.
16. Nazi I, Arnold DM, Warkentin TE, Smith JW, Staibano P, Kelton JG. Distinguishing between anti-platelet factor 4/heparin antibodies that can and cannot cause heparin-induced thrombocytopenia. J Thromb Haemost. 2015;13(10):1900–7.
17. Rollin J, Pouplard C, Sung HC, Leroux D, Saada A, Gouilleux-Gruart V, et al. Increased risk of thrombosis in FcγRIIA 131RR patients with HIT due to defective control of platelet activation by plasma IgG2. Blood. 2015;125(15):2397–404.
18. Greinacher A, Farner B, Kroll H, Kohlmann T, Warkentin TE, Eichler P. Clinical features of heparin-induced thrombocytopenia including risk factors for thrombosis. A retrospective analysis of 408 patients. Thromb Haemost. 2005;94:132–5.
19. Warkentin TE. An overview of the heparin-induced thrombocytopenia syndrome. Semin Thromb Hemost. 2004;30(3):273–83.
20. Schindewolf M, Lindhoff-Last E, Ludwig RJ, Boehncke WH. Heparin-induced skin lesions. Lancet. 2012;380(9856):1867–79.
21. Warkentin TE, Sikov WM, Lillicrap DP. Multicentric warfarin-induced skin necrosis complicating heparin-induced thrombocytopenia. Am J Hematol. 1999;62(1):44–8.
22. Warkentin TE, Elavathil LJ, Hayward CP, Johnston MA, Russett JI, Kelton JG. The pathogenesis of venous limb gangrene associated with heparin-induced thrombocytopenia. Ann Intern Med. 1997;127(9):804–12.
23. Singla A, Amini MR, Alpert MA, Gornik HL. Fatal anaphylactoid reaction associated with heparin-induced thrombocytopenia. Vasc Med. 2013;18(3):136–8.
24. Rosenberger LH, Smith PW, Sawyer RG, Hanks JB, Adams RB, Hedrick TL. Bilateral adrenal hemorrhage: the unrecognized cause of hemodynamic collapse associated with heparin-induced thrombocytopenia. Crit Care Med. 2011;39(4):833–8.
25. Lo GK, Juhl D, Warkentin TE, Sigouin CS, Eichler P, Greinacher A. Evaluation of pretest clinical score (4 T's) for the diagnosis of heparin-induced thrombocytopenia in two clinical settings. J Thromb Haemost. 2006;4(4):759–65.
26. Cuker A, Arepally G, Crowther MA, Rice L, Datko F, Hook K, et al. The HIT Expert Probability (HEP) Score: a novel pre-test probability model for heparin-induced thrombocytopenia based on broad expert opinion. J Thromb Haemost. 2010;8(12):2642–50.
27. Joseph L, Gomes MPV, Al Solaiman F, St John J, Ozaki A, Raju M, et al. External validation of the HIT expert probability (HEP) score. Thromb Haemost. 2015;113(3):633–40.
28. Warkentin TE. Scoring systems for heparin-induced thrombocytopenia (HIT): Whither now? Thromb Haemost. 2015;113(3):437–8.

29. Lillo-Le Louët A, Boutouyrie P, Alhenc-Gelas M, Le Beller C, Gautier I, Aiach M, et al. Diagnostic score for heparin-induced thrombocytopenia after cardiopulmonary bypass. J Thromb Haemost. 2004;2(11):1882–8.
30. Nagler M, Bakchoul T. Clinical and laboratory tests for the diagnosis of heparin-induced thrombocytopenia. Thromb Haemost. 2016;116(5):823–34.
31. Warkentin TE, Sheppard JI, Moore JC, Sigouin CS, Kelton JG. Quantitative interpretation of optical density measurements using PF4-dependent enzyme-immunoassays. J Thromb Haemost. 2008;6(8):1304–12.
32. Cuker A, Cines DB. How I treat heparin-induced thrombocytopenia. Blood. 2012;119(10):2209–18.
33. Tardy B, Lillo le Louet A, Presles E. Predictive factors for thrombosis and major bleeding in an observational study including patients with heparin-induced-thrombocytopenia treated with lepirudin. Fundam Clin Pharmacol. 2007;21(5):36.
34. Berlex. Lepirudin package insert. Montville, NJ; 2004. p 1–22.
35. Greinacher A, Janssens U, Berg G, Böck M, Kwasny H, Kemkes-Matthes B, et al. Lepirudin (recombinant hirudin) for parenteral anticoagulation in patients with heparin-induced thrombocytopenia. Heparin-Associated Thrombocytopenia Study (HAT) investigators. Circulation. 1999;100(6):587–93.
36. Eichler P, Friesen HJ, Lubenow N, Jaeger B, Greinacher A. Antihirudin antibodies in patients with heparin-induced thrombocytopenia treated with lepirudin: incidence, effects on aPTT, and clinical relevance. Blood. 2000;96(7):2373–8.
37. Song X, Huhle G, Wang L, Hoffmann U, Harenberg J. Generation of anti-hirudin antibodies in heparin-induced thrombocytopenic patients treated with r-hirudin. Circulation. 1999;100(14):1528–32.
38. Greinacher A, Lubenow N, Eichler P. Anaphylactic and anaphylactoid reactions associated with lepirudin in patients with heparin-induced thrombocytopenia. Circulation. 2003;108(17):2062–5.
39. Greinacher A, Völpel H, Janssens U, Hach-Wunderle V, Kemkes-Matthes B, Eichler P, et al. Recombinant hirudin (lepirudin) provides safe and effective anticoagulation in patients with heparin-induced thrombocytopenia: a prospective study. Circulation. 1999;99(1):73–80.
40. Lubenow N, Eichler P, Lietz T, Farner B, Greinacher A. Lepirudin for prophylaxis of thrombosis in patients with acute isolated heparin-induced thrombocytopenia: an analysis of 3 prospective studies. Blood. 2004;104(10):3072–7.
41. Lubenow N, Eichler P, Lietz T, Greinacher A. Lepirudin in patients with heparin-induced thrombocytopenia – results of the third prospective study (HAT-3) and a combined analysis of HAT-1, HAT-2, and HAT-3. J Thromb Haemost. 2005;3(11):2428–36.
42. Iprivask [package insert]. Hunt Valley, MD: Canyon Pharmaceuticals, Inc; 2010.
43. Eriksson BI, Ekman S, Lindbratt S, Baur M, Bach D, Torholm C, et al. Prevention of thromboembolism with use of recombinant hirudin. Results of a double-blind, multicenter trial comparing the efficacy of desirudin (Revasc) with that of unfractionated heparin in patients having a total hip replacement. J Bone Joint Surg Am. 1997;79(3):326–33.
44. Eriksson BI, Wille-Jørgensen P, Kälebo P, Mouret P, Rosencher N, Bösch P, et al. A comparison of recombinant hirudin with a low molecular-weight heparin to prevent thromboembolic complications after total hip replacement. N Engl J Med. 1997;337(19):1329–35.
45. Boyce SW, Bandyk DF, Bartholomew JR, Frame JN, Rice L. A randomized, open-label pilot study comparing desirudin and argatroban in patients with suspected heparin-induced thrombocytopenia with or without thrombosis: PREVENT-HIT Study. Am J Ther. 2011;18(1):14–22.
46. Duncan L, Kurz M, Levy J. Use of the subcutaneous direct thrombin inhibitor desirudin in patients with heparin-induced thrombocytopenia (HIT) requiring venous thromboembolic event (VTE) prophylaxis. 40th Annual Meeting of the Society of Critical Care Medicine. San Diego, CA; 2011.
47. Levy J, Koster A. Safety of perioperative bridging with desirudin and intraoperative bivalirudin in patients with heparin antibodies undergoing coronary artery bypass surgery (CABG). 33rd Annual Meeting and Workshops of the Society of Cardiovascular Anesthesiologists. Savannah, GA; 2011.
48. Bittl JA, Chaitman BR, Feit F, Kimball W, Topol EJ. Bivalirudin versus heparin during coronary angioplasty for unstable or postinfarction angina: final report reanalysis of the Bivalirudin Angioplasty Study. Am Heart J. 2001;142(6):952–9.
49. Dyke CM, Smedira NG, Koster A, Aronson S, McCarthy HL, Kirshner R, et al. A comparison of bivalirudin to heparin with protamine reversal in patients undergoing cardiac surgery with cardiopulmonary bypass: the EVOLUTION-ON study. J Thorac Cardiovasc Surg. 2006;131(3):533–9.
50. Koster A, Spiess B, Jurmann M, Dyke CM, Smedira NG, Aronson S, et al. Bivalirudin provides rapid, effective, and reliable anticoagulation during off-pump coronary revascularization: Results of the "EVOLUTION OFF" trial. Anesth Analg. 2006;103(3):540–4.
51. Seybert AL, Coons JC, Zerumsky K. Treatment of heparin-induced thrombocytopenia: is there a role for bivalirudin? Pharmacotherapy. 2006;26(2):229–41.
52. Francis JL, Drexler A, Gwyn G, Moroose R. Successful use of bivalirudin in the treatment of patients suspected, or at risk of, heparin-induced thrombocytopenia. Blood. 2015;104(11):4077.
53. Joseph L, Casanegra AI, Dhariwal M, Smith MA, Raju MG, Militello MA, et al. Bivalirudin for the treatment of patients with confirmed or suspected heparin-induced thrombocytopenia. J Thromb Haemost. 2014;12(7):1044–53.

54. Kiser TH, Fish DN. Evaluation of bivalirudin treatment for heparin-induced thrombocytopenia in critically ill patients with hepatic and/or renal dysfunction. Pharmacotherapy. 2006;26(4):452–60.
55. Wisler JW, Washam JB, Becker RC. Evaluation of dose requirements for prolonged bivalirudin administration in patients with renal insufficiency and suspected heparin-induced thrombocytopenia. J Thromb Thrombolysis. 2012;33(3):287–95.
56. Augoustides JGT. Update in hematology: heparin-induced thrombocytopenia and bivalirudin. J Cardiothorac Vasc Anesth. 2011;25(2):371–5.
57. Kiser TH, Burch JC, Klem PM, Hassell KL. Safety, efficacy, and dosing requirements of bivalirudin in patients with heparin-induced thrombocytopenia. Pharmacotherapy. 2008;28(9):1115–24.
58. Dang CH, Durkalski VL, Nappi JM. Evaluation of treatment with direct thrombin inhibitors in patients with heparin-induced thrombocytopenia. Pharmacotherapy. 2006;26(4):461–8.
59. Skrupky LP, Smith JR, Deal EN, Arnold H, Hollands JM, Martinez EJ, et al. Comparison of bivalirudin and argatroban for the management of heparin-induced thrombocytopenia. Pharmacotherapy. 2010;30(12):1229–38.
60. Vo QAT, Lin JK, Tong LM. Efficacy and safety of argatroban and bivalirudine in patients with suspected heparin-induced thrombocytopenia. Ann Pharmacother. 2015;49(2):178–84.
61. Bain J, Meyer A. Comparison of bivalirudin to lepirudin and argatroban in patients with heparin-induced thrombocytopenia. Am J Health Syst Pharm. 2015;72(17):S104–9.
62. Lee MS, Liao H, Yang T, Dhoot J, Tobis J, Fonarow G, et al. Comparison of bivalirudin versus heparin plus glycoprotein IIb/IIIa inhibitors in patients undergoing an invasive strategy: a meta-analysis of randomized clinical trials. Int J Cardiol. 2011;152(3):369–74.
63. Mahaffey KW, Lewis BE, Wildermann NM, Berkowitz SD, Oliverio RM, Turco MA, et al. The anticoagulant therapy with bivalirudin to assist in the performance of percutaneous coronary intervention in patients with heparin-induced thrombocytopenia (ATBAT) study: main results. J Invasive Cardiol. 2003;15(11):611–6.
64. Arixtra [package insert]. Research Triangle Park, NC: GlaxoSmithKline Pharmaceuticals, Inc.; 2010.
65. Babin JL, Traylor KL, Witt DM. Laboratory monitoring of low-molecular-weight heparin and fondaparinux. Semin Thromb Hemost. 2017; 43(3):261–9.
66. Savi P, Chong BH, Greinacher A, Gruel Y, Kelton JG, Warkentin TE, et al. Effect of fondaparinux on platelet activation in the presence of heparin-dependent antibodies: a blinded comparative multicenter study with unfractionated heparin. Blood. 2005;105(1):139–44.
67. Aljabri A, Huckleberry Y, Karnes JH, Gharaibeh M, Kutbi HI, Raz Y, et al. Cost-effectiveness of anticoagulants for suspected heparin-induced thrombocytopenia in the United States. Blood. 2016;128(26):3043–51.
68. Kang M, Alahmadi M, Sawh S, Kovacs MJ, Lazo-Langner A. Fondaparinux versus argatroban and danaparoid for the treatment of suspected or confirmed heparin-induced thrombocytopenia: a propensity score analysis. Blood. 2012;120(21):924–30.
69. Link A, Girndt M, Selejan S, Mathes A, Böhm M, Rensing H. Argatroban for anticoagulation in continuous renal replacement therapy. Crit Care Med. 2009;37(1):105–10.
70. Reddy BV, Grossman EJ, Trevino SA, Hursting MJ, Murray PT. Argatroban anticoagulation in patients with heparin-induced thrombocytopenia requiring renal replacement therapy. Ann Pharmacother. 2005;39(10):1601–5.
71. Warkentin TE, Kelton JG. Temporal aspects of heparin-induced thrombocytopenia. N Engl J Med. 2001;344(17):1286–92.
72. Koster A, Hansen R, Kuppe H, Hetzer R, Crystal GJ, Mertzlufft F. Recombinant hirudin as an alternative for anticoagulation during cardiopulmonary bypass in patients with heparin-induced thrombocytopenia type II: a 1-year experience in 57 patients. J Cardiothorac Vasc Anesth. 2000;14(3):243–8.
73. Greer IA, Nelson-Piercy C. Low-molecular-weight heparins for thromboprophylaxis and treatment of venous thromboembolism in pregnancy: a systematic review of safety and efficacy. [Review] [108 refs]. Blood. 2005;106(2):401–7.
74. Magnani HN. An analysis of clinical outcomes of 91 pregnancies in 83 women treated with danaparoid (Orgaran®). Thromb Res. 2010;125(4):297–302.
75. Knol HM, Schultinge L, Erwich JJHM, Meijer K. Fondaparinux as an alternative anticoagulant therapy during pregnancy. J Thromb Haemost. 2010; 8(8):1876–9.
76. Winger EE, Reed JL. A retrospective analysis of fondaparinux versus enoxaparin treatment in women with infertility or pregnancy loss. Am J Reprod Immunol. 2009;62(4):253–60.
77. Dempfle C-EH. Minor transplacental passage of fondaparinux in vivo. N Engl J Med. 2004; 350(18):1914–5.
78. Bartholomew JR, Hursting MJ. Transitioning from argatroban to warfarin in heparin-induced thrombocytopenia: an analysis of outcomes in Patients with elevated international normalized ratio (INR). J Thromb Thrombolysis. 2005;19(3):183–8.
79. Sheth SB, DiCicco RA, Hursting MJ, Montague T, Jorkasky DK. Interpreting the international normalized ratio (INR) in individuals receiving argatroban and warfarin. Thromb Haemost. 2001;85(3):435–40.
80. Austin JH, Stearns CR, Winkler AM, Paciullo CA. Use of the chromogenic factor X assay in patients transitioning from argatroban to warfarin therapy. Pharmacotherapy. 2012;32(6):493–501.
81. Warkentin TE. Fondaparinux: does it cause HIT? Can it treat HIT? Expert Rev Hematol. 2010;3(5):567–81.
82. Baroletti S, Labreche M, Niles M, Fanikos J, Goldhaber SZ. Prescription of fondaparinux in hospitalised patients. Thromb Haemost. 2009;101(6):1091–4.

83. Ekbatani A, Asaro LR, Malinow AM. Anticoagulation with argatroban in a parturient with heparin-induced thrombocytopenia. Int J Obstet Anesth. 2010;19(1):82–7.
84. Krauel K, Hackbarth C, Furll B, Greinacher A. Heparin-induced thrombocytopenia: in vitro studies on the interaction of dabigatran, rivaroxaban, and low-sulfated heparin, with platelet factor 4 and anti-PF4/heparin antibodies. Blood. 2012;119(5):1248–55.
85. Kunk PR, Brown J, McShane M, Palkimas S, Gail MB. Direct oral anticoagulants in hypercoagulable states. J Thromb Thrombolysis. 2016;43(1):1–7.
86. Sharifi M, Bay C, Vajo Z, Freeman W, Sharifi M, Schwartz F. New oral anticoagulants in the treatment of heparin-induced thrombocytopenia. Thromb Res. 2015;135(4):607–9.
87. Linkins LA, Warkentin TE, Pai M, Shivakumar S, Manji RA, Wells PS, et al. Rivaroxaban for treatment of suspected or confirmed heparin-induced thrombocytopenia study. J Thromb Haemost. 2016; 14(6):1206–10.
88. Refaai MA, Chuang C, Menegus M, Blumberg N, Francis CW. Outcomes after platelet transfusion in patients with heparin-induced thrombocytopenia. J Thromb Haemost. 2010;8(6):1419–21.
89. Hopkins CK, Goldfinger D. Platelet transfusions in heparin-induced thrombocytopenia: a report of four cases and review of the literature. Transfusion. 2008;48(10):2128–32.
90. Rice L. Heparin-induced thrombocytopenia: myths and misconceptions (that will cause trouble for you and your patient). Arch Intern Med. 2004;164(18):1961–4.
91. Jung M, McCarthy JJ, Baker KR, Rice L. Safety of IVC filters with heparin-induced thrombocytopenia: a retrospecive study. Blood. 2015; 118(21):2225.
92. Warkentin TE, Greinacher A. Heparin-induced thrombocytopenia and cardiac surgery. Ann Thorac Surg. 2003;76:2121–31.
93. Downs E, Johnston LE, Magno-Padron D, Patton S, Schaheen B, Ailawadi G, et al. Utility of a clinical risk score to limit therapeutic anticoagulation in suspected cases of heparin-induced thrombocytopenia (HIT) after cardiac surgery. Society for Vascular Medicine Annual Scientific Meeting; 2016.
94. Warkentin TE. Heparin-induced thrombocytopenia: pathogenesis and management. Br J Haematol. 2003;121(4):535–55.
95. Welsby IJ, Um J, Milano CA, Ortel TL, Arepally G. Plasmapheresis and heparin reexposure as a management strategy for cardiac surgical patients with heparin-induced thrombocytopenia. Anesth Analg. 2010;110(1):30–5.

Anticoagulation Therapy in Pregnant Patients

18

Steven A. Savella, Jessica A. Kvasic, and Joe F. Lau

Clinical Vignette

A 30-year-old woman G1P0 who is 23 weeks pregnant presents to her primary care physician with left lower extremity pain, swelling, and erythema for the last 2–3 weeks. She is otherwise healthy. Her only medication is prenatal vitamins, and her family history is significant for hyperlipidemia and hypertension in her father. She denies any recent travel, periods of immobility, trauma to her legs, chest pain, dyspnea, and other associated symptoms. She does not smoke or drink. A venous duplex ultrasound of her left lower extremity reveals an acute deep vein thrombosis in her left common femoral, popliteal, and posterior tibial veins.

Which type of anticoagulant should be started and for how long should it be continued? If the venous duplex ultrasound of her lower extremities had been negative and a pulmonary embolism is suspected, what imaging modality should be ordered? Will she be able to breastfeed her child while receiving anticoagulant therapy? If this woman is to become pregnant again, should she receive prophylactic anticoagulation? The following review will address these questions, with an emphasis on the diagnosis and management of VTE in pregnant patients.

S. A. Savella
Department of Cardiology, Zucker School of Medicine at Hofstra/Northwell, Northwell Health, Manhasset, NY, USA
e-mail: ssavella@northwell.edu

J. A. Kvasic
Department of Medicine, Zucker School of Medicine at Hofstra/Northwell, Northwell Health, Manhasset, NY, USA
e-mail: jkvasic@northwell.edu

J. F. Lau (✉)
Department of Cardiology, Zucker School of Medicine at Hofstra/Northwell, Northwell Health, Manhasset, NY, USA
e-mail: JLau@northwell.edu

Introduction and Epidemiology

Pregnancy remains a well-known risk factor for venous thromboembolism (VTE) which consists of deep vein thrombosis (DVT) and pulmonary embolism (PE). It is currently estimated that symptomatic VTE occurs in 5–12 women per 10,000 pregnancies during the antepartum period and in 3–7 women per 10,000 deliveries during the postpartum period [1]. Although these numbers may appear low, they represent a five- to tenfold increase in risk for pregnant women as compared to age-matched nonpregnant females [2].

J. F. Lau et al. (eds.), *Anticoagulation Therapy*, https://doi.org/10.1007/978-3-319-73709-6_18

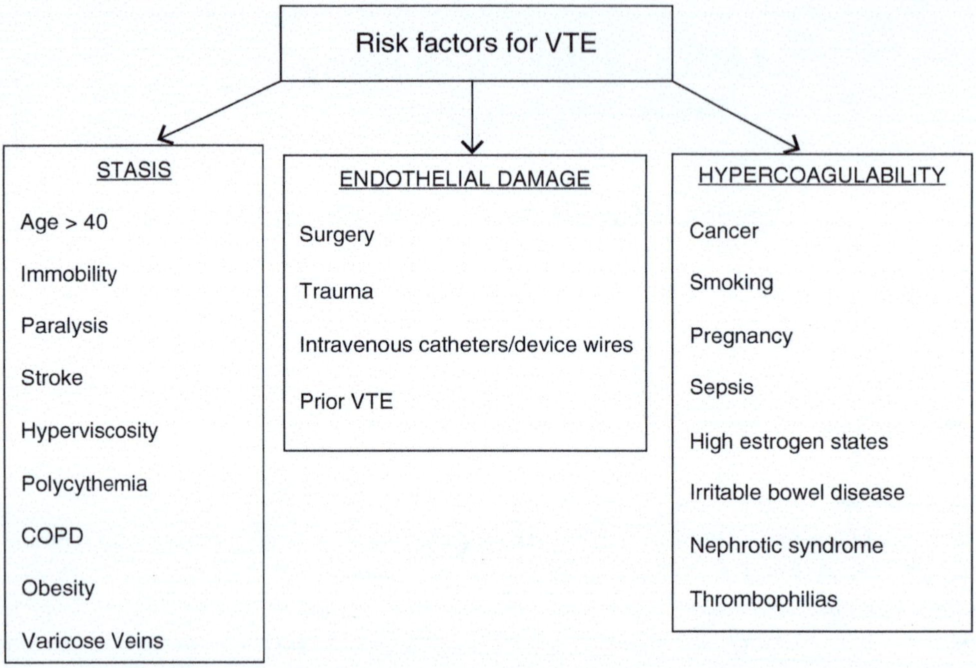

Fig. 18.1 Risk factors for VTE (venous thromboembolism). Various risk factors and comorbid conditions can lead to increased venous stasis, endothelial wall damage, or hypercoagulability

Thromboembolic disease accounts for 1 death in 100,000 births which is equal to 10% of maternal deaths, only after complications of preeclampsia (16%), amniotic fluid embolism (14%), obstetric hemorrhage (12%), and cardiac disease (11%). Surprisingly, an upward trend in the number of DVTs seen in pregnancy from 1979 to 1999 has been noted. This is believed to be from increased clinical awareness and improved overall surveillance as well as improved diagnostic imaging modalities (Fig. 18.1).

During pregnancy, VTE events are four times more common than arterial thrombotic events. Of those, around 80% are DVTs and the other 20% are PE. A meta-analysis demonstrated that two-thirds of DVTs occur during the antepartum period. In contrast, 43–60% of pregnancy-related PEs occur during the immediate postpartum period, particularly within the first 4–6 weeks after delivery, with the highest risk being within the first week postpartum and a steady decline to baseline 6–12 weeks thereafter. Based on a population-based cohort study over a 30-year period, the relative risk for developing VTE during pregnancy was 4.29 (95% CI, 3.49–5.22, $p < 0.001$) [3]. The annual incidence of VTE was five times higher for postpartum than pregnant women, which is why the postpartum weeks are considered the highest risk period. Pulmonary embolisms were relatively uncommon during pregnancy, but much more commonly seen postpartum (10.6 *versus* 159.7 per 100,000) [4]. In a Danish cohort study from 1995 to 2005, the risk of DVT was seen to increase throughout pregnancy and was the greatest right after delivery [5]. Available data also suggests that VTE risk is higher after Cesarean rather than vaginal delivery [6].

Risk Factors Contributing to VTE in Pregnant Patient

The risk of VTE may be more common in the third trimester, but the increased risk starts with the beginning of the first trimester [7]. Venous stasis, vascular damage, and changes in coagulation factors are all responsible for the increased risk [8].

The most important risk factors during pregnancy are thrombophilias (either acquired or inherited) and a prior history of thrombosis [9]. Prior thrombosis increases the risk for VTE by 2–12%. Other statistically significant medical risk factors during pregnancy include heart disease, anemia, lupus, and obesity [10]. A UK cohort study suggested that varicose veins, inflammatory bowel disease, urinary tract infections, and preexisting diabetes mellitus were all associated with a slightly increased risk of thromboembolic disease [11]. This was compared to a postpartum analysis, which suggested that stillbirth, the above medical comorbidities, obstetric hemorrhage, Cesarean delivery, and a BMI >30 kg/m^2 were all associated with increased postpartum VTE risk [11].

Acquired and inherited thrombophilias both increase the risk for maternal thrombosis. Thrombophilias are typically present in 20–50% of women who experience VTE during pregnancy in the postpartum period. However, overall probabilities of developing VTE still remain low. According to Gerhardt and colleagues, the individual probability of gestational VTE was 0.5% for women aged <35 years old with heterozygous factor V Leiden (FVL) mutations, 2.2% in homozygous FVL, 0.4% for heterozygous prothrombin G20210A, 5.5% in compound heterozygotes for prothrombin and FVL, 6.1% in antithrombin deficiencies, and 0.7% for protein C and S deficiencies [12]. These absolute risks as discussed are detailed in the table below, comparing patients below and above the ages of 35, with the different thrombophilias.

In addition to inherited thrombophilias, women with antiphospholipid antibody syndrome (APS) are at increased risk of VTE as well and should be considered for anticoagulation [13, 14]. Patients with hyperhomocysteinemia have also been found to have increased risks of VTE as compared to nonpregnant subjects [15]. However, patients with homozygosity for methylene-tetrahydrofolate reductase (MTHFR) gene mutation, which is most commonly associated with hyperhomocysteinemia, do not have an increased risk of developing VTE [16] (Table 18.1).

Table 18.1 Absolute risk of venous thromboembolism in pregnancy and puerperium associated with thrombophilias

Coagulation defect	Probability of VTE in pts <35 years old (%)	Probability of VTE in pts >35 years old (%)
Genetic defects		
FVL (heterozygous)	0.5	0.7
FVL (homozygous)	2.2	3.4
Prothrombin G20210A heterozygous	0.4	0.6
FVL and prothrombin G20210A (compound heterozygous)	5.5	8.2
Antithrombin deficiency (activity)		
Mild deficiency (cutoff <90%)	0.2	0.3
Severe deficiency (cutoff <60%)	6.1	9.0
Protein C deficiency (activity)		
Mild deficiency (cutoff <76%)	0.3	0.5
Severe deficiency (cutoff <40%)	0.7	1.0
Protein S deficiency (activity)		
Mild deficiency (cutoff <57%)	0.3	0.5
Severe deficiency (cutoff <40%)	0.3	0.5

VTE venous thromboembolism, *FVL* factor V Leiden mutation, *Pt* patient
The absolute risks are listed for the various inherited and acquired thrombophilias, comparing patients below and above the ages of 35 [12]

Pregnant women are at an increased risk of venous stasis because of hormonally induced decreased venous capacitance and decreased venous outflow from presumed mechanical obstruction of the inferior vena cava and pelvic veins by the enlarging uterus [17]. Overall, there is a decrease in natural anticoagulants and an increase in procoagulant factors and inhibitors of fibrinolysis. During pregnancy, there is a documented increase in the levels of factors VII, VIII, and X, von Willebrand factor (vWF), and fibrinogen, while factors II and V are relatively unchanged [18]. Factor VII may increase as much as tenfold, whereas vWF and factor VIII increase twofold later in pregnancy. Factor XI is the only procoagulant factor that decreases [18, 19].

There is also a decrease in the level of free and total protein S due to increased levels of its binding protein, C4b binding protein. Plasma fibrinolytic activity is reduced during pregnancy because of increased levels of plasminogen activator inhibitor-2 (PAI-2) from the placenta but returns to normal values shortly after placental delivery [18, 19]. Thrombomodulin, an endothelial cell expressed protein cofactor responsible for inhibiting thrombin, also increases during pregnancy [19]. The overall hypercoagulable state and hemostatic changes do not return to pre-pregnancy state until around 8 weeks after delivery [20].

Several other risk factors for VTE in pregnancy have been identified including multiple pregnancies, preeclampsia, heavy smoking, and blood group type A, despite limited data [21]. Whether advanced maternal age greater than 35 years old is a risk factor remains to be determined, as there are conflicting data [22]. Limited data are also available for assisted reproduction as a risk factor.

Thromboembolism Prophylaxis During Pregnancy

Despite having an overall increased risk of thrombosis, most pregnant patients do not require anticoagulation. The overall incidence of VTE is approximately 2 per 1000 births, and VTE is the cause of death in 1 out of 100,000 births [2, 3, 7]. Important risk factors for VTE in pregnancy, as discussed before, are a history of thrombosis and thrombophilias. A history of thrombosis in general increases the VTE recurrence risk by 2–12% [23].

If postpartum prophylaxis is indicated, the general recommendation is to anticoagulate for 6 weeks. Therapy may include either prophylactic or intermediate-dose low-molecular-weight heparin (LMWH) or vitamin K antagonists (VKAs), such as warfarin, with a goal INR of 2.0–3.0.

Anticoagulation is not typically required for those with inherited thrombophilias if there is no personal history of VTE or no previous complications during pregnancy. The exceptions to this recommendation include women with a very high risk of thrombosis, including those with *known* antithrombin deficiency, homozygosity for factor V Leiden (FVL) mutation, homozygosity for Prothrombin gene G20210A mutation, or antiphospholipid antibody syndrome (APS) [24]. If pregnant females are homozygous for FVL or prothrombin gene G20210A mutations and have a positive family history of VTE, then both antepartum and postpartum prophylaxis should be considered as per current guidelines [25]. An observational study performed by Tormene and colleagues suggested that LMWH prophylaxis reduced obstetric complications in carriers of FVL or prothrombin variant mutation [26].

Although current evidence is limited, available studies suggest that antepartum prophylaxis may be beneficial, and decreases the rates of fetal loss in women with deficiencies of protein C, protein S, and antithrombin [27]. In a randomized clinical trial published by Gris and colleagues, there were improved fetal outcomes when women with inherited thrombophilia and a history of a single fetal loss were treated with prophylactic enoxaparin (40 mg/day) versus low-dose aspirin [28]. For patients who meet criteria for antiphospholipid antibody syndrome (APS), guidelines recommend antepartum administration of unfractionated heparin or low-molecular-weight heparin combined with low-dose aspirin (75–100 mg/day) [24–26].

In conjunction with the above, current guidelines suggest that for women with prior VTEs which were associated with a transient risk factor and did not have an inherited or acquired thrombophilia, no antepartum prophylaxis is required [29]. Postpartum prophylaxis for 6 weeks with LMWH or VKA is usually recommended for any woman with a prior DVT, regardless if unprovoked or estrogen dependent [25, 30].

In a prospective study performed by Brill-Edwards and colleagues, the recurrence rate of VTE during pregnancy was assessed to be low overall (3 events during 125 pregnancies), but a comparison with periods outside pregnancy was not performed. A limitation to this study was that patients in their first trimester were not enrolled, which could have caused an underestimated result [31]. In a retrospective study conducted by Pabinger and colleagues, women with prior VTEs were once again studied to assess for risk of recurrent episodes during pregnancy. This study included women in all three trimesters and also included those that ended prematurely. Out of 109 studied women, 43 had recurrent VTEs, but only eight events were during pregnancy (35 occurred outside of pregnancy). The relative risk was calculated to be 4.3% (95% confidence interval, 1.6–7.8; $P = 0.002$) [23].

Key Points

- Patients with a history of unprovoked VTE, which were treated in the past, should be anticoagulated with LMWH or VKA during the postpartum period.
- Patients with history of single episode of provoked VTE with a resolved risk factor and no thrombophilia can be clinically monitored during antepartum and prophylactically anticoagulated postpartum.
- Patients with thrombophilias but no prior VTE need to be risk-assessed by the clinician rather than automatically using routine antepartum prophylaxis.
- Patients with thrombophilias with one previous VTE episode and not on long-term anticoagulation should be placed on prophylactic anticoagulation during antepartum and postpartum periods.
- Patients with antithrombin deficiency with no previous VTE are recommended to have antepartum and postpartum prophylaxis.
- Patients who are homozygous for FVL or prothrombin gene G20210A mutations and have a positive family history of VTE should undergo both antepartum and postpartum prophylaxis.
- Pregnant females with history of APS and recurrent pregnancy loss (> 3) with no history of VTE should be anticoagulated prophylactically during the antepartum period in addition to continuing aspirin.

Clinical Presentation and Diagnostic Evaluation of DVT and PE in Pregnant Patient

The two most common presenting symptoms of DVT in pregnancy are extremity pain and swelling. As in the nonpregnant patient, the initial recommended test for a suspected DVT is a duplex ultrasound of the veins [32]. DVTs in pregnancy are more likely to involve the left lower extremity, and as high as 70–90% are occurring in the more proximal (i.e., iliofemoral) veins of the left leg [33]. This is assumed to occur because of extrinsic compression of the left common iliac vein by the gravid uterus.

The Wells rule for diagnosing DVT and PE has not been validated in pregnant patients. Instead, three clinical variables are noted to be highly predictive of a DVT in the pregnant patient: (1) left leg symptoms, (2) >2 cm calf circumference difference, and (3) first trimester presentation as seen in Table 18.2 [8, 34]. The sensitivity and negative predictive value were determined to be near 100%, for first time DVT [8]. None of the patients without any of the three clinical variables had a DVT (0%; 95% CI 0–4.2%) The predictive value of this clinical prediction rule warrants validation in a prospective management study.

A VTE risk assessment score in pregnancy was created that utilized three main criteria: (1) personal history of DVT, (2) known thrombophilia, and (3) contemporary risk factors dependent on the pregnancy. This score was created to decide who requires antepartum prophylaxis and to tailor anticoagulation during this period and can be seen in Table 18.3. If the total score is <3, no antenatal prophylaxis is required. For scores between 3 and 5, LMWH was only prescribed in the third trimester [36].

Table 18.2 Clinical findings predictive of DVT in pregnancy

1. Left leg symptoms (e.g., pain, erythema, etc.)
2. >2 cm circumferential size difference
3. Patient in first trimester of pregnancy

DVT deep vein thrombosis

Table 18.3 Venous thromboembolism (VTE) risk assessment score in pregnancy and corresponding prophylaxis strategy

Personal history of VTE	History of VTE related to pregnancy (during antepartum) or CVT or VTE in childhood (<16 y.o.)	6
	Spontaneous or estrogen-induced PE or proximal DVT	3
	Spontaneous or estrogen-induced distal calf DVT	2
	Transient risk factor-induced PE or proximal DVT	2
	Transient risk factor-induced distal calf DVT	1
If + personal history of VTE	Recurrent VTE history	3
	Residual venous thrombi	3
	Recent VTE history (<2 years)	2
Thrombophilia	Homozygous mutations, combined thrombophilia risk factors	3
	Protein C deficiency, protein S deficiency, heterozygous *F5* G1691A mutation, heterozygous *F2* G20210A mutation	1
	If no hypercoagulability detected, family history of severe or recurrent VTE	1
Other risk factors	Bed rest, immobilization	2
	Twin pregnancy	1
	Age >35 years	1
	Body mass index >30	1

VTE venous thromboembolism, *CVT* central venous thrombosis, *PE* pulmonary embolism, *DVT* deep vein thrombosis, *LMWH* low-molecular-weight heparin

No antenatal prophylaxis if score is <3. Early heparin prophylaxis in patients with a score ≥6. LMWH was prescribed only in the third trimester to patients with a score between 3 and 5

A VTE risk assessment score in pregnancy was created that utilized three main criteria: (1) personal history of DVT, (2) known thrombophilia, and (3) contemporary risk factors dependent on the pregnancy. This score was created to decide who requires antepartum prophylaxis and to tailor anticoagulation during this period. If the total score is <3, no antenatal prophylaxis is required. For pregnant patients with a score ≥6, early LMWH was prescribed. For scores between 3 and 5, LMWH was only prescribed in the third trimester [35]. (Reprinted with permission from Dargaud Y, Rugeri L, Vergnes MC, et al., A risk score for the management of pregnant women with increased risk of venous thromboembolism: a multicentre prospective study, British Journal of Haematology, Vol. 145, pages 825-835, © 2009, with permission from John Wiley and Sons)

The value of this prediction rule in identifying patients in need of antenatal thromboprophylaxis was recently demonstrated in a prospective management trial [35].

D-Dimer Testing

D-dimer levels may be helpful for ruling out VTE in low-risk nonpregnant patients, but D-dimer levels are usually elevated in pregnancy and are not diagnostic of a DVT [6]. The rise in D-dimers occurs as early as the first trimester and peaks in the third trimester. Raising the D-dimer level cut-off may overcome difficulties in testing and standardization, but this requires further research [8]. A red blood cell agglutination D-dimer test known as SimpliRED suggested a 100% sensitivity and 100% negative predictive value for excluding DVT in pregnant patient [36]. Despite this result, it should not be utilized alone to rule out a DVT given varying confidence intervals, high rates of false negatives, and subjectivity of visual interpretation that is required for diagnosis.

Activated Protein C Sensitivity

It has been suggested that response to activated protein C (APC) can be a diagnostic marker of VTE during pregnancy. Sensitivity to APC was reduced in pregnant patients diagnosed with VTE with a clinically significant odds ratio of 31.9 [37]. Despite this result, more research is required to confirm this finding.

Venous Duplex Ultrasonography

Duplex ultrasonography is considered an accurate, noninvasive, radiation-free, and cost-effective method of diagnosing a DVT in pregnant patient. In nonpregnant patients, duplex ultrasound is considered to be highly sensitive (97%) and highly specific (94%) for detecting symptomatic proximal DVT [38]. Considerably less data on the diagnostic utility of duplex ultrasound is available for pregnant patients, but it remains the first-line imaging test for DVT.

Bilateral lower extremity venous duplex ultrasound should also be the initial test ordered in a pregnant patient with suspected PE with associated leg symptoms. If the venous duplex ultrasound is positive, then the clinician can consider initiating treatment without further immediate imaging. Iliac vein thrombosis is more common in pregnancy, and visualization with ultrasound can be difficult because of uterine size and changes in blood flow [33]. These thromboses are more likely to present with back or buttocks pain and/or upper leg swelling [8]. If the results of duplex ultrasound are equivocal and an iliac vein thrombosis is expected, a magnetic resonance venography (MRV) without gadolinium can be performed [39].

Other Imaging Modalities (CT/VQ)

In the absence of leg symptoms and negative duplex ultrasound, either computed tomography angiography or ventilation/perfusion scanning should be performed. These are also the two most common imaging methods for diagnosing a PE in a nonpregnant patient. Both of these modalities involve the use of some radiation [8]. Radiation exposure for the mother and the fetus may vary. In a survey performed in the UK in 2006, a typical CTA dose for mothers was calculated to be 2.2–6.0 mSv as compared to the radiation for a V/Q scan which was measured to be roughly 1.4 mSv. Compared to maternal exposure, the fetus would have a much larger exposure to radiation with the V/Q scintigraphy (640–800 μGy) as compared to CTA (3–131 μGy) [39–41]. Fetal malformations occur with a threshold of 100–200 mSv. Therefore, confirmatory diagnostic imaging should not be withheld in pregnant patients with a high clinical suspicion of PE.

CT scanning has both advantages and disadvantages in pregnant patient. Radiation can be limited with the use of an abdominopelvic shield, without loss of image quality [42]. CT scanning may also confer alternative diagnoses if a PE is excluded. Despite this, CT scanning has had higher diagnostic inadequacy in pregnant patients (35%) likely because of the hyperdynamic pregnant state and interruption of contrast by unopacified blood [43] (Fig. 18.2).

Concerns about radiation exposure with CT angiography must be compared against consequences of withholding imaging. A chest radiograph performed prior to V/Q scanning may reduce likelihood of non-diagnostic scans [44]. This suggests that V/Q scanning should be used in pregnant patients with a negative CXR, and CT scanning may be preferred in those with a positive CXR findings and/or a history of lung disease [8].

Key Points

- Patients with suspected DVT should undergo a venous duplex ultrasound.
- D-dimers are not diagnostic of DVT as they are often elevated at baseline in pregnant patients.
- If proximal lower extremity vein (*i.e.*, iliofemoral) thrombosis is suspected, the study of choice is magnetic resonance venography.

If no lower extremity symptoms are found and ultrasound is negative, CTA of the chest or V/Q scan should be performed in patients with high clinical suspicion for PE.

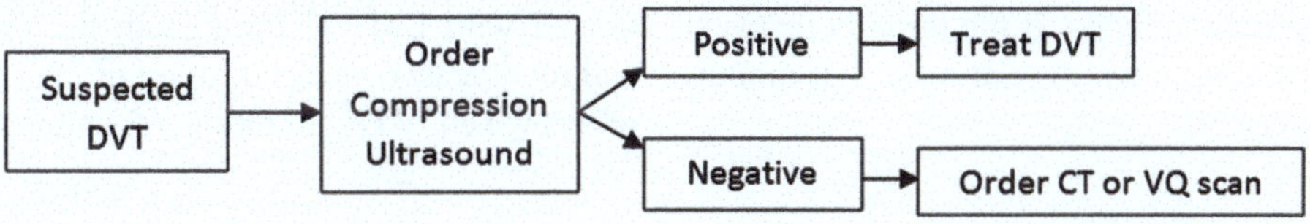

Fig. 18.2 Algorithm for suspected lower extremity DVT in pregnant patient. *DVT* deep vein thrombosis, *CT* computed tomography, *V/Q* ventilation/perfusion

Management of DVT and PE in Pregnancy and the Puerperium

If a DVT or PE is discovered, the patient should be admitted to the hospital and started on intravenous unfractionated heparin (UFH) or subcutaneous low-molecular-weight heparin (LMWH). LMWH is administered twice daily; however, the half-life is shorter in pregnancy and increased dosing may be needed. If the patient is hemodynamically unstable, thrombolysis can be considered, but is associated with a 6% rate of fetal loss and an even higher rate of maternal hemorrhage. Thrombolysis should only be considered in life-threatening VTE [45]. Thrombectomy is another option that may be necessary when DVTs involve the iliofemoral veins and/or inferior vena cava. Studies have demonstrated that thrombectomy may be a safe surgical option (when thrombolysis is contraindicated) and can restore venous patency in those with massive DVTs [46]. Emergent pulmonary embolectomies have also been successfully performed with the use of an intra-aortic balloon pump to maintain placental blood flow [47].

At about 36–37 weeks of gestation, patients are usually switched from LMWH to unfractionated heparin. LMWH and UFH should be stopped at least 24–48 h prior to delivery, especially if epidural anesthesia is desired. Intravenous unfractionated heparin should be held for 6 h prior to delivery. If spontaneous labor ensues, epidural anesthesia should not be implemented in order to prevent any negative anticoagulation effects during delivery. Resumption of prophylactic dose LMWH can be considered 12 h after vaginal delivery and 24 h after Cesarean delivery and, if prophylactic dose UFH/LMWH is tolerated, then at 24 h after vaginal delivery and 48–72 h after Cesarean delivery. Either LMWH or warfarin should be continued for at least 6 weeks postpartum and, if the thrombotic event occurred during pregnancy, at least 3–6 months after delivery [9].

Pneumatic Compression

At time of labor and delivery, pneumatic compression devices are recommended, even though their benefit in prevention of pregnancy related VTE is unknown [48]. Compression stockings were studied during pregnancy in patients diagnosed with DVT on therapeutic anticoagulation, and it is believed that they along with early mobilization (and concurrent anticoagulation) lead to a faster improvement in symptoms [49].

Key Points

- If DVT/PE is diagnosed, hospitalize the patient and begin IV UFH/LMWH.
- Thrombolysis is reserved for life-threatening VTE given the high rate of fetal death/maternal hemorrhage.
- Thrombectomy is the choice of treatment when the DVT involves the iliofemoral veins or inferior vena cava.
- Switch patients from LMWH to UFH at 36–37 weeks gestation.
- Hold UFH 6–24 h prior to delivery.
- Hold LMWH at least 24 h prior to delivery.
- Resume anticoagulation 12 h after vaginal delivery or 24 h after C-section.
- If the patient had a DVT/PE during pregnancy, anticoagulation should be continued for 3–6 months postpartum.

Treatment

Although the evidence base supporting treatment of VTE in pregnant patients is limited, guidelines recommend that pregnant patients with VTE be treated with LMWH throughout the pregnancy and for at least 6 weeks postpartum. For this type of provoked VTE, duration of anticoagulation should be continued for 3–6 months postpartum [13, 50]. For women on anticoagulation who become pregnant, LMWH is recommended over vitamin K antagonists during all trimesters.

Vitamin K Antagonists

Successful treatment of VTE in pregnancy remains difficult because of risk to both patient and developing fetus. Vitamin K antagonists including warfarin cross the placenta and pose increased risk to the fetus with potential teratogenicity [13]. Weeks 6–12 are recognized as a period of fetal synthesis of proteins crucial for bone and cartilage formation, which can be impaired by warfarin [51]. These embryopathies, most commonly mid-facial hypoplasia and stippled epiphysis, usually occur within the first trimester of pregnancy [52]. When vitamin K antagonists are used throughout pregnancy, congenital abnormalities are estimated to occur in 3.7% of live births [53]. Because of this risk, it is recommended that heparin be substituted for vitamin K antagonists at or prior to 6 weeks gestation to eliminate the risk of embryopathy. When taking warfarin during the period of organogenesis alone, it is associated with a 14.6–56% reported risk of miscarriage and up to a 30% risk of congenital abnormalities [54]. The fetal and maternal effects are also presumed to be dose dependent, as the frequency of fetal complications (spontaneous abortion and congenital heart disease) was higher when the mean daily dose of warfarin exceeded 5 mg/day [55–57]. In a meta-analysis of studies on anticoagulation agents in pregnancy, it was shown that the rate of spontaneous abortion, stillbirth, and neonatal death was 19.2% in a low-dose (<5 mg) warfarin group as compared to 63.9% in the high-dose group [58, 59].

Unfractionated and Low-Molecular-Weight Heparin

In contrast to warfarin, unfractionated heparin (UFH) does not cross the placenta nor is it considered a teratogen. Its use may be associated with heparin-induced thrombocytopenia and heparin-associated osteoporosis [13]. Therapeutic doses must also be frequently monitored, and larger doses may be necessary because of accelerated clearance during pregnancy. UFH can be used for both the prevention and treatment of VTE. It is usually administered subcutaneously for prophylaxis and intravenously by continuous infusion with dose adjustment to achieve target therapeutic aPTT for successful treatment. In cases where aPTT is markedly prolonged, protamine sulfate may be utilized to reduce the risk of bleeding [57].

Low-molecular-weight heparin (LMWH) does not cross the placenta, and there is no evidence of increased risk of fetal bleeding. It also has superior subcutaneous absorption and bioavailability as compared to UFH. It also has a two- to fourfold longer half-life as well. An improved safety profile and more predictable dose response are also noted, which have made LMWH the recommended treatment for acute VTE during pregnancy [60] despite limited data on recurrent VTE or bleeding during treatment. Both UFH and LMWH are presumed not to enter breast milk, as clinically relevant amounts have not been found of these heparins or warfarin [61]. According to the 2012 CHEST guidelines, LMWH is recommended over vitamin K antagonists during the first, second, and third trimesters and around the time of delivery [13].

The LMWHs used in the treatment of VTE during pregnancy are enoxaparin, dalteparin, and tinzaparin. Enoxaparin is preferred [50]. A systematic review confirms the safety and efficacy of LMWH in the pregnant population [62]. Studies confirm that it is the preferred option because of its better bioavailability, longer plasma half-life, and improved maternal safety profile. It is also more convenient than UFH because it can be given once to twice daily and does not require monitoring of the activated partial thromboplastin time (aPTT) [13]. The once-daily dosing regimen is often used for convenience, even though research comparing dosing regimens is limited. If LMWH is used, a weight-adjusted dosing regimen is recommended. LMWH requirements may change because of increases in the glomerular filtration rate and change in the volume of distribution/increase in maternal blood volume during pregnancy. Lower peak plasma concentrations of both UFH and LMWH have been noted because of increased renal excretion during pregnancy [7]. Despite this, anti-factor Xa monitoring is not usually recommended on a continuous basis.

Maternal complications of anticoagulant therapy are similar to those seen in their nonpregnant counterparts and include bleeding, heparin-induced thrombocytopenia (HIT), heparin-associated osteoporosis, bruising, local allergic reaction, and pain at the injection site. In a recent meta-analysis, the use of anticoagulant therapy was associated with an antepartum incidence of hemorrhagic complications of 3.28% [63]. A total of 260 postpartum hemorrhages were recorded, with only 14 being described as major hemorrhages, which corresponded with an incidence of 1.9%.

Thrombocytopenia is common during pregnancy and HIT, which occurs in around 3% of nonpregnant patients receiving UFH, and must be distinguished from gestational and pregnancy-related thrombocytopenia [64]. HIT is uncommon in pregnancy affecting only 1 of 1167 pregnancies in three clinical series and 0 of 2227 pregnancies in a systematic review [65]. In pregnant patients who do develop HIT, danaparoid (although withdrawn from the US market) is recommended because it does not cross the placenta and has low cross-reactivity with UFH. Fondaparinux has also been used successfully to treat nonpregnant patients with HIT and could be considered if danaparoid is not available [65].

Direct Thrombin Inhibitors, Fondaparinux, and HIT

Several cases of HIT during pregnancy have been documented, usually occurring after UFH therapy [66]. Treatment of HIT requires withdrawal of all heparin exposure and replacement with an alternative anticoagulant including one of the direct thrombin inhibitors. The direct thrombin inhibitors include argatroban, bivalirudin, and lepirudin and are all considered pregnancy Category B drugs despite limited safety data [67]. Utilization of argatroban in pregnant patient has been limited but was successfully used as early as the first trimester [68]. It has also been utilized in the third trimester, specifically in a 33-week pregnant female with a portal vein thrombosis and HIT [67]. While there are reports of fondaparinux being used for HIT during pregnancy, experience with this remains limited.

Use of fondaparinux and direct thrombin inhibitors should be limited to those with severe allergic reactions to heparin (Grade 2C recommendation). Fondaparinux, a selective factor Xa inhibitor that requires daily dosing, has insufficient data to justify its routine use in pregnant patients who do not have a reason to use this drug, such as severe cutaneous allergies or HIT. The FDA had previously categorized this drug as a Class B medication, meaning that there were no risks demonstrated in animal reproductive studies, but human controlled studies may be lacking (Note: Since December 2014, the FDA has changed the labeling requirements for pregnancy and lactation sections on prescription drugs. More descriptive labeling, rather than the previously used letter categories, will be used for new medications, and previously approved drugs will also eventually use the new classification system) [67].

Direct Oral Anticoagulants (DOACs)

No published data exists for the use of the direct oral anticoagulants in pregnant patients. These agents are believed to cross the placenta and may hinder fetal development [69]. Thus, DOACs are generally contraindicated in this patient population. Newer studies are needed to determine concentrations of these anticoagulants secreted by lactating women. Thus, the use of direct thrombin inhibitors like dabigatran and factor Xa inhibitors like rivaroxaban, edoxaban, and apixaban cannot be recommended [13] (Table 18.4).

Table 18.4 Previous FDA drug classifications in pregnancy

Drug	Classification for use in pregnancy
Argatroban	B
Fondaparinux	B
Low-molecular-weight heparin	B
Unfractionated heparin	C
Warfarin	X
Dabigatran	C
Rivaroxaban	C
Apixaban	C

Pregnancy categories of various anticoagulants and the risk of fetal injury using the previous FDA classification. Pregnancy category B: no risk in animal reproduction studies, but no adequate, well-controlled human studies; C: risk not ruled out as animal reproductive studies have demonstrated an adverse effect on the fetus, and there are no adequate, well-controlled human studies; X: contraindicated in pregnancy, studies in animals or humans have demonstrated fetal abnormalities and/or positive evidence of human fetal risk. Since December 2014, the FDA has changed the labeling requirements for pregnancy and lactation sections on prescription drugs and now employs more descriptive labeling rather than letter categories [24]

IVC Filters as Prophylaxis Around Delivery

The use of retrievable inferior vena cava (IVC) filters should only be considered in those with a proximal DVT diagnosed near term (within 1 month of delivery) or who have a major contraindication to anticoagulation [50]. In a 2005 review of patients receiving IVC filters during the perinatal period, no complications were described and no symptomatic PE occurred during or after delivery [70].

Superficial Vein Thrombosis

While the traditional therapeutic approach was to use local symptomatic control measures that consists of nonsteroidal anti-inflammatory medications (NSAIDs) and warm compress therapy, findings from the CALISTO trial suggest that a short course of anticoagulation for patients with symptomatic proximal lower extremity superficial vein thrombosis (SVT) may reduce the risk for progression and development of DVT or PE [71]. In the CALISTO study, symptomatic patients were treated with 45 days of fondaparinux 2.5 mg daily, which reduced the relative risk of thromboembolic complications by 85% compared with placebo (0.9 versus 5.9%) [72]. Pregnant patients with symptomatic proximal lower extremity superficial vein thrombosis should consider therapy with LMWH [50]. Patients with limited (<5 cm in length), distal (below the knee) clots can be managed conservatively, which includes application of warm compresses to the affected areas and the judicious use of nonsteroidal anti-inflammatory drugs (NSAIDs).

Duration of Therapy

Although it has been determined that UFH and LMWH are the preferred therapies for VTE during pregnancy, the length of therapy has never been formally studied. In general, 3–6 months of therapy is appropriate with continuation until at least 6 weeks postpartum.

Key Points

- Vitamin K antagonists (warfarin) are contraindicated in pregnancy as they cross the placenta and are potentially teratogenic.
- However, for those with mechanical heart valves, current AHA/ACC guidelines state that it may be reasonable to use warfarin during the first trimester if the dose required to achieve therapeutic INR is less than 5 mg/day (Class IIa recommendation).
- Unfractionated heparin (UFH) and low-molecular-weight heparin (LMWH) do not cross the placenta, nor are they teratogenic. In addition, neither anticoagulant has been found in breast milk.
- LMWH is the recommended treatment for acute VTE in pregnancy because of its better bioavailability, longer half-life, and improved maternal safety profile.

- Symptomatic superficial vein thrombosis (*i.e.*, extensive thrombus by the sapheno-femoral junction) can be treated with LMWH.
- In cases of HIT, argatroban, bivalirudin, and lepirudin are all Grade B drugs.
- Fondaparinux and direct thrombin inhibitors should only be used in patients with severe allergic reactions to heparin.
- Direct oral anticoagulants (DOACs) are contraindicated as they cross the placenta and may hinder fetal development.
- Inferior vena cava (IVC) filters should only be considered for patients with extensive DVT diagnosed near term or those who have major contraindications to anticoagulation.

Pregnant Patients with Mechanical Valves

Management of pregnant patients with mechanical heart valves can be both challenging and confusing, as guideline recommendations for the use of VKAs such as warfarin in this cohort continue to evolve [13]. Indeed, for pregnant patients, several anticoagulant agents are available for use, but all options carry risk for both the mother and fetus. Warfarin is the preferred anticoagulant for preventing mechanical valve thrombosis, but its teratogenic effects on the fetus substantially limit its utility during pregnancy.

In a recent retrospective study comparing warfarin and LMWH in pregnant women with mechanical valves, there were significant side effects in all groups, ranging from fetal loss to valve thrombosis, maternal death, and postpartum hemorrhage [73]. A systematic review of literature performed by Chan and colleagues showed that the overall pooled maternal mortality rate was 2.9% with major bleeding occurring in 2.5% of all pregnancies, primarily at the time of delivery [74]. It was also seen that the lowest risk of valve thrombosis/systemic embolism occurred when patients were continued on vitamin K antagonists (3.9%). The use of LWMH/UFH only during weeks 6–12 of gestation was associated with increased risk of valve thrombosis (9.2%), and the highest risk of thromboembolism was when heparin was used as the sole anticoagulant (33.3%) [59].

Steinberg and colleagues recently conducted a meta-analysis of 18 studies evaluating maternal outcomes that included death, valve failure, thromboembolism, spontaneous abortion, and congenital defects in those who received VKA versus LMWH during pregnancy. The composite maternal risk was found to be the lowest with VKA (5%) as compared to LMWH (16%). In contrast, there was a dose-dependent relationship between fetal risk and warfarin use. Higher doses of VKA, particularly greater than 5 mg of warfarin, led to greater fetal risk (39%), as compared to LMWH (13%). However, no difference in fetal risk was seen in patients on ≤5 mg warfarin daily and those on LMWH [75].

Thus, current AHA/ACC guidelines state that it may be reasonable to continue anticoagulation therapy with warfarin during the first trimester if the daily dose needed to achieve a therapeutic INR is 5 mg or less (Class IIa recommendation). For women whose daily dose of warfarin exceeds 5 mg, the recommendation is to use dose-adjusted LMWH during the first trimester, specifically targeting serum anti-Xa levels to be 0.8–1.2 U/mL at 4–8 h post dose administration) [76]. However, evaluation of European registry data by van Hagen and colleagues found that ~50% of the mechanical valve thromboses occurred during the transition from VKA to LMWH during the first trimester. This finding suggests the need to use even higher doses of LMWH during the transition period [77].

The American College of Chest Physicians (ACCP) Evidence-Based Clinical Practice Guidelines have outlined different options that may be offered to pregnant females with mechanical heart valves who were diagnosed with acute VTE [32]. The first option is dose-adjusted LMWH dosing with testing of anti-factor Xa level to ensure that the peak level (1.0–1.2 U/mL) was achieved 4 h after administration [59, 74].

The second option is dose-adjusted UFH with dosing every 12 h, with close monitoring of aPTT. The final option is to initiate LMWH/UFH until the 13th week of gestation and then substituting with warfarin until the immediate peripartum period just before delivery which is when LMWH/UFH would be reinitiated for delivery. The addition of aspirin (75–100 mg/d) can also be considered to reduce the risk of thrombosis. The use of direct oral anticoagulants (i.e., dabigatran) is not supported given the high risk of mechanical valve thrombosis [59].

Conclusion

Despite advances in diagnosis and treatment, VTE remains an important cause of morbidity and mortality. All pregnant patients are at increased risk for thrombosis given the hemodynamic and prothrombotic changes associated with pregnancy. A history of a prior VTE remains the most significant risk factor, and those with prior VTE all require 6 weeks of postpartum prophylaxis with LMWH or vitamin K antagonists. Depending on the presence of inherited or acquired thrombophilias, as well as family history of VTE, antepartum and/or postpartum prophylaxis may or may not be recommended. Diagnosis with duplex ultrasound is ideal, but further imaging involving potentially harmful radiation may be necessary to confirm the diagnosis. For those diagnosed with VTE, LMWH is recommended over vitamin K antagonists during all trimesters. Because of the high risk of maternal and fetal complications, the management of VTE in pregnant patient remains a difficult task for all physicians.

Overall Clinical Practice Guidelines and Grade Recommendations

- Vitamin K antagonists should be substituted with LMWH/UFH, except under special circumstances for women with mechanical heart valves (Grade 1A).
- Pregnant patients should get treated with LMWH or UFH for prevention and treatment of VTE (Grade 2C).
- Acute VTE in pregnancy should have continued LMWH/UFH therapy throughout the pregnancy (Grade 1B).
- Anticoagulants should be continued for at least 6 weeks postpartum for a total minimal duration of therapy of 3 months (Grade 2C).
- Patients with antithrombin deficiency should have antepartum and postpartum anticoagulation regardless of VTE history (Grade 2C).
- Pregnant patients with history of VTE with transient risk factors which are no longer present and no thrombophilias should be clinically assessed antepartum and anticoagulant prophylaxis postpartum (Grade 1C).
- Patients with recurrent fetal loss should undergo APS screening (Grade 1A) and if positive, antepartum prophylactic anticoagulation in addition to aspirin therapy is recommended (Grade 1B).
- Patients with mechanical heart valves need to review the risks and benefits of different anticoagulation strategies prior to pregnancy.

Self-Assessment Questions

1. A 25-year-old woman G2P1, who is currently 8 weeks pregnant, presents to the emergency department with progressively worsening dyspnea on exertion over the last week. Her history is notable for a right lower extremity DVT diagnosed during her first pregnancy, 3 years ago. She was treated with low-molecular-weight heparin for the duration of this pregnancy and for a short period after her scheduled uncomplicated Cesarean section. On arrival, her vital signs are BP 122/88, HR 119, RR 20, and O2sat 94% on room air.

Physical exam is notable for a regular tachycardia and left lower extremity swelling. Her lungs are clear to auscultation and there are no murmurs, rubs, or gallops. What is the next best step to make a diagnosis?

   (a) Check a D-dimer level
   (b) Low-dose CT angiogram
   (c) Ventilation-perfusion scan
   (d) Lower extremity venous duplex ultrasound
   (e) High-sensitivity troponin level

2. The above patient has a lower extremity venous duplex ultrasound that demonstrated the presence of a left popliteal DVT. Using standard precautions, CT angiography of her chest was performed which demonstrated the presence of bilateral subsegmental PE. Which of the following is the anticoagulant of choice with appropriate dosing for the duration of her pregnancy?
   (a) Warfarin 6 mg PO daily to a goal INR of 2–3
   (b) Enoxaparin 1.5 mg/kg subcutaneous daily
   (c) Enoxaparin 1 mg/kg subcutaneous BID
   (d) Unfractionated heparin IV infusion to a goal PTT 60–90
   (e) Rivaroxaban 20 mg PO daily
3. She returns to the hospital as recommended at 37 weeks of gestation. Enoxaparin is switched to IV unfractionated heparin (UFH), which is then held 6 h prior to a scheduled delivery via Cesarean section. LMWH is resumed 24 h post-surgery, at which point there are no signs of bleeding. She returns to the outpatient office in 1–2 weeks, after an uneventful recovery, and requests to discontinue her anticoagulation. She plans to breastfeed if possible. Which of the following is the appropriate recommendation for her?
   (a) She can stop her anticoagulation at this time.
   (b) She can stop anticoagulation in 1 week if a lower extremity venous duplex ultrasound is normal.
   (c) Anticoagulation should be continued for at least 3–6 months postpartum, and lifelong anticoagulation can be considered given her two VTE events.
   (d) Anticoagulation should be continued for at least 3–6 months, but breastfeeding is contraindicated.
4. A 32-year-old woman is referred to you because she was previously told that she had a clotting disorder and is considering becoming pregnant in the near future. She has no history of PE, DVT, or miscarriages. This will be her first pregnancy. Her mother had three miscarriages but no documented history of PE or DVT. She is unaware of her mother's diagnosis. Another physician has informed her that she may need some "blood thinner" during her pregnancy, because of her past history. Which of the following inherited thrombophilias would not warrant consideration of postpartum anticoagulation?
   (a) Antithrombin deficiency
   (b) Homozygosity for factor V Leiden mutation
   (c) Homozygosity for prothrombin gene G20210A mutation
   (d) Antiphospholipid antibody syndrome
   (e) Heterozygosity for factor V Leiden mutation
   (f) All of the above inherited thrombophilias should warrant some anticoagulation.
5. It is determined that the above 32-year-old woman is homozygous for a factor V Leiden mutation. She is again wondering if she will need anticoagulation during and/or after her pregnancy, even though she has never had a DVT or PE. You recommend:
   (a) Periodic risk assessment alone is sufficient.
   (b) Antepartum and postpartum prophylactic anticoagulation.
   (c) Clinical surveillance during the antepartum period with prophylactic anticoagulation in the postpartum period.
   (d) Antepartum prophylactic anticoagulation and aspirin.
   (e) No anticoagulation will likely be needed because there is no personal history of DVT or PE.

Self-Assessment Answers

1. (d) Lower extremity venous duplex ultrasound

   The next best step to confirm the diagnosis of a suspected DVT is to perform a lower extremity venous duplex ultrasound. Duplex ultrasonography is considered an accurate, noninvasive, radiation-free, and cost-effective method of diagnosing a DVT in pregnant patient. CT angiography and V/Q scans are not the initial tests of choice but may be considered if compression ultrasound is negative while suspicion for VTE remains high. D-dimers may be elevated in pregnant patient. High sensitivity troponins are not utilized in the initial diagnosis and evaluation for DVT but may be elevated in the setting of a hemodynamically significant pulmonary embolisms.

2. (c) Enoxaparin 1 mg/kg subcutaneous BID

   Current guidelines recommend that pregnant patient with VTE should be treated with low-molecular-weight heparin (LMWH) throughout the pregnancy and for at least 6 weeks postpartum. LMWH at a dose of 1 mg/kg subcutaneously twice daily has an improved safety profile and more predictable dose response, making it the treatment of choice. Vitamin K antagonists, like warfarin, cross the placenta and are known to pose increased risk to the fetus with potential teratogenicity. The frequency of fetal complications was found to be higher when the mean daily dose exceeded 5 mg/day. The use of factor Xa inhibitors, like apixaban and rivaroxaban, is not well studied in the pregnant population and should currently be avoided. Unfractionated heparin is another short-term treatment option for this patient but would not be the optimal longer-term option for the remaining months of her pregnancy.

3. (c) Anticoagulation should be continued for at least 3–6 months postpartum, and lifelong anticoagulation can be considered given her two VTE events.

   Anticoagulation should be continued for 3–6 months postpartum and should not be stopped at current visit, even if a lower extremity duplex is normal. Given the fact that she has had two isolated VTE events, lifelong anticoagulation should be considered. Both LMWH and warfarin are presumed not to enter breast milk and are considered safe for the use in women who breastfeed.

4. (e) Heterozygosity for factor V Leiden mutation

   Anticoagulation is not usually required for those with inherited thrombophilias, if there is no personal history of VTE or complication during a previous pregnancy. The exception to this includes women with a very high risk of thrombosis, including those with antithrombin deficiency, homozygosity for factor V Leiden mutation, homozygosity for prothrombin gene G20210A mutation, or antiphospholipid syndrome. Postpartum prophylaxis for 6 weeks is recommended for all of these thrombophilias, except for heterozygosity for factor V Leiden mutation, which is associated with lower risks of gestational VTE.

5. (c) Clinical surveillance during the antepartum period with prophylactic anticoagulation in the postpartum period

   If pregnant women are homozygous for factor V Leiden or prothrombin gene G20210A mutation and have a positive family history of VTE or a prior VTE episode, then both antepartum and postpartum prophylaxis should be considered per current guidelines. If there is no prior VTE nor family history of VTE, then these patients hould undergo clinical surveillance during the antepartum period plus prophylactic anticoagulation in the postpartum period. Periodic risk assessment alone is not sufficient. Women with APS and recurrent pregnancy loss should receive antepartum prophylactic anticoagulation, in addition to the continuation of aspirin.

References

1. McColl MD, Ramsay JE, Tait RC, et al. Risk factors for pregnancy associated venous thromboembolism. Thromb Haemost. 1997;78(4):1183–8.
2. Ray JG, Chan WS. Deep vein thrombosis during pregnancy and the puerperium: a meta-analysis of the

period of risk and leg of presentation. Obstet Gynecol Surv. 1999;54:254–71.

3. Romualdi E, Dentali F, Rancan E, Squizzato A, Steidl L, et al. Anticoagulant therapy for venous thromboembolism during pregnancy: a systematic review and a meta-analysis of the literature. J Thromb Haemost. 2013;11(4):788–9.
4. Heit JA, Kobbervig CE, James AH, Petterson TM, Bailey KR, Melton LJ. Trends in the incidence of venous thromboembolism during pregnancy or postpartum: a 30-year population-based study. Ann Intern Med. 2005;143:697–706.
5. Virkus RA, Lokkegaard EC, Bergholt T, Mogensen U, Langhoff-Roos J, Lidegaard O. Venous thromboembolism in pregnant and puerperal women in Denmark 1995-2005. A national cohort study. Thromb Haemost. 2011;106:304–9.
6. Damodaram M, Kaladindi M, Luckit J, Yoong W. D-dimers are a screening test of venous thromboembolism in pregnancy: is it of any use? J Obstet Gynaecol. 2009;29:101–3.
7. James A, Committee on Practice B-O. Practice bulletin no. 123: thromboembolism in pregnancy. Obstet Gynecol. 2011;118:718–29.
8. Tan M, Huisman MV. The diagnostic management of acute venous thromboembolism during pregnancy: recent advancements and unresolved issues. Thromb Res. 2011;127(Suppl 3):S13–6.
9. James AH. Prevention and treatment of venous thromboembolism in pregnancy. Clin Obstet Gynecol. 2012;55:774–87.
10. James AH, Jamison MG, Brancazio LR, Myers ER. Venous thromboembolism during pregnancy and the postpartum period: incidence, risk factors, and mortality. Am J Obstet Gynecol. 2006;194:1311–5.
11. Sultan AA, West J, Tata LJ, Fleming KM, Nelson-Piercy C, Grainge MJ. Risk of first venous thromboembolism in and around pregnancy: a population-based cohort study. Br J Haematol. 2012;156:366–73.
12. Gerhardt A, Scharf RE, Greer IA, Zotz RB. Hereditary risk factors of thrombophilia and probability of venous thromboembolism during pregnancy and the puerperium. Blood. 2016;128(19):2343–9.
13. Yarrington CD, Valente AM, Economy KE. Cardiovascular management in pregnancy: antithrombotic agents and antiplatelet agents. Circulation. 2015;132:1354–64.
14. Long AA, Ginsberg JS, Brill-Edwards P, et al. The relationship of antiphospholipid antibodies to thromboembolic disease in systemic lupus erythematosus: a cross-sectional study. Thromb Haemost. 1991;66:520–4.
15. Den Heijer M, Rosendaal FR, Blom HJ, et al. Hyperhomocysteinemia as a risk for deep-vein thrombosis. N Engl J Med. 1995;334:759–62.
16. Robertson L, Wu O, Langhorne P, et al. Thrombosis risk and economic assessment of thrombophilia screening (treats) study. Thrombophilia in pregnancy; a systematic review. Br J Haematol. 2005;132:171–96.
17. Gordon M. Maternal physiology in pregnancy. In: Gabbe S, Niebyl J, Simpson J, editors. Normal and problem pregnancies. 4th ed. New York: Churchill Livingstone; 2002. p. 63–92.
18. Bremme KA. Haemostatic changes in pregnancy. Best Pract Res Clin Haematol. 2003;16:153–68.
19. Hellgren M. Hemostasis during normal pregnancy and puerperium. Semin Thromb Hemost. 2003;29:125–30.
20. James AH. Pregnancy-associated thrombosis. Hematology Am Soc Hematol Educ Program. 2009;2009:277–85.
21. Lindqvist P, Dahlback B, Marsal K. Thrombotic risk during pregnancy: a population study. Obstet Gynecol. 1999;94:595–9.
22. Jacobsen AF, Skjeldestad FE, Sandset PM. Incidence and risk patterns of venous thromboembolism in pregnancy and puerperium--a register-based case-control study. Am J Obstet Gynecol. 2008;198:233.e1–7.
23. Pabinger I, Grafenhofer H, Kyrle PA, et al. Temporary increase in the risk for recurrence during pregnancy in women with a history of venous thromboembolism. Blood. 2002;100:1060–2.
24. Bates SM, Greer IA, Middeldorp S, Veenstra DL, Prabulos A-M, Vandvik PO. VTE, thrombophilia, antithrombotic therapy, and pregnancy: antithrombotic therapy and prevention of thrombosis, 9th ed: American College of Chest Physicians evidence-based clinical practice guidelines. Chest. 2012;141(2 suppl):e691S–736S.
25. James AH, Brancazio LR, Ortel TL. Thrombosis, thrombophilia, and thromboprophylaxis in pregnancy. Clin Adv Hematol Oncol. 2005;3:187–97.
26. Tormene D, Grandone E, De Stefano V, et al. Obstetric complications and pregnancy-related venous thromboembolism: the effect of low-molecular-weight heparin on their prevention in carriers of factor V Leiden or prothrombin G20210A mutation. Thromb Haemost. 2012;107:477–84.
27. Folkeringa N, Brouwer JL, Korteweg FJ, et al. Reduction of high fetal loss rate by anticoagulant treatment during pregnancy in antithrombin, protein C or protein S deficient women. Br J Haematol. 2007;136:656–61.
28. Gris JC, Mercier E, Quere I, Lavigne-Lissalde G, Cochery-Nouvellon E, Hoffet M, et al. Low-molecular-weight heparin versus low-dose aspirin in women with one fetal loss and a constitutional thrombophilic disorder. Blood. 2004;103:3695–9.
29. Johnston JA, Brill-Edwards P, Ginsberg JS, Pauker SG, Eckman MH. Cost-effectiveness of prophylactic low molecular weight heparin in pregnant women with a prior history of venous thromboembolism. Am J Med. 2005;118:503–14.
30. Okoroh EM, Azonobi IC, Grosse SD, Grant AM, Atrash HK, James AH. Prevention of venous thromboembolism in pregnancy: a review of guidelines, 2000-2011. J Women's Health. 2012;21:611–5.

31. Brill-Edwards P, Ginsberg JS, Gent M, et al. Safety of withholding heparin in pregnant women with a history of venous thromboembolism. N Engl J Med. 2000;343:1439–44.
32. Bates SM, Ginsberg JS. How we manage venous thromboembolism during pregnancy. Blood. 2002;100:3470–8.
33. Chan WS, Spencer FA, Ginsberg JS. Anatomic distribution of deep vein thrombosis in pregnancy. CMAJ. 2010;182:657–60.
34. Chan WS, Lee A, Spencer FA, et al. Predicting deep venous thrombosis in pregnancy: out in "LEFt" field? Ann Intern Med. 2009;151:85–92.
35. Dargaud Y, Rugeri L, Vergnes MC, et al. A risk score for the management of pregnant women with increased risk of venous thromboembolism: a multicentre prospective study. Br J Haematol. 2009;145:825–35.
36. Chan WS, Chunilal S, Lee A, Crowther M, Rodger M, Ginsberg JS. A red blood cell agglutination D-dimer test to exclude deep venous thrombosis in pregnancy. Ann Intern Med. 2007;147:165–70.
37. Hirai K, Sugimura M, Ohashi R, et al. A rapid activated protein C sensitivity test as a diagnostic marker for a suspected venous thromboembolism in pregnancy and puerperium. Gynecol Obstet Investig. 2011;72:55–62.
38. Kearon C, Julian JA, Newman TE, Ginsberg JS. Noninvasive diagnosis of deep venous thrombosis. McMaster diagnostic imaging practice guidelines initiative. Ann Intern Med. 1998;128:663–77.
39. Nijkeuter M, Ginsberg JS, Huisman MV. Diagnosis of deep vein thrombosis and pulmonary embolism in pregnancy: a systematic review. J Thromb Haemost. 2006;4:496–500.
40. Groves AM, Yates SJ, Win T, Kayani I, Gallagher FA, et al. CT pulmonary angiography versus ventilation-perfusion scintigraphy in pregnancy: implications from a UK survey of doctors' knowledge of radiation exposure. Radiology. 2006;240:765–70.
41. Hunsaker AR, MT L, Goldhaber SZ, Rybicki FJ. Imaging in acute pulmonary embolism with special clinical scenarios. Circ Cardiovasc Imaging. 2010;3:491–500.
42. Litmanovich D, Boiselle PM, Bankier AA, Kataoka ML, Pianykh O, Raptopoulos V. Dose reduction in computed tomographic angiography of pregnant patients with suspected acute pulmonary embolism. J Comput Assist Tomogr. 2009;33(6):961.
43. Ridge CA, McDermott S, Freyne BJ, Brennan DJ, Collins CD, Skehan SJ. Pulmonary embolism in pregnancy: comparison of pulmonary CT angiography and lung scintigraphy. Am J Roentgenol. 2009;193:1223–7.
44. Cahill AG, Stout MJ, Macones GA, Bhalla S. Diagnosing pulmonary embolism in pregnancy using computed tomographic angiography or ventilation-perfusion. Obstet Gynecol. 2009;114:124–9.
45. Turrentine MA, Braems G, Ramirez MM. Use of thrombolytics for the treatment of thromboembolic disease during pregnancy. Obstet Gynecol Surv. 1995;50:534–41.
46. Pillny M, Sandmann W, Luther B, et al. Deep venous thrombosis during pregnancy and after delivery: indications for and results of thrombectomy. J Vasc Surg. 2003;37:528–32.
47. Taniguchi S, Fukuda I, Minakawa M, Watanabe K, Daitoku K, Suzuki Y. Emergency pulmonary embolectomy during the second trimester of pregnancy: report of a case. Surg Today. 2008;38:59–61.
48. Baker WH, Mahler DK, Foldes MS, et al. Pneumatic compression devices for prophylaxis of deep venous thrombosis (DVT). Am Surg. 1986;52:371–3.
49. Ratiu A, Motoc A, Pascut D, Crisan DC, Anca T, Pascut M. Compression and walking compared with bed rest in the treatment of proximal deep venous thrombosis during pregnancy. Rev Med Chir Soc Med Nat Iasi. 2009;113:795–8.
50. Arya R. How I manage venous thromboembolism in pregnancy. Br J Haemotol. 2011;153:698–708.
51. Walfisch A, Koren G. The "warfarin window" in pregnancy: the importance of half-life. J Obstet Gynaecol Can. 2010;32:988–9.
52. Hall JG, Pauli RM, Wilson KM. Maternal and fetal sequelae of anticoagulation during pregnancy. Am J Med. 1980;68(1):122–40.
53. Hassouna A, Allam H. Anticoagulation of pregnant women with mechanical heart valve prosthesis: a systematic review of the literature (2000-2009). J Coagul Disord. 2010;2(1):81–8.
54. Blickstein D, Blickstein I. The risk of fetal loss associated with warfarin anticoagulation. Int J Gynaecol Obstet. 2002;78:221–5.
55. Vitale N, De Eeo M, De Santo LS, et al. Dose-dependent fetal complications of warfarin in pregnant women with mechanical heart valves. J Am Coll Cardiol. 1999;33:1637–41.
56. Cotrufo M, De Feo M, De Santo LS, et al. Risk of warfarin during pregnancy with mechanical valve prostheses. Obstet Gynecol. 2002;99:35–40.
57. Massonnet-Castel S, Pelissier E, Bara L, et al. Partial reversal of low molecular-weight heparin (PK 101699) anti-Xa activity by protamine sulfate: in vitro and in vivo study during cardiac surgery with extracorporeal circulation. Haemostasis. 1986;16:139–46.
58. Xu Z, Fan J, Luo X, et al. Anticoagulation regimens during pregnancy in patients with mechanical heart valves: a systematic review and meta-analysis. Can J Cardiol. 2016;32(10):1248.e1–9.
59. Alshawabkeh L, Economy KE, Valente AM. Anticoagulation during pregnancy: evolving strategies with a focus on mechanical valves. J Am Coll Cardiol. 2016;68:1804–13.
60. Chunilal SD, Bates SM. Venous thromboembolism in pregnancy: diagnosis, management and prevention. Thromb Haemost. 2009;101:428–43.

61. Stone SE, Morris TA. Pulmonary embolism during and after pregnancy. Crit Care Med. 2005;33(Suppl. 10):S294–300.
62. Greer IA, Nelson-Piercy C. Low-molecular-weight heparins for thromboprophylaxis and treatment of venous thromboembolism in pregnancy: a systematic review of safety and efficacy. Blood. 2005;106(2):401–7.
63. Romualdi E, Dentali F, Rancan E, Squizzato A, Steidl L, et al. Anticoagulant therapy for venous thromboembolism during pregnancy: a systematic review and a meta-analysis of the literature. J Thromb Haemost. 2013;11(2):270–81.
64. Warkentin TE, Levine MN, Hirsh J, et al. Heparin-induced thrombocytopenia in patients treated with low-molecular-weight heparin or unfractionated heparin. N Engl J Med. 1995;332(20):1330–5.
65. Linkins L-A, Dans AL, Moores LK, et al. Treatment and prevention of heparin-induced thrombocytopenia: antithrombotic therapy and prevention of thrombosis, 9th ed: American College of Chest Physicians Evidence- Based Clinical Practice Guidelines. Chest. 2012;141:e495S–530S.
66. Mehta R, Golichowski A. Treatment of heparin induced thrombocytopenia and thrombosis during the first trimester of pregnancy. J Thromb Haemost. 2004;2:1665–6.
67. Young SK, Al-Mondhiry HA, Vaida SJ, Ambrose A, Botti JJ. Successful use of argatroban during the third trimester of pregnancy: case report and review of the literature. Pharmacotherapy. 2008;28:1531–6.
68. Tanimura K, Ebina Y, Sonoyama A, Morita H, Miyata S, Yamada H. Argatroban therapy for heparin-induced thrombocytopenia during pregnancy in a woman with hereditary antithrombin deficiency. J Obstet Gynaecol Res. 2012;38:749–52.
69. Jacobsen AF, Sandset PM. Venous thromboembolism associated with pregnancy and hormonal therapy. Best Pract Res Clin Haematol. 2012;25:319–32.
70. Kawamata K, Chiba Y, Tanaka R, Higashi M, Nishigami K. Experience of temporary inferior vena cava filters inserted in the perinatal period to prevent pulmonary embolism in pregnant women with deep vein thrombosis. J Vasc Surg. 2005;41:652–6.
71. Decousus H, Quéré I, Presles E, et al. POST (prospective observational superficial thrombophlebitis). Superficial venous thrombosis and venous thromboembolism: a large, prospective epidemiologic study. Ann Intern Med. 2010;152(4):218–24.
72. Decousus H, Prandoni P, Mismetti P, CALISTO Study Group CALISTO Study Group, et al. Fondaparinux for the treatment of superficial-vein thrombosis in the legs. N Engl J Med. 2010;363(13):1222–32.
73. Basude S, Hein C, Curtis S, Clark A, Trinder J. Low-molecular-weight heparin or warfarin for anticoagulation in pregnant women with mechanical heart valves: what are the risks? A retrospective observational study. BJOG. 2012;119:1008–13.
74. Pauli RM, Haun J. Intrauterine effects of coumadin derivatives. Dev Brain Dysfunct. 1993;6:229–47.
75. Steinberg ZL, Dominguez-Islas CP, Otto CM, Stout KK, Krieger EV. Maternal and fetal outcomes of anticoagulation in pregnant women with mechanical heart valves. J Am Coll Cardiol. 2017;69:2681–91.
76. Nishimura RA, Otto CM, Bonow RO, Carabello BA, Erwin JP, Guyton RA, ACC/AHA Task Force Members, et al. 2014 AHA/ACC guideline for the management of patients with valvular heart disease: a report of the American College of Cardiology/American Heart Association Task Force on Practice Guidelines. Circulation. 2014;129:e521–643.
77. van Hagen IM, Roos-Hesselink JW, Ruys TPE, Merz WM, Goland S, et al. Pregnancy in women with a mechanical heart valve: data of the European Society of Cardiology Registry Of Pregnancy And Cardiac disease (ROPAC). Circulation. 2015;132:132–42.

Anticoagulation in the Elderly

19

Ruchika Harisingani, Ibrahim M. Ali, Bhakti Shah, and Salonie Pereira

Clinical Vignettes

Case 1: *An 89-year-old woman with a history of prior stroke, dementia, chronic atrial fibrillation, hypertension, coronary artery disease, and systolic heart failure with an ejection fraction of 40% comes to your office accompanied by her daughter who states that she has been increasingly fatigued with episodes of exertional dyspnea over the past several weeks. Her medications include aspirin 81 mg and dabigatran 75 mg BID. At her baseline, the patient is ambulatory with a walker, but requires assistance performing several activities of daily living. With the exception of moderate kyphosis, her physical exam was unremarkable. Labs are significant for a drop in hemoglobin to 8.0 g/dL from a baseline of 12.1 g/dL last assessed 4 months ago. Fecal occult blood testing is positive. The patient's last colonoscopy was 10 years ago, which was "normal." Her family states that she would not want to undergo another colonoscopy at this age. The daughter asks you whether her mother should continue taking aspirin and dabigatran, fully aware of her risk of embolic stroke.*

Case 2: *A 69-year-old man with a history of seizures and chronic kidney disease was brought in to the Emergency Department for unresponsiveness. He was found to have a systolic BP of 90 mmHg, was started on IV pressor support, and admitted to MICU. Bedside echocardiogram revealed severely decreased right ventricular systolic function and acutely increased pulmonary artery systolic pressures supportive of right heart strain. CT angiogram of the chest confirmed extensive bilateral segmental pulmonary emboli. He was given tPA and started on an unfractionated heparin drip. His mental status improved and his clinical course stabilized. He was*

Author contributed equally with all other contributors.
Ruchika Harisingani and Salonie Pereira

R. Harisingani (✉) · B. Shah · S. Pereira
Department of Medicine, Northwell Health, Zucker School of Medicine at Hofstra/Northwell, Manhasset, NY, USA
e-mail: rharisin@northwell.edu; bshah4@northwell.edu; spereira3@northwell.edu

I. M. Ali
Department of Cardiology, Northwell Health, Zucker School of Medicine at Hofstra/Northwell, Manhasset, NY, USA
e-mail: iali@northwell.edu;

J. F. Lau et al. (eds.), *Anticoagulation Therapy*, https://doi.org/10.1007/978-3-319-73709-6_19

transferred to an inpatient medicine floor, where he was started on anticoagulation with warfarin. The next day, he began complaining of a headache and developed significant mental status changes. Head CT revealed an acute intracranial hemorrhage involving the body of the left lateral ventricle and the posterior horn of right lateral ventricle. Anticoagulation was stopped and serial follow-up MRI scans showed stability of the bleed. Neurosurgery evaluated the patient and recommended no urgent surgical intervention. The house staff team involved with his care consults you for your recommendation on anticoagulation management in this patient.

Case 3: *An 85-year-old woman with type II diabetes mellitus, paroxysmal atrial fibrillation, and coronary artery disease (CAD) with recent percutaneous intervention using a drug-eluting stent 8 months ago is brought into clinic by her family for a routine follow-up visit. Her medications include aspirin, clopidogrel, warfarin, insulin, metoprolol, and atorvastatin. Of note, the patient has fallen twice in the past month. The patient and her son deny any history of syncope or bleeding. The patient uses a cane to ambulate and requires assistance with her activities of daily living. Her physical exam is notable for ecchymosis on the extremities. Laboratory tests are unremarkable. Her son is concerned about his mother's history of frequent falls while being on "blood thinners," and is asking if they can be safely discontinued.*

Introduction

Between 2012 and 2050, the United States will see considerable growth in the number of older Americans. In 2050, the population aged 65 and over is projected to be 83.7 million, almost double the current estimate of 43.1 million in 2012 (Refer to: www.census.gov/prod/2014pubs/p25-1140.pdf). The aging body undergoes significant pharmacokinetic and pharmacodynamic changes. Drug metabolism—absorption, distribution, metabolism, and excretion—all change with age. Despite an age-related decrease in small-bowel surface area, slowed gastric emptying, and an increase in gastric pH, changes in drug absorption tend to be clinically inconsequential for most drugs. With age, body fat generally increases and total body water decreases. Increased fat increases the volume of distribution for highly lipophilic drugs like diazepam and may increase their elimination half-lives. In patients with an acute critical illness or malnutrition, rapid reductions in serum albumin may enhance drug effects because serum levels of unbound (free) drug may increase (only unbound drug has a pharmacologic effect). One of the medications that places patients at high risk for toxic effects is warfarin, due to the age-related decrease in albumin levels and in the hepatic metabolism of many drugs through the cytochrome P-450 enzyme system. Theoretically, maintenance doses of drugs should be decreased accordingly; however, the rate of drug metabolism varies greatly from person to person, so individual dose adjustment is required [1].

One of the most important pharmacokinetic changes associated with aging is decreased renal elimination of drugs. Serum creatinine levels often remain within normal limits despite a decrease in glomerular filtration rate (GFR) because elderly patients typically have less muscle mass, are less physically active, and therefore produce less creatinine. A "normal" serum creatinine level in an elderly patient may be misleading, and may not reflect true kidney function. To guide drug dosing in this patient population, one can either estimate or calculate creatinine clearance using the Cockcroft–Gault formula. Since renal function is dynamic, maintenance doses of drugs may need periodic readjustment, particularly when the patient's intravascular volume status fluctuates, as in the case during illness or dehydration [1]. The elderly patient presents a unique challenge in the realm of anticoagulation because of the complex interactions between the physical, cognitive, and social domains. Frailty, risk of falls, polypharmacy, altered drug metabolism, cognitive impairment, decline in functional status, and issues with adherence to the care plan are several concerns that are important to highlight. Thus, the approach to the care of the older patient must be individualized.

Due to pharmacodynamic changes as well as the increasing prevalence of comorbid conditions with advanced age, the elderly are at higher risk of bleeding with anticoagulants. Risk factors associated with bleeding include: (1) prior history of bleeding, perhaps the most potent predictor of recurrent bleeding; (2) anemia; (3) prior stroke; (4) uncontrolled hypertension (systolic blood pressure >140 mmHg), and; (5) hepatic and renal impairment [2]. Congestive heart failure and diabetes mellitus have also been shown to be associated with bleeding in patients on anticoagulation therapy for atrial fibrillation [2]. Antiplatelet therapy (i.e., aspirin and clopidogrel) used with anticoagulants concomitantly increases risk of bleeding [2]. NSAIDs and concurrent excessive alcohol intake also elevate bleeding risk [2]. Advanced age (>80-years-old) has been cited as an independent risk factor for major bleeding during warfarin monotherapy. Of note, this age group had a 15% higher incidence of stroke as compared to the 70 to 79-year-olds [2], which suggests the increased benefit of anticoagulation therapy in elderly patients to decrease risk of stroke. Physicians are constantly struggling with the risk versus benefit trade-off when considering anticoagulation for older patients with complex comorbid conditions [3]. In a retrospective cohort study, physician barriers to anticoagulation therapy in older adults (mean age 79) were explored. Despite high stroke risk, more than 40% of patients were not started on an oral anticoagulant due to fall risk, poor prognosis, older age, and dementia [4].

Assessing Thromboembolic and Bleeding Risks in the Elderly Patient

Age is a significant risk factor for venous thromboembolism (VTE) as well as atrial fibrillation. In fact, a third of patients who have atrial fibrillation are 80 years or older [5]. Age is also a risk factor for thrombotic complications associated with these conditions, as it represents an important factor in the CHA_2DS_2-VASc scoring system to assess thromboembolic risk [6]. One study demonstrated that approximately 24% of strokes in the elderly were due to atrial fibrillation [7]. Therefore, anticoagulation should not be withheld from older patients solely due to their advanced age and concern for increased bleeding complications. Instead, clinicians should carefully evaluate elderly patients to identify the safest approach to minimize disease related complications as well as those due to its treatment.

Several risk assessment tools are available to assist clinicians. The CHA_2DS_2-VASc score is an extensively validated risk assessment tool that has been demonstrated to be useful in assessing patients' risk of thromboembolism. Similarly, the HAS-BLED score has been demonstrated to be useful in the assessment of bleeding risk in patients being evaluated for anticoagulant thromboprophylaxis for atrial fibrillation. A thorough history and physical exam can identify potential bleeding risks. Elderly patients have a higher risk of gastrointestinal bleeding as they have a high prevalence of diverticulosis and angiodysplasia than the general population [6]. The CHA_2DS_2-VASc and HAS-BLED scores are depicted below in Table 19.1 [7, 8].

Table 19.1 Assessment of Stroke (CHA_2DS_2-VASc) and Bleeding Risk (HAS-BLED) in Atrial Fibrillation Patients [8]

CHA_2DS_2-VASc	Score	HAS-BLED	Score
Congestive heart failure	1	Hypertension (systolic blood pressure >160 mmHg)	1
Hypertension	1	Abnormal renal (dialysis, renal transplant, or Creatinine >2.26 mg/dL) and liver function (cirrhosis or bilirubin greater than 2-3× the normal in association with elevated transaminases or alkaline phosphatase greater than 3× the normal (1 point for each)	1 or 2
Age ≥75 years	2	Stroke	1
Diabetes mellitus	1	Bleeding tendency/predisposition	1
Stroke/transient ischemic attack	2	Labile INRs (if on warfarin) (i.e., time in therapeutic range <60%)	1
Vascular disease (prior myocardial infarction, peripheral arterial disease, or aortic plaque)	1	Elderly (e.g., age >65 years)	1
		Drugs or alcohol (1 point each) concomitant antiplatelets or nonsteroidal anti-inflammatory drugs, or excess alcohol.	1 or 2
Age 65–74 years	1		
Female sex	1		
Maximum score	9	Maximum score	9

For a CHA_2DS_2-VASc score of 0 in males or 1 in females: no antithrombotic therapy is recommended. CHA_2DS_2-VASc score-1: oral anticoagulation or antiplatelet therapy should be considered but oral anticoagulation is preferred. For a CHA_2DS_2-VASc score ≥2: oral anticoagulation is indicated. A HAS-BLED score of ≥3 indicates that caution is warranted when prescribing oral anticoagulation and regular review for signs or symptoms of bleeding is recommended [8]
Reprinted with permission from Lane DA, Lip GY. Use of the CHA_2DS_2-VASc and HAS-BLED scores to aid decision making for thromboprophylaxis in nonvalvular atrial fibrillation. Circulation. Vol. 126/Issue number 7, pages 860–865, © 2012, http://circ.ahajournals.org/content/126/7/860, with permission of Wolters Kluwer Health, Inc
The HAS-BLED score is also recommended as a tool to identify reversible factors associated with bleeding risk

The HAS-BLED score is also recommended as a tool to identify reversible factors associated with bleeding risk.

Selecting an Appropriate Anticoagulant for the Elderly Patient

The next step the clinician must take is to decide *if* their elderly patient should be started on an oral anticoagulant such as a vitamin K antagonist (VKA) or DOAC. The use of DOACs in elderly patients has been met with controversy. There are no clinical trials comparing the safety profile of DOACs to that of VKAs in elderly patients, although one meta-analysis which compared the use of dabigatran, apixaban, and rivaroxaban to conventional anticoagulation therapy (VKAs, low-molecular-weight heparin, aspirin, and placebo) demonstrated that the use of DOACs in the elderly population was not associated with a significant increase in major or clinically relevant bleeding (6.4% with NOAC versus 6.3% with conventional anticoagulants) [9]. However, in a separate study, dabigatran was associated with an increased risk of gastrointestinal bleeding in the elderly (3.42% with dabigatran versus 2.65% with VKAs) [Office2]. It is important for clinicians to keep this in mind when choosing the right agent to anticoagulate an elderly person [10].

Renal function and the patient's GFR are important considerations in the decision towards prescribing DOACs to elderly patients. DOACs such as dabigatran and rivaroxaban are predominantly cleared through the kidneys, while apixaban and edoxaban are renally cleared to a lesser extent. If a patient has diminished renal function, there will be an accumulation of active drug, which in turn will lead to an increased risk for bleeding [7]. Because elderly patients frequently have fluctuations in renal function, there is greater unpredictability with regard to the serum bioavailability of anticoagulants. In addition, elderly patients consume less water and have decreased muscle mass, so it is important for the clinician to monitor an elderly patient's creatinine clearance on a regular basis [7].

Direct oral anticoagulants (DOACs) have provided clinicians additional choices for oral anticoagulation. Moreover, the ease of use for the DOACs makes them an ideal first choice for anticoagulation. DOACs can be used in the elderly population (75 or older); however, many factors make use of DOACs in the elderly a controversial subject [5, 7]. For example, elderly patients have lower body mass, altered body composition, lower muscle mass, renal impairment, as well as other comorbidities [5–7, 9]. Furthermore, certain DOACs have been associated with increased risk of bleeding in the elderly, particularly dabigatran [7, 11].

Intracranial Bleeding Risk in the Elderly

Anticoagulation-related intracranial hemorrhage is a serious complication that is becoming more common as more elderly patients are prescribed anticoagulation for atrial fibrillation or venous thromboembolism. DVTs and PEs have an estimated incidence annually of 0.1–0.27%, affecting up to 5% of the population during their lifetime [12]. The most recent American College of Chest Physicians (ACCP) guidelines recommend anticoagulation treatment be limited to 3 months for patients with provoked DVT or PE and for a minimum of 3 months for patients with unprovoked DVT or PE. The ACCP guidelines recommend a DOAC as first line therapy, but also support using warfarin with an INR goal of 2–3 [13]. Treatment for atrial fibrillation calls for lifelong anticoagulation therapy either with a DOAC or with warfarin titrated to an INR goal of 2–3 for patients at intermediate to high risk of stroke [14]. Mechanical aortic valve and mechanical mitral valve require lifelong warfarin therapy with goal INR 2–3 and 2.5–3.5, respectively [15]. Since elderly patients are at increased risk of VTE and AF, the use of oral anticoagulants and their associated bleeding risks are increasing as well. Prior studies have shown mortality rates of 20–57% following anticoagulation associated ICH [16]. In the ARISTOTLE trial, 18,201 patients with non-valvular AF and at least 1 additional risk factor for stroke (age ≥75 years, previous stroke/transient ischemic attack (TIA), symptomatic heart failure or left ventricular ejection fraction <40%, diabetes, or hypertension) were randomized to receive either apixaban 5 mg twice daily or dose-adjusted warfarin with a target INR of 2.0–3.0. A secondary analysis of all patients who received at least 1 dose of study drug (n = 18,140) with follow-up until death or end of the study noted that independent risk factors associated with ICH were older age, prior stroke or TIA, aspirin use at baseline and if the patient lived in Asia or Latin America [16]. The findings of this analysis were similar to other studies-crude annual rates of ICH around 1.0% in patients with AF treated with oral anticoagulants over a 1- to 2-year time frame and high associated 30-day mortality rates following an ICH event [16].

Although extracranial hemorrhages, predominantly gastrointestinal in origin, are much more common, intracranial hemorrhages result in significantly more morbidity and mortality. Only 5.1% of extracranial hemorrhages associated with warfarin result in death within 30 days, compared to nearly 50% in patients with warfarin-associated intracranial hemorrhage [17, 18]. A recent study evaluated 2727 patients who received thrombolytic therapy for PE. The prevalence of intracranial hemorrhage was 1.8% (48 patients); of the patients who developed ICH, most tended to be older, had a history of prior CVA, and had a longer hospital stay [19]. An analysis of 52,993 patients with ICH admitted to a US hospital demonstrated in-patient mortality from warfarin-associated ICH of approximately 40%, while non-warfarin associated ICH was associated with mortality of 25–29% [12]. Sixty percent of patients with anticoagulant-associated ICH were discharged with a major functional neurological deficit. The annual incidence of warfarin-related ICH ranges nationally averages about 0.6–1.0% [12].

Management strategies for warfarin-associated ICH thereby focus on restoring normal levels of the vitamin K dependent factors affected by warfarin. The current treatment options include vitamin K, fresh frozen plasma, prothrombin complex concentrate, and recombinant activated factor VIIa [20].

For years, physicians have been trying to develop a risk stratification tool to identify patients at higher risk for anticoagulation-associated ICH. A cohort evaluated in 2008 noted that a majority of patients who developed ICH while on warfarin were within the therapeutic range at the time of presentation [21]. While an INR greater than 3.5 doubles the risk of a fatal ICH [21], INR levels cannot be a used as a reliable tool in determining which patients are at increased risk for bleeding. Researchers have also evaluated whether educating patients on anticoagulant-related adverse effects improves outcomes. A study conducted in September 2016 found no association between education level and anticoagulation quality or clinical outcomes in elderly patients with acute VTE who were treated with warfarin [22].

A number of bleeding risk assessment tools have been developed to identify patients at higher risk for bleeding, including HAS-BLED, $HEMORR_2HAGES$, and ATRIA for patients with AF. For patients with VTE, the ACCP or Kuijer bleeding risk scores may be used. However, these tools have only been demonstrated to be of modest value in predicting bleeding in clinical practice [15]. There is a need to develop more predictive clinical decision-making tools to evaluate the risks and benefits of anticoagulation specifically for the elderly population (Table 19.2).

A Dutch study showed that the risk of bleeding with vitamin K antagonists was not significantly increased in patients aged 80–89 years and only mildly increased in patients 90 years or older as compared with patients aged 70–79 years. The risk of thrombosis was higher for patients in their 80s and 90s than for those in their 70s [24]. Despite these findings, several renowned geriatricians have expressed concerns with the study, noting that patients who can get anticoagulation were identified, but not the patients who cannot be safely treated. They also raised concerns about polypharmacy, cognitive impairment, lack of social support and the risks of falls as they each relate to bleeding risk [25]. Another study looked at the competing risk of stroke against other causes of death in a cohort of older individuals with atrial fibrillation over 7 years and it showed that although the death rate was higher in those taking warfarin, once the cause specific hazard ratio was adjusted, the association was substantially attenuated. In other words, patients may not be living long enough to get the substantial benefit from anticoagulation treatment [26]. Therefore, the decision to prescribe anticoagulation in patients 80 years and older must carefully consider the risk of bleeding and thrombosis on a case-by-case basis.

Table 19.2 ATRIA TABLE—If the score is <4 low risk, >4 then high risk for bleeding with warfarin [23]

Risk factor	No history of stroke	Positive history of stroke
Age > 85	6	9
Age 75–84	5	7
Age 65–74	3	7
Age < 65	0	8
Female	1	1
Diabetes	1	1
Hypertension	1	1
CHF	1	1
GFR < 45 or ESRD	1	1
Proteinuria	1	1

Table adapted from Singer DE, Chang Y, Borowsky LH, et al. A New Risk Scheme to Predict Ischemic Stroke and Other Thromboembolism in Atrial Fibrillation: The ATRIA Study Stroke Risk Score. J Am Heart Assoc. 2013 Jun; 2(3): e000250

Triple Antithrombotic Therapy in the Elderly

About 5–10% of patients who undergo coronary artery stenting and require dual antiplatelet therapy (DAPT) are also on long-term oral anticoagulants (OAC) for conditions such as atrial fibrillation, venous thromboembolism (VTE), or mechanical heart valves [27]. With an increased prevalence of atrial fibrillation and thromboem-

Table 19.3 Key points regarding triple antithrombotic therapy in the elderly

1.	Physicians should conduct a comprehensive and objective assessment of patients' risk of stroke and bleeding
2.	For patients receiving triple therapy, the lowest effective dose of aspirin (75–100 mg) should be used to reduce the risk of gastrointestinal bleeding [28]
3.	Clinicians must balance the risk of stroke or thromboembolism against bleeding risk to determine if triple therapy is appropriate and for what duration it should be given [29]. Triple therapy should be planned for the shortest possible duration with a focus on the presence or absence of acute coronary syndrome, individual bleeding risk, and type of stent [30]
4.	Clopidogrel is the thienopyridine of choice in combination with aspirin and warfarin [30]
5.	Warfarin should be closely monitored, with a target INR between 2 and 2.5 [30]
6.	Based on the results of the WOEST trial, dual therapy with warfarin and clopidogrel can be considered in those at high risk of bleeding [31]
7.	The prophylactic administration of gastric acid suppressing agents to reduce GI bleeding, preferably a PPI, should be given. Proton-pump inhibitors, other than omeprazole should be given [32]

bolism as well ischemic events in the elderly, it is not infrequent to encounter geriatric patients taking triple antithrombotic therapy with aspirin, clopidogrel, and oral anticoagulant (OAC). Although the use of triple antithrombotic therapy is the cornerstone in preventing the combined incidence of death, stroke, major adverse cardiovascular events (MACE) including stent thrombosis and thromboembolism in these patients, it poses a significant dilemma for the clinician as it has been associated with an increased risk of major bleeding events and mortality (Table 19.3).

Though both the 2014 European revascularization guidelines and an older 2011 North American expert consensus document recommend triple antithrombotic therapy in patients with atrial fibrillation and on OAC undergoing PCI (Class IIa, level of evidence C) [29, 33], this strategy was not studied prospectively until recently. The focus is now shifting to decrease the intensity (with the omission of aspirin) and duration of antithrombotic therapy as well as to explore regimens using the novel anticoagulants instead of warfarin.

The results of the recent WOEST trial demonstrate that a combination of OAC plus clopidogrel, with the exclusion of aspirin, is associated with less bleeding and similar, or even superior, ischemic protection with a significant reduction in mortality [31]. Similarly, a Danish group published results of a real-life nationwide retrospective registry of 12,165 patients that supported the findings of the WOEST trial and suggested that the combination of OAC plus clopidogrel is sufficient to reduce the risk of thrombotic events [34]. Following the results of the WOEST trial, the American Heart Association/American College of Cardiology/Heart Rhythm Society issued a Class IIb (Level of Evidence: B) recommendation for the combination of VKA and clopidogrel after PCI in patients with atrial fibrillation [14].

The optimal duration of triple therapy after PCI is established—on the basis of observational data—minimum of 4 weeks of triple therapy after bare-metal stent (BMS) implantation and 1–12 months of therapy after drug-eluting stent (DES) implantation is recommended [35]. In the first open label ISAR-TRIPLE trial evaluating a 6-week versus a 6-month clopidogrel treatment regimen in patients treated with DES with concomitant aspirin and OAC, there was no significant difference in the primary endpoint of death, myocardial infarction (MI), definite stent thrombosis, stroke, or major bleeding at 9 months (9.8% in the 6-week group versus 8.8% in the 6-month group). The results of ISAR-TRIPLE provide new evidence that the discontinuation of clopidogrel instead of aspirin and the reduction in the duration of triple therapy to 6 weeks neither lessened the incidence of major bleeding nor increased the incidence of ischemic events and could be reasonable option [36].

The PIONEER AF-PCI study is the first randomized trial which compared standard therapy with a Vitamin K antagonist to a direct oral anticoagulant, rivaroxaban-based regimen. In the trial, 2124 stented patients with AF were randomized to 1 of 3 groups: reduced-dose rivaroxaban 15 mg daily plus a P2Y12 antagonist for

12 months (Group 1); rivaroxaban 2.5 mg twice a day with stratification to a pre-specified duration of DAPT of 1, 6, or 12 months (Group 2); or the control arm of dose-adjusted vitamin K antagonists daily with a similar DAPT stratification as above (Group 3). The trial demonstrated that the rivaroxaban-based strategy was associated with a significant reduction in the composite outcome of all-cause mortality or hospitalization and a significant reduction in bleeding hospitalization and cardiovascular hospitalizations [37].

Ongoing studies with dabigatran and apixaban are focused on redefining the use of direct anticoagulant agents in triple therapy [38].

Special Considerations When Prescribing "Triple Therapy" to the Elderly

Hemorrhagic Risk

Although several studies have reported a high annual risk (4–16%) of bleeding episodes, consistently linked with hospitalization, increased morbidity, and death [39], most of these trials excluded elderly patients. Hess and colleagues conducted one of the largest studies on antithrombotic treatment and outcomes in older individuals with acute myocardial infarction (MI) treated with PCI who also had concomitant AF on OAC. They found that compared to DAPT, triple therapy was associated with a significantly higher risk of early and long-term bleeding, including intracranial hemorrhage, and higher mortality [39]. In a study performed by Buresly and colleagues 21,443 elderly patients were followed for an average of 22 months after acute MI and evaluated for bleeding complications associated with combination therapies including aspirin, thienopyridine derivatives, and warfarin. The study demonstrated rates of bleeding were higher among patients receiving the 3-drug combination (0.09 per patient-year) compared with anticoagulant-antiplatelet combined therapy (0.08 per patient-year) and dual antiplatelet therapy (0.07 per patient-year). They concluded that although the antiplatelet and anticoagulant combinations lead to modest increases in bleeding risk in elderly patients, the overall risk is small and in the order of 0.06–0.08 events per patient-year [40].

The Risk of Falls While on Antithrombotic Therapy

Approximately 32–42% of community dwelling individuals 70 years and older fall each year. This incidence increases with age and frailty level [41]. In addition, those who fall once are at increased risk of additional falls, and approximately 10% of these falls result in serious injury. Given the concerns of head trauma and intracranial bleeding associated with falls while on OAC, many physicians are reluctant to prescribe antithrombotic therapy, especially warfarin, to elderly whom they consider at risk for falls [36]. However, a meta-analysis conducted on elderly patients with atrial fibrillation and an average annual stroke of 6% who are also at risk for falls showed that the derived relative risk of developing a fall-related subdural hematoma compared to those who did not is 1.4 and is completely overshadowed by the benefit of stroke protection provided by warfarin [42]. Using the Markov decision model, the authors of this study also calculated that a person taking warfarin must fall about 295 times in 1 year for warfarin not to be the optimal therapy [42]. In a prospective trial of 515 elderly patients on oral anticoagulants, the 304 patients (59.8%) who were at high risk of fall did not have a higher crude incidence rate of major bleeding than patients at lower risk of falls (8.0 versus 6.8 per 100 patient-years, $P = 0.64$) [43]. In multivariate analysis, a high falls risk was not statistically significantly associated with the risk of a major bleeding [43].

These findings suggest that risk of falls is not a valid reason to avoid oral anticoagulants in the elderly patients who are at high risk of stroke and other thromboembolic events. Management of fall risk, however, should be an important part of anticoagulation management and every effort should be made to minimize fall risk (Table 19.3).

When to Discontinue or Withhold Anticoagulation in the Elderly

Determining which patients receive anticoagulation therapy is perhaps one of the most difficult choices clinicians make [25]. Clinicians must weigh the risks versus benefits of any anticoagulant. Current treatment guidelines were developed on the basis of observations from younger populations and mainly provide general considerations applicable to the older patients—the management and outcomes of this subgroup are often uncertain [44]. Adding to the paucity of evidence for the aging population, there are safety concerns as well regarding antithrombotic therapy [44].

Historical data has shown underutilization of anticoagulation therapy in the elderly, with approximately half of all patients with atrial fibrillation not receiving treatment [45]. Contraindications to anticoagulation therapy are often relative and subject to provide interpretation; there remain few consistent, absolute contraindications. Based on the study of Medicare claims in 2009 for patients with atrial fibrillation, the authors identified beneficiaries with absolute contraindications to any anticoagulation therapy based on ICD-9 diagnoses of intracranial hemorrhage, intracranial mass, or end-stage liver disease (defined as ICD-9 codes for chronic liver disease like cirrhosis in combination with an acute hepatic decompensation event of spontaneous bacterial peritonitis, hepatic encephalopathy, ascites, variceal bleeding, hepatorenal syndrome). Patients with dementia and history of bleeding had the lowest rates of warfarin use. The authors pointed out that physicians are left to make highly subjective judgments of risk vs. benefit when deciding about these therapies [45]. In a large, real-world cardiac outpatient population of atrial fibrillation patients with a moderate to high risk of stroke, 1 in 3 were treated with aspirin alone [46]. After multivariable adjustment, hypertension, dyslipidemia, coronary artery disease, prior MI, unstable and stable angina, recent coronary artery bypass graft, and peripheral arterial disease were associated with prescription of aspirin only, whereas male sex, higher body mass index, prior stroke/transient ischemic attack, prior systemic embolism, and congestive heart failure were associated with more frequent prescription of oral anticoagulants [46].

Although numerous risk factors have been linked to a higher bleeding risk, noting the presence of these risk factors is not sufficiently informative to help clinicians gauge a patient's hemorrhage risk [17]. In response, a number of risk stratification tools, such as OBRI (Outpatient Bleeding Risk Index), RIETE, HAS-BLED, and ATRIA, have been developed to quantify a patient's risk of hemorrhage. Most of these risk assessment tools were developed in cohorts of patients newly prescribed or already taking anticoagulants, and thus reflect populations already suitable for anticoagulation therapy [17]. Patients with high risk for bleeding may not be represented in these risk tools [17]. There is considerable overlap in the risk factors included in these risk scores, as most account for traits such as older age (the definition varied amongst the different tools), renal disease, history of bleeding, anemia, and labile INR [17]. Unfortunately, none of the bleeding risk tools are highly predictive, especially of intracranial bleeding. The authors suggested that the bleeding risk tools could be of help in patients at the lower end of thrombotic risk, where the benefits of anticoagulation are smaller and the risk of bleeding higher; bleeding risk tools can also be useful in identifying low risk groups of patients who can be reassured that they are unlikely to have significant bleeding complications [17].

The benefits of anticoagulation to decrease stroke and to improve quality of life by minimizing hospitalizations in the elderly are well-recognized [44]. However, the clinician has to weigh the pros and cons of the drug individually for the patient and the caregiver. Although there is no clear definition of frailty, the syndrome is recognized as age-related decline in physiological systems that increases the risk of dramatic changes in health and functional status, often provoked by minor incidences such as medications [44]. A frail 70-year-old patient with dementia, declining performance status, malnutrition might not be the ideal candidate for anticoagulation for new onset or even established atrial fibrillation, due to higher mortality risk, whereas an 85-year-old patient who lives independently and is physically active would warrant treatment.

There are no established guidelines on when drug therapy should be stopped. There have been several attempts to create a "hit list" of medications that should be avoided in the elderly. The Beers list and Canadian criteria are not all encompassing as they do not include drug interactions [47]. The START/STOPP (Screening Tool to Alert doctors to Right Treatment/Screening Tool of Older Persons') criteria address some of these concerns (Refer to: http://www.alzforum.org/news/research-news/are-too-many-meds-given-end-stage-dementia-patients). However, there is no convincing evidence that using these lists helps reduce morbidity, mortality, or cost [47].

Preventing polypharmacy will improve the quality of life for patients with advanced dementia. In a study of patients with advanced dementia, more than half of the participants received at least one medication that was deemed questionable with regard to the patients' conditions (http://www.alzforum.org/news/research-news/are-too-many-meds-given-end-stage-dementia-patients). Of note, 22% of participants were taking statin, and 7% were on an antithrombotic agent other than aspirin, such as clopidogrel (http://www.alzforum.org/news/research-news/are-too-many-meds-given-end-stage-dementia-patients). For this particular group of patients with advanced comorbid conditions and overall decreased life expectancy, many medications may be unnecessary as the patients will not live long enough to derive benefits (http://www.alzforum.org/news/research-news/are-too-many-meds-given-end-stage-dementia-patients). The author postulated that it is difficult for physicians to stop these drugs as there is concern for harm when the treatment is discontinued or the caregivers might not be ready to talk about it. Nonetheless, caretakers should perform periodic reviews of medication lists, particularly for those with dementia (Refer to: http://www.alzforum.org/news/research-news/are-too-many-meds-given-end-stage-dementia-patients). Involving a specialist such as a geriatrician or palliative care clinician may help provide additional insight to align therapeutic options with the patient's goals of care.

Non-Pharmacologic Management of Atrial Fibrillation

Left atrial appendage (LAA) closure has emerged as a minimally-invasive mechanical alternative to pharmacologic stroke prevention, especially in those patients for whom oral anticoagulants are perceived as contraindicated [48]. Autopsy and surgical data suggest that anywhere from 35–91% of atrial thrombi are found in the left atrial appendage, a remnant structure of the primordial left atrium, resembling a blind pouch [48]. LAA closure might be an option for patients who remain high risk for stroke despite oral anticoagulation [48]. The closure can be accomplished via surgical or percutaneous approaches. As per the European Society of Cardiology and AHA/ACC guidelines, surgical LAA excision should be considered in patients already undergoing cardiac surgery or thoracoscopic AF surgery [48].

The Watchman device, a nitinol device implanted percutaneously to seal the LAA, has emerged as a therapeutic option for those with atrial fibrillation who may not be able to tolerate long-term anticoagulation therapy. In the multicenter PROTECT AF trial, a majority of participants were over 70 years old (average age of 71-year-old in the device arm and 72-year-old in the warfarin arm) [49]. Patients were randomized to warfarin, then aspirin and clopidogrel for 6 months, then aspirin alone indefinitely [49]. The ASAP study showed that LAA closure with Watchman can be done with antiplatelet therapy, mitigating the need for anticoagulants [49]. While randomized controlled trials of these methods have enrolled patients who are eligible for anticoagulation, the clinical need is greatest in patients who are not candidates for anticoagulation [48]. Piccini and colleagues postulated that the closure of LAA would be beneficial for patients with atrial fibrillation who at high risk for bleeding based on HAS-BLED scores, those with concomitant end-stage renal disease due to high risk of thromboembolic and bleeding events, and those that remain at high risk for stroke despite anticoagulation. LAA closure presents several challenges, as no clinical studies to compare the various percutaneous closure methods with each other; the need for long-term antiplatelet therapy after LAA closure in patients who are at high risk for bleeding; risks of leak and thrombus formation around devices, while uncommon, have been reported [48].

Radiofrequency catheter ablation of atrial fibrillation has evolved as an important treatment option for selected patients with atrial fibrillation [50]. The pulmonary veins (PV) have been shown to play a major role in the initiation of atrial fibrillation. However, isolation and ablation of PV alone is insufficient for restoration and maintenance of sinus rhythm. Several other sites for ablation have been studied, such as complex fragmented atrial electrograms which did not show reduction in rate of recurrent atrial fibrillation and the ablation of patient specific sources— focal impulse and rotor modulation (FIRM)—which helps improve long-term success of PV ablation [50]. The assessment of efficacy of catheter ablation with various techniques can be complex and is dependent on multiple variables including patient characteristics, chronicity of atrial fibrillation, and intensity of follow-up [50]. Catheter ablation is not without risks, as major complications have been reported in as many as 6% of patients worldwide. These include phrenic nerve injury, cardiac tamponade, pulmonary vein stenosis, systemic thromboembolism post-procedure and, most significantly, atrioesophageal fistula formation [50].

The clinician must not only weigh the risks and benefits, but also consider the applicability of non-pharmacologic approaches such as catheter-based ablation and LAA closure in patients of advanced age. LAA closure has become an increasingly utilized option, particularly for those who are not ideal candidates for anticoagulation. However, these patients will still require antiplatelet therapy after device implantation [49]. Technical improvements in catheter-based ablation techniques and improved efficacy have offered alternative strategies for the treatment of atrial fibrillation. Compared to radiofrequency ablation, cryoballoon ablation may involve lower risk of pulmonary stenosis or esophageal injury [49]. For the older patients, especially those in whom anticoagulation poses a challenge, these options need to be discussed, together, with the patient and a cardiologist or an electrophysiologist. These techniques, with their risks and benefits, have to be weighed in the context of the patient's functional and psychosocial status and their other co-morbidities.

Conclusion

Given the broad spectrum of patients in the geriatric age group with their diverse stages of functional, physical, and cognitive decline, it behooves the provider to carefully assess the clinical indication for anticoagulant therapy in the elderly patient, who are greatly susceptible to adverse events from polypharmacy. A discussion with the patient and their families must take place to review both the risks and benefits of anticoagulation therapy, vis-a-vis the overall goals of care.

Self-Assessment Questions

1. An 87-year-old woman comes to the geriatric clinic for a follow-up visit. She has a history of atrial fibrillation, chronic kidney disease (CKD) with an estimated glomerular filtration rate (eGFR) of 45 mL/min, hypertension, and type 2 diabetes. She lives alone in a 2-story walk-up apartment and performs her activities of daily living on her own. Her current medications include warfarin, lisinopril, metoprolol, metformin, amlodipine, and aspirin. She comes to clinic every 2 weeks for an INR check because her INR has been labile. In addition, she has had recurrent urinary tract infections over the past 6 months requiring antibiotics, which has made management of her INR even more difficult. On physical

exam her vitals are normal and her heart sounds are irregularly irregular. The remainder of her exam is unremarkable. Her laboratory results including her kidney function are within normal limits. Her INR today is 1.7. The patient mentions to you that it is getting increasingly difficult for her to come to get her blood work done every 2 weeks. Which of the following is the most appropriate way to manage this patient's anticoagulation?

(a) Stop all anticoagulation, because she is at low thrombotic risk.
(b) Continue warfarin as other oral anticoagulants have been shown to be dangerous in the elderly.
(c) Stop warfarin and start a direct oral anticoagulant
(d) Stop all anticoagulation, because the bleeding risk outweighs the anticoagulation benefit.

2. The patient eagerly agrees to try a direct oral anticoagulant if it will save her trips to the doctor's office. She is advised on the risks and benefits of the direct oral anticoagulants. She is told that she will still have to come in regularly to get her kidney function monitored. She agrees to do so.

   Which of the following is true in regard to choosing a direct oral anticoagulant for the patient?

   (a) In patients with CKD, the safest DOAC to use is Dabigatran owing to low renal clearance
   (b) Although the DOAC will save the patient trips to the office, warfarin is still overall a safer drug in the elderly with moderate-severe chronic kidney disease
   (c) There is no need for dose adjustment for DOAC in patients with chronic kidney disease.
   (d) Apixaban is associated with a better safety profile in patients with moderate renal impairment.

3. An 80-year-old woman with Alzheimer's dementia, atrial fibrillation, remote history of CAD, HTN is brought in by family for change in mental status. At baseline, she is nonverbal, bed bound, and dependent on all her activities of daily living. She is on warfarin 2.5 mg daily, aspirin 81 mg daily, simvastatin 40 mg daily, donepezil 5 mg daily, and amlodipine 5 mg daily. The daughter mentions that patient is having considerable trouble with swallowing and her condition is progressively deteriorating. The patient's wishes were not to receive artificial nutrition and hydration. The daughter wishes to take her mother home with hospice once she is discharged from the hospital. In order to optimize her drug regimen so patient what should be done next?

   (a) Discontinue aspirin
   (b) Discontinue simvastatin
   (c) Change to aspirin suppository.
   (d) Discontinue warfarin
   (e) a, b, and d

4. A 75-year-old man with a history of stroke with no residual deficits, diabetes mellitus, and atrial fibrillation on apixaban is seen in the office for evaluation of an unsteady gait. His wife mentions that he falls occasionally, especially when he forgets to use his walker. She also notes that he is becoming forgetful and she has to help him with his medications. On physical exam, the patient has stable vitals with no orthostasis. What is the next step in management?

   (a) Physical therapy referral for gait evaluation
   (b) Discontinue apixaban
   (c) Encourage use of a walker
   (d) Visiting nurse referral

5. A 58-year-old woman is evaluated during a routine physical examination. She has a history of paroxysmal atrial fibrillation, transient ischemic attack (TIA), hypertension, and hyperlipidemia. Her medications are warfarin, metoprolol, candesartan, and simvastatin. On physical examination, the patient is afebrile, blood pressure is 130/80 mmHg, pulse rate is 64/min, and respiration rate is 16/min. BMI is 30. Heart rate and rhythm are regular.

An electrocardiogram shows normal sinus rhythm.

   (a) Continue warfarin
   (b) Continue warfarin and add aspirin
   (c) Discontinue warfarin

(d) Discontinue warfarin and start aspirin
(e) Discontinue warfarin and start aspirin and clopidogrel

Self-Assessment Answers

1. (c) Stop warfarin and start a direct oral anticoagulant

   The patient's CHA_2DS_2-VASc score is five which puts her at moderate to high risk for developing a stroke. She will benefit from DOAC therapy for stroke prevention. Warfarin has a narrow therapeutic range and requires frequent monitoring to avoid potentially life-threatening complications from both under- and over-coagulation. Despite frequent visits for INR check, the patient's INR control with warfarin continues to be labile. One reason for the lability in INRs could be the concomitant use of antibiotics for recurrent UTI due to the drug–drug interactions. The patient has already expressed difficulty in getting to the clinic As several studies comparing DOACs with VKAs have showed that DOACs are associated with equal or greater efficacy than VKAs in the prevention of stroke and systemic embolism in elderly patients with non-valvular atrial fibrillation, a reasonable option would be to stop warfarin and start a direct oral anticoagulant. Some of the advantages of DOACs are their predictable therapeutic effect, fewer drug interactions, and the decreased need for frequent monitoring.

2. (d) Apixaban is associated with a better safety profile in patients with moderate renal impairment.

   In CKD patients with an estimated glomerular filtration rate (eGFR) above 60 mL/min, DOACs can be used safely with greater efficacy and safety as compared to VKAs. In patients with CKD 3, DOACs are as effective as VKAs with a lower bleeding rate. As the renal function declines, the risk of bleeding increases with DOACs. All DOACs need dose adjustment in CKD population because of their renal clearance, ranging from 25% (apixaban) to 80% (dabigatran). Dabigatran should be used at a dose of 75 mg twice-daily for creatinine clearance (CrCl) 15–30 mL/min, Rivaroxaban at 15 mg once-daily for CrCl of 15–50 mL/min, Edoxaban at 30 mg once-daily for CrCl 15–50 mL/min, and Apixaban at 2.5 mg twice-daily for patients with two of the following three criteria: serum creatinine greater than 1.5 mg/dL, age 80 years or older, or a weight less than 60 kg. The 2014 American Heart Association (AHA)/American College of Cardiology (ACC)/Heart Rhythm Society (HRS) Guideline for the Management of Patients with Atrial Fibrillation recommends against the use of dabigatran and rivaroxaban in patients with end-stage renal disease (ESRD) (CrCl less than 15 mL/min). Apixaban, on the other hand, with its lower renal clearance, has a better safety profile compared to other DOACS in patients with moderate renal impairment and is the only DOAC which is FDA approved for use in patients requiring dialysis. The above recommendation was based on a single dose pharmacokinetic and pharmacodynamic (anti-factor Xa activity) study involving only 8 patients. Clinical efficacy and long-term safety studies have not been done in this population; therefore, it should be used with caution in the dialysis population.

3. (e) a, b, and d

   The patient should discontinue aspirin, simvastatin, and warfarin. She has considerable difficulty swallowing and her treatment plan should take into account her goals including hospice and avoidance of artificial nutrition and hydration. When a patient with a terminal illness continues to deteriorate, the patient (and/or representative) may decide to stop medications for a chronic nonterminal illness especially when taking these drugs cause significant distress due to swallowing problems or when these medications are no longer effective. At this stage, the patient may not even absorb medications due to dehydration as well as liver and other organ failure, and giving medications may be more troublesome than any benefit they could offer. The focus at this point would be to offer medications that optimize comfort, for example those that relieve dyspnea and pain.

4. (a) Physical therapy referral for gait evaluation

   Falls are a major public health problem in the elderly population with accidental falls occurring in nearly one-third of those aged more than 65 years every year. Many physicians are reluctant to use OAC in these patients given the risk of head trauma and subsequent subdural/intracranial bleeds associated with falls. However, the risk of falls alone should not automatically disqualify a patient with AF from being treated with oral anticoagulant. Three risk–benefit analyses have been performed, and all found that despite risks associated with OACs, their benefits outweigh risks even in patients who fall. Assessment and management of fall risk including a physical therapy referral for gait evaluation should be an important part of anticoagulation management. Multidisciplinary falls—prevention strategies such as muscle strengthening and balance retraining have been shown to be effective
5. (a) Continue warfarin

   The patient should continue taking warfarin. Though the patient is in sinus rhythm at the time of the physical exam, given her history of paroxysmal atrial fibrillation and comorbidities, her CHA_2DS_2-VASc score is 4 (2 points for TIA, 1 point each for hypertension and female sex). Her annual stroke risk ranges from 4.8% to 6.7% and she must be continued on warfarin. Several studies demonstrated the risk of thromboembolic complications for PAF may be similar or even less than that of permanent AF. The 2014 AHA/ACC/HRS Guideline recommends antithrombotic therapy should be based on the risk of thromboembolism irrespective of whether the AF pattern is paroxysmal, persistent, or permanent.

References

1. Capodanno D, Angiolillo D. Antithrombotic therapy in the elderly. J Am Coll Cardiol. 2010;56:1683–92.
2. Myat A, Yousif A, Shouvik H, et al. Is bleeding a necessary evil? The inherent risk of antithrombotic pharmacotherapy used for stroke prevention in atrial fibrillation. Expert Rev Cardiovasc Ther. 2013;11(8):1029–49.
3. Gurwitz J. Warfarin in complex older patients: have we reached a tipping point? JAGS. 2017;65:236–7.
4. McGrath ER, Go AS, Chang Y, et al. Use of oral anticoagulant therapy in older adults with atrial fibrillation after acute ischemic stroke. JAGS. 2017;65:241–8.
5. Go AS, Hylek EM, Phillips KA, et al. Prevalence of diagnosed atrial fibrillation in adults: national implications for rhythm management and stroke prevention: the Anticoagulation and Risk Factors in Atrial Fibrillation (ATRIA) study. JAMA. 2001;285(18):2370–5.
6. Lip GY, Halperin JL. Improving stroke risk stratification in atrial fibrillation. Am J Med. 2010;123:484–8.
7. Wolf PA, Abbott RD, Kannel WB. Atrial fibrillation as an independent risk factor for stroke: The Framingham Study. Stroke. 1991;22:983–8.
8. Lane DA, Lip GY. Use of the CHA(2)DS(2)-VASc and HASBLED scores to aid decision making for thromboprophylaxis in nonvalvular atrial fibrillation. Circulation. 2012;126(7):860–5.
9. Sardar P, Chatterjee S, Chaudhari S, et al. New oral anticoagulants in elderly adults: evidence from a meta-analysis of randomized trials. J Am Geriatr Soc. 2014;62(5):857–64.
10. Graham DJ, Reichman ME, Wernecke M, Zhang R, Southworth MR, Levenson M, et al. Cardiovascular, bleeding, and mortality risks in elderly medicare patients treated with dabigatran or warfarin for nonvalvular atrial fibrillation. Circulation. 2015;131:157–64.
11. Coppens M, Eikelboom J, Ezekowitz M, et al. Dabigatran versus warfarin in very elderly patients with atrial fibrillation: results from the RE-LY trail. Circulation. 2012;126:A151537.
12. Becattini C, Sembolini A, Paciaroni M. Resuming anticoagulant therapy after intracerebral bleeding. Vasc Pharmacol. 2016;84:15–24.
13. Kearon C, Akl EA, Ornealas J, et al. Antithrombotic therapy for VTE disease: chest guidelines expert panel report. Chest. 2016;149(2):315–52.
14. January CT, Wann LS, Alpert JS, et al. 2014 AHA/ACC/HRS guideline for the management of patients with atrial fibrillation: a report of the American College of Cardiology/American Heart Association Task Force on practice guidelines and the Heart Rhythm Society. Circulation. 2014;130(23):2071–104.
15. Nishimura RA, Otto CM, Bonow RO, Carabello BA, Erwin JP 3rd, Guyton RA, et al. American College of Cardiology/American Heart Association Task Force on Practice Guidelines. 2014 AHA/ACC guideline for the management of patients with valvular heart disease: a report of the American College of Cardiology/American Heart Association Task Force on Practice Guidelines. J Am Coll Cardiol. 2014;63(22):e57–185.
16. Lopes RD, Guimaraes PO, Kolls BJ, et al. Intracranial hemorrhage in patients with atrial fibrillation receiving anticoagulation therapy. Blood. 2017; 129(22):2980–7.

17. Shoeb M, Fang MC. Assessing bleeding risk in patients taking anticoagulants. J Thromb Thrombolysis. 2013; 35(3):312–9.
18. Strate LL. Lower GI bleeding: epidemiology and diagnosis. Gastroenterol Clin North Am. 2005;34(4):643–64.
19. Chatterjee S, Lip GY, Giri J. HAS-BLED versus ATRIA risk scores for intracranial hemorrhage in patients receiving thrombolytics for pulmonary embolism. J Am Coll Cardiol. 2016;67(24):2904–5.
20. Appelboam R, Thomas EO. Warfarin and intracranial haemorrhage. Blood Rev. 2009;23(1):1–9.
21. Jeffree R, Gordon DH, Sivasubramaniam R, Chapman A. Warfarin related intracranial haemorrhage: a case-controlled study of anticoagulation monitoring prior to spontaneous subdural or intracerebral haemorrhage. J Clin Neurosci. 2009;16(7):882–5.
22. Hoffman E, Faller N, Limacher A. Educational level, anticoagulation quality, and clinical outcomes in elderly patients with acute venous thromboembolism: a prospective cohort study. PLoS One. 2016;11(9):e0162108.
23. Singer DE, Chang Y, Borowsky LH, et al. A new risk scheme to predict ischemic stroke and other thromboembolism in atrial fibrillation: the ATRIA study stroke risk score. J Am Heart Assoc. 2013;2(3):e000250.
24. Kooistra HA, Calf AH, Piersma-Wichers M, et al. Venous thromboembolism in very elderly patients: findings from a prospective registry (RIETE). Haematologica. 2006;91(8):1046–51.
25. Yasgur BS. Weighing benefits and risks of anticoagulation in the elderly. The cardiology advisor Oct 24, 2016. http://www.thecardiologyadvisor.com/stroke/anticogulation-stroke-prevention-in-elderly/article/567835/2/.
26. Ashburner JM, Go AS, Chang Y, et al. Influence of competing risks on the association between warfarin and ischemic stroke in atrial fibrillation: the anticoagulation and risk factors in atrial fibrillation (ATRIA) study. Circulation. 2015;132:A11900.
27. Rossini R, Musumeci G, Lettieri C, et al. Long-term outcomes in patients undergoing coronary stenting on dual oral antiplatelet treatment requiring oral anticoagulant therapy. Am J Cardiol. 2008;102:1618–23.
28. Mehta SR on behalf of the CURRENT Steering Committee. A randomized comparison of a clopidogrel high loading and maintenance dose regimen versus standard dose and high versus low dose aspirin in 25,000 patients with acute coronary syndromes: results of the CURRENT OASIS 7 Trial. Presented at: European Society of Cardiology Congress 2009; August 30, 2009; Barcelona, Spain. Presentation No. 177.
29. Faxon DP, Eikelboom JW, Berger PB, et al. Antithrombotic therapy in patients with atrial fibrillation undergoing coronary stenting: a North American perspective: executive summary. Circ Cardiovasc Interv. 2011;4:522–34.
30. King SB III, Smith SC Jr, Hirshfeld JW Jr, et al. 2005 Writing Committee Members. 2007 Focused update of the ACC/AHA/SCAI 2005 guideline update for percutaneous coronary intervention: a report of the American College of Cardiology/American Heart Association task force on practice guidelines: 2007 writing group to review new evidence and update the ACC/AHA/SCAI 2005 guideline update for percutaneous coronary intervention, writing on behalf of the 2005 writing committee [published correction appears in Circulation. 2008; 117:e161]. Circulation. 2008;117:261–95.
31. Dewilde W, Oirbans T, Verheugt FW, et al. Use of clopidogrel with or without aspirin in patients taking oral anticoagulant therapy and undergoing percutaneous coronary intervention: an open-label, randomised, controlled trial. Lancet. 2013;381(9872):1107–15.
32. Juurlink DN, Gomes T, Ko DT, et al. A population-based study of the drug interaction between proton pump inhibitors and clopidogrel. CMAJ. 2009;180:713–8.
33. Lip GY, Windecker S, Huber K, et al. Management of antithrombotic therapy in atrial fibrillation patients presenting with acute coronary syndrome and/or undergoing percutaneous coronary or valve interventions: a joint consensus document of the European Society of Cardiology Working Group on Thrombosis, European Heart Rhythm Association (EHRA), European Association of Percutaneous Cardiovascular Interventions (EAPCI) and European Association of Acute Cardiac Care (ACCA) endorsed by the Heart Rhythm Society (HRS) and Asia-Pacific Heart Rhythm Society (APHRS). Eur Heart J. 2014;35(45):3155–79.
34. Lamberts M, Gislason GH, Olesen JB, et al. Oral anticoagulation and antiplatelets in atrial fibrillation patients after myocardial infarction and coronary intervention. J Am Coll Cardiol. 2013;62:981–9.
35. Amsterdam EA, Wenger NK, Brindis RG, et al. 2014 AHA/ACC guideline for the management of patients with non–ST-elevation acute coronary syndromes: a report of the American College of Cardiology/American Heart Association Task Force on Practice Guidelines. J Am Coll Cardiol. 2014;64(24):e139–228.
36. Fiedler KA, Maeng M, Mehilli J, Schulz-Schüpke S, Byrne RA, Sibbing D, et al. Duration of triple therapy in patients requiring oral anticoagulation after drug-eluting stent implantation: the ISAR-TRIPLE trial. J Am Coll Cardiol. 2015;65(16):1619–29.
37. Gibson CM, Mehran R, Bode C, Halperin J, Verheugt FW, Wildgoose P, et al. Prevention of bleeding in patients with atrial fibrillation undergoing PCI. N Engl J Med. 2016;375(25):2423–34.
38. Cannon CP, Gropper S, Bhatt DL, et al. RE-DUAL PCI steering committee and investigators. Design and rationale of the RE-DUAL PCI Trial: a prospective, randomized, phase 3b study comparing the safety and efficacy of dual antithrombotic therapy with dabigatran etexilate versus warfarin triple therapy in patients with nonvalvular atrial fibrillation who have undergone percutaneous coronary intervention with stenting. Clin Cardiol. 2016;39(10):555–64.

39. Hess CN, Peterson ED, Peng SA, et al. Use and outcomes of triple therapy among older patients with acute myocardial infarction and atrial fibrillation. J Am Coll Cardiol. 2015;66:616–27.
40. Buresly K, Eisenberg MJ, Zhang X, et al. Bleeding complications associated with combinations of aspirin, thienopyridine derivatives, and warfarin in elderly patients following acute myocardial infarction. Arch Intern Med. 2005;165(7):784–9.
41. Sellers MB, Newby KL. Atrial fibrillation, anticoagulation, fall risk, and outcomes in elderly patients. Am Heart J. 2011;161(2):241–6.
42. Man-Son-Hing M, Nichol G, Lau A, Laupacis A. Choosing antithrombotic therapy for elderly patients with atrial fibrillation who are at risk for falls. Arch Intern Med. 1999;159:677–85.
43. Sorensen R, Hansen ML. Risk of bleeding in patients with acute myocardial infarction treated with different combinations of aspirin, clopidogrel, and vitamin K antagonists in Denmark: a retrospective analysis of nationwide registry data. Lancet. 2009;374:1967–74.
44. Steinberg B, Greiner M, Hammill B, et al. Contraindications to anticoagulation therapy and eligibility for novel anticoagulants in older patients with atrial fibrillation. Cardiovasc Ther. 2015;33(4):177–83.
45. Hsu JC, Maddox TM, Kennedy K, et al. Aspirin is being used instead of oral anticoagulation in atrial fibrillation patients at risk for stroke. J Am Coll Cardiol. 2016;67(925):2913–23.
46. Gordon SF, Dainty C, Smith T. Why and when to withdraw drugs in the elderly and frail. Prescriber. 2012;23:47–51.
47. Pharmacist's letter/Prescriber's letter September 2011.
48. Piccini JP, Horst S, Patel M. Left atrial appendage occlusion: rationale, evidence, devices, and patient selection. Eur Heart J. 2016;38(12):869–76.
49. Karamichalakis N, Letsas K, Vlachos K, et al. Managing atrial fibrillation in the very elderly patient: challenges and solutions. Vasc Health Risk Manag. 2015;11:555–62.
50. Khaji A, Kowey PR. Update on atrial fibrillation. Trends Cardiovasc Med. 2016;27(1):14–25.

Check for updates

20 Anticoagulation in the Patient with Cancer

Simon Mantha, Dipti Gupta, Chadi Salmane, Mansour Khaddr, Gerald A. Soff, and Richard Steingart

Clinical Vignette

Ms. White was diagnosed with metastatic pancreatic adenocarcinoma 3 months ago when she presented with painless jaundice. She is 57 years old and has no other major medical problems. On endoscopy, the tumor was found to be invading the duodenum and laboratory testing revealed mild iron deficiency. Liver metastases were demonstrated on imaging. She was started on chemotherapy with fluorouracil, leucovorin, oxaliplatin, and irinotecan 2 months ago.

She is seen in the clinic today for a new complaint of progressive left lower extremity swelling and pain. She denies having chest pain, dyspnea, palpitations, or syncope. On exam, the leg is warm to the touch and markedly edematous with associated pitting. Venous duplex ultrasound reveals extensive deep vein thrombosis involving the left popliteal vein, deep femoral vein, and common femoral vein. Hemoglobin has improved compared to 3 months prior, at which time the patient had received intravenous iron sucrose. She denies any melena or overt red blood per rectum.

After discussion of bleeding risk associated with anticoagulation therapy, treatment is started with enoxaparin 1 mg/kg administered subcutaneously every 12 h. Teaching is given on how to perform injections and precautions, including avoidance of aspirin or nonsteroidal anti-inflammatory drugs. The patient is sent home from the clinic with instructions to follow up in the anticoagulation clinic 2 weeks later. She knows to call her oncologist should there be any onset of black stools or rectorrhagia.

Introduction

The French physician Armand Trousseau associated migratory thrombophlebitis with cancer in the late-nineteenth century, and accordingly, the association of venous thromboembolism (VTE) with cancer is known as Trousseau's syndrome [1]. In spite of advances in cancer care afforded by modern medical knowledge, VTE remains a common and difficult-to-manage problem in

S. Mantha (✉) · D. Gupta · C. Salmane · M. Khaddr
G. A. Soff · R. Steingart
Department of Medicine, Memorial Sloan Kettering Cancer Center, New York, NY, USA
e-mail: manthas@mskcc.org; guptad@mskcc.org; soffg@mskcc.org; steingar@mskcc.org

J. F. Lau et al. (eds.), *Anticoagulation Therapy*, https://doi.org/10.1007/978-3-319-73709-6_20

oncology practice. Arterial thromboembolism can also occur, and both disorders tend to be treated with anticoagulation. There are a number of challenges to anticoagulation management for patients with cancer. In the following text we will be discussing different aspects of this paradigm.

Treatment of Venous Thromboembolism: VKA and LMWH

The pathophysiology of cancer-associated thrombosis (CAT) is multifactorial. In addition to decreased mobility, the cancer itself often induces a hypercoagulable state [2]. In this regard, it has been well demonstrated that many tumors release tissue factor in the form of microparticles which have been associated with an increased systemic risk of thrombosis [3]. Other tumor-secreted mediators may also contribute, but such a discussion would be beyond the scope of this text. Lastly, some chemotherapy agents can clearly be thrombogenic, with some agents having more effect than others [4–21] (Table 20.1).

Cancer surgery has been associated with a substantial rate of VTE complications [22]. The risk of VTE is highest in the first months after diagnosis and can be estimated with the Khorana risk score which has been validated in multiple independent large cohorts [23].

In view of these cancer-specific characteristics, it is not surprising that VTE treatment differs in patients with cancer compared to the general population. In the pivotal CLOT trial, the LMWH dalteparin was shown to be more effective than a VKA comparator [24]. Other studies have shown a trend toward improved efficacy or safety of LMWH versus VKA, although no other study reached statistical significance (Table 20.2) [25–28]. LMWH has been recommended as the anticoagulant of choice for treatment of CAT, although VKA remain widely used [29].

The CLOT trial demonstrated a 50% reduction in the risk of recurrent VTE with dalteparin compared with VKA with no significant difference in the risk of major bleeding. Although the CLOT trial only followed patients for the first 6 months of therapy and scant data exist beyond this initial period, current guidelines recommend continuing anticoagulation indefinitely [30]. Surprisingly, the larger CATCH trial did not show a significant reduction in recurrent VTE for tinzaparin versus VKA. INR time in the therapeutic range (TTR) was 46% for patients allocated to the coumarin arm in CLOT compared to 47% for CATCH, so the quality of anticoagulation in the comparator arm probably does not explain the lower relative effectiveness in the bigger study. Switching to a VKA may be acceptable depending on patient wishes and physician discretion [31, 32]. These data apply mostly to patients with proximal, lower extremity deep vein thrombosis (DVT) or pulmonary embolism (PE), even though individuals with a distal DVT are usually treated as well due to a perceived high risk of progression. Indefinite treatment is also suggested, at least as long as there is evidence of active malignancy or the patient remains on therapy. Interestingly, retrospective data suggest that asymptomatic PE and very small emboli (i.e., subsegmental) portend a similar risk of recurrent VTE, so they should be treated similarly to symptomatic events [33]. A synthesis of data from available randomized trials suggests that there is no survival benefit for LMWH versus VKA in the setting of CAT [34].

Recurrence of VTE in cancer patients is common, even with LMWH, and occurred in 9% of patients on dalteparin in the CLOT cohort. The appropriate strategy to manage recurrent CAT is unknown, as little data exists [35]. Increasing the dose of LMWH by 25% has been advocated [30]. It is also reasonable to try a different class of anticoagulant, although this has never been prospectively studied.

The risk of bleeding on anticoagulation is increased in cancer patients [36]. In the CLOT trial, the risk of major bleeding at 6 months was 6%. Possible factors contributing to the higher bleeding risk in the cancer setting include a range of comorbidities, older age, generalized weakness with the associated risk of falls, decreased renal clearance of LMWH, the presence of GI primary or secondary tumors, and frequent thrombocytopenia associated with chemotherapy.

Table 20.1 Risk of venous thromboembolism associated with chemo- and immunotherapeutic agents [4–21]

Chemotherapy agent	Patient population	Venous thromboembolism
VEGF receptor monoclonal antibody—bevacizumab [4]	6055 cancer patients in phase 2 and 3 RCTs	Bevacizumab 18.5 per 100 patient-years vs. controls 20.3 per 100 patient-years (rate ratio 0.91; 95% CI, 0.77–1.06; $P = 0.23$)
VEGF receptor monoclonal antibody—aflibercept [5]	1226 metastatic colorectal cancer patients in phase 3 RCT	Aflibercept/FOLFIRI 9.3% vs. placebo/FOLFIRI 7.3%
VEGF receptor tyrosine kinase inhibitors (sunitinib, sorafenib, pazopanib, vandetanib, axitinib) [6]	Meta-analysis of 7441 cancer patients in phase 2 and 3 RCT	RR 1.10 (95% CI 0.73–1.66, $p = 0.64$)
EGF receptor inhibitors (cetuximab, panitumumab, erlotinib, gefitinib) [7]	Meta-analysis of 11 RCT comprising 7073 patients	Monoclonal antibody EGF receptor antagonists (cetuximab and panitumumab) 5.9% RR 1.34 (95% CI 1.07–1.68) EGF receptor tyrosine kinase inhibitors (erlotinib and gefitinib) 2.6% RR 1.16 (95% CI 0.61–2.18)
L-asparaginase [8]	548 acute lymphocyte leukemia patients	27/501 (5%) pediatric patients and 16/47 (34%) adult patients
Tamoxifen [9–12]	13,888 women in the Breast Cancer Prevention Trial	Tamoxifen vs. placebo Risk ratio for PE 3.0 (95% CI 1.1–11.2) Risk ratio for DVT 1.6 (95% CI 0.9–2.9)
	7145 women in the International Breast Cancer Prevention study	Tamoxifen vs. placebo Risk ratio = 2.26 (95% CI = 1.36–3.87)
	20,878 breast cancer patients in 13 RCT	African-American Tamoxifen + chemo Risk ratio 10.70 (95% CI 5.94–19.28) Tamoxifen alone Risk ratio 2.16 (1.26–3.71) White Tamoxifen + chemo Risk ratio 15.49 (95% CI 9.53–25.17) Tamoxifen alone Risk ratio 3.13 (95% CI 2.04–4.79)
	30,023 patients with breast cancer from RCT of aromatase inhibitors and tamoxifen	VTE aromatase inhibitors 1.6% vs. tamoxifen 2.8% (OR = 0.55, 95% CI = 0.46–0.64, $P < 0.001$)
Thalidomide [13–16]	Systematic review of 1672 patients in phase 2 RCT of thalidomide monotherapy	VTE 18/752 (2.4%)
	470 patients in RCT of dexamethasone vs. thalidomide + dexamethasone	Dexamethasone alone 5.6% vs. thalidomide + dexamethasone 18.8%
	255 patients with newly diagnosed myeloma randomized to melphalan, prednisone, and thalidomide (MPT) or melphalan and prednisone (MP)	MPT 15 (12%) vs. MP 2 (2%), $P = 0.001$
	100 patients with newly diagnosed myeloma randomized to anthracycline- and cyclophosphamide-based regimens with or without thalidomide	Thalidomide 14/50 (28%) vs. no thalidomide 2/50 (4%), $P = 0.002$
Lenalidomide [17–19]	7764 MDS patients on single-agent lenalidomide	41/7764 (0.53%)
	Two RCTs of lenalidomide plus dexamethasone vs. dexamethasone alone for MM	Lenalidomide + dexamethasone vs. dexamethasone alone *or* 3.5 (1.77–6.97)

(continued)

Table 20.1 (continued)

Chemotherapy agent	Patient population	Venous thromboembolism
	Lenalidomide plus high-dose dexamethasone (480 mg/cycle) vs. lenalidomide plus low-dose dexamethasone (160 mg/cycle) for multiple myeloma	Lenalidomide + high-dose dexamethasone 26% vs. lenalidomide + low-dose dexamethasone 12%
Pomalidomide [20]	Trial of pomalidomide plus low-dose dexamethasone	1/60 (1.6%) (all patients given aspirin thromboprophylaxis)
Cisplatin [21]	8216 patients in phase 2 and 3 RCT of cisplatin-based and non-cisplatin-based chemotherapy regimens	VTE incidence Cisplatin-containing regimens: 1.92% (95% CI, 1.07–2.76) vs. non-cisplatin-containing regimens 0.79% (95% CI, 0.45–1.13) RR 1.67 (95% CI, 1.25–2.23; $P = 0.01$)

VEGF vascular endothelial growth factor, *EGF* epidermal growth factor, *RCT* randomized controlled trial, *FOLFIRI* irinotecan 180 mg/m^2 IV over 90 min, with leucovorin 400 mg/m^2 IV over 2 h, followed by FU 400 mg/m^2 bolus and FU 2400 mg/m^2 continuous infusion over 46 h), *RR* relative risk, *95% CI* 95% confidence interval, *VTE* venous thromboembolism, *OR* odds ratio, *MDS* myelodysplastic syndrome

Table 20.2 Major randomized studies of a LMWH versus vitamin K antagonist for the treatment of cancer-associated thrombosis (>100 patients)

Study	Year published	LWMH	*N*	RR of recurrent VTE (95% CI)	RR of major bleeding (95% CI)
CANTHANOX [28]	2002	Enoxaparin	146	0.71 (0.12–4.10)	0.44 (0.16–1.19)
CLOT [24]	2003	Dalteparin	672	0.51 (0.33–0.79)[a]	1.57 (0.77–3.18)
LITE[b] [26]	2006	Tinzaparin	200	0.44 (0.19–1.02)	1.00 (0.36–2.75)
ONCENOX [25]	2006	Enoxaparin	122	0.81 (0.19–3.37)	3.62 (0.46–28.74)
CATCH [27]	2015	Tinzaparin	900	0.69 (0.45–1.07)	1.10 (0.49–2.46)

LMWH low-molecular-weight heparin, *N* total number of randomized patients, *RR* relative risk, *VTE* venous thromboembolism, *CI* confidence interval

[a]The only significant result noted was a reduction in the risk of recurrent VTE with dalteparin for the CLOT study ($p = 0.002$)

[b]This study was criticized due to the longer planned duration of treatment in the LMWH group compared with the VKA control arm

Fondaparinux is a pentasaccharide. While it is technically not a LMWH, fondaparinux works in a similar fashion as an anticoagulant. Little information exists as to the effectiveness of fondaparinux in the cancer population. Notably, some retrospective data suggest that first-line fondaparinux is less effective than LMWH in this population [37].

Treatment of Venous Thromboembolism: Direct Oral Anticoagulants

No clinical trial directly comparing DOACs with LMWH in CAT has been published, although trials are ongoing for rivaroxaban, apixaban, and edoxaban [38–40]. Currently available data consist of post hoc analyses of the landmark VTE trials for dabigatran [41], rivaroxaban [42], apixaban [27], and edoxaban [43], along with dedicated prospective [44, 45] and retrospective [46–48] cohort studies, totaling over 1200 evaluable patients who received DOACs for CAT (Table 20.3). Some of these studies were included in a meta-analysis of DOAC versus VKA for CAT, showing trends toward less recurrent VTE (OR = 0.63, 95% CI = 0.37–1.10) and less major bleeding (OR = 0.77, 95% CI = 0.41–1.44) for the DOACs, with no statistically significant difference noted however [49]. Rivaroxaban is by far the agent for which there is the most accumulated data in this setting. The available information suggests that this drug appears to be safe and effective for the treatment of CAT with 6-month cumulative incidences of recurrent VTE and major bleeding estimated at 4.4 % (95% CI = 1.4–7.4%) and 2.2 % (95% CI = 0–4.2%), respectively, in one report [45], with similar results noted at a different center [44]. Due to poor patient compliance with LMWH as well as the marked quality of life improvement with DOACs, a growing number of cancer patients are receiving rivaroxaban or other DOACs for the treatment of CAT [29].

There are important limitations to possible use of DOACs in some cancer patients. These drugs are present and active in the gastrointestinal (GI) and genitourinary tracts, which confer a higher risk of bleeding at these locations [50, 51]. This is a concern for individuals with neoplastic lesions at these anatomical sites that DOACs may be associated with an increased risk of bleeding. The presence of stents and other hardware in the genitourinary tract can also be a source of bleeding, for example, urinary stents or nephrostomy tubes. In theory, prior surgery of the GI tract like a Whipple procedure could impact absorption negatively. *Thus, we recommend against the use of DOACs in patients with active genitourinary or GI pathology or altered upper GI anatomy.* Possible drug interactions must also be considered, particularly drugs involving the CYP3A4 and/or P-glycoprotein pathways. For example, the use of new azole antifungals after allogeneic stem cell transplant in the case of rivaroxaban and apixaban. For these reasons and others, cancer patients need to be carefully selected before administering rivaroxaban or apixaban, while the use of enoxaparin is more straightforward albeit associated with substantial discomfort for the patient.

To this point, only indirect comparisons have been made between the DOACs and LMWH for the treatment of CAT. In a meta-analysis evaluating 10 RCTs evaluating 3242 cancer patients who were treated with anticoagulation for VTE, the estimated relative risks of recurrent VTE (1.08, 95% CI = 0.59–1.95) and major bleeding (0.67, 95% CI = 0.31–1.46) for DOAC versus LMWH did not differ significantly and suggest that the efficacy and safety of these two drug classes in cancer patients may be comparable [52].

Prevention of Venous Thromboembolism

The National Comprehensive Cancer Network guidelines currently recommend pharmacological prophylaxis unless a contraindication to anticoagulation is present, in which case mechanical prophylaxis with intermittent pneumatic compression can be used. Unfractionated heparin and LMWH are both acceptable drug regimens. Patients undergoing abdominal or pelvic cancer surgery are at particularly high risk, and preoperative as well as postoperative prophylaxis should be given, up to 4 weeks after the procedure [30]. In this regard, the @RISTOS registry reported that a substantial proportion of VTE episodes occurred late after the surgery (40% were diagnosed more than 21 days following surgery) [53]. Outpatients receiving cancer chemotherapy are also at substantial risk of developing a VTE episode, the risk of which can be assessed using the Khorana risk score [23]. There is substantial evidence that primary anticoagulation prophylaxis is effective for the prevention of VTE in this setting. The largest study looking at this question was the SAVE-ONCO trial [54]. Patients in the study had locally advanced or metastatic solid tumor, were starting chemotherapy, and were randomized to semuloparin (an ultra-LMWH) or placebo. Semuloparin resulted in a decrease in the risk of VTE from 3.4% in the control arm to 1.2% in the semuloparin arm. While this represented a relative risk reduction of 64%, the number needed to

Table 20.3 Cohorts of patients with cancer-associated thrombosis treated with a DOAC

Cohort	Year published	DOAC	Duration of treatment	Risk of recurrent VTE *n*/*N* (%)	Risk of major bleeding *n*/*N* (%)
Pooled EINSTEIN-DVT and EINSTEIN-PE[a] [42]	2013	Rivaroxaban	Mean ± SD = 179 ± 96.9 days	16/316 (5.1)	9/316 (2.8)
AMPLIFY[a] [27]	2015	Apixaban	NA[b]	3/81 (3.7)	2/87 (2.3)
Huntsman Cancer Institute[c] [48]	2015	Rivaroxaban	NA	4/92 (4.3)	10/92 (10.8)
Moffitt Cancer Center[c] [47]	2015	Rivaroxaban	NA	2/107(1.9)[d]	0/107 (0)
Pooled RE-COVER and RE-COVER II[a] [41]	2015	Dabigatran	NA	9/173 (5.2)	6/159 (3.8)
Yale New Haven Hospital[c] [46]	2015	Rivaroxaban	NA	5/75 (6.7)	NA[e]
HOKUSAI-VTE[a] [43]	2016	Edoxaban	Median (IQR) = 199 (110–352) days	4/109 (3.7)	5/109 (4.6)
Mayo Clinic[f] [44]	2016	Rivaroxaban	Mean ± SD = 1.36 ± 0.5 years	4/118 (3.3)	
Memorial Sloan Kettering Cancer Center[f] [45]	2016	Rivaroxaban	NA[b]	8/200 (4.0)	4/200 (2.0)

DOAC direct oral anticoagulant, *VTE* venous thromboembolism, *SD* standard deviation, *IQR* interquartile range
[a]Post hoc analysis of a randomized trial comparing a DOAC to a vitamin K antagonist. "Cohort" designates the name of the original study
[b]Patients followed for up to 6 months of treatment
[c]Retrospective cohort study (abstract only). "Cohort" designates the originating institution
[d]Evaluated at 30 days
[e]Risk of "clinically relevant bleeding" was 19/75 (25.3)
[f]Prospective cohort study. "Cohort" designates the originating institution

treat to prevent a VTE episode was 46. Considering the cost and burden of a parenteral anticoagulant for primary VTE prophylaxis, semuloparin was not approved.

Importantly, prophylactic anticoagulation did not result in a survival benefit in the SAVE-ONCO study or in other similar studies [55–58]. Consequently, primary pharmacological VTE thromboprophylaxis in ambulatory cancer patients undergoing chemotherapy has not entered mainstream practice. A primary thromboprophylaxis trial with rivaroxaban, the CASSINI study, is ongoing [59]. The CASSINI study is specifically targeting patients at increased risk of VTE based on the Khorana risk score, which may help reduce the NNT. In addition, by using a DOAC, the burden of thromboprophylaxis should be more acceptable to the patient, if successful.

One cancer situation where primary anticoagulation prophylaxis is widely used is in medical oncology patients receiving immunomodulatory drugs like thalidomide or lenalidomide for multiple myeloma. When used in conjunction with high-dose dexamethasone or cytotoxic chemotherapy, these medications have been associated with a substantial risk of thromboembolism [60]. National Comprehensive Cancer Network guidelines recommend the use of thromboprophylaxis with an anticoagulant (LMWH or VKA) or aspirin based on an assessment of the individual patient's risk factors [30]. At present there is insufficient evidence to recommend use of a DOAC for thromboprophylaxis in this setting [59].

Postoperative subcutaneous low-dose unfractionated heparin has been demonstrated to decrease the risk of fatal PE in meta-analysis [61], and prophylactic doses of LMWH has been shown to be at least as safe and effective in general or orthopedic surgery [62]. Because of this and additional data specific to surgical oncology patients, LMWH is widely used in the setting of cancer surgery [63].

Thrombocytopenia

One important factor complicating anticoagulation therapy is the frequent occurrence of thrombocytopenia. This is most often secondary to chemotherapy but can also result from bone marrow involvement by cancer, infection, liver disease, or noncytotoxic drugs. Scant data exists about the best approach to dose management in this setting, and all published series feature a LMWH [64–66]. The largest such cohort originated from Memorial Sloan Kettering Cancer Center and featured 101 individuals with 144 episodes of thrombocytopenia of at least 7 days duration. Based on institutional guidelines, patients were kept on full-dose enoxaparin (1 mg/kg BID or 1.5 mg/kg daily) as long as the platelet count remained above 50,000/mcl, since the bleeding risk at this platelet count is perceived to be similar to that of individuals with a normal platelet count. For platelet counts of 25,000–50,000/mcl, the dose of enoxaparin dose was reduced by half, and for platelet counts of <25,000/mcl, enoxaparin was temporarily held because the bleeding risk was considered to be prohibitive. This approach resulted in no recurrent thrombosis or major bleeding when the enoxaparin dose had been adjusted. There was one trauma-associated major bleeding episode, which occurred in an individual prior to identification of thrombocytopenia, and therefore the enoxaparin dose had not been adjusted [66].

There are no data yet to guide DOAC management in the setting of thrombocytopenia, and VKA therapy would be anticipated to be particularly difficult to manage given its long effective half-life and prolonged time to fill anticoagulant effect when restarted. For these reasons, patients who undergo chemotherapy with myelosuppressive regimens associated with a high incidence of thrombocytopenia below 50,000/mcl are probably better served by treatment with LMWH when they need anticoagulation.

Primary and Metastatic Brain Tumors

Intracranial hemorrhage (ICH) is one of the most feared complications of anticoagulation therapy. Its incidence and risk factors have been well documented for patients on a VKA [67, 68]. The presence of primary or metastatic brain lesions certainly raises concern over an increased risk of

ICH; however, in carefully selected patients, it has been shown that anticoagulation therapy can be safely administered.

There is a general perception that some tumors have been associated with an increased risk of spontaneous bleeding, including melanoma, choriocarcinoma, and thyroid and renal carcinoma [69]. However, retrospective data specific to cases of melanoma or renal cell carcinoma suggest that anticoagulation with a LMWH is not associated with a significant increase in the risk of ICH [70, 71]. The later studies are limited by potential bias from factors influencing clinician decision-making as to start or not start a LMWH. A meta-analysis did not note an increase in ICHs in patients with brain metastases on LMWH or a VKA, although a possible increased risk was identified in patients with primary brain gliomas [72]. In contrast, a matched cohort study of glioma patients on LMWH did not note an increased risk of ICH [72]. Given these data, brain metastases from tumors not considered at higher risk of bleeding are not an absolute contraindication to treatment with full-dose LMWH. Data are needed to conform that DOACs are a viable option for treatment of CAT in patients with primary or metastatic brain tumors. In the recently published prospective cohort study of rivaroxaban for CAT, patients with untreated primary or metastatic brain tumors were excluded [45].

If there is any history of prior ICH or even small amounts of blood products in the metastases on brain MRI, treatment should be individualized based on other risk factors for bleeding and an assessment of thrombotic risk. The same considerations apply for melanoma, choriocarcinoma, and thyroid and renal carcinoma. Twice daily prophylactic-dose LWMH may be an acceptable treatment approach for CAT in patients with brain metastases at higher risk of ICH, based on the notion that this regimen has not been associated with an increased risk of ICH but may potentially reduce the risk of recurrent VTE. In these authors' practice, the BID regimen is favored due to the short half-life of LMWH and the expected gap in coverage with daily dosing. Importantly, the presence of active ICH would be considered by most to be an absolute contraindication to the administration of any amount of an anticoagulant. In this case and for patients with a recent VTE episode (less than 3-month-old), placement of an IVC filter should be considered, especially if the residual venous thrombus burden is substantial.

Atrial Fibrillation

Atrial fibrillation (AF) is the most common tachyarrhythmia and is associated with a fivefold increased thromboembolic stroke risk in the general population [73–75]. AF is encountered frequently in patients with malignancy likely due to shared risk factors for disease, comorbid states such as infection and hypoxia, direct tumor effects (local invasion and exocrine), arrhythmogenic chemotherapy, and cancer surgery [75]. Atrial fibrillation is a poor prognostic factor that impacts cancer treatment and affects its outcomes [76].

The association between atrial fibrillation and malignancy is particularly common in the oncologic thoracic surgery setting [75, 77, 78]. While the risk of atrial fibrillation with non-thoracic cancer surgery is lower than with thoracic cancer surgery, it is still higher than with non-cancer surgery [79]. It is also worth noting that there is greater prevalence of atrial fibrillation in cancer patients even prior to chemotherapy or surgery compared with patients without cancer [80]. A recent study showed that women with new-onset cancer have ≈fivefold increased risk of developing atrial fibrillation in the first 3 months after diagnosis compared with a non-cancer cohort [81]. In addition, there is a growing list of arrhythmogenic chemotherapeutic agents that increase the risk of atrial fibrillation [75, 77].

Defining an appropriate anticoagulation strategy to reduce stroke risk is a key aspect of AF management. Cancer and its therapeutics make the patient vulnerable to increased thrombotic and bleeding risk. Recent preliminary data from the cancer subset of the ORBIT-AF trial showed that cancer patients with AF treated with antithrombotic/antiplatelet therapy had higher risk of major bleeding compared with non-cancer patients [82]. There is lack of data addressing the impact, if any, of cancer on stroke risk in patients with atrial fibrillation.

There are many available scoring systems to predict the stroke and bleeding risk in patients with AF including but not limited to the HAS-BLED score for bleeding risk and the $CHADS_2$ and CHA_2DS_2-VASc for stroke risk [83, 84]. These prediction models have not been validated in the cancer population and may not be reliable predictors of adverse events in this unique cohort [67].

Warfarin is superior to aspirin in decreasing stroke risk in AF (64 versus 22% risk reduction) in the general population [85]. However, warfarin use is challenging in the cancer population. In a retrospective study of 2168 AF patients with newly diagnosed cancer, the optimal therapeutic warfarin level was achieved only in 12% of the treatment cohort during the first year after cancer diagnosis [74]. Warfarin necessitates regular blood monitoring, and its myriad drug-drug and drug-food interactions as well as its unpredictable pharmacokinetics limit its use in the cancer population [86, 87]. While LMWH is preferred over VKA in the cancer population for the treatment of VTE, it should be noted that such data are lacking in atrial fibrillation and cancer. Warfarin is still the only oral anticoagulant recommended in patients with valvular disease [88]. DOACs have more predictable pharmacokinetics, fewer drug-drug and drug-food interactions, rapid onset of action, and no need for regular monitoring with exception of dose adjustment according to kidney function. Over the past decade, the efficacy and safety of DOAC has been established in nonvalvular atrial fibrillation for stroke prevention in the general population, and emerging data suggests a promising role for these agents in the treatment of venous thromboembolism in patients with cancer [89]. Preliminary data has shown encouraging results on the safety and efficacy of rivaroxaban in cancer patients with AF; however, confirmation of these findings in larger studies is needed [90].

Due to lack of high-quality data in cancer patients, the current management of cancer-related AF is based on extrapolation of the current guidelines from non-cancer patients. The increased thrombotic and bleeding risk related to the underlying malignancy or its treatment and the dynamic nature of the clinical course make the anticoagulation decisions for AF challenging.

The decision to initiate or interrupt anticoagulation treatment in atrial fibrillation in cancer should be individualized with emphasis on shared decision-making in a multidisciplinary collaborative environment.

Management of Line-Associated Thrombosis

The use of central venous catheters is ubiquitous in oncology. In the general population, they have been associated with varying rates of deep venous thrombosis, with a higher risk noted for patients with cancer [91, 92]. Compression by tumor, tumor-induced thrombophilia, and infusion of chemotherapeutic drugs irritating the vascular endothelium are thrombotic risk factors specific to this population. Peripherally inserted central catheters (PICCs) portend a higher risk of thrombotic event, as do lines with a bigger lumen and those inserted in the subclavian vein as opposed to the internal jugular vein [93, 94].

There is a dearth of hard evidence to guide the management of line-associated thrombosis in the cancer patient. General recommendations are to anticoagulate for thrombi involving the axillary line or more proximal segments. It is also considered acceptable to keep the central catheter in place as long as it is functional and anticoagulation is administered [31, 32]. The agent of choice in the oncology setting is not clear; however, the use of a VKA has been discouraged, and treatment with a LMWH is favored, based on results of studies for lower extremity DVT and PE. Rivaroxaban was reported as being safe and effective in a small group of cancer patients; however, those results need to be replicated in a larger cohort [95].

Nonbacterial Thrombotic Endocarditis

Nonbacterial thrombotic endocarditis (NBTE) is an uncommon and underdiagnosed entity characterized by the presence of noninfectious cardiac valvular vegetations consisting of fibrin and platelet aggregates typically associated with hypercoagulable states in patients with advanced malignancy [96]. Adenocarcinoma is the most common histologic type of malignancy associated with NBTE [97, 98]. NBTE affects patients usually between the fourth and eighth decade of life without any sex predilection. Left-sided heart valves (aortic > mitral) are more commonly involved [96]. Several pathogenic mechanisms have been reported including elevated cytokine levels, hypercoagulable state/disseminated intravascular coagulation (DIC), hypoxia/increased tissue factor levels, blood flow velocity, and oncogene activation [96, 99, 100]. Patients with NBTE are often asymptomatic. While the precise incidence of systemic embolization is not known, on average as many as 50% of patients present with an embolic event [99]. However, it is also possible that multiorgan infarcts are the consequence of in situ arterial thrombosis as we have seen patients with bland splenic, brain, and kidney infarcts who have never been shown to have valvular vegetations. *Antemortem* diagnosis can be challenging. A focused workup based on high clinical suspicion is prudent to establish a diagnosis. In addition to routine blood work and serial blood cultures, hypercoagulable states and disseminated intravascular coagulation should also be ruled out [99]. In cases of unrevealing transthoracic echocardiography, transesophageal echocardiography is the diagnostic modality of choice due to its high sensitivity for smaller valvular lesions [100]. Diffusion-weighted MRI is able to detect evidence of embolic cerebrovascular events [101]. Cardiac MRI and transcranial Doppler may play larger roles in the future [102, 103]. The definitive diagnosis can be made from a pathological specimen obtained at autopsy or post-operation.

The cornerstone of treatment of NBTE is antitumor therapy and systemic anticoagulation. In the absence of contraindications, systemic anticoagulation should be started in all patients with NBTE even in the absence of systemic emboli [96, 99]. Unfractionated heparin is the most effective anticoagulant in preventing recurrent emboli and is the agent of choice. LMWH may be a reasonable alternative. VKA are not recommended due to a high risk of recurrent thromboembolic events [96, 104]. Anticoagulation should be continued indefinitely due to the risk of recurrence [104]. The safety and efficacy of DOAC has not been established in patients with NBTE. Early diagnosis and management can improve the quality of life and prognosis, but NBTE signals a later stage of disease with a poor prognosis.

Conclusion

The field of anticoagulation therapy has evolved substantially over the last few years, most remarkably with the advent of the DOAC which has an improved safety profile and greater convenience when compared to VKA. On the other hand, prospective data with DOAC in the treatment of CAT are limited. Early single-arm studies of DOAC in the treatment of VTE and atrial fibrillation are promising. However, an accurate assessment of the comparative efficacy and safety of DOAC compared with LMWH for CAT awaits the completion of ongoing randomized controlled trials. Preliminary data suggest that rivaroxaban is safe and effective for CAT and atrial fibrillation. Anticoagulation with a LMWH can be safely given to carefully selected patients with intracranial neoplasms.

Key Points

- Low-molecular-weight heparin (LMWH) has been shown to be superior to vitamin K antagonists (VKA) for the treatment of cancer-associated venous thromboembolism (CAT).
- Accumulating data suggests that direct oral anticoagulants may be effective in

patients with cancer, although randomized trial data directly comparing DOACs to low-molecular-weight heparin are lacking.

- Rivaroxaban appears to be safe and effective for the treatment of CAT, although a definitive assessment of its comparative efficacy and safety vis-à-vis LMWH is pending completion of randomized controlled trials.
- Enoxaparin can be safely administered to patients experiencing frequent episodes of thrombocytopenia, provided a simple dose-adjustment algorithm is applied.
- Thrombocytopenia and brain tumors do not necessarily constitute absolute contraindications to anticoagulation, as long as special precautions are taken.
- Atrial fibrillation is frequently encountered in patients with malignancy. It is associated with a fivefold stroke risk, increases mortality, and significantly impacts therapeutic decision-making and the quality of life of the cancer patient.
- Traditional thromboembolic and bleeding risk scores for atrial fibrillation have not been validated in the cancer patients and may not be accurate.
- Nonbacterial thrombotic endocarditis is characterized by the formation of sterile vegetations on cardiac valves and is seen in patients with advanced malignancy. Antitumor therapy and anticoagulation with unfractionated or low-molecular-weight heparins are recommended, but prognosis is poor.
- Atrial fibrillation is commonly encountered in the setting of cancer or cancer therapies, particularly in patients undergoing thoracic surgery. Traditionally used risk scores for thromboembolic and bleeding risk may not be applicable, and anticoagulation decisions have to be individualized after careful evaluation of thrombotic and bleeding risk.

Self-Assessment Questions

Questions 1 and 2: A 55-year-old man with pancreatic adenocarcinoma metastatic to liver presented with transient right facial numbness. The patient denied any recent trauma, fever, joint pains, rash, or seizures. His medical history was otherwise unremarkable. Vitals were stable and physical exam was unremarkable. Head CT scan was normal. Over the next few hours, the patient developed sudden aphasia and dizziness. Neurology was consulted and a diffusion-weighted brain MRI showed multiple lesions at the border zones and an acute infarct at the right temporal zone. Laboratory studies showed anemia with a hemoglobin level of 11g/dl and hematocrit of 31%; platelet count, renal function, and electrolytes were within the normal range.

An embolic stroke workup included a transthoracic echocardiogram, which revealed an ejection fraction of >55% without obvious cardiac valvular abnormalities. Transesophageal echocardiography demonstrated multiple subcentimeter nodular, mobile echodensities on the atrial surface of the anterior mitral valve leaflet associated with mild mitral regurgitation without evidence of leaflet destruction. A CT scan of the abdomen and pelvis showed a pancreatic mass with metastatic liver lesions and splenic infarcts. An extensive hypercoagulable workup and serial blood cultures were negative.

1. What is the most likely diagnosis?
   (a) Fibroelastoma
   (b) Degenerative valve disease
   (c) Infective endocarditis
   (d) Nonbacterial thrombotic endocarditis
2. What is the best treatment option?
   (a) Start warfarin and target INR 2–3.
   (b) Start rivaroxaban.
   (c) Start intravenous unfractionated heparin.
   (d) No anticoagulation.
3. Which anticoagulant is currently considered first-line therapy for cancer-associated venous thromboembolism based on published randomized controlled trials?
   (a) Unfractionated heparin
   (b) Direct oral anticoagulant

   (c) Low-molecular-weight heparin
   (d) Vitamin K antagonist
4. Above which platelet count threshold is the adjustment of enoxaparin dose usually not required?
   (a) 25,000
   (b) 50,000
   (c) 75,000
   (d) 100,000
5. Which anticoagulant would be most problematic for a patient with a newly diagnostic malignant stomach ulcer?
   (a) Fondaparinux
   (b) Enoxaparin
   (c) Rivaroxaban
   (d) Unfractionated heparin

Self-Assessment Answers

1. (d) Nonbacterial thrombotic endocarditis

   The most likely diagnosis is nonbacterial thrombotic endocarditis because of the characteristic appearance of vegetations on transesophageal echocardiography (TEE) (subcentimeter vegetations without significant valve destruction) seen in this patient with advanced pancreatic cancer presenting with embolic strokes with a negative infectious workup. Papillary fibroelastomas are benign tumors with a characteristic echocardiographic appearance; they are usually pedunculated and mobile, with a homogeneous speckled pattern and characteristic stippling along their edges on TEE. Degenerative valve disease is likely to result in calcification of the valve with resultant functional perturbations like regurgitation or stenosis without discrete valvular vegetations. Infectious endocarditis is usually associated with positive blood cultures, and vegetations can be differentiated on TEE. Unlike NBTE, the other entities are not associated with hypercoagulable states or advanced malignancy.
2. (c) Start intravenous unfractionated heparin

   Management of NBTE consists of treatment of the underlying malignancy and indefinite systemic anticoagulation with unfractionated heparin or low-molecular-weight heparin. Warfarin is not recommended due to high rates of recurrent thromboembolism. The efficacy of rivaroxaban is not known.
3. (c) Low-molecular-weight heparin

   In the CLOT trial, dalteparin was associated with about half the risk of recurrent VTE compared to the use of a VKA.
4. (b) 50,000

   Retrospective cohort data suggests that thrombocytopenia above 50,000 is not associated with an increased risk of bleeding in individuals on full-dose enoxaparin.
5. (c) Rivaroxaban

   DOACs are present at high concentrations and have anti-hemostatic activity in the GI tract, so they are a suboptimal choice in patients with GI lesions with bleeding potential. In this setting, heparinoids while not devoid of risk remain a better alternative.

References

1. Khorana AA, Streiff MB, Farge D, Mandala M, Debourdeau P, Cajfinger F, et al. Venous thromboembolism prophylaxis and treatment in cancer: a consensus statement of major guidelines panels and call to action. J Clin Oncol. 2009;27(29):4919–26.
2. Dipasco PJ, Misra S, Koniaris LG, Moffat FL Jr. Thrombophilic state in cancer, part I: biology, incidence, and risk factors. J Surg Oncol. 2011;104(3):316–22.
3. Zwicker JI, Liebman HA, Neuberg D, Lacroix R, Bauer KA, Furie BC, et al. Tumor-derived tissue factor-bearing microparticles are associated with venous thromboembolic events in malignancy. Clin Cancer Res. 2009;15(22):6830–40.
4. Hurwitz HI, Saltz LB, Van Cutsem E, Cassidy J, Wiedemann J, Sirzén F, et al. Venous thromboembolic events with chemotherapy plus bevacizumab: a pooled analysis of patients in randomized phase II and III studies. J Clin Oncol. 2011;29(13):1757–64.
5. Van Cutsem E, Tabernero J, Lakomy R, Prenen H, Prausová J, Macarulla T, et al. Addition of aflibercept to fluorouracil, leucovorin, and irinotecan improves survival in a phase III randomized trial in patients with metastatic colorectal cancer previously treated with an oxaliplatin-based regimen. J Clin Oncol. 2012;30(28):3499–506.
6. Sonpavde G, Je Y, Schutz F, Galsky MD, Paluri R, Rosenberg JE, et al. Venous thromboembolic events with vascular endothelial growth factor receptor tyrosine kinase inhibitors: a systematic review and

meta-analysis of randomized clinical trials. Crit Rev Oncol Hematol. 2013;87(1):80–9.
7. Petrelli F, Cabiddu M, Borgonovo K, Barni S. Risk of venous and arterial thromboembolic events associated with anti-EGFR agents: a meta-analysis of randomized clinical trials. Ann Oncol. 2012;23(7):1672–9.
8. Grace RF, Dahlberg SE, Neuberg D, Sallan SE, Connors JM, Neufeld EJ, et al. The frequency and management of asparaginase-related thrombosis in paediatric and adult patients with acute lymphoblastic leukaemia treated on Dana-Farber Cancer Institute consortium protocols. Br J Haematol. 2011; 152(4):452–9.
9. Fisher B, Costantino JP, Wickerham DL, Redmond CK, Kavanah M, Cronin WM, et al. Tamoxifen for prevention of breast cancer: report of the National Surgical Adjuvant Breast and Bowel Project P-1 study. J Natl Cancer Inst. 1998;90(18):1371–88.
10. Cuzick J, Forbes JF, Sestak I, Cawthorn S, Hamed H, Holli K, Howell A. International Breast Cancer Intervention Study I Investigators Long-term results of tamoxifen prophylaxis for breast cancer--96-month follow-up of the randomized IBIS-I trial. J Natl Cancer Inst. 2007;99(4):272–82.
11. McCaskill-Stevens W, Wilson J, Bryant J, Mamounas E, Garvey L, James J, et al. Contralateral breast cancer and thromboembolic events in African American women treated with tamoxifen. J Natl Cancer Inst. 2004;96(23):1762–9.
12. Amir E, Seruga B, Niraula S, Carlsson L, Ocaña A. Toxicity of adjuvant endocrine therapy in postmenopausal breast cancer patients: a systematic review and meta-analysis. J Natl Cancer Inst. 2011; 103(17):1299–309.
13. Glasmacher A, Hahn C, Hoffmann F, Naumann R, Goldschmidt H, von Lilienfeld-Toal M, et al. A systematic review of phase-II trials of thalidomide monotherapy in patients with relapsed or refractory multiple myeloma. Br J Haematol. 2006;132(5):584–93.
14. Rajkumar SV, Blood E, Vesole D, Fonseca R, Greipp PR. Eastern Cooperative Oncology Group Phase III clinical trial of thalidomide plus dexamethasone compared with dexamethasone alone in newly diagnosed multiple myeloma: a clinical trial coordinated by the Eastern Cooperative Oncology Group. J Clin Oncol. 2006;24(3):431–6.
15. Palumbo A, Bringhen S, Caravita T, Merla E, Capparella V, Callea V, et al. Italian Multiple Myeloma Network, GIMEMA. Oral melphalan and prednisone chemotherapy plus thalidomide compared with melphalan and prednisone alone in elderly patients with multiple myeloma: randomised controlled trial. Lancet. 2006;367(9513):825–31.
16. Zangari M, Anaissie E, Barlogie B, Badros A, Desikan R, et al. Increased risk of deep-vein thrombosis in patients with multiple myeloma receiving thalidomide and chemotherapy. Blood. 2001;98(5): 1614–5.
17. Yang X, Brandenburg NA, Freeman J, Salomon ML, Zeldis JB, Knight RD, Bwire R. Venous thromboembolism in myelodysplastic syndrome patients receiving lenalidomide: results from postmarketing surveillance and data mining techniques. Clin Drug Investig. 2009;29(3):161–71.
18. Rajkumar SV, Blood E. Lenalidomide and venous thrombosis in multiple myeloma. N Engl J Med. 2006;354(19):2079–80.
19. Rajkumar SV, Jacobus S, Callender N, et al. Phase III trial of lenalidomide plus high-dose dexamethasone versus lenalidomide plus low-dose dexamethasone in newly diagnosed multiple myeloma (E4A03): a trial coordinated by the Eastern Cooperative Oncology Group (abstract). J Clin Oncol. 2007;25 (18 Suppl):LBA8025.
20. Lacy MQ, Hayman SR, Gertz MA, Dispenzieri A, Buadi F, Kumar S, et al. Pomalidomide (CC4047) plus low-dose dexamethasone as therapy for relapsed multiple myeloma. J Clin Oncol. 2009;27(30):5008–14.
21. Seng S, Liu Z, Chiu SK, Proverbs-Singh T, Sonpavde G, Choueiri TK, et al. Risk of venous thromboembolism in patients with cancer treated with Cisplatin: a systematic review and meta-analysis. J Clin Oncol. 2012;30(35):4416–26.
22. Falanga A, Marchetti M. Anticancer treatment and thrombosis. Thromb Res. 2012;129(3):353–9.
23. Khorana AA, Kuderer NM, Culakova E, Lyman GH, Francis CW. Development and validation of a predictive model for chemotherapy-associated thrombosis. Blood. 2008;111(10):4902–7.
24. Lee AY, Levine MN, Baker RI, Bowden C, Kakkar AK, Prins M, et al. Low-molecular-weight heparin versus a coumarin for the prevention of recurrent venous thromboembolism in patients with cancer. N Engl J Med. 2003;349(2):146–53.
25. Deitcher SR, Kessler CM, Merli G, Rigas JR, Lyons RM, Fareed J, et al. Secondary prevention of venous thromboembolic events in patients with active cancer: enoxaparin alone versus initial enoxaparin followed by warfarin for a 180-day period. Clin Appl Thromb Hemost. 2006;12(4):389–96.
26. Hull RD, Pineo GF, Brant RF, Mah AF, Burke N, Dear R, et al. Long-term low-molecular-weight heparin versus usual care in proximal-vein thrombosis patients with cancer. Am J Med. 2006;119(12):1062–72.
27. Agnelli G, Buller HR, Cohen A, Gallus AS, Lee TC, Pak R, et al. Oral apixaban for the treatment of venous thromboembolism in cancer patients: results from the AMPLIFY trial. J Thromb Haemost. 2015;13(12):2187–91.
28. Meyer G, Marjanovic Z, Valcke J, Lorcerie B, Gruel Y, Solal-Celigny P, et al. Comparison of low-molecular-weight heparin and warfarin for the secondary prevention of venous thromboembolism in patients with cancer: a randomized controlled study. Arch Intern Med. 2002;162(15):1729–35.
29. Khorana AA, McCrae K, Milentijevic D, Fortier J, Nelson W, Laliberté F, et al. Current practice patterns and patient persistence on anticoagulant treatments for cancer-associated thrombosis (abstract). Blood. 2015;126:626.

30. Streiff MB. Cancer-associated venous thromboembolic disease, version 1.2016 of NCCN Guidelines. 2016. Available from: www.nccn.org.
31. Kearon C, Akl EA, Comerota AJ, Prandoni P, Bounameaux H, Goldhaber SZ, et al. Antithrombotic therapy for VTE disease: antithrombotic therapy and prevention of thrombosis, 9th ed: American College of Chest Physicians Evidence-Based Clinical Practice Guidelines. Chest. 2012;141(2 Suppl):e419S–94S.
32. Kearon C, Akl EA, Ornelas J, Blaivas A, Jimenez D, Bounameaux H, et al. Antithrombotic therapy for VTE disease: CHEST guideline and expert panel report. Chest. 2016;149(2):315–52.
33. Deng K, Parameswaran R, Soff BP, Soff GA. Incidental versus symptomatic pulmonary embolism in cancer patients: a multivariate analysis of recurrent VTE and mortality (abstract). Blood. 2012;120:2257.
34. Akl EA, Kahale L, Barba M, Neumann I, Labedi N, Terrenato I, et al. Anticoagulation for the long-term treatment of venous thromboembolism in patients with cancer. Cochrane Database Syst Rev. 2014;7:CD006650.
35. Carrier M, Le Gal G, Cho R, Tierney S, Rodger M, Lee AY. Dose escalation of low molecular weight heparin to manage recurrent venous thromboembolic events despite systemic anticoagulation in cancer patients. J Thromb Haemost. 2009;7(5):760–5.
36. Prandoni P, Lensing AW, Piccioli A, Bernardi E, Simioni P, Girolami B, et al. Recurrent venous thromboembolism and bleeding complications during anticoagulant treatment in patients with cancer and venous thrombosis. Blood. 2002;100(10):3484–8.
37. van Doormaal FF, Raskob GE, Davidson BL, Decousus H, Gallus A, Lensing AW, Piovella F, Prins MH, Büller HR. Treatment of venous thromboembolism in patients with cancer: subgroup analysis of the Matisse clinical trials. Thromb Haemost. 2009;101(4):762–9.
38. NIH. Cancer associated thrombosis, a pilot treatment study using rivaroxaban (CASTA-DIVA) NCT02746185. Available from: www.clinicaltrials.gov.
39. NIH. Apixaban or dalteparin in reducing blood clots in patients with cancer related venous thromboembolism NCT02585713.
40. van Es N, Di Nisio M, Bleker SM, Segers A, Mercuri MF, Schwocho L, et al. Edoxaban for treatment of venous thromboembolism in patients with cancer. Rationale and design of the Hokusai VTE-cancer study. Thromb Haemost. 2015;114(6):1268–76.
41. Schulman S, Goldhaber SZ, Kearon C, Kakkar AK, Schellong S, Eriksson H, et al. Treatment with dabigatran or warfarin in patients with venous thromboembolism and cancer. Thromb Haemost. 2015;114(1):150–7.
42. Prins MH, Lensing AW, Bauersachs R, van Bellen B, Bounameaux H, Brighton TA, et al. Oral rivaroxaban versus standard therapy for the treatment of symptomatic venous thromboembolism: a pooled analysis of the EINSTEIN-DVT and PE randomized studies. Thromb J. 2013;11(1):21.
43. Raskob GE, van Es N, Segers A, Angchaisuksiri P, Oh D, Boda Z, et al. Edoxaban for venous thromboembolism in patients with cancer: results from a non-inferiority subgroup analysis of the Hokusai-VTE randomised, double-blind, double-dummy trial. Lancet Haematol. 2016;3(8):e379–87.
44. Bott-Kitslaar DM, Saadiq RA, McBane RD, Loprinzi CL, Ashrani AA, Ransone TR, et al. Efficacy and safety of rivaroxaban in patients with venous thromboembolism and active malignancy: a single-center registry. Am J Med. 2016;129(6):615–9.
45. Mantha S, Laube E, Miao Y, Sarasohn DM, Parameswaran R, Stefanik S, et al. Safe and effective use of rivaroxaban for treatment of cancer-associated venous thromboembolic disease: a prospective cohort study. J Thromb Thrombolysis. 2017;43(2):166–71.
46. Cambareri C, Yao X, Merl MY, Pham T, Lee AI. The use of oral anticoagulants for the treatment of venous thromboembolism in cancer patients (abstract). Blood. 2015;126:4728.
47. Chaudhury A, Balakrishnan A, Thai C, Holmstrom B, Jaglal MV. Evaluation of rivaroxaban and dalteparin in cancer associated thrombosis (abstract). Blood. 2015;126:432.
48. Win KZ, Wilson N, Stenehjem DD, Tanner N, Rodgers GM, Gilreath J. Effectiveness and safety of rivaroxaban in treatment of venous thromboembolism in cancer patients (abstract). Blood. 2015;126:2319.
49. Vedovati MC, Germini F, Agnelli G, Becattini C. Direct oral anticoagulants in patients with VTE and cancer: a systematic review and meta-analysis. Chest. 2015;147(2):475–83.
50. Sherwood MW, Nessel CC, Hellkamp AS, Mahaffey KW, Piccini JP, Suh EY, et al. Gastrointestinal bleeding in patients with atrial fibrillation treated with rivaroxaban or warfarin: ROCKET AF trial. J Am Coll Cardiol. 2015;66(21):2271–81.
51. Goodman SG, Wojdyla DM, Piccini JP, White HD, Paolini JF, Nessel CC, et al. Factors associated with major bleeding events: insights from the ROCKET AF trial (rivaroxaban once-daily oral direct factor Xa inhibition compared with vitamin K antagonism for prevention of stroke and embolism trial in atrial fibrillation). J Am Coll Cardiol. 2014;63(9):891–900.
52. Posch F, Konigsbrugge O, Zielinski C, Pabinger I, Ay C. Treatment of venous thromboembolism in patients with cancer: a network meta-analysis comparing efficacy and safety of anticoagulants. Thromb Res. 2015;136(3):582–9.
53. Agnelli G, Bolis G, Capussotti L, Scarpa RM, Tonelli F, Bonizzoni E, et al. A clinical outcome-based prospective study on venous thromboembolism after cancer surgery: the @RISTOS project. Ann Surg. 2006;243(1):89–95.
54. Agnelli G, George DJ, Kakkar AK, Fisher W, Lassen MR, Mismetti P, et al. Semuloparin for thrombopro-

phylaxis in patients receiving chemotherapy for cancer. N Engl J Med. 2012;366(7):601–9.
55. Maraveyas A, Waters J, Roy R, Fyfe D, Propper D, Lofts F, et al. Gemcitabine versus gemcitabine plus dalteparin thromboprophylaxis in pancreatic cancer. Eur J Cancer. 2012;48(9):1283–92.
56. Vadhan-Raj S, Zhou X, Varadhachary GR, Milind J, Fogelman D, Shroff R, et al. Randomized controlled trial of dalteparin for primary thromboprophylaxis for venous thromboembolism (VTE) in patients with advanced pancreatic cancer (APC): risk factors predictive of VTE (abstract). Blood. 2013;122:580.
57. Zwicker JI, Liebman HA, Bauer KA, Caughey T, Campigotto F, Rosovsky R, et al. Prediction and prevention of thromboembolic events with enoxaparin in cancer patients with elevated tissue factor-bearing microparticles: a randomized-controlled phase II trial (the Microtec study). Br J Haematol. 2013;160(4):530–7.
58. Pelzer U, Opitz B, Deutschinoff G, Stauch M, Reitzig PC, Hahnfeld S, et al. Efficacy of prophylactic low-molecular weight heparin for ambulatory patients with advanced pancreatic cancer: outcomes from the CONKO-004 trial. J Clin Oncol. 2015;33(18):2028–34.
59. Bach M, Bauersachs R. Spotlight on advances in VTE management: CALLISTO and EINSTEIN CHOICE. Thromb Haemost. 2016;116(Suppl. 2): S24–32.
60. Palumbo A, Rajkumar SV, Dimopoulos MA, Richardson PG, San Miguel J, Barlogie B, et al. Prevention of thalidomide- and lenalidomide-associated thrombosis in myeloma. Leukemia. 2008; 22(2):414–23.
61. Collins R, Scrimgeour A, Yusuf S, Peto R. Reduction in fatal pulmonary embolism and venous thrombosis by perioperative administration of subcutaneous heparin. Overview of results of randomized trials in general, orthopedic, and urologic surgery. N Engl J Med. 1988;318(18):1162–73.
62. Nurmohamed MT, Rosendaal FR, Buller HR, Dekker E, Hommes DW, Vandenbroucke JP, et al. Low-molecular-weight heparin versus standard heparin in general and orthopaedic surgery: a meta-analysis. Lancet. 1992;340(8812):152–6.
63. Akl EA, Terrenato I, Barba M, Sperati F, Sempos EV, Muti P, et al. Low-molecular-weight heparin vs unfractionated heparin for perioperative thromboprophylaxis in patients with cancer: a systematic review and meta-analysis. Arch Intern Med. 2008; 168(12):1261–9.
64. Herishanu Y, Misgav M, Kirgner I, Ben-Tal O, Eldor A, Naparstek E. Enoxaparin can be used safely in patients with severe thrombocytopenia due to intensive chemotherapy regimens. Leuk Lymphoma. 2004;45(7):1407–11.
65. Ibrahim RB, Peres E, Dansey R, Abidi MH, Abella EM, Gumma MM, et al. Safety of low-dose low-molecular-weight-heparins in thrombocytopenic stem cell transplantation patients: a case series and review of the literature. Bone Marrow Transplant. 2005;35(11):1071–7.
66. Mantha S, Miao Y, Wills J, Parameswaran R, Soff GA. Enoxaparin dose reduction for thrombocytopenia in patients with cancer: a quality assessment study. J Thromb Thrombolysis. 2017;43(4):514–8.
67. Garcia-Rodriguez LA, Gaist D, Morton J, Cookson C, Gonzalez-Perez A. Antithrombotic drugs and risk of hemorrhagic stroke in the general population. Neurology. 2013;81(6):566–74.
68. Fang MC, Chang YC, Hylek EM, Rosand J, Greenberg SM, Go AS, et al. Advanced age, anticoagulation intensity, and risk for intracranial hemorrhage among patients taking warfarin for atrial fibrillation. Ann Intern Med. 2004;141(10):745–52.
69. Mandybur TI. Intracranial hemorrhage caused by metastatic tumors. Neurology. 1977;27(7):650–5.
70. Alvarado G, Noor R, Bassett R, Papadopoulos NE, Kim KB, Hwu WJ, et al. Risk of intracranial hemorrhage with anticoagulation therapy in melanoma patients with brain metastases. Melanoma Res. 2012;22(4):310–5.
71. Donato J, Campigotto F, Uhlmann EJ, Coletti E, Neuberg D, Weber GM, et al. Intracranial hemorrhage in patients with brain metastases treated with therapeutic enoxaparin: a matched cohort study. Blood. 2015;126(4):494–9.
72. Mantia C, Uhlmann E, Puligandla M, Neuberg DS, Weber GM, Zwicker JI. Intracranial hemorrhage in patients with primary brain tumors treated with therapeutic enoxaparin: a matched cohort study (abstract). Blood. 2016;128:142.
73. Boriani G, Pettorelli D. Atrial fibrillation burden and atrial fibrillation type: clinical significance and impact on the risk of stroke and decision making for long-term anticoagulation. Vasc Pharmacol. 2016;83:26–35.
74. Lee YJ, Park JK, Uhm JS, Kim JY, Pak HN, Lee MH, et al. Bleeding risk and major adverse events in patients with cancer on oral anticoagulation therapy. Int J Cardiol. 2016;203:372–8.
75. Farmakis D, Parissis J, Filippatos G. Insights into onco-cardiologyatrial fibrillation in cancer. J Am Coll Cardiol. 2014;63(10):945–53.
76. Cheng WL, Kao YH, Chen SA, Chen YJ. Pathophysiology of cancer therapy-provoked atrial fibrillation. Int J Cardiol. 2016;219:186–94.
77. Zamorano JL, Lancellotti P, Rodriguez Munoz D, Aboyans V, Asteggiano R, Galderisi M, et al. 2016 ESC Position Paper on cancer treatments and cardiovascular toxicity developed under the auspices of the ESC Committee for Practice Guidelines: The Task Force for cancer treatments and cardiovascular toxicity of the European Society of Cardiology (ESC). Eur Heart J. 2016;37(36):2768–801.
78. Onaitis M, D'Amico T, Zhao Y, O'Brien S, Harpole D. Risk factors for atrial fibrillation after lung cancer surgery: analysis of the society of thoracic surgeons general thoracic surgery database. Ann Thorac Surg. 2010;90(2):368–74.

79. Guzzetti S, Costantino G, Vernocchi A, Sada S, Fundaro C. First diagnosis of colorectal or breast cancer and prevalence of atrial fibrillation. Intern Emerg Med. 2008;3(3):227–31.
80. O'Neal WT, Lakoski SG, Qureshi W, Judd SE, Howard G, Howard VJ, et al. Relation Between Cancer and Atrial Fibrillation (from the REasons for Geographic And Racial Differences in Stroke Study). Am J Cardiol. 2010;115(8):1090–4.
81. Conen D, Wong JA, Sandhu RK, et al. Risk of malignant cancer among women with new-onset atrial fibrillation. JAMA Cardiol. 2016;1(4):389–96.
82. Melloni C, Shrader P, Carver J, Piccini J, Fonarow G, Ansell J, et al. Management and outcomes of patients with atrial fibrillation and cancer: The ORBIT-AF registry. Eur Heart J Qual Care Clin Outcomes. 2017;3(3):192–7.
83. Apostolakis S, Lane DA, Guo Y, Buller H, Lip GY. Performance of the HEMORR(2)HAGES, ATRIA, and HAS-BLED bleeding risk-prediction scores in patients with atrial fibrillation undergoing anticoagulation: the AMADEUS (evaluating the use of SR34006 compared to warfarin or acenocoumarol in patients with atrial fibrillation) study. J Am Coll Cardiol. 2012;60(9):861–7.
84. Gage BF, Waterman AD, Shannon W, Boechler M, Rich MW, Radford MJ. Validation of clinical classification schemes for predicting stroke: results from the National Registry of Atrial Fibrillation. JAMA. 2001;285(22):2864–70.
85. Hart RG, Pearce LA, Aguilar MI. Meta-analysis: antithrombotic therapy to prevent stroke in patients who have nonvalvular atrial fibrillation. Ann Intern Med. 2007;146(12):857–67.
86. Olesen JB, Sorensen R, Hansen ML, Lamberts M, Weeke P, Mikkelsen AP, et al. Non-vitamin K antagonist oral anticoagulation agents in anticoagulant naive atrial fibrillation patients: Danish nationwide descriptive data 2011-2013. Europace. 2015;17(2):187–93.
87. Steinberg B, Shrader P, Thomas L, Fonarow G, Hylek E, Ansell J, et al. Oral anticoagulant selection in community patients with new-onset atrial fibrillation: results from the ORBIT-AF registry (abstract). J Am Coll Cardiol. 2016;67(13_S):885.
88. January CT, Wann LS, Alpert JS, Calkins H, Cigarroa JE, Cleveland JJC, et al. 2014 AHA/ACC/HRS guideline for the management of patients with atrial fibrillation: executive summarya report of the American College of Cardiology/American Heart Association Task Force on Practice Guidelines and the Heart Rhythm Society. J Am Coll Cardiol. 2014;64(21):2246–80.
89. Larsen TB, Nielsen PB, Skjoth F, Rasmussen LH, Lip GY. Non-vitamin K antagonist oral anticoagulants and the treatment of venous thromboembolism in cancer patients: a semi systematic review and meta-analysis of safety and efficacy outcomes. PLoS One. 2014;9(12):e114445.
90. Laube ES, Yu A, Gupta D, Miao Y, Samedy P, Wills J, et al. Rivaroxaban for stroke prevention in patients with non-valvular atrial fibrillation and active cancer (abstract). Blood. 2016;128:2621.
91. Rooden CJ, Tesselaar ME, Osanto S, Rosendaal FR, Huisman MV. Deep vein thrombosis associated with central venous catheters - a review. J Thromb Haemost. 2005;3(11):2409–19.
92. King MM, Rasnake MS, Rodriguez RG, Riley NJ, Stamm JA. Peripherally inserted central venous catheter-associated thrombosis: retrospective analysis of clinical risk factors in adult patients. South Med J. 2006;99(10):1073–7.
93. Saber W, Moua T, Williams EC, Verso M, Agnelli G, Couban S, et al. Risk factors for catheter-related thrombosis (CRT) in cancer patients: a patient-level data (IPD) meta-analysis of clinical trials and prospective studies. J Thromb Haemost. 2011;9(2):312–9.
94. O'Brien J, Paquet F, Lindsay R, Valenti D. Insertion of PICCs with minimum number of lumens reduces complications and costs. J Am Coll Radiol. 2013;10(11):864–8.
95. Laube ES, Mantha S, Samedy P, Wills J, Harnicar S, Soff GA. Treatment of central venous catheter-associated deep venous thrombosis in cancer patients with rivaroxaban. Am J Hematol. 2017;92(1):E9–E10.
96. Lopez JA, Ross RS, Fishbein MC, Siegel RJ. Nonbacterial thrombotic endocarditis: a review. Am Heart J. 1987;113(3):773–84.
97. Deppisch LM, Fayemi AO. Non-bacterial thrombotic endocarditis: clinicopathologic correlations. Am Heart J. 1976;92(6):723–9.
98. Gonzalez Quintela A, Candela MJ, Vidal C, Roman J, Aramburo P. Non-bacterial thrombotic endocarditis in cancer patients. Acta Cardiol. 1991;46(1):1–9.
99. el-Shami K, Griffiths E, Streiff M. Nonbacterial thrombotic endocarditis in cancer patients: pathogenesis, diagnosis, and treatment. Oncologist. 2007; 12(5):518–23.
100. Dutta T, Karas MG, Segal AZ, Kizer JR. Yield of transesophageal echocardiography for nonbacterial thrombotic endocarditis and other cardiac sources of embolism in cancer patients with cerebral ischemia. Am J Cardiol. 2006;97(6):894–8.
101. Singhal AB, Topcuoglu MA, Buonanno FS. Acute ischemic stroke patterns in infective and nonbacterial thrombotic endocarditis a diffusion-weighted magnetic resonance imaging study. Stroke. 2002; 33(5):1267–73.
102. Sievers B, Brandts B, Franken U, Trappe H-J. Cardiovascular magnetic resonance imaging demonstrates mitral valve endocarditis. Am J Med. 2003;115(8):681–2.
103. Schulte-Altedorneburg G, Nam E-M, Ritter M, Magyar T, Dittrich R, Csiba L, et al. On the origin of microembolic signals. J Neurol. 2003;250(9):1044–9.
104. Rogers LR, Cho ES, Kempin S, Posner JB. Cerebral infarction from non-bacterial thrombotic endocarditis. Clinical and pathological study including the effects of anticoagulation. Am J Med. 1987; 83(4):746–56.

Index

J. F. Lau et al. (eds.), *Anticoagulation Therapy*, https://doi.org/10.1007/978-3-319-73709-6

E

M

N

The manufacturer's authorised representative in the EU is Springer Nature Customer Service Centre GmbH, Europaplatz 3, 69115 Heidelberg, Germany. If you have any concerns regarding our products, please contact ProductSafety@springernature.com

Printed and bound by CPI Group (UK) Ltd, Croydon, CR0 4YY
30/09/2026
02225236-0002